Statistical Methods in Medical Research

To J.O. Irwin

Mentor and friend

Statistical Methods in Medical Research

P. Armitage
MA, PhD
Emeritus Professor of Applied Statistics
University of Oxford

G. Berry
MA, PhD
Professor in Epidemiology and Biostatistics
University of Sydney

J.N.S. Matthews
MA, PhD
Professor of Medical Statistics
University of Newcastle upon Tyne

FOURTH EDITION

Blackwell
Science

First published 1971
Reprinted 1973, 1974, 1977, 1980, 1983, 1985
Second edition 1987
Reprinted 1988 (twice), 1990, 1991, 1993
Thrid edition 1994
Reprinted 1995, 1996
Fourth edition 2002
Reprinted 2002

Library of Congress Cataloging-in-Publication Data

Armitage, P.
Statistical methods in medical research / P. Armitage,
G. Berry, J.N.S. Matthews.—4th ed.
    p. cm.
    Includes bibliographical references and indexes.
    ISBN 0-632-05257-0
    1. Medicine—Research—Statistical methods.
I. Berry, G (Geoffrey) II. Matthews, J.N.S. III. Title.
    [DNLM: 1. Biometry. 2. Research—methods.
WA 950 A 733s 2001] R852 A75 2001 610′ .7′27—dc21

                                                                        00–067992

ISBN 0-632-05257-0

A catalogue record for this title is available from the British Library

Set by Kolam Information Services Pvt. Ltd., Pondicherry, India
Printed and bound in the United Kingdom by MPG Books Ltd, Bodmin, Cornwall

Commissioning Editor: Alison Brown
Production Editor: Fiona Pattison
Production Controller: Kylie Ord

For further information on Blackwell Science, visit our website:
www.blackwell-science.com

Contents

Preface to the fourth edition

In the prefaces to the first three editions of this book, we set out our aims as follows: to gather together the majority of statistical techniques that are used at all frequently in medical research, and to describe them in terms accessible to the non-mathematician. We expressed a hope that the book would have two special assets, distinguishing it from other books on applied statistics: the use of examples selected almost entirely from medical research projects, and a choice of statistical topics reflecting the extent of their usage in medical research.

These aims are equally relevant for this new edition. The steady sales of the earlier editions suggest that there was a gap in the literature which this book has to some extent filled. Why then, the reader may ask, is a new edition needed? The answer is that medical statistics (or, synonymously, *biostatistics*) is an expanding subject, with a continually developing body of techniques, and a steadily growing number of practitioners, especially in medical research organizations and the pharmaceutical industry, playing an increasingly influential role in medical research. New methods, new applications and changing attitudes call for a fresh approach to the exposition of our subject.

The first three editions followed much the same infrastructure, with little change to the original sequence of chapters—essentially an evolutionary approach to the introduction of new topics. In planning this fourth edition we decided at an early stage that the structure previously adopted had already been stretched to its limits. Many topics previously added wherever they would most conveniently fit could be handled better by a more radical rearrangement. The changing face of the subject demanded new chapters for topics now being treated at much greater length, and several areas of methodology still under active development needed to be described much more fully.

The principal changes from the third edition can be summarized as follows.
- Material on descriptive statistics is brought together in Chapter 2, following a very brief introductory Chapter 1.
- The basic results on sampling variation and inference for means, proportions and other simple measures are presented, in Chapters 4 and 5, in a more homogeneous way. For example, the important results for a mean are treated together in §4.2, rather than being split, as before, across two chapters.

- The important and influential approach to statistical inference using Bayesian methods is now dealt with much more fully—in Chapters 6 and 16, and in shorter references elsewhere in the book.
- Chapter 10 covers distribution-free methods and transformations, and also the new topics of permutation and Monte Carlo tests, the bootstrap and jackknife.
- Chapter 12 describes a wide range of special regression problems not covered in previous editions, including non-parametric and non-linear regression models, the construction of reference ranges for clinical test measurements, and multilevel models to take account of dependency between observations.
- In the treatment of categorical data primary emphasis is placed, in Chapter 14, on the use of logistic and related regression models. The older, and more empirical, methods based on χ^2 tests, are described in Chapter 15 and now related more closely to the model-based methods.
- Clinical trials, which now engage the attention of medical statisticians more intensively than ever, were allotted too small a corner in earlier editions. We now have a full treatment of the organizational and statistical aspects of trials in Chapter 18. This includes material on sequential methods, which find a natural home in §18.7.
- Chapter 19, on epidemiological statistics, includes topics previously treated separately, such as survey design and vital statistical rates.
- A new Chapter 20 on laboratory assays includes previous material on biological assay, and, in §§20.5 and 20.6, new topics such as dilution assays and tumour incidence studies.

The effect of this radical reorganization is, we hope, to improve the continuity and cohesion of the presentation, and to extend the scope to cover many new ideas now being introduced into the analysis of medical research data. We have tried to maintain the modest level of mathematical exposition which characterized earlier editions, essentially confining the mathematics to the statement of algebraic formulae rather than pursuing mathematical proofs. However, some of the newer methods involve formulae that cannot be expressed in simple algebraic terms, typically because they are most naturally explained by means of matrix algebra and/or calculus. We have attempted to ease the reader's route through these passages, but some difficulties will inevitably arise. When this happens the reader is strongly encouraged to skip the detail: continuity will not normally be lost, and the general points under discussion will usually emerge without recourse to advanced mathematics.

In the last two editions we included a final chapter on computing. Its omission from the present edition does not in any way indicate a downplaying of the role of computers in modern statistical analysis—rather the reverse. Few scientists, whether statisticians, clinicians or laboratory workers, would nowadays contemplate an analysis without recourse to a computer and a set of statistical programs, typically in the form of a standard statistics package.

However, descriptions of the characteristics of different packages quickly go out of date. Most potential users will have access to one or more packages, and probably to sources of advice about them. Detailed descriptions and instructions can, therefore, readily be obtained elsewhere. We have confined our descriptions to some general remarks in §2.2 and brief comments on specific programs at relevant points throughout the book.

As with earlier editions, we have had in mind a very broad class of readership. A major purpose of the book has always been to guide the medical research worker with no particular mathematical expertise but with the ability to follow algebraic formulae and, more particularly, the concepts behind them. Even the more advanced methods described in this edition are being extensively used in medical research and they find their way into the reports subsequently published in the medical press. It is important that the medical research worker should understand the gist of these methods, even though the technical details may remain something of a mystery.

Statisticians engaged in medical work or interested in medical applications will, we hope, find many points of interest in this new review of the subject. We hope especially that newly qualified medical statisticians, faced with the need to respond to the demands of unfamiliar applications, will find the book to be of value. Although the book developed from material used in courses for postgraduate students in the medical sciences, we have always regarded it primarily as a resource for research workers rather than as a course book. Nevertheless, much of the book would provide a useful framework for courses at various levels, either for students trained in medical or biological sciences or for those moving towards a career in medical statistics. The statistics teacher would have little difficulty in making appropriate selections for particular groups of students.

For much of the material included in the book, both illustrative and general, we owe our thanks to our present and former colleagues. We have attempted to give attributions for quoted data, but the origins of some are lost in the mists of time, and we must apologize to authors who find their data put to unsuspected purposes in these pages.

In preparing each of these editions for the press we have had much secretarial and other help from many people, to all of whom we express our thanks. We appreciate also the encouragement and support given by Stuart Taylor and his colleagues at Blackwell Science. Two of the authors (P.A. and G.B.) are grateful to the third (J.N.S.M.) for joining them in this enterprise, and all the authors thank their wives and families for their forbearance in the face of occasionally unsocial working practices.

P. Armitage
G. Berry
J.N.S. Matthews

1 The scope of statistics

In one sense medical statistics are merely numerical statements about medical matters: how many people die from a certain cause each year, how many hospital beds are available in a certain area, how much money is spent on a certain medical service. Such facts are clearly of administrative importance. To plan the maternity-bed service for a community we need to know how many women in that community give birth to a child in a given period, and how many of these should be cared for in hospitals or maternity homes. Numerical facts also supply the basis for a great deal of medical research; examples will be found throughout this book. It is no purpose of the book to list or even to summarize numerical information of this sort. Such facts may be found in official publications of national or international health departments, in the published reports of research investigations and in textbooks and monographs on medical subjects. This book is concerned with the general rather than the particular, with methodology rather than factual information, with the general principles of statistical investigations rather than the results of particular studies.

Statistics may be defined as the discipline concerned with the treatment of numerical data derived from groups of individuals. These individuals will often be people—for instance, those suffering from a certain disease or those living in a certain area. They may be animals or other organisms. They may be different administrative units, as when we measure the case-fatality rate in each of a number of hospitals. They may be merely different occasions on which a particular measurement has been made.

Why should we be interested in the numerical properties of groups of people or objects? Sometimes, for administrative reasons like those mentioned earlier, statistical facts are needed: these may be contained in official publications; they may be derivable from established systems of data collection such as cancer registries or systems for the notification of congenital malformations; they may, however, require specially designed statistical investigations.

This book is concerned particularly with the uses of statistics in medical research, and here—in contrast to its administrative uses—the case for statistics has not always been free from controversy. The argument occasionally used to be heard that statistical information contributes little or nothing to the progress of medicine, because the physician is concerned at any one time with the treatment of a single patient, and every patient differs in important respects from every other patient. The clinical judgement exercised by a physician in the choice of treatment for an individual patient is based to an extent on theoretical considerations derived from an understanding of the nature of the illness. But it is based also on an appreciation of statistical information about diagnosis, treatment and prognosis acquired either through personal experience or through medical education. The important argument is whether such information should be stored in a rather informal way in the physician's mind, or whether it should be collected and reported in a systematic way. Very few doctors acquire, by personal experience, factual information over the whole range of medicine, and it is partly by the collection, analysis and reporting of statistical information that a common body of knowledge is built and solidified.

The phrase *evidence-based medicine* is often applied to describe the compilation of reliable and comprehensive information about medical care (Sackett *et al.*, 1996). Its scope extends throughout the specialties of medicine, including, for instance, research into diagnostic tests, prognostic factors, therapeutic and prophylactic procedures, and covers public health and medical economics as well as clinical and epidemiological topics. A major role in the collection, critical evaluation and dissemination of such information is played by the Cochrane Collaboration, an international network of research centres (http://www.cochrane.org/).

In all this work, the statistical approach is essential. The variability of disease is an argument *for* statistical information, not *against* it. If the bedside physician finds that on one occasion a patient with migraine feels better after drinking plum juice, it does not follow, from this single observation, that plum juice is a useful therapy for migraine. The doctor needs statistical information showing, for example, whether in a group of patients improvement is reported more frequently after the administration of plum juice than after the use of some alternative treatment.

The difficulty of arguing from a single instance is equally apparent in studies of the aetiology of disease. The fact that a particular person was alive and well at the age of 95 and that he smoked 50 cigarettes a day and drank heavily would not convince one that such habits are conducive to good health and longevity. Individuals vary greatly in their susceptibility to disease. Many abstemious non-smokers die young. To study these questions one should look at the morbidity and mortality experience of groups of people with different habits: that is, one should do a statistical study.

The second chapter of this book is concerned mainly with some of the basic tools for collecting and presenting numerical data, a part of the subject usually called *descriptive statistics*. The statistician needs to go beyond this descriptive task, in two important respects. First, it may be possible to improve the quality of the information by careful planning of the data collection. For example, information on the efficacy of specific treatments is most reliably obtained from the experimental approach provided by a *clinical trial* (Chapter 18), and questions about the aetiology of disease can be tackled by carefully designed *epidemiological surveys* (Chapter 19). Secondly, the methods of *statistical inference* provide a largely objective means of drawing conclusions from the data about the issues under research. Both these developments, of planning and inference, owe much to the work of R.A. (later Sir Ronald) Fisher (1890–1962), whose influence is apparent throughout modern statistical practice.

Almost all the techniques described in this book can be used in a wide variety of branches of medical research, and indeed frequently in the non-medical sciences also. To set the scene it may be useful to mention four quite different investigations in which statistical methods played an essential part.

1 MacKie *et al.* (1992) studied the trend in the incidence of primary cutaneous malignant melanoma in Scotland during the period 1979–89. In assessing trends of this sort it is important to take account of such factors as changes in standards of diagnosis and in definition of disease categories, changes in the pattern of referrals of patients in and out of the area under study, and changes in the age structure of the population. The study group was set up with these points in mind, and dealt with almost 4000 patients. The investigators found that the annual incidence rate increased during the period from 3·4 to 7·1 per 100 000 for men, and from 6·6 to 10·4 for women. These findings suggest that the disease, which is known to be affected by high levels of ultraviolet radiation, may be becoming more common even in areas where these levels are relatively low.

2 Women who have had a pregnancy with a neural tube defect (NTD) are known to be at higher than average risk of having a similar occurrence in a future pregnancy. During the early 1980s two studies were published suggesting that vitamin supplementation around the time of conception might reduce this risk. In one study, women who agreed to participate were given a mixture of vitamins including folic acid, and they showed a much lower incidence of NTD in their subsequent pregnancies than women who were already pregnant or who declined to participate. It was possible, however, that some systematic difference in the characteristics of those who participated and those who did not might explain the results. The second study attempted to overcome this ambiguity by allocating women randomly to receive folic acid supplementation or a placebo, but it was too small to give clear-cut results. The Medical Research Council (MRC) Vitamin Study Research Group (1991) reported a much larger randomized trial, in which the separate effects could be studied of both folic acid and other vitamins. The outcome was clear. Of 593 women receiving folic acid and becoming pregnant, six had NTD; of 602 not receiving folic acid, 21 had NTD. No effect of other vitamins was apparent. Statistical methods confirmed the immediate impression that the contrast between the folic acid and control

groups is very unlikely to be due to chance and can safely be ascribed to the treatment used.

3   The World Health Organization carried out a collaborative case–control study at 12 participating centres in 10 countries to investigate the possible association between breast cancer and the use of oral contraceptives (WHO Collaborative Study of Neoplasia and Steroid Contraceptives, 1990). In each hospital, women with breast cancer and meeting specific age and residential criteria were taken as cases. Controls were taken from women who were admitted to the same hospital, who satisfied the same age and residential criteria as the cases, and who were not suffering from a condition considered as possibly influencing contraceptive practices. The study included 2116 cases and 13 072 controls. The analysis of the association between breast cancer and use of oral contraceptives had to consider a number of other variables that are associated with breast cancer and which might differ between users and non-users of oral contraceptives. These variables included age, age at first live birth (2·7-fold effect between age 30 or older and less than 20 years), a socio-economic index (twofold effect), year of marriage and family history of breast cancer (threefold effect). After making allowance for these possible confounding variables as necessary, the risk of breast cancer for users of oral contraceptives was estimated as 1·15 times the risk for non-users, a weak association in comparison with the size of the associations with some of the other variables that had to be considered.

4   A further example of the use of statistical arguments is a study to quantify illness in babies under 6 months of age reported by Cole *et al.* (1991). It is important that parents and general practitioners have an appropriate method for identifying severe illness requiring referral to a specialist paediatrician. Whether this is possible can only be determined by the study of a large number of babies for whom possible signs and symptoms are recorded, and for whom the severity of illness is also determined. In this study the authors considered 28 symptoms and 47 physical signs. The analysis showed that it was sufficient to use seven of the symptoms and 12 of the signs, and each symptom or sign was assigned an integer score proportional to its importance. A baby's illness score was then derived by adding the scores for any signs or symptoms that were present. The score was then considered in three categories, 0–7, 8–12 and 13 or more, indicating well or mildly ill, moderate illness and serious illness, respectively. It was predicted that the use of this score would correctly classify 98% of the babies who were well or mildly ill and correctly identify 92% of the seriously ill.

These examples come from different fields of medicine. A review of research in any one branch of medicine is likely to reveal the pervasive influence of the statistical approach, in laboratory, clinical and epidemiological studies. Consider, for instance, research into the human immunodeficiency virus (HIV) and the acquired immune deficiency syndrome (AIDS). Early studies extrapolated the trend in reported cases of AIDS to give estimates of the future incidence. However, changes in the incidence of clinical AIDS are largely determined by the trends in the incidence of earlier events, namely the original HIV infections. The timing of an HIV infection is usually unknown, but it is possible to use estimates of the incubation period to work backwards from the AIDS incidence to that of HIV infection, and then to project forwards to obtain estimates of future trends in AIDS. Estimation of duration of survival of AIDS patients is complicated by the fact that, at any one time, many are still alive, a standard situation in the analysis of survival data (Chapter 17). As possible methods of treatment became available, they were subjected to carefully controlled clinical trials, and reliable evidence was produced for the efficacy of various forms of combined therapy. The progression of disease in each patient may be assessed both by clinical symptoms and signs and by measurement of specific markers. Of these, the most important are the CD4 cell count, as a measure of the patient's immune status, and the viral load, as measured by an assay of viral RNA by the polymerase chain reaction (PCR) method or some alternative test. Statistical questions arising with markers include their ability to predict clinical progression (and hence perhaps act as surrogate measures in trials that would otherwise require long observation periods); their variability, both between patients and on repeated occasions on the same patient; and the stability of the assay methods used for the determinations.

Statistical work in this field, as in any other specialized branch of medicine, must take into account the special features of the disease under study, and must involve close collaboration between statisticians and medical experts. Nevertheless, most of the issues that arise are common to work in other branches of medicine, and can thus be discussed in fairly general terms. It is the purpose of this book to present these general methods, illustrating them by examples from different medical fields.

Statistical investigations

The statistical investigations described above have one feature in common: they involve observations of a similar type being made on each of a group of individuals. The individuals may be people (as in **1-4** above), animals, blood samples, or even inanimate objects such as birth certificates or parishes. The need to study groups rather than merely single individuals arises from the presence of random, unexplained variation. If all patients suffering from the common cold experienced well-defined symptoms for precisely 7 days, it might be possible to demonstrate the merits of a purported drug for the alleviation of symptoms by administering it to one patient only. If the symptoms lasted only 5 days, the reduction could safely be attributed to the new treatment. Similarly, if blood pressure were an exact function of age, varying neither from person to person nor between occasions on the same person, the blood pressure at age 55 could be determined by one observation only. Such studies would not be statistical in nature and would not call for statistical analysis. Those situations, of course, do not hold. The duration of symptoms from the common cold varies from one attack to another; blood pressures vary both between individuals and between occasions. Comparisons of the effects of different medical treatments must therefore be made on groups of patients; studies of physiological norms require population surveys.

In the planning of a statistical study a number of administrative and technical problems are likely to arise. These will be characteristic of the particular field of research and cannot be discussed fully in the present context. Two aspects of the planning will almost invariably be present and are of particular concern to the statistician. The investigator will wish the inferences from the study to be sufficiently precise, and will also wish the results to be relevant to the questions being asked. Discussions of the statistical design of investigations are concerned especially with the general considerations that bear on these two objectives. Some of the questions that arise are: (i) how to select the individuals on which observations are to be made; (ii) how to decide on the numbers of observations falling into different groups; and (iii) how to allocate observations between different possible categories, such as groups of animals receiving different treatments or groups of people living in different areas.

It is useful to make a conceptual distinction between two different types of statistical investigation, the *experiment* and the *survey*. Experimentation involves a planned interference with the natural course of events so that its effect can be observed. In a survey, on the other hand, the investigator is a more passive observer, interfering as little as possible with the phenomena to be recorded. It is easy to think of extreme examples to illustrate this antithesis, but in practice the distinction is sometimes hard to draw. Consider, for instance, the following series of statistical studies:

1   A register of deaths occurring during a particular year, classified by the cause of death.
2   A survey of the types of motor vehicle passing a checkpoint during a certain period.
3   A public opinion poll.
4   A study of the respiratory function (as measured by various tests) of men working in a certain industry.
5   Observations of the survival times of mice of three different strains, after inoculation with the same dose of a toxic substance.
6   A clinical trial to compare the merits of surgery and conservative treatment for patients with a certain condition, the subjects being allotted randomly to the two treatments.

Studies **1** to **4** are clearly surveys, although they involve an increasing amount of interference with nature. Study **6** is equally clearly an experiment. Study **5** occupies an equivocal position. In its statistical aspects it is conceptually a survey, since the object is to observe and compare certain characteristics of three strains of mice. It happens, though, that the characteristic of interest requires the most extreme form of interference—the death of the animal—and the non-statistical techniques are more akin to those of a laboratory experiment than to those required in most survey work.

The general principles of experimental design will be discussed in §9.1, and those of survey design in §§19.2 and 19.4.

2 Describing data

2.1 **Diagrams**

One of the principal methods of displaying statistical information is the use of diagrams. Trends and contrasts are often more readily apprehended, and perhaps retained longer in the memory, by casual observation of a well-proportioned diagram than by scrutiny of the corresponding numerical data presented in tabular form. Diagrams must, however, be simple. If too much information is presented in one diagram it becomes too difficult to unravel and the reader is unlikely even to make the effort. Furthermore, details will usually be lost when data are shown in diagrammatic form. For any critical analysis of the data, therefore, reference must be made to the relevant numerical quantities.

Statistical diagrams serve two main purposes. The first is the presentation of statistical information in articles and other reports, when it may be felt that the reader will appreciate a simple, evocative display. Official statistics of trade, finance, and medical and demographic data are often illustrated by diagrams in newspaper articles and in annual reports of government departments. The powerful impact of diagrams makes them also a potential means of misrepresentation by the unscrupulous. The reader should pay little attention to a diagram unless the definition of the quantities represented and the scales on which they are shown are all clearly explained. In research papers it is inadvisable to present basic data solely in diagrams because of the loss of detail referred to above. The use of diagrams here should be restricted to the emphasis of important points, the detailed evidence being presented separately in tabular form.

The second main use is as a private aid to statistical analysis. The statistician will often have recourse to diagrams to gain insight into the structure of the data and to check assumptions which might be made in an analysis. This informal use of diagrams will often reveal new aspects of the data or suggest hypotheses which may be further investigated.

Various types of diagrams are discussed at appropriate points in this book. It will suffice here to mention a few of the main uses to which statistical diagrams are put, illustrating these from official publications.

1 *To compare two or more numbers.* The comparison is often by bars of different lengths (Fig. 2.1), but another common method (the *pictogram*) is

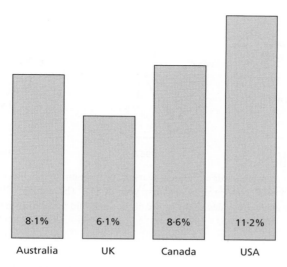

Fig. 2.1 A bar diagram showing the percentages of gross domestic product spent on health care in four countries in 1987 (reproduced with permission from Macklin, 1990).

to use rows of repeated symbols; for example, the populations of different countries may be depicted by rows of 'people', each 'person' representing 1 000 000 people. Care should be taken not to use symbols of the same shape but different sizes because of ambiguity in interpretation; for example, if exports of different countries are represented by money bags of different sizes the reader is uncertain whether the numerical quantities are represented by the linear or the areal dimensions of the bags.

2 *To express the distribution of individual objects or measurements into different categories.* The frequency distribution of different values of a numerical measurement is usually depicted by a histogram, a method discussed more fully in §2.3 (see Figs 2.6–2.8). The distribution of individuals into non-numerical categories can be shown as a *bar diagram* as in **1**, the length of each bar representing the number of observations (or *frequency*) in each category. If the frequencies are expressed as percentages, totalling 100%, a convenient device is the *pie chart* (Fig. 2.2).

3 *To express the change in some quantity over a period of time.* The natural method here is a graph in which points, representing the values of the quantity at successive times, are joined by a series of straight-line segments (Fig. 2.3). If the time intervals are very short the graph will become a smooth curve. If the variation in the measurement is over a small range centred some distance from zero it will be undesirable to start the scale (usually shown vertically) at zero for this will leave too much of the diagram completely blank. A non-zero origin should be indicated by a break in the axis at the

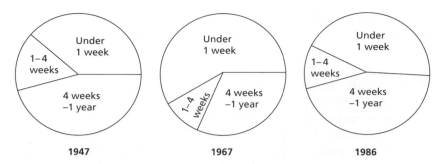

Fig. 2.2 A pie chart showing for three different years the proportions of infant deaths in England and Wales that occur in different parts of the first year of life. The amount for each category is proportional to the angle subtended at the centre of the circle and hence to the area of the sector.

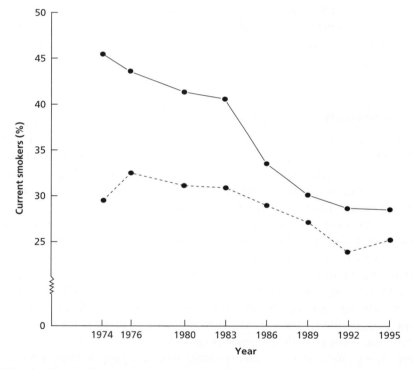

Fig. 2.3 A line diagram showing the changes between six surveys in the proportion of men (solid line) and women (dashed line) in Australia who were current smokers (adapted from Hill *et al.*, 1998).

lower end of the scale, to attract the readers' attention (Fig. 2.3). A slight trend can, of course, be made to appear much more dramatic than it really is by the judicious choice of a non-zero origin, and it is unfortunately only too easy for the unscrupulous to support a chosen interpretation of a time trend by a careful choice of origin. A sudden change of scale over part of the range of variation is even more misleading and should almost always be avoided. Special scales based on logarithmic and other transformations are discussed in §§2.5 and 10.8.

4 *To express the relationship between two measurements, in a situation where they occur in pairs.* The usual device is the *scatter diagram* (see Fig. 7.1), which is described in detail in Chapter 7 and will not be discussed further here. Time trends, discussed in **3**, are of course a particular form of relationship, but they called for special comment because the data often consist of one measurement at each point of time (these times being often equally spaced). In general, data on relationships are not restricted in this way and the continuous graph is not generally appropriate.

Modern computing methods provide great flexibility in the construction of diagrams, by such features as interaction with the visual display, colour printing and dynamic displays of complex data. For extensive reviews of the art of graphical display, see Tufte (1983), Cleveland (1985, 1993) and Martin and Welsh (1998).

2.2 **Tabulation and data processing**

Tabulation

Another way of summarizing and presenting some of the important features of a set of data is in the form of a table. There are many variants, but the essential features are that the structure and meaning of a table are indicated by headings or labels and the statistical summary is provided by numbers in the body of the table. Frequently the table is two-dimensional, in that the headings for the horizontal rows and vertical columns define two different ways of categorizing the data. Each portion of the table defined by a combination of row and column is called a *cell*. The numerical information may be counts of numbers of individuals in different cells, mean values of some measurements (see §2.4) or more complex indices.

Some useful guidelines in the presentation of tables for publication are given by Ehrenberg (1975, 1977). Points to note are the avoidance of an unnecessarily large number of digits (since shorter, rounded-off numbers convey their message to the eye more effectively) and care that the layout allows the eye easily to compare numbers that need to be compared.

Table 2.1, taken from a report on assisted conception (AIH National Perinatal Statistics Unit, 1991), is an example of a table summarizing counts. It summarizes information on 5116 women who conceived following *in vitro* fertilization (IVF), and shows that the proportion of women whose pregnancy

Table 2.1 Outcome of pregnancies according to maternal age (adapted from AIH National Perinatal Statistics Unit, 1991).

Age		Live birth	Spontaneous abortion	Ectopic pregnancy	Stillbirth	Termination of pregnancy	Total
< 25	No.	94	21	10	2	0	127
	%	74·0	16·5	7·9	1·6	0·0	100·0
25–29	No.	962	272	96	36	2	1368
	%	70·3	19·9	7·0	2·6	0·1	99·9
30–34	No.	1615	430	143	58	8	2254
	%	71·7	19·1	6·3	2·6	0·4	100·1
35–39	No.	789	338	66	27	6	1226
	%	64·4	27·6	5·4	2·2	0·5	100·1
40 +	No.	69	60	6	1	5	141
	%	48·9	42·6	4·3	0·7	3·5	100·0
Total	No.	3529	1121	321	124	21	5116
	%	69·0	21·9	6·3	2·4	0·4	100·0

resulted in a live birth was related to age. How is such a table constructed? With a small quantity of data a table of this type could be formed by manual sorting and counting of the original records, but if there were many observations (as in Table 2.1) or if many tables had to be produced the labour would obviously be immense.

Data collection and preparation

We may distinguish first between the problems of preparing the data in a form suitable for tabulation, and the mechanical (or electronic) problems of getting the computations done. Some studies, particularly small laboratory experiments, give rise to relatively few observations, and the problems of data preparation are correspondingly simple. Indeed, tabulations of the type under discussion may not be required, and the statistician may be concerned solely with more complex forms of analysis.

Data preparation is, in contrast, a problem of serious proportions in many large-scale investigations, whether with complex automated laboratory measurements or in clinical or other studies on a 'human' scale. In large-scale therapeutic and prophylactic trials, in prognostic investigations, in studies in epidemiology and social medicine and in many other fields, a large number of people may be included as subjects, and very many observations may be made on each subject. Furthermore, much of the information may be difficult to obtain in unambiguous form and the precise definition of the variables may require careful thought. This subsection and the two following ones are concerned primarily with data from these large studies.

In most investigations of this type it will be necessary to collect the information on specially designed record forms or questionnaires. The design of forms and questionnaires is considered in some detail by Babbie (1989). The following points may be noted briefly here.

1 There is a temptation to attempt to collect more information than is clearly required, in case it turns out to be useful in either the present or some future study. While there is obviously a case for this course of action it carries serious disadvantages. The collection of data costs money and, although the cost of collecting extra information from an individual who is in any case providing some information may be relatively low, it must always be considered. The most serious disadvantage, though, is that the collection of marginally useful information may detract from the value of the essential data. The interviewer faced with 50 items for each subject may take appreciably less care than if only 20 items were required. If there is a serious risk of non-cooperation of the subject, as perhaps in postal surveys using questionnaires which are self-administered, the length of a questionnaire may be a strong disincentive and the list of items must be severely pruned. Similarly, if the data are collected by telephone interview, cooperation may be reduced if the respondent expects the call to take more than a few minutes.

2 Care should be taken over the wording of questions to ensure that their interpretation is unambiguous and in keeping with the purpose of the investigation. Whenever possible the various categories of response that are of interest should be enumerated on the form. This helps to prevent meaningless or ambiguous replies and saves time in the later classification of results. For example,

What is your working status? (circle number)

1 Domestic duties with no paid job outside home.
2 In part-time employment (less than 25 hours per week).
3 In full-time employment.
4 Unemployed seeking work.
5 Retired due to disability or illness (please specify cause)..
6 Retired for other reasons.
7 Other (please specify)...

If the answer to a question is a numerical quantity the units required should be specified. For example,

Your weight: ....kg.

In some cases more than one set of units may be in common use and both should be allowed for. For example,

Your height:....... cm.

         Or....... feet....... inches.

In other cases it may be sufficient to specify a number of categories. For example,

How many years have you lived in this town? (circle number)

1   Less than 5.
2   5–9.
3   10–19.
4   20–29.
5   30–39.
6   40 or more.

When the answer is qualitative but may nevertheless be regarded as a grada-tion of a single dimensional scale, a number of ordered choices may be given. For example,

How much stress or worry have you had in the last month with:

		None	A little	Some	Much	Very much
1	Your spouse?	1	2	3	4	5
2	Other members of your family?	1	2	3	4	5
3	Friends?	1	2	3	4	5
4	Money or finance?	1	2	3	4	5
5	Your job?	1	2	3	4	5
6	Your health?	1	2	3	4	5

Sometimes the data may be recorded directly into a computer. Biomedical data are often recorded on automatic analysers or other specialized equipment, and automatically transferred to a computer. In telephone interviews, it may be possible to dispense with the paper record, so that the interviewer reads a question on the computer screen and enters the response directly from the keyboard.

In many situations, though, the data will need to be transferred from data sheets to a computer, a process described in the next subsection.

Data transfer

The data are normally entered via the keyboard and screen on to disk, either the computer's own hard disk or a floppy disk (diskette) or both. Editing facilities allow amendments to be made directly on the stored data. As it is no longer necessary to keep a hard copy of the data in computer-readable form, it is essential to maintain back-up copies of data files to guard against computer malfunctions that may result in a particular file becoming unreadable.

There are two strategies for the entry of data. In the first the data are regarded as a row of characters, and no interpretation occurs until a data file has been created. The second method is much more powerful and involves using the computer interactively as the data are entered. Questionnaires often contain items that are only applicable if a particular answer has been given to an earlier item. For example, if a detailed smoking history is required, the first question might be 'Have you smoked?' If the answer was 'yes', there would follow several questions on the number of years smoked, the amount smoked, the brands of cigarettes, etc. On the other hand, if the answer was 'no', these questions would not be applicable and should be skipped. With screen-based data entry the controlling program would automatically display the next applicable item on the screen.

There are various ways in which information from a form or questionnaire can be represented in a computer record. In the simplest method the reply to each question is given in one or more specific columns and each column contains a digit from 0 to 9. This means that non-numerical information must be 'coded'. For example, the coding of the first few questions might be as in Fig. 2.4. In some systems leading zeros must be entered, e.g. if three digits were allowed for a variable like diastolic blood pressure, a reading of 88 mmHg would be recorded as 088, whereas other systems allow blanks instead. For a subject with study number 122 who was a married woman aged 49, the first eight columns of the record given in Fig. 2.4 would be entered as the following codes:

Column	1	2	3	4	5	6	7	8
Code	0	1	2	2	2	4	9	2

Clearly the person entering the data must know which code to enter for any particular column. Two different approaches are possible. The information may

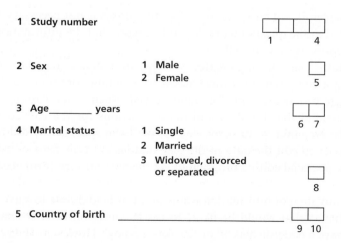

Fig. 2.4 An example of part of a questionnaire with coding indicated.

be transferred from the original record to a 'coding sheet' which will show for each column of each record precisely which code is to be entered. This may be a sheet of paper, ruled as a grid, in which the rows represent the different individuals and the vertical columns represent the columns of the record. Except for small jobs it will usually be preferable to design a special coding form showing clearly the different items; this will reduce the frequency of transcription errors. Alternatively, the coding may be included on the basic record form so that the transfer may be done direct from this form and the need for an intermediate coding sheet is removed. If sufficient care is given to the design of the record form, this second method is preferable, as it removes a potential source of copying errors. This is the approach shown in Fig. 2.4, where the boxes on the right are used for coding. For the first four items the codes are shown and an interviewer could fill in the coding boxes immediately. For item 5 there are so many possibilities that all the codes cannot be shown. Instead, the response would be recorded in open form, e.g. 'Greece', and the code looked up later in a detailed set of coding instructions.

It was stated above that it is preferable to use the record form or questionnaire also for the coding. One reservation must, however, be made. The purpose of the questionnaire is to obtain accurate information, and anything that detracts from this should be removed. Particularly with self-administered questionnaires the presence of coding boxes, even though the respondent is not asked to use them, may reduce the cooperation a subject would otherwise give. This may be because of an abhorrence of what may be regarded as looking like an 'official' form, or it may be simply that the boxes have made the form appear cramped and less interesting. This should not be a problem where a few interviewers are being used but if there is any doubt, separate coding sheets should be used.

With screen-based entry the use of coding boxes is not necessary but care is still essential in the questionnaire design to ensure that the information required by the operator is easy to find.

The statistician or investigator wishing to tabulate the data in various ways using a computer must have access to a suitable program, and statistical packages are widely available for standard tasks such as tabulation.

It is essential that the data and the instructions for the particular analysis required be prepared in, or converted to, the form specified by the package. It may be better to edit the data in the way that leads to the fewest mistakes, and then to use a special editing program to get the data into the form needed for the package.

When any item of information is missing, it is inadvisable to leave a blank in the data file as that would be likely to cause confusion in later analyses. It is better to have a code such as '9' or '99' for 'missing'. However, when the missing information is numerical, care must be taken to ensure that the code cannot be mistaken for a real observation. The coding scheme shown in Fig. 2.4 would be deficient in a survey of elderly people, since a code of '99' for an unknown age could be confused with a true age of 99 years, and indeed there is no provision for centenarians. A better plan would have been to use three digits for age, and to denote a missing reading by, say, '999'.

Data cleaning

Before data are subjected to further analyses, they should be carefully checked for errors. These may have arisen during data entry, and ideally data should be transferred by *double entry*, independently by two different operators, the two files being checked for consistency by a separate computer program. In practice, most data-processing organizations find this system too expensive, and rely on single entry by an experienced operator, with regular monitoring for errors, which should be maintained at a very low rate.

Other errors may occur because inaccurate information appeared on the initial record forms. Computer programs can be used to detect implausible values, which can be checked and corrected where necessary. Methods of data checking are discussed further in §2.7.

With direct entry of data, as in a telephone interview, logical errors or implausible values could be detected by the computer program and queried immediately with the respondent.

Statistical computation

Most of the methods of analysis described later in this book may be carried out using standard statistical packages or languages. Widely available packages include *BMDP* (BMDP, 1993), *SPSS* (SPSS, 1999), *Stata* (Stata, 2001) *MINITAB* (Minitab, 2000), *SAS* (SAS, 2000) and *SYSTAT* (SYSTAT, 2000). The scope of such packages develops too rapidly to justify any detailed descriptions here, but summaries can be found on the relevant websites, with fuller descriptions and operating instructions in the package manuals. Goldstein (1998) provides a useful summary. Many of these packages, such as *SAS*, offer facilities for the data management tasks described earlier in this section. *S-PLUS* (S-PLUS, 2000) provides an interactive data analysis system, together with a programming language, *S*. For very large data sets a database management system such as *Oracle* may be needed (Walker, 1998). *StatsDirect* (StatsDirect, 1999) is a more recent package covering many of the methods for medical applications that are described in this book.

Some statistical analyses may be performed on small data sets, or on compact tables summarizing larger data sets, and these may be read, item by item, directly into the computer. In larger studies, the analyses will refer to data extracted from the full data file. In such cases it will be useful to form a derived file containing the subset of data needed for the analysis, in whatever form is required by the package program. As Altman (1991) remarks, the user is well advised as far as possible to use the same package for all his or her analyses, 'as it takes a considerable effort to become fully acquainted with even one package'.

In addition to the major statistical computing packages, which cover many of the standard methods described in this book, there are many other packages or programs suitable for some of the more specialized tasks. Occasional references to these are made throughout the book.

Although computers are increasingly used for analysis, with smaller sets of data it is often convenient to use a calculator, the most convenient form of which is the pocket calculator. These machines perform at high speed all the basic arithmetic operations, and have a range of mathematical functions such as the square, square root, exponential, logarithm, etc. An additional feature particularly useful in statistical work is the automatic calculation and accumulation of sums of squares of numbers. Some machines have a special range of extended facilities for statistical analyses. It is particularly common for the automatic calculation of the mean and standard deviation to be available. Programmable calculators are available and these facilitate repeated use of statistical formulae.

The user of a calculator often finds it difficult to know how much rounding off is permissible in the data and in the intermediate or final steps of the computations. Some guidance will be derived from the examples in this book, but the following general points may be noted.

1   Different values of any one measurement should normally be expressed to the same degree of precision. If a series of children's heights is generally given to the nearest centimetre, but a few are expressed to the nearest millimetre, this extra precision will be wasted in any calculations done on the series as a whole. All the measurements should therefore be rounded to the nearest centimetre for convenience of calculation.

2   A useful rule in rounding mid-point values (such as a height of 127·5 cm when rounding to whole numbers) is to round to the nearest even number. Thus 127·5 would be rounded to 128. This rule prevents a slight bias which would otherwise occur if the figures were always rounded up or always rounded down.

3   It may occasionally be justifiable to quote the results of calculations to a little more accuracy than the original data. For example, if a large series of heights is measured to the nearest centimetre the mean may sometimes be quoted to one decimal point. The reason for this is that, as we shall see, the effect of the rounding errors is reduced by the process of averaging.

4   If any quantity calculated during an intermediate stage of the calculations is quoted to, say, n significant digits, the result of any multiplication or division

of this quantity will be valid to, at the most, n digits. The significant digits are those from the first non-zero digit to the last meaningful digit, irrespective of the position of the decimal point. Thus, 1·002, 10·02, 100 200 (if this number is expressed to the nearest 100) all have four significant digits. Cumulative inaccuracy arises with successive operations of multiplication or division.

5   The result of an addition or subtraction is valid to, at most, the number of decimal digits of the least accurate figure. Thus, the result of adding 101 (accurate to the nearest integer) and 4·39 (accurate to two decimal points) is 105 (to the nearest integer). The last digit may be in error by one unit; for example, the exact figure corresponding to 101 may have been 101·42, in which case the result of the addition now should have been 105·81, or 106 to the nearest integer. These considerations are particularly important in subtraction. Very frequently in statistical calculations one number is subtracted from another of very similar size. The result of the subtraction may then be accurate to many fewer significant digits than either of the original numbers. For example, $3212·78 - 3208·44 = 4·34$; three digits have been lost by the subtraction. For this reason it is essential in some early parts of a computation to keep more significant digits than will be required in the final result.

A final general point about computation is that the writing down of intermediate steps offers countless opportunities for error. It is therefore important to keep a tidy layout on paper, with adequate labelling and vertical and horizontal alignment of digits, and without undue crowding.

2.3 **Summarizing numerical data**

The raw material of all statistical investigations consists of individual observations, and these almost always have to be summarized in some way before any use can be made of them. We have discussed in the last two sections the use of diagrams and tables to present some of the main features of a set of data. We must now examine some particular forms of table, and the associated diagrams, in more detail. As we have seen, the aim of statistical methods goes beyond the mere presentation of data to include the drawing of inferences from them. These two aspects—description and inference—cannot be entirely separated. We cannot discuss the descriptive tools without some consideration of the purpose for which they are needed. In the next few sections, we shall occasionally have to anticipate questions of inference which will be discussed in more detail later in the book.

Any class of measurement or classification on which individual observations are made is called a *variable* or *variate*. For instance, in one problem the variable might be a particular measure of respiratory function in schoolboys, in another it might be the number of bacteria found in samples of water. In most problems many variables are involved. In a study of the natural history of a certain disease, for example, observations are likely to be made, for each patient, on a number of variables measuring the clinical state of the patient at various times throughout the illness, and also on certain variables, such as age, not directly relating to the patient's health.

It is useful first to distinguish between two types of variable, *qualitative* (or *categorical*) and *quantitative*. Qualitative observations are those that are not characterized by a numerical quantity, but whose possible values consist of a number of categories, with any individual recorded as belonging to just one of these categories. Typical examples are sex, hair colour, death or survival in a certain period of time, and occupation. Qualitative variables may be subdivided into *nominal* and *ordinal* observations. An ordinal variable is one where the categories have an unambiguous natural order. For example, the stage of a cancer at a certain site may be categorized as state A, B, C or D, where previous observations have indicated that there is a progression through these stages in sequence from A to D. Sometimes the fact that the stages are ordered may be indicated by referring to them in terms of a number, stage 1, 2, 3 or 4, but the use of a number here is as a label and does not indicate that the variable is quantitative. A nominal variable is one for which there is no natural order of the categories. For example, certified cause of death might be classified as infectious disease, cancer, heart disease, etc. Again, the fact that cause of death is often referred to as a number (the International Classification of Diseases, or ICD, code) does not obscure the fact that the variable is nominal, with the codes serving only as shorthand labels.

The problem of summarizing qualitative nominal data is relatively simple. The main task is to count the number of observations in various categories, and perhaps to express them as proportions or percentages of appropriate totals. These counts are often called *frequencies* or *relative frequencies*. Examples are shown in Tables 2.1 and 2.2. If relative frequencies in certain subgroups are shown, it is useful to add them to give 1·00, or 100%, so that the reader can easily see which total frequencies have been subdivided. (Slight discrepancies in these totals, due to rounding the relative frequencies, as in Tables 2.1 and 2.3, may be ignored.)

Ordinal variables may be summarized in the same way as nominal variables. One difference is that the order of the categories in any table or figure is predetermined, whereas it is arbitrary for a nominal variable. The order also allows the calculation of *cumulative relative frequencies*, which are the sums of all relative frequencies below and including each category.

A particularly important type of qualitative observation is that in which a certain characteristic is either present or absent, so that the observations fall into one of two categories. Examples are sex, and survival or death. Such variables are variously called *binary, dichotomous* or *quantal*.

Table 2.2 Result of sputum examination 3 months after operation in group of patients treated with streptomycin and control group treated without streptomycin.

	Streptomycin		Control	
	Frequency	%	Frequency	%
Smear negative, culture negative	141	45·0	117	41·8
Smear negative, not cultured	90	28·8	67	23·9
Smear or culture positive	82	26·2	96	34·3
Total with known sputum result	313	100·0	280	100·0
Results not known	12		17	
Total	325		297	

Table 2.3 Frequency distribution of number of lesions caused by smallpox virus in egg membranes.

Number of lesions	Frequency (number of membranes)	Relative frequency (%)
0–	1	1
10–	6	8
20–	14	18
30–	14	18
40–	17	21
50–	8	10
60–	9	11
70–	3	4
80–	6	8
90–	1	1
100–	0	0
110–119	1	1
Total	80	101

Quantitative variables are those for which the individual observations are numerical quantities, usually either measurements or counts. It is useful to subdivide quantitative observations into *discrete* and *continuous* variables. Discrete measurements are those for which the possible values are quite distinct and separated. Often they are counts, such as the number of times an individual has been admitted to hospital in the last 5 years.

Continuous variables are those which can assume a continuous uninterrupted range of values. Examples are height, weight, age and blood pressure. Continuous measurements usually have an upper and a lower limit. For instance, height cannot be less than zero, and there is presumably some lower limit above zero and some upper limit, but it would be difficult to say exactly what these limits are. The distinction between discrete and continuous variables is not always clear, because all continuous measurements are in practice rounded off; for instance, a series of heights might be recorded to the nearest centimetre and so appear discrete. Any ambiguity rarely matters, since the same statistical methods can often be safely applied to both continuous and discrete variables, particularly if the scale used for the latter is fairly finely subdivided. On the other hand, there are some special methods applicable to counts, which as we have seen must be positive whole numbers. The problems of summarizing quantitative data are much more complex than those for qualitative data, and the remainder of this chapter will be devoted almost entirely to them.

Sometimes a continuous or a discrete quantitative variable may be summarized by dividing the range of values into a number of categories, or *grouping intervals*, and producing a table of frequencies. For example, for age a number of age groups could be created and each individual put into one of the groups. The variable, age, has then been transformed into a new variable, age group, which has all the characteristics of an ordered categorical variable. Such a variable may be called an *interval* variable.

A useful first step in summarizing a fairly large collection of quantitative data is the formation of a *frequency distribution*. This is a table showing the number of observations, or frequency, at different values or within certain ranges of values of the variable. For a discrete variable with a few categories the frequency may be tabulated at each value, but, if there is a wide range of possible values, it will be convenient to subdivide the range into categories. An example is shown in Table 2.3. (In this example the reader should note the distinction between two types of count—the variable, which is the number of lesions on an individual chorioallantoic membrane, and the frequency, which is the number of membranes on which the variable falls within a specified range.) With continuous measurements one *must* form grouping intervals (Table 2.4). In Table 2.4 the cumulative relative

Table 2.4 Frequency distribution of age for 1357 male patients with lung cancer.

Age (years)	Frequency (number of patients)	Relative frequency (%)	Cumulative relative frequency (%)
25–	17	1·3	1·3
35–	116	8·5	9·8
45–	493	36·3	46·1
55–	545	40·2	86·3
65–74	186	13·7	100·0
Total	1357	100·0	

frequencies are also tabulated. These give the percentages of the total who are younger than the lower limit of the following interval, that is, 9·8% of the subjects are in the age groups 25–34 and 35–44 and so are younger than 45.

The advantages in presenting numerical data in the form of a frequency distribution rather than a long list of individual observations are too obvious to need stressing. On the other hand, if there are only a few observations, a frequency distribution will be of little value since the number of readings falling into each group will be too small to permit any meaningful pattern to emerge.

We now consider in more detail the practical task of forming a frequency distribution. If the variable is to be grouped, a decision will have to be taken about the end-points of the groups. For convenience these should be chosen, as far as possible, to be 'round' numbers. For distributions of age, for example, it is customary to use multiples of 5 or 10 as the boundaries of the groups. Care should be taken in deciding in which group to place an observation falling on one of the group boundaries, and the decision must be made clear to the reader. Usually such an observation is placed in the group of which the observation is the lower limit. For example, in Table 2.3 a count of 20 lesions would be placed in the group 20–, which includes all counts between 20 and 29, and this convention is indicated by the notation used for the groups.

How many groups should there be? No clear-cut rule can be given. To provide a useful, concise indication of the nature of the distribution, fewer than five groups will usually be too few and more than 20 will usually be too many. Again, if too large a number of groups is chosen, the investigator may find that many of the groups contain frequencies which are too small to provide any regularity in the shape of the distribution. For a given size of grouping interval this difficulty will become more acute as the total number of observations is reduced, and the choice of grouping interval may, therefore, depend on this number. If in doubt, the grouping interval may be chosen smaller than that to be finally used, and groups may be amalgamated in the most appropriate way after the distribution has been formed.

If the original data are contained in a computer file, a frequency distribution can readily be formed by use of a statistical package. If the measurements are available only as a list on paper, the counts should be made by going systematically through the list, 'tallying' each measurement into its appropriate group. The whole process should be repeated as a check. The alternative method of taking each group in turn and counting the observations falling into that group is not to be recommended, as it requires the scanning of the list of observations once for each group (or more than once if a check is required) and thus encourages mistakes.

If the number of observations is not too great (say, fewer than about 50), a frequency distribution can be depicted graphically by a diagram such as Fig. 2.5. Here each individual observation is represented by a dot or some other mark

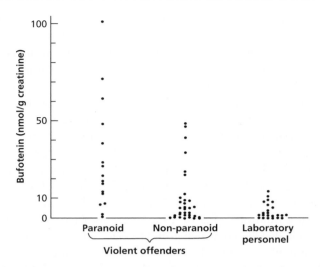

Fig. 2.5 Dot diagram showing the distribution of urinary excretion of bufotenin in three groups of subjects (reprinted from Räisänen *et al.*, 1984, by permission of the authors and the editor of *The Lancet*).

opposite the appropriate point on a scale. The general shape of the distribution can be seen at a glance, and it is easy to compare visually two or more distributions of the same variable (Fig. 2.5). With larger numbers of observations this method is unsuitable because the marks tend to become congested, and a *box-and-whisker* plot is more suitable (see p. 38).

When the number of observations is large the original data may be grouped into a frequency distribution table and the appropriate form of diagram is then the *histogram*. Here the values of the variable are by convention represented on the horizontal scale, and the vertical scale represents the frequency, or relative frequency, at each value or in each group. If the variable is discrete and ungrouped (Fig. 2.6), the frequencies may be represented by vertical lines. The more general method, which must be applied if the variable is grouped, is to draw rectangles based on the different groups (Figs 2.7 and 2.8). It may happen that the grouping intervals are not of constant length. In Table 2.3, for example, suppose we decided to pool the groups 60–, 70– and 80–. The total frequency in these groups is 18, but it would clearly be misleading to represent this frequency by a rectangle on a base extending from 60 to 90 and with a height of 18. The correct procedure would be to make the height of the rectangle 6, the average frequency in the three groups (as indicated by the dashed line in Fig. 2.7). One way of interpreting this rule is to say that the height of the rectangle in a histogram is the frequency per standard grouping of the variable (in this example the standard grouping is 10 lesions). Another way is to say that the frequency for

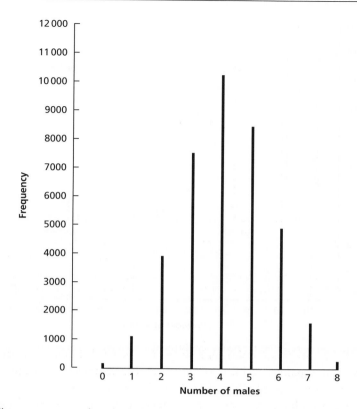

Fig. 2.6 Histogram representing the frequency distribution for an ungrouped discrete variable (number of males in sibships of eight children).

a group is proportional to the *area* rather than the height of the rectangle (in this example the area of any of the original rectangles, or of the composite rectangle formed by the dashed line, is 10 times the frequency for the group). If there is no variation in length of grouping interval, areas are, of course, proportional to heights, and frequencies are represented by either heights or areas.

The cumulative relative frequency may be represented by a line diagram (Fig. 2.9). The positioning of the points on the age axis needs special care, since in the frequency distribution (Table 2.4) the cumulative relative frequencies in the final column are plotted against the start of the age group in the next line. That is, since none of the men are younger than 25, zero is plotted on the vertical axis at age 25, 1·3% are younger than 35 so 1·3% is plotted at age 35, 9·8% at age 45, and so on to 100% at age 75.

The *stem-and-leaf display*, illustrated in Table 2.5, is a useful way of tabulating the original data and, at the same time, depicting the general shape of the frequency distribution. In Table 2.5, the first column lists the initial digit in

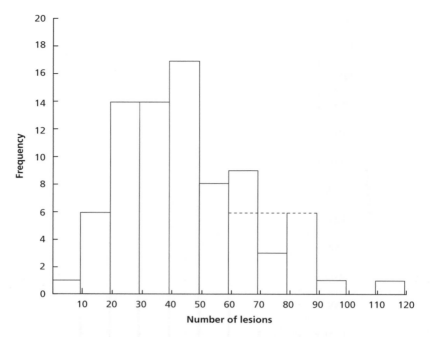

Fig. 2.7 Histogram representing the frequency distribution for a grouped discrete variable (Table 2.3).

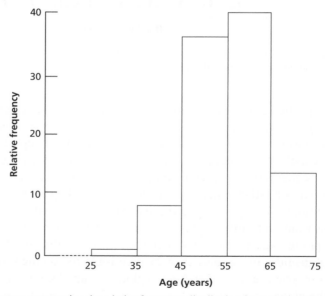

Fig. 2.8 Histogram representing the relative frequency distribution for a continuous variable (age of 1357 men with lung cancer, Table 2.4). Note that the variable shown here is exact age. The age at last birthday is a discrete variable and would be represented by groups displaced half a year to the left from those shown here; see p. 32.

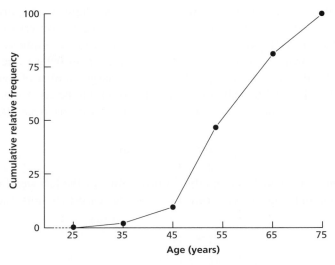

Fig. 2.9 Cumulative frequency plot for age of 1357 men with lung cancer (Table 2.4 and Fig. 2.8).

Table 2.5 Stem-and-leaf display for distribution of number of lesions caused by smallpox virus in egg membranes (see Table 2.3).

Number of lesions	
0*	7
1	024779
2	11122266678999
3	00223456788999
4	01233346677888999
5	11234478
6	014567779
7	057
8	023447
9	8
10	
11	2

the count, and in each row (or 'stem') the numbers to the right (the 'leaves') are the values of the second digit for the various observations in that group. Thus, the single observation in the first group is 7, and the observations in the second group are 10, 12, 14, 17, 17 and 19. The leaves have been ordered on each stem. The similarity in the shape of the stem-and-leaf display and the histogram in Fig. 2.7 is apparent.

The number of asterisks (*) indicates how many digits are required for each leaf. Thus, in Table 2.5, one asterisk is shown because the observations require only one digit from the leaf in addition to the row heading. Suppose that, in the distribution shown in Table 2.5, there had been four outlying values over 100: say, 112, 187, 191 and 248. Rather than having a large number of stems with no leaves and a few with only one leaf, it would be better to use a wider group interval for these high readings. The observations over 100 could be shown as:

$$1** \quad 12, \quad 87, \quad 91$$
$$2 \quad \quad 48$$

Sometimes it might be acceptable to drop some of the less significant digits. Thus, if such high counts were needed only to the nearest 10 units, they could be displayed as:

$$1** \quad 199$$
$$2 \quad \quad 5$$

representing 110, 190, 190 and 250.

For other variants on stem-and-leaf displays, see Tukey (1977).

If the main purpose of a visual display is to compare two or more distributions, the histogram is a clumsy tool. Superimposed histograms are usually confusing, and spatially separated histograms are often too distant to provide a means of comparison. The dot diagram of Fig. 2.5 or the box-and-whisker plot of Fig. 2.14 (p. 39) is preferable for this purpose.

Alternatively, use may be made of the representation of three-dimensional figures now available in some computer programs; an example is shown in Fig. 2.10 of a bar diagram plotted against two variables simultaneously. With this representation care must be taken not to mislead because of the effects of perspective. Some computer packages produce a three-dimensional effect even for bar charts (such as Fig. 2.1), histograms and pie charts. While the third dimension provides no extra information here, the effect can be very attractive.

The frequency in a distribution or in a histogram is often expressed not as an absolute count but as a relative frequency, i.e. as a proportion or percentage of the total frequency. If the standard grouping of the variable in terms of which the frequencies are expressed is a single unit, the total area under the histogram will be 1 (or 100% if percentage frequencies are used), and the area between any two points will be the relative frequency in this range.

Suppose we had a frequency distribution of heights of 100 men, in 1 cm groups. The relative frequencies would be rather irregular, especially near the extremes of the distribution, owing to the small frequencies in some of the groups. If the number of observations were increased to, say, 1000, the trend of the frequencies would become smoother and we might then reduce the grouping

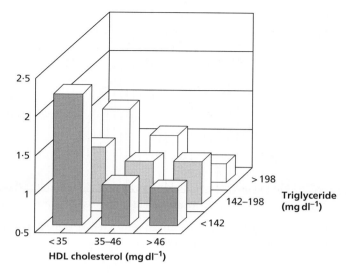

Fig 2.10 A 'three-dimensional' bar diagram showing the relative risk of coronary heart disease in men, according to high-density lipoprotein (HDL) cholesterol and triglyceride (reproduced from Simons *et al.*, 1991, by permission of the authors and publishers).

to 0·5 cm, still making the vertical scale in the histogram represent the relative frequency per cm. We could imagine continuing this process indefinitely if there were no limit to the fineness of the measurement of length or to the number of observations we could make. In this imaginary situation the histogram would approach closer and closer to a smooth curve, the *frequency curve*, which can be thought of as an idealized form of histogram (Fig. 2.11). The area between the ordinates erected at any two values of the variable will represent the relative frequency of observations between these two points. These frequency curves are useful as models on which statistical theory is based, and should be regarded as idealized approximations to the histograms which might be obtained in practice with a large number of observations on a variable which can be measured extremely accurately.

We now consider various features which may characterize frequency distributions. Any value of the variable at which the frequency curve reaches a peak is called a *mode*. Most frequency distributions encountered in practice have one peak and are described as *unimodal*. For example, the distribution in Fig. 2.6 has a mode at four males, and that in Table 2.3 at 40–49 lesions. Usually, as in these two examples, the mode occurs somewhere between the two extremes of the distribution. These extreme portions, where the frequency becomes low, are called *tails*. Some unimodal distributions have the mode at one end of the range. For instance, if the emission of γ-particles by some radioactive material

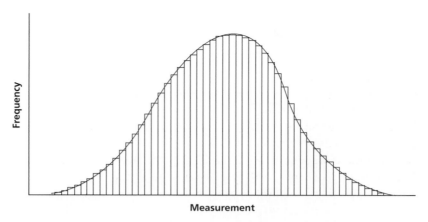

Fig. 2.11 Histogram representing the frequency distribution for a very large number of measurements finely subdivided, with an approximating frequency curve.

is being studied, the frequency distribution of the time interval between successive emissions is shaped like a letter *J* (or rather its mirror image), with a mode at zero. Similarly, if we take families with four children and record the numbers of families in which there have been 0, 1, 2, 3 or 4 cases of poliomyelitis, we shall find a very pronounced mode at zero.

Some distributions will appear to have more than one mode owing to the inevitable random fluctuations of small numbers. In Table 2.3, for example, the observed frequencies show subsidiary modes at 60–69, 80–89 and 110–119, although we should be inclined to pay no great attention to these. Occasionally, even with very large numbers of observations, distributions with more than one mode are found. There has been a great deal of discussion as to whether the distribution of casual blood pressure in a large population free from known circulatory diseases is *bimodal*, i.e. has two modes, because the presence of a second mode at blood pressures higher than the principal mode might indicate that a substantial proportion of the population suffered from essential hypertension.

Another characteristic of some interest is the symmetry or lack of symmetry of the distribution. An asymmetric distribution is called *skew*. The distribution in Fig. 2.6 is fairly symmetrical about the mode. That in Table 2.3 and Fig. 2.7, in which the upper tail is longer than the lower, would be called *positively* skew. The distribution in Table 2.4 and Fig. 2.8 has a slight negative skewness.

Two other characteristics of distributions are of such importance that separate sections will be devoted to them. They are the general location of the distribution on the scale of the variable, and the degree of variation of the observations about the centre of the distribution. Indeed, measures of location and variation are of such general importance that we shall discuss them first in relation to the original, ungrouped, observations, before referring again to frequency distributions.

2.4 **Means and other measures of location**

It is often important to give, in a single figure, some indication of the general level of a series of measurements. Such a figure may be called a *measure of location*, a *measure of central tendency*, a *mean* or an *average*. The most familiar of these measures is the *arithmetic* mean, and is customarily referred to as the 'average'. In statistics the term is often abbreviated to 'mean'.

The mean is the sum of the observations divided by the number of observations. It is awkward to have to express rules of calculation verbally in this way, and we shall therefore digress a little to discuss a convenient notation. A single algebraic symbol, like x or y, will often be used to denote a particular variable. For each variable there may be one or more observations. If there are n observations of variable x they will be denoted by

$$x_1, x_2, x_3, \ldots, x_{n-1}, x_n.$$

The various xs are not necessarily or even usually arranged in order of magnitude. They may be thought of as arranged in the order in which they were calculated or observed. It is often useful to refer to a typical member of the group in order to show some calculation which is to be performed on each member. This is done by introducing a 'dummy' suffix, which will often be i or j. Thus, if x is the height of a schoolchild and $x_1, x_2, \ldots, x_n$ are n values of x, a typical value may be denoted by x_i.

The arithmetic mean of the xs will be denoted by $\bar{x}$ (spoken 'x bar'). Thus,

$$\bar{x} = \frac{x_1 + x_2 + \ldots + x_n}{n}.$$

The summation occurring in the numerator can be denoted by use of the *summation sign* $\sum$ (the capital Greek letter 'sigma'), which means 'the sum of'. The range of values taken by the dummy suffix is indicated above and below the summation sign. Thus,

$$\sum_{i=1}^{n} x_i = x_1 + x_2 + \ldots + x_n$$

and

$$\bar{x} = \frac{\sum_{i=1}^{n} x_i}{n}.$$

If, as in this instance, it is clear which values the dummy suffix assumes throughout the summation, the range of the summation, and even occasionally the dummy suffix, may be omitted. Thus,

$$\sum_{i=1}^{n} x_i$$

may be abbreviated to $\sum x_i$ or to $\sum x$. Sometimes the capital letter S is used instead of $\sum$. It is important to realize that $\sum$ stands for an operation (that of obtaining the sum of quantities which follow), rather than a quantity itself.

The mean of a series of observations can be calculated readily on a pocket calculator or computer. Occasionally data may be presented merely in the form of a frequency distribution such as those shown in Tables 2.3 and 2.4. If the original data are available they should certainly be retrieved for calculation of the mean. If the original data are not retrievable, the mean may be estimated (although not with complete accuracy) by assuming that the observations are all clustered at the centres of their grouping intervals. Thus, in Table 2.3, the observations in the group 20–, ranging potentially from 20 to 29, could all be assumed to be 24·5; in Table 2.4, those in the group 45– years, ranging from 45 to 54, could be assumed to be 49·5. The calculated mean is then a *weighted mean* of the mid-points of the age groups (see §8.2). The reference to Table 2.4 draws attention to an unusual feature of ages, which are commonly given as integers, showing the age at last birthday. If the intention were to measure the exact age (which is not usually the case), the mean could be estimated (but again with incomplete accuracy) by adding half a year; in the frequency distribution the mid-point of the group 45– would then be taken to be 50.

Another useful measure of location is the *median*. If the observations are arranged in increasing or decreasing order, the median is the middle observation. If the number of observations, n, is odd, there will be a unique median—the $\frac{1}{2}(n+1)$th observation from either end. If n is even, there is strictly no middle observation, but the median is defined by convention as the mean of the two middle observations—the $\frac{1}{2}n$th and the $(\frac{1}{2}n+1)$th from either end.

The median has several disadvantages in comparison with the mean.

1   It takes no account of the precise magnitude of most of the observations, and is therefore usually less efficient than the mean because it wastes information.
2   If two groups of observations are pooled, the median of the combined group cannot be expressed in terms of the medians of the two component groups. This is not so with the mean. If groups containing n_1 and n_2 observations have means of $\bar{x}_1$ and $\bar{x}_2$, respectively, the mean of the combined group is the weighted mean:

$$(n_1\bar{x}_1 + n_2\bar{x}_2)/(n_1 + n_2).$$

3   The median is much less amenable than the mean to mathematical treatment, and is not much used in the more elaborate statistical techniques.

For descriptive work, however, the median is occasionally useful. Consider the following series of durations (in days) of absence from work owing to sickness:

1, 1, 2, 2, 3, 3, 4, 4, 4, 4, 5, 6, 6, 6, 6, 7, 8, 10, 10, 38, 80.

From a purely descriptive point of view the mean might be said to be misleading. Owing to the highly skew nature of the distribution the mean of 10 days is not really typical of the series as a whole, and the median of 5 days might be a more useful index. Another point is that in skew distributions of this type the mean is very much influenced by the presence of isolated high values. The median is therefore more stable than the mean in the sense that it is likely to fluctuate less from one series of readings to another.

The median of a grouped frequency distribution may be estimated (with incomplete accuracy) from the cumulative frequency plot or from the tabulated cumulative frequencies. In Fig. 2.9, for example, the median is the point on the age axis corresponding to 50% on the cumulative scale. In this example, based on the data from Table 2.4, the mean (of actual age, rather than age last birthday) is estimated as 55·7 years, and the median as 56·0 years.

The median and mean are equal if the series of observations is symmetrically distributed about their common value (as is nearly the case in Table 2.4). For a positively skew distribution (as in Table 2.3) the mean will be greater than the median, while if the distribution is negatively skew the median will be the greater.

A third measure of location, the mode, was introduced in §2.3. It is not widely used in analytical statistics, mainly because of the ambiguity in its definition as the fluctuations of small frequencies are apt to produce spurious modes.

Finally, reference should be made to two other forms of average, which are occasionally used for observations taking positive values only. The *geometric mean* is used extensively in microbiological and serological research. It involves the use of logarithms, and is dealt with in §2.5. The *harmonic mean* is much more rarely used. It requires the replacement of each observation by its reciprocal (i.e. 1 divided by the observation), and the calculation of the arithmetic mean of these reciprocals; the harmonic mean is then the reciprocal of this quantity.

2.5 **Taking logs**

When a variable is restricted to positive values and can vary over a wide range, its distribution is often positively skew. The distribution of numbers of lesions shown in Table 2.3 provides an example. Other examples commonly occurring in medical statistics are concentrations of chemical substances in the blood or urine; and time intervals between two events. Intuitively, the skewness is unsurprising: the lower bound of zero prevents an unduly long left-hand tail, whereas no such constraint exists for the right-hand tail.

We noted in §2.4 that for skewly distributed variables, such as the duration of absence of work used as an illustration on p. 32, the mean may be a less satisfactory measure of location than the median. More generally, many of the methods of analysis to be described later in this book are more appropriate for variables following an approximately symmetric distribution than for those with skew distributions.

A useful device in such situations is the *logarithmic* (or *log*) *transformation* (or *transform*). Logarithms are readily obtainable by a keystroke on a pocket calculator or as a simple instruction on a computer. In practical work it is customary to use *common* logarithms, to base 10, usually denoted by the key marked 'log' on a calculator. In purely mathematical work, and in many formulae arising in statistics, the *natural* logarithm, denoted by 'ln', may be more convenient (see p. 126).

The essential point about logs is that, when numbers are multiplied together, their logs are added. If a series of numbers increases by a constant multiplying factor, their logs must increase by a constant difference. This is shown by the following series of values of a variable x, and the corresponding values of $y = \log x$.

x	2	20	200	2000
y	0·3	1·3	2·3	3·3

These four values of x are highly skew, with increasing differences between the higher values, whereas the values of y are symmetrically distributed, with equal differences between adjacent values.

Observations made in microbiological and serological research are sometimes expressed as *titres*, which are the dilutions of certain suspensions or reagents at which a specific phenomenon, like agglutination of red cells, first takes place. If repeated observations are made during the same investigation, the possible values of a titre will usually be multiples of the same dilution factor: for example, 2, 4, 8, 16, etc., for twofold dilutions. It is commonly found that a series of titres, obtained, for example, from different sera, is distributed with marked positive skewness on account of the increasingly wide intervals between possible values. A series of titres 2, 4, 8, 16, etc., has logarithms very nearly equal to 0·3, 0·6, 0·9, 1·2, etc., which increase successively by an increment of 0·3 ($= \log 2$). As in the earlier example, the use of log titres is likely to give a series of observations which is more symmetrically distributed than were the original titres.

As an alternative to the median, as a measure of location for this type of variable, the *geometric mean* is widely used. Denote the original readings by x, and the transformed values by y ($= \log x$). The arithmetic mean, $\bar{y}$, is, like the individual values of y, measured on a logarithmic scale. To get back to the original scale of x, we take $\bar{x}_g = $ antilog $\bar{y}$. (The antilog is often marked '10^{x}' on a calculator.) The quantity $\bar{x}_g$ is the geometric mean of x. It can never be greater than the arithmetic mean, and the two means will be equal only if all the xs are the same. Note that the geometric mean cannot be used if any of the original observations are negative, since a negative number has no logarithm. Nor can it be used if any of the original readings are zero, since $\log 0 = $ minus infinity.

Figures 2.12 and 2.13 illustrate the effect of the log transform in reducing positive skewness. The distribution of serum creatinine levels shown in Fig. 2.12 has considerable positive skewness, as is characteristic of this type of measurement. The distribution of logs shown in Fig. 2.13 is more nearly symmetric. The arithmetic mean of the original data, calculated from the individual readings, is

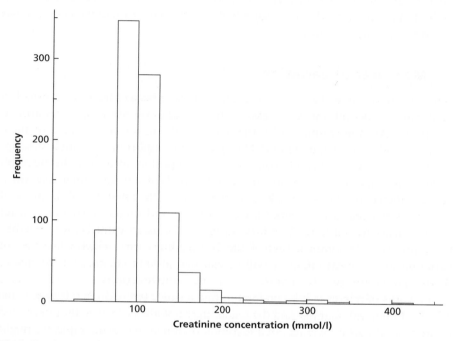

Fig. 2.12 Histogram showing the distribution of serum creatinine levels in a group of 901 subjects.

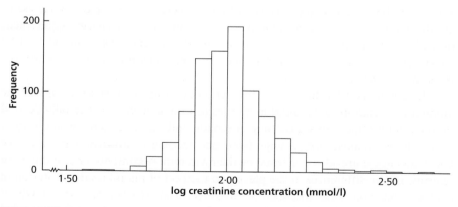

Fig. 2.13 Histogram showing the distribution of the logarithms of creatinine levels, the original values being depicted in Fig. 2.12.

107·01. The geometric mean, calculated from the logs and then transformed back to the original scale, is 102·36. The median is 100·00, closer to the geometric mean than to the arithmetic mean, as one might expect.

The log transform is one example of the way in which raw data can often usefully be transformed to a new scale of measurement before analyses are carried out. The use of transformations is described in more detail in §§10.8 and 11.10. In particular, the log transform will be seen to have other uses besides that of reducing positive skewness.

2.6 **Measures of variation**

When the mean value of a series of measurements has been obtained, it is usually a matter of considerable interest to express the degree of variation or scatter around this mean. Are the readings all rather close to the mean or are some of them scattered widely in each direction? This question is important for purely descriptive reasons, as we shall emphasize below. It is important also since the measurement of variation plays a central part in the methods of statistical inference which are described in this book. To take a simple example, the reliability of the mean of 100 values of some variable depends on the extent to which the 100 readings differ among themselves; if they show little variation the mean value is more reliable, more precisely determined, than if the 100 readings vary widely. The role of variation in statistical inference will be clarified in later chapters of this book. At present we are concerned more with the descriptive aspects.

In works of reference it is common to find a single figure quoted for the value of some biological quantity and the reader may not always realize that the stated figure is some sort of average. In a textbook on nutrition, for example, we might find the vitamin A content of Cheddar cheese given as 390 micrograms per 100 grams of cheese. Clearly, not all specimens of Cheddar cheese contain precisely 390 µg per 100 g; how much variation, then, is there from one piece of cheese to another? To take another example from nutrition, the daily energy requirement of a physically active man aged 25 years, of 180 cm and 73 kg, should be 12·0 megajoules. This requirement must vary from one person to another; how large is the variation?

There is unlikely to be a single answer to questions of this sort, because the amount of variation to be found in a series of measurements will usually depend on the circumstances in which they are made and, in particular, on the way in which these circumstances change from one reading to another. Specimens of Cheddar cheese are likely to vary in their vitamin A content for a number of reasons: major differences in the place and method of manufacture; variation in composition from one specimen to another even within the same batch of manufacture; the age of the cheese, and so on. Variation in the recorded measurement may be partly due to measurement error—in the method of assay, for example, or because of observer errors. Similarly, if reference is made to the variation in systolic blood pressure it must be made clear what sort of comparison is envisaged. Are we considering differences between various types of individual (for example, groups defined by age or by clinical state); differences between individuals classified in the same group; or variation from one occasion to another in the same individual? And are the instrument and the observer kept constant throughout the series?

We now consider some methods of measuring the variation or scatter of a series of continuous measurements.

This scatter is, of course, one of the features of the data which is elucidated by a frequency distribution. It is, however, convenient to use some single quantity to measure this feature of the data, first for economy of presentation, secondly because the statistical methods to be described later require such an index, and thirdly because the data may be too sparse to enable a distribution to be formed. We therefore require what is variously termed a measure of *variation, scatter, spread* or *dispersion*.

An obvious candidate is the *range*, which is defined as the difference between the maximum value and the minimum value. Note that the range is a definite quantity, measured in the same units as the original observations; if the highest and lowest of a series of diastolic blood pressures are 95 and 65 mmHg, we may say not only (as in conversation) that the readings range from 65 to 95 mmHg, but also that the range is 30 mmHg. There are three main difficulties about the use of the range as a measure of variation. The first is that the numerical value assumed by the range is determined by only two of the original observations. It is true that, if we say that the minimum and maximum readings have the values 65 and 95, we are saying something about the other readings—that they are between these extremes—but apart from this, their exact values have no effect on the range. In this example, the range would be 30 whether: (i) all the other readings were concentrated between 75 and 80; or (ii) they were spread rather evenly between 65 and 95. A desirable measure of the variation of the whole set of readings should be greater in case (ii) than in case (i). Secondly, the interpretation of the range depends on the number of observations. If observations are selected serially from a large group (for example, by taking the blood pressures of one individual after another), the range cannot possibly decrease; it will increase whenever a new reading falls outside the interval between the two previous extremes. The interpretation of the range as a measure of variation of the group as a whole must therefore depend on a knowledge of the number of observations on which it is based. This is an undesirable feature; no such allowance is required, for instance, in the interpretation of a mean value as a measure of location. Thirdly, calculations based on extreme values are rather unreliable because big differences in these extremes are liable to occur between two similar investigations.

If the number of observations is not too small, a modification may be introduced which avoids the use of the absolute extreme values. If the readings are arranged in ascending or descending order, two values may be ascertained which cut off a small fraction of the observations at each end, just as the median breaks the distribution into two equal parts. The value below which a quarter of the observations fall is called the *lower quartile*, that which is exceeded by a quarter of the observations is called the *upper quartile*, and the distance between them is called the *interquartile range*. This measure is not subject to the second disadvantage of the range and is less subject to the other disadvantages.

The evaluation of the quartiles for a set of n values is achieved by first calculating the corresponding ranks by

$$r_l = \tfrac{1}{4}n + \tfrac{1}{2}$$

and

$$r_u = \tfrac{3}{4}n + \tfrac{1}{2}$$

and then calculating the quartiles as the corresponding values in the orderd set of values, using interpolation if necessary. For example, in the data on duration of absence from work (p. 32) where n is 21, $r_l = 5\tfrac{3}{4}$ and $r_u = 16\tfrac{1}{4}$. The lower quartile is then obtained by interpolation between the 5th and 6th values; these are both 3 days, so the lower quartile is also 3 days. The upper quartile is obtained by interpolation between the 16th and 17th values, 7 and 8 days. The interpolation involves moving $\tfrac{1}{4}$ of the way from the 16th value towards the 17th value, to give $7 + \tfrac{1}{4}(8 - 7) = 7\tfrac{1}{4}$ days. It should be noted that there is not a single standard convention for calculating the quartiles. Some authors define the quartiles in terms of the ranks $r_l = \tfrac{1}{4}(n + 1)$ and $r_u = \tfrac{3}{4}(n + 1)$. It is also common to round $\tfrac{1}{4}$ and $\tfrac{3}{4}$ to the nearest integer and to use interpolation only when this involves calculation of the mid-point between two values. Differences between the results using the different conventions are usually small and unimportant in practice.

The quartiles are particular examples of a more general index, the *percentile* (or *centile*). The value below which $P\%$ of the values fall is called the Pth percentile. Thus, the lower and upper quartiles are the 25th and 75th percentiles, respectively. The quartiles or any other percentiles could be read off a plot of cumulative relative frequency such as Fig. 2.9. The term *quantile* is used when the proportion is expressed as a fraction rather than a percentage: thus, the 30th percentile is the same as the 0·3 quantile.

A convenient method of displaying the location and variability of a set of data is the box-and-whisker plot. The basic form of this plot shows a box defined by the lower and upper quartiles and with the median marked by a subdivision of the box. The whiskers extend from both ends of the box to the minimum and maximum values. Elaborations of this plot show possible outlying values (§2.7) separately beyond the ends of the whiskers by redefining the whiskers to have a maximum length in terms of the interquartile range. Box-and-whisker plots facilitate a visual comparison of groups. Figure 2.14 shows a comparison of birth weight between two groups of migrant Vietnamese mothers, one group following a traditional diet and the other a non-traditional diet. In this plot the whiskers extend to the most extreme observations within $\pm 1 \cdot 5$ interquartile ranges of the quartiles and more extreme points are plotted individually. The higher median and quartiles for the group with the non-traditional diet show clearly, as also does the lower variability associated with this diet.

An alternative approach is to make some use of all the deviations from the mean, $x_i - \bar{x}$. Clearly, the greater the scatter of the observations the greater will the magnitude of these deviations tend to be. It would be of no use to take the mean of the deviations $x_i - \bar{x}$, since some of these will be negative and some positive. In fact,

$$\sum (x_i - \bar{x}) = \sum x_i - \sum \bar{x}$$
$$= \sum x_i - n\bar{x}$$
$$= 0 \quad \text{since } \bar{x} = \sum x_i / n.$$

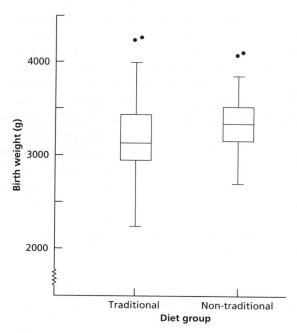

Fig. 2.14 Box-and-whisker plot comparing the distributions of birth weight of babies between two groups of Vietnamese mothers (data of Mitchell and Mackerras, 1995).

Therefore the mean of the deviations $x_i - \bar{x}$ will always be zero. We could, however, take the mean of the deviations ignoring their sign, i.e. counting them all as positive. These quantities are called the absolute values of the deviations and are denoted by $|x_i - \bar{x}|$. Their mean, $\sum |x_i - \bar{x}|/n$, is called the *mean deviation*. This measure has the drawback of being difficult to handle mathematically, and we shall not consider it any further in this book.

Another way of getting over the difficulty caused by the positive and negative signs is to square them. The mean value of the squared deviations is called the *variance* and is a most important measure in statistics. Its formula is

$$\text{Variance} = \frac{\sum (x_i - \bar{x})^2}{n}. \tag{2.1}$$

The numerator is often called the *sum of squares about the mean*. The variance is measured in the square of the units in which x is measured. For example, if x is height in cm, the variance will be measured in cm^2. It is convenient to have a measure of variation expressed in the original units of x, and this can be easily done by taking the square root of the variance. This quantity is known as the *standard deviation*, and its formula is

$$\text{Standard deviation} = \sqrt{\left[\frac{\sum (x_i - \bar{x})^2}{n}\right]}. \tag{2.1a}$$

In practice, in calculating variances and standard deviations, the n in the denominator is almost always replaced by $n - 1$. The reason for this is that in applying the methods of statistical inference, developed later in this book, it is useful to regard the collection of observations as being a *sample* drawn from a much larger group of possible readings. The large group is often called a *population*. When we calculate a variance or a standard deviation we may wish not merely to describe the variation in the sample with which we are dealing, but also to estimate as best we can the variation in the population from which the sample is supposed to have been drawn. In a certain respect (see §5.1) a better estimate of the population variance is obtained by using a divisor $n - 1$ instead of n. Thus, we shall almost always use the formula for the *estimated variance* or *sample variance*:

$$\text{Estimated variance}, s^2 = \frac{\sum (x_i - \bar{x})^2}{n - 1}, \tag{2.2}$$

and, similarly,

$$\text{Estimated standard deviation}, s = \sqrt{\left[\frac{\sum (x_i - \bar{x})^2}{n - 1}\right]}. \tag{2.2a}$$

Having established the convention we shall very often omit the word 'estimated' and refer to s^2 and s as 'variance' and 'standard deviation', respectively.

The modification of the divisor from n to $n - 1$ is clearly not very important when n is large. It is more important for small values of n. Although the theoretical justification will be discussed more fully in §5.1, two heuristic arguments may be used now which may make the divisor $n - 1$ appear more plausible. First, consider the case when $n = 1$; that is, there is a single observation. Formula (2.1) with a divisor n gives a variance $0/1 = 0$. Now, this is a reasonable expression of the complete absence of variation in the available observation: it cannot differ from itself. On the other hand, a single observation provides no information at all about the variation in the population from which it is drawn, and this fact is reflected in the calculation of the estimated variance, s^2, from (2.2), which becomes $0/0$, an indeterminate quantity.

Secondly, in the general case when n takes any value, we have already seen that $\sum(x_i - \bar{x}) = 0$. This means that if $n - 1$ of these deviations $x_i - \bar{x}$ are chosen arbitrarily, the nth is determined automatically. (It is the sum of the $n - 1$ chosen values of $x_i - \bar{x}$ with the sign changed.) In other words, only $n - 1$ of the n deviations which are squared in the numerator of (2.1) or (2.2) are *independent*. The divisor $n - 1$ in (2.2) may be regarded as the number of independent quantities among the sum of squared deviations in the numerator. The divisor $n - 1$ is, in fact, a particular case of a far-reaching concept known as the *degrees of freedom* of an estimate of variance, which will be developed in §5.1.

The direct calculation of the estimated variance is illustrated in Table 2.6. In this particular example the calculation is fairly straightforward. In general, two features of the method are likely to cause trouble. Errors can easily arise in the subtraction of the mean from each reading. Further, if the mean is not a 'round' number, as it was in this example, it will need to be rounded off. The deviations

Table 2.6 Calculation of estimated variance and standard deviation: direct formula.

x_i	$x_i - \bar{x}$	$(x_i - \bar{x})^2$
8	0	0
5	−3	9
4	−4	16
12	4	16
15	7	49
5	−3	9
7	−1	1

$\sum x_i = 56$ $\sum(x_i - \bar{x})^2 = 100$

$n = 7$

$\bar{x} = 56/7 = 8$

$s^2 = 100/6 = 16{\cdot}67$

$s = \sqrt{16{\cdot}67} = 4{\cdot}08$

$x_i - \bar{x}$ will then need to be written with several significant digits and doubt will arise as to whether an adequate number of significant digits was retained for $\bar{x}$. These difficulties have led to the widespread use of an alternative method of calculating the sum of squares about the mean, $\sum(x_i - \bar{x})^2$. It is based on the fact that

$$\sum(x_i - \bar{x})^2 = \sum x_i^2 - \frac{(\sum x_i)^2}{n}. \tag{2.3}$$

This is called the short-cut formula for the sum of squares about the mean.

The important point about (2.3) is that the computation is performed without the need to calculate individual deviations from the mean, $x_i - \bar{x}$. The sum of squares of the original observations, x_i, is corrected by subtraction of a quantity dependent only on the mean (or, equivalently, the total) of the x_i. This second term is therefore often called the *correction term*, and the whole expression a *corrected* sum of squares.

The previous example is reworked in Table 2.7. We again have the result $\sum(x_i - \bar{x})^2 = 100$, and the subsequent calculations follow as in Table 2.6.

The short-cut formula avoids the need to square individual deviations with many significant digits, but involves the squares of the x_i, which may be large numbers. This rarely causes trouble using a calculator, although care must be taken to carry sufficient digits in the correction term to give the required number of digits in the difference between the two terms. (For example, if $\sum x_i^2 = 2025$ and $(\sum x_i)^2/n = 2019 \cdot 3825$, the retention of all these decimals will give

Table 2.7 Calculation of estimated variance and standard deviation: short-cut formula (same data as in Table 2.6).

x_i	x_i^2
8	64
5	25
4	16
12	144
15	225
5	25
7	49
56	548

$$\sum(x_i - \bar{x})^2 = \sum x_i^2 - (\sum x_i)^2/n$$
$$= 548 - 56^2/7$$
$$= 548 - 448$$
$$= 100$$

Subsequent steps as in Table 2.6

$\sum(x_i - \bar{x})^2 = 5\cdot6175$; if the correction term had been rounded off to the nearest whole number it would have given $\sum(x_i - \bar{x})^2 = 6$—an accuracy of only 1 significant digit.) Indeed, this rounding error can cause problems in high-speed computing, and computer programs should use the direct rather than the short-cut formula for the sum of squares about the mean.

Most scientific calculators have a summation key which accumulates n, $\sum x$ and $\sum x^2$ in stores and then the mean and standard deviation are each calculated by successive keystrokes, the latter invoking calculation of (2.3). Calculators usually have separate keys for (2.1a) and (2.2a), often called σ_n and σ_{n-1}, respectively.

If the observations are presented in the form of a frequency distribution, and the raw data are not retrievable, the standard deviation may be obtained, as indicated earlier for the calculation of the mean, by assuming that all observations are clustered at the mid-points of their grouping intervals. As with the mean, the true standard deviation can then only be estimated, with some loss of accuracy. There is an additional problem with the standard deviation and variance, in that the calculation from grouped data tends to give somewhat too high a value. An appropriate correction for this effect, called *Sheppard's correction*, is to subtract $\frac{1}{12}h^2$ from the calculated variance, h being the size of the grouping interval. (If the grouping interval is not constant an average value may be used.) The correction is rather small unless the grouping is quite crude, and for this reason is often ignored. In the example based on the data of Table 2.4, for which $h = 10$, the standard deviation is estimated as 8·76 years, or 8·27 years after applying Sheppard's correction.

The standard deviation of a set of measurements is expressed in the same units as the measurements and hence in the same units as the mean. It is occasionally useful to describe the variability by expressing the standard deviation as a proportion, or a percentage, of the mean. The resulting measure, called the *coefficient of variation*, is thus a dimensionless quantity—a pure number. In symbols,

$$\mathrm{CV}(x) = \frac{s}{\bar{x}} \times 100\%. \qquad (2.4)$$

The coefficient of variation is most useful as a descriptive tool in situations in which a change in the conditions under which measurements are made alters the standard deviation in the same proportion as it alters the mean. The coefficient of variation then remains unchanged and is a useful single measure of variability. It is mentioned again in a more substantive context in §5.3.

In §2.5 we described the geometric mean. By analogy, the *geometric standard deviation* may be obtained by calculating the standard deviation of the logarithmically transformed measurements and converting back to the original scale by taking the antilog. The resulting quantity is a factor by which the geometric mean may be multiplied or divided to give a typically deviant value, and is most useful for skew distributions where the variation may be more symmetric after logarithmic transformation (as in Figs 2.12 and 2.13).

2.7 **Outlying observations**

Occasionally, as noted in §2.2, a single observation is affected by a gross error, either of measurement or recording, or due to a sudden lapse from the general standards of investigation applying to the rest of the data. It is important to detect such errors if possible, partly because they are likely to invalidate the assumptions underlying standard methods of analysis and partly because gross errors may seriously distort estimates such as mean values.

Some errors will result in recorded observations that are entirely plausible, and they are likely to be very difficult to detect. The position is more hopeful if (as is often the case) the error leads to an outlying observation, far distant from other comparable observations. Of course, such outliers are not necessarily the result of error. They may give valuable information about a patient's health at the time of the observation. In any case, outliers should be investigated and the reasons for their appearance should be sought. We therefore need methods for detecting outlying observations so that appropriate action can be taken.

Recording errors can often be reduced by careful checking of all the steps at which results are copied on to paper, and by minimizing the number of transcription steps between the original record and the final data. Frequently the original measurement will come under suspicion. The measurement may be repeatable (for example, the height of an individual if a short time has elapsed since the first measurement), or one may be able to check it by referring to an authoritative document (such as a birth certificate, if age is in doubt). A much more difficult situation arises when an observation is strongly suspected of being erroneous but no independent check is available. Possible courses of action are discussed below, at (b) and (c). First we discuss some methods of detecting gross errors.

(a) Logical checks

Certain values may be seen to be either impossible or extremely implausible by virtue of the meaning of the variable. Frequently the range of variation is known sufficiently well to enable upper and/or lower limits to be set; for example, an adult man's height below, say, 140 cm or above 205 cm would cause suspicion. Other results would be impossible because of relationships between variables; for example, in the UK a child aged 10 years cannot be married. Checks of this sort can be carried out routinely, once the rules of acceptability have been defined. They can readily be performed by computer, possibly when the data are being entered (p.17); indeed, editing procedures of this sort should form a regular part of the analysis of large-scale bodies of data by computer.

(b) Statistical checks

Certain observations may be found to be unusual, not necessarily on a priori grounds, but at least by comparison with the rest of the data. Whether or not they are to be rejected or amended is a controversial matter to be discussed below; at any rate, the investigator will probably wish to have his/her attention drawn to them.

A good deal of statistical checking can be done quite informally by graphical exploration and the formation of frequency distributions. If most of the observations follow a simple bell-shaped distribution such as the *normal* (§3.8), with one or two aberrant values falling well away from the main distribution, the *normal plot* described in §11.9 is a useful device. Sometimes, observations are unusual only when considered in relation to other variables; for example, in an anthropometric survey of schoolchildren, a weight measurement may be seen to be unusually low or high in relation to the child's height; checking rules for weights in terms of heights will be much more effective than rules based on weights alone (Healy, 1952; see also §12.3). The detection of outliers that are apparent only when other variables are considered forms part of the diagnostic methods used in multiple regression (§11.9).

Should a statistically unusual reading be rejected or amended? If there is some external reason for suspicion, for example that an inexperienced technician made the observation in question, or that the air-conditioning plant failed at a certain point during an experiment, common sense would suggest the omission of the observation and (where appropriate) the use of special techniques for making adjustments for the missing data (§18.6). When there is no external reason for suspicion there are strong arguments for retaining the original observations. Clearly there are some observations which no reasonable person would retain—for example, an adult height recorded as 30 cm. However, the decision will usually have to be made as a subjective judgement on ill-defined criteria which depend on one's knowledge of the data under study, the purpose of the analysis and so on. A full treatment of this topic, including descriptions of more formal methods of dealing with outliers, is given by Barnett and Lewis (1994).

(c) Robust estimation

In some analyses the question of rejection or correction may not arise, and yet it may be suspected or known that occasional outliers occur, and some safeguard against their effect may be sought. We shall discuss in §4.2 the idea of estimating the mean of a large population from a sample of observations drawn from it. In most situations we should be content to do this by calculating the mean of the sample values, but we might sometimes seek an estimator that is less influenced than the sample mean by occasional outliers. This approach is called *robust estimation*, and a wide range of such estimators has been suggested. In §2.4 we commended the sample median as a measure of location on the grounds that it is less influenced by outliers than is the mean. For positive-valued observations, the logarithmic transformation described in §2.5, and the use of the geometric mean, would have a similar effect in damping down the effect of outlying high values, but unfortunately it would have the opposite effect of exaggerating the effect of outlying low values. One of the most widely used robust measures of location is the *trimmed mean*, obtained by omitting some of the most extreme observations (for example, a fixed proportion in each tail) and taking the mean of the rest. These estimators are remarkably efficient for samples from normal distributions (§3.8), and better than the sample mean for distributions 'contaminated' with a moderate proportion of outliers. The choice of method (e.g. the proportion to be trimmed from the tails) is not entirely straightforward, and the precision of the resulting estimator may be difficult to determine.

Similar methods are available for more complex problems, although the choice of method is, as in the simpler case of the mean, often arbitrary, and the details of the analysis may be complicated. See Draper and Smith (1998, Chapter 25) for further discussion in the case of multiple regression (§11.6).

3 Probability

3.1 **The meaning of probability**

A clinical trial shows that 50 patients receiving treatment A for a certain disease fare better, on the average, than 50 similar patients receiving treatment B. Is it safe to assume that treatment A is really better than treatment B for this condition? Should the investigator use A rather than B for future patients? These are questions typical of those arising from any statistical investigation. The first is one of inference: what conclusions can reasonably be drawn from this investigation? The second question is one of decision: what is the rational choice of future treatment, taking into account the information provided by the trial and the known or unknown consequences of using an inferior treatment? The point to be emphasized here is that the answers to both questions, and indeed those to almost all questions asked about statistical data, are in some degree couched in uncertainty. There may be a very strong suggestion indeed that A is better than B, but can we be entirely sure that the patients receiving B were not more severely affected than those on A and that this variability between the patients was not a sufficient reason for their different responses to treatment? This possibility may, in any particular instance, seem unlikely, but it can rarely, if ever, be completely ruled out. The questions that have to be asked, therefore, must receive an answer phrased in terms of uncertainty. If the uncertainty is low, the conclusion will be firm, the decision will be safe. If the uncertainty is high, the investigation must be regarded as inconclusive. It is thus important to consider the measurement of uncertainty, and the appropriate tool for this purpose is the *theory of probability*. Initially the approach will be rather formal; later chapters are concerned with the application of probability theory to statistical problems of various types.

If a coin is tossed a very large number of times and the result of each toss written down, the results may be something like the following (*H* standing for heads and *T* for tails):

$$TTHTHHTHTTTHTHHTHHHHTTH\ldots$$

Such a sequence will be called a *random sequence* or *random series*, each place in the sequence will be called a *trial*, and each result will often be called an *event* or *outcome*. A random sequence of binary outcomes, such as *H* and *T* in this example, is sometimes called a *Bernoulli sequence* (James Bernoulli, 1654–1705). A random sequence is characterized by a complete lack of pattern or of predictability. In coin tossing the chance of finding *H* at any one stage is just the same as at any other stage, and is quite uninfluenced by the outcomes of the previous tosses. (Contrary to some people's intuition, the chance of getting a head would be neither raised nor lowered by a knowledge that there had just occurred a run of, say, six tails.)

In such a sequence it will be found that as the sequence gets larger and larger the proportion of trials resulting in a particular outcome becomes less and less variable and settles down closer to some limiting value. This long-run proportion is called the *probability* of the particular outcome. Figure 3.1 shows the proportion of heads after various numbers of tosses, in an actual experiment. Clearly the proportion is settling down close to $\frac{1}{2}$, and it would be reasonable to say that the probability of a head is about $\frac{1}{2}$. Considerations of symmetry would, of course, have led us to this conclusion before seeing the experimental results. The slight differences between the indentations on the two sides of a coin, possibly variations in density, and even some minor imbalance in the tossing method, might make the probability very slightly different from $\frac{1}{2}$, but we should be unlikely ever to do a tossing experiment sufficiently long to distinguish between a probability of 0·5 and one of, say, 0·5001.

The reader will observe that this definition of probability is rather heuristic. We can never observe a sequence of trials and say unambiguously 'This is a

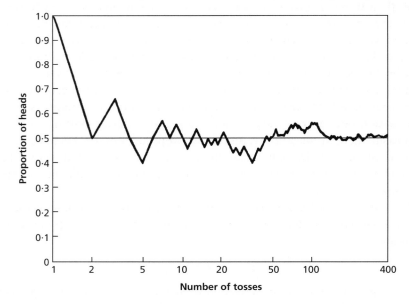

Fig. 3.1 Proportion of heads in a sequence of tosses of a coin with a logarithmic scale for the number of tosses (reprinted from Cramér, 1946, by permission of the author and publishers).

random sequence'; we observe only a finite portion of the sequence and there may be underlying patterns in the outcomes which cannot readily be discerned. Nor can we observe a sequence and state precisely the probability of a certain outcome; the probability is a long-run property and again an insufficient portion of the sequence is observed. Nevertheless, there are many phenomena which apparently behave in this way, and the concept of a random sequence should be regarded as an idealistic concept which apparently describes these phenomena very faithfully indeed. Here are some other examples of empirical 'random' (Bernoulli) sequences.

1   *The throws of a dice.* If the dice is well made, the probability of each outcome, 1–6, will be very close to $\frac{1}{6}$.

2   *The sex of successive live births occurring in a large human population.* The probability of a male is known to vary from population to population (for example, it depends on the stillbirth rate) but it is usually a little over $\frac{1}{2}$. In England and Wales it is currently about 0·515; the probability of a female birth is correspondingly about $1 - 0·515 = 0·485$.

3   *A sequence of outcomes of antenatal screening examinations, each classified by whether or not a specific fetal abnormality is present.* Thus, the probability that open spina bifida is present might be about 0·0012.

A consequence of this definition of probability is that it is measured by a number between 0 and 1. If an event never occurs in any of the trials in a random sequence, its probability is zero. If it occurs in every trial, its probability is unity.

A further consequence is that probability is not defined for sequences in which the succession of events follows a manifestly non-random pattern. If a machine were invented which tossed heads and tails in strict alternation ($H, T, H, T, H, T, \ldots$, etc.), the long-run proportions of heads and tails would both be $\frac{1}{2}$, but it would be incorrect to say that the probabilities of these events were $\frac{1}{2}$. The sequence is non-random because the behaviour of the odd-numbered trials is different from that of the even-numbered trials. It would be better to think of the series as a mixture of two separate series: the odd-numbered trials, in which the probability of H is 1, and the even-numbered trials, in which this probability is 0.

This concept of probability provides a measure of uncertainty for certain types of phenomena which occur in nature. There is a fairly high degree of certainty that any one future birth will not exhibit spina bifida because the probability for that event is low. There is considerable uncertainty about the sex of a future birth because the probabilities of both outcomes are about $\frac{1}{2}$. The definition is, however, much more restrictive than might be wished. What is the probability that smoking is a contributory cause of lung cancer? This question uses the word 'probability' in a perfectly natural conversational way. It does not, however, accord with our technical definition, for it is impossible to think of a random sequence of trials, in some of which smoking is a contributory cause of lung cancer and in some of which it is not.

It will appear in due course that the so-called 'frequency' definition of probability, which has been put forward above, can be used as the basis of statistical inference, and often some rewording of the question can shed some light on the plausibility of hypotheses such as 'Smoking is a contributory cause of lung cancer.' However, many theoretical statisticians, probabilitists and logicians advocate a much wider interpretation of the concept of probability than is permitted in the frequency definition outlined above. On this broader view, one should interpret probability as a measure of one's degree of belief in a proposition, and direct statements about the probability that a certain scientific hypothesis is true are quite in order. We return to this point of view in Chapter 6, but until that chapter is reached we shall restrict our attention to the frequency definition.

3.2 Probability calculations

The main purpose of allotting numerical values to probabilities is to allow calculations to be performed on these numbers. The two basic operations which concern us here are *addition* and *multiplication*, and we consider first the addition of probabilities.

Consider a random sequence of trials with more than one possible outcome for each trial. In a series of throws of a dice, for example, we might ask for the probability of *either* a 1 *or* a 3 being thrown. The answer is fairly clear. If the dice is perfectly formed, the probability of a 1 is $\frac{1}{6}$, and the probability of a 3 is $\frac{1}{6}$. That is, a 1 will appear in $\frac{1}{6}$ of trials in the long run, and a 3 will appear in the same proportion of a long series of trials. In no trial will a 1 *and* a 3 appear together. Therefore the compound event 'either a 1 or a 3' will occur in $\frac{1}{6} + \frac{1}{6}$, or $\frac{1}{3}$, of the trials in the long run. The probabilities for the two separate events have been added together.

Note the importance of the observation that a 1 and a 3 cannot both occur together; they are, in other words, *mutually exclusive*. Without this condition the simple form of the addition rule could not be valid. For example, if a doctor's name is chosen haphazardly from the *British Medical Register*, the probability that the doctor is male is about 0·8. The probability that the doctor qualified at an English medical school is about 0·6. What is the probability that the doctor either is male or qualified in England, or both? If the two separate probabilities are added the result is $0\cdot8 + 0\cdot6 = 1\cdot4$, clearly a wrong answer since probabilities cannot be greater than 1. The trouble is that the probability of the double event—male and qualified in England—has been counted twice, once as part of the probability of being male and once as part of the probability of being qualified in England. To obtain the right answer, the probability of the double event must be subtracted. Thus, denoting the two events by *A* and *B*, we have the more general form of the *addition rule*:

Probability of *A* or *B* or both = (Probability of *A*)
+ (Probability of *B*)
− (Probability of *A* and *B*).

It will be convenient to write this as

$$P(A \text{ or } B \text{ or both}) = P(A) + P(B) - P(A \text{ and } B). \qquad (3.1)$$

In this particular example the probability of the double event has not been given, but it must clearly be greater than 0·4, to ensure that the right side of the equation (3.1) is less than 1.

If the two events are mutually exclusive, the last term on the right of (3.1) is zero, and we have the *simple form of the addition rule*:

$$P(A \text{ or } B) = P(A) + P(B).$$

Suppose now that two random sequences of trials are proceeding simultaneously; for example, at each stage a coin may be tossed and a dice thrown. What is the *joint probability* of a particular combination of results, for example a head (*H*) on the coin and a 5 on the dice? The result is given by the *multiplication rule*:

$$P(H \text{ and } 5) = P(H) \times P(5, \text{ given } H). \qquad (3.2)$$

That is, the long-run proportion of pairs of trials in which both *H* and 5 occur is equal to the long-run proportion of trials in which *H* occurs on the coin, multiplied by the long-run proportion of those trials which occur with 5 on the dice. The second term on the right of (3.2) is an example of a *conditional probability*, the first event, 5, being 'conditional' on the second, *H*. A common notation is to replace 'given' by a vertical line, that is, $P(5 \mid H)$.

In this particular example, there would be no reason to suppose that the probability of 5 on the dice was in the least affected by whether or not *H* occurred on the coin. In other words,

$$P(5, \text{ given } H) = P(5).$$

The conditional probability is equal to the unconditional probability. The two events are now said to be *independent*, and we have the *simple form of the multiplication rule*:

$$P(H \text{ and } 5) = P(H) \times P(5)$$
$$= \tfrac{1}{2} \times \tfrac{1}{6}$$
$$= \tfrac{1}{12}.$$

Effectively, in this example, there are 12 combinations which occur equally often in the long run: *H1, H2,..., H6, T1, T2,..., T6*.

In general, pairs of events need not be independent, and the general form of the multiplication rule (3.2) must be used. In the earlier example we referred to the probability of a doctor being male and having qualified in England. If these events were independent, we could calculate this as

$$0.8 \times 0.6 = 0.48,$$

and, denoting the events by A and B, (3.1) would give

$$P(A \text{ or } B \text{ or both}) = 0.80 + 0.60 - 0.48$$
$$= 0.92.$$

These events may not be independent, however, since some medical schools are more likely to accept women than others. The correct value for $P(A \text{ and } B)$ could only be ascertained by direct investigation.

As another example of the lack of independence, suppose that in a certain large community 30% of individuals have blue eyes. Then

$$P(\text{blue right eye}) = 0.3$$
$$P(\text{blue left eye}) = 0.3.$$

P(blue right eye and blue left eye) is not given by

$$P(\text{blue right eye}) \times P(\text{blue left eye}) = 0.09.$$

It is obtained by the general formula (3.2) as

$$P(\text{blue right eye}) \times P(\text{blue left eye, given blue right eye})$$
$$= 0.3 \times 1.0$$
$$= 0.3.$$

Addition and multiplication may be combined in the same calculation. In the double sequence with a coin and a dice, what is the probability of getting either heads and 2 *or* tails and 4? Each of these combinations has a probability of $\frac{1}{12}$ (by the multiplication rule for independent events). Each combination is a possible outcome in the double sequence and the outcomes are mutually exclusive. The two probabilities of $\frac{1}{12}$ may therefore be added to give a final probability of $\frac{1}{6}$ that either one or the other combination occurs.

As a slightly more complicated example, consider the sex composition of families of four children. As an approximation, let us assume that the proportion of males at birth is 0.51, that all the children in the families may be considered as independent random selections from a sequence in which the probability of a boy is 0.51, and that the question relates to all liveborn infants so that differential survival does not concern us. The question is, what are the probabilities that a family of four contains no boys, one boy, two boys, three boys and four boys?

The probability that there will be no boys is the probability that each of the four children will be a girl. The probability that the first child is a girl is $1 - 0.51 = 0.49$. By successive applications of the multiplication rule for independent events, the probability that the first two are girls is $(0.49)^2$; the probability that the first three are girls is $(0.49)^3$; and the probability that all four are girls is $(0.49)^4 = 0.0576$. About 1 in 17 of all families of four will consist of four girls. Write this

$$P(GGGG) = 0.0576.$$

A family with one boy and three girls might arise in any of the following ways, $BGGG$, $GBGG$, $GGBG$, $GGGB$, according to which of the four children is the boy. Each of these ways has a probability of $(0.49)^3(0.51) = 0.0600$. The total probability of one boy is therefore, by the addition rule,

$$0.0600 + 0.0600 + 0.0600 + 0.0600$$
$$= 4(0.0600)$$
$$= 0.2400.$$

A family with two boys and two girls might arise in any of the following ways: $BBGG$, $BGBG$, $BGGB$, $GBBG$, $GBGB$, $GGBB$. Each of these has a probability of $(0.49)^2(0.51)^2$, and the total probability of two boys is

$$6(0.49)^2(0.51)^2 = 0.3747.$$

Similarly for the other family composition types. The complete results are shown in Table 3.1.

Note that the five probabilities total to 1, as they should since this total is the probability that one or other of the five family composition types arises (these being mutually exclusive). Since these five types exhaust all the possibilities, the total probability must be unity. If one examined the records of a very large number of families experiencing four live births, would the proportions of

Table 3.1 Calculation of probabilities of families with various sex compositions.

Composition		Probability
Boys	Girls	
0	4	$(0.49)^4 = 0.0576$
1	3	$4(0.49)^3(0.51) = 0.2400$
2	2	$6(0.49)^2(0.51)^2 = 0.3747$
3	1	$4(0.49)(0.51)^3 = 0.2600$
4	0	$(0.51)^4 = 0.0677$
		1.0000

the five types be close to the values shown in the last column? Rather close, perhaps, but it would not be surprising to find some slight but systematic discrepancies because the formal assumptions underlying our argument may not be strictly correct. For one thing, the probability of a male birth may vary slightly from family to family (as pointed out in §3.1). More importantly, families that start in an unbalanced way, with several births of the same sex, are more likely to be continued than those that are better balanced. The first two births in families that are continued to the third stage will then not be representative of all two-birth families. A similar bias may exist in the progression from three births to four. The extent of these biases would be expected to differ from one community to another, and this seems to be borne out by actual data, some of which agree more closely than others with the theoretical probabilities.

It is sometimes convenient to express a probability in terms of the *odds*, which equal the probability that the event occurs divided by the probability that it does not occur. Thus, the odds of throwing a 6 with a dice are $\frac{1}{5}$.

3.3 **Bayes' theorem**

It was pointed out in §3.1 that the frequency definition of probability does not normally permit one to allot a numerical value to the probability that a certain proposition or hypothesis is true. We shall discuss in Chapter 6 the 'Bayesian' approach of assigning numerical values to probabilities of hypotheses, to represent degrees of belief. In the present section we introduce one of the basic tools of Bayesian statistics, Bayes' theorem, entirely within a frequentist framework.

There are some situations in which the relevant alternative hypotheses can be thought of as presenting themselves in a random sequence so that numerical probabilities can be associated with them. For instance, a doctor in charge of a clinic may be interested in the hypothesis: 'This patient has disease A.' By regarding the patient as a random member of a large collection of patients presenting themselves at the clinic the doctor may be able to associate with the hypothesis a certain probability, namely the long-run proportion of patients with disease A. This may be regarded as a *prior probability*, since it can be ascertained (or at least estimated roughly) from retrospective observations.

Suppose the doctor now makes certain new observations, after which the probability of the hypothesis: 'This patient has disease A' is again considered. The new value may be called a *posterior probability* because it refers to the situation after the new observations have been made. Intuitively one would expect the posterior probability to exceed the prior probability if the new observations were particularly common on the hypothesis in question and relatively uncommon on any alternative hypothesis. Conversely, the posterior probability would be expected to be less than the prior probability if the observations were not often observed in disease A but were common in other situations.

Consider a simple example in which there are only three possible diseases (A, B and C), with prior probabilities π_A, π_B and π_C (with $\pi_A + \pi_B + \pi_C = 1$). Suppose that the doctor's observations fall conveniently into one of four categories 1, 2, 3, 4, and that the probability distributions of the various outcomes for each disease are as follows:

	Outcome				
Disease	1	2	3	4	Total
A	$l_{1|A}$	$l_{2|A}$	$l_{3|A}$	$l_{4|A}$	1
B	$l_{1|B}$	$l_{2|B}$	$l_{3|B}$	$l_{4|B}$	1
C	$l_{1|C}$	$l_{2|C}$	$l_{3|C}$	$l_{4|C}$	1

Suppose the doctor observes outcome 2. The total probability of this outcome is

$$\pi_A l_{2|A} + \pi_B l_{2|B} + \pi_C l_{2|C}.$$

The three terms in this expression are in fact the probabilities of disease A and outcome 2, disease B and outcome 2, disease C and outcome 2. Once the doctor has observed outcome 2, therefore, the posterior probabilities of A, B and C, $\pi_{A|2}$, $\pi_{B|2}$ and $\pi_{C|2}$, are

$$\frac{\pi_A l_{2|A}}{\pi_A l_{2|A} + \pi_B l_{2|B} + \pi_C l_{2|C}}, \frac{\pi_B l_{2|B}}{\pi_A l_{2|A} + \pi_B l_{2|B} + \pi_C l_{2|C}}, \frac{\pi_C l_{2|C}}{\pi_A l_{2|A} + \pi_B l_{2|B} + \pi_C l_{2|C}}.$$

The prior probabilities have been multiplied by factors proportional to $l_{2|A}$, $l_{2|B}$ and $l_{2|C}$. Although these three quantities are straightforward probabilities, they do not form part of the same distribution, being entries in a column rather than a row of the table above. Probabilities of a particular outcome on different hypotheses are called *likelihoods* of these hypotheses.

This is an example of the use of Bayes' theorem (named after an English clergyman, Thomas Bayes, *c.* 1701–61). More generally, if the hypothesis H_i has a prior probability π_i and outcome y has a probability $l_{y|i}$ when H_i is true, the posterior probability of H_i after outcome y has been observed is

$$\pi_{i|y} = \frac{\pi_i l_{y|i}}{\sum_h \pi_h l_{y|h}}. \tag{3.3}$$

An alternative form of this equation concerns the ratio of probabilities of two hypotheses, H_i and H_j:

$$\frac{\pi_{i|y}}{\pi_{j|y}} = \frac{\pi_i}{\pi_j} \times \frac{l_{y|i}}{l_{y|j}}. \tag{3.4}$$

In (3.4), the left-hand side is the ratio of posterior probabilities, and the terms on the right-hand side are the ratio of prior probabilities and the likelihood ratio for the outcome y. In other words, a ratio of prior probabilities is converted to a ratio of posterior probabilities by multiplication by the likelihood ratio.

A third form of Bayes' theorem concerns the odds in favour of hypothesis H_i:

$$\frac{\pi_{i|y}}{1 - \pi_{i|y}} = \frac{\pi_i}{1 - \pi_i} \times \frac{l_{y|i}}{P(y \,|\, \text{not } H_i)}. \qquad (3.5)$$

In (3.5), the posterior odds are derived from the prior odds by multiplication by a ratio called the *Bayes factor*. The denominator $P(y \,|\, \text{not } H_i)$ is not a pure likelihood, since it involves the prior probabilities for hypotheses other than H_i.

In some examples, the outcomes will be continuous variables such as weight or blood pressure, in which case the likelihoods take the form of *probability densities*, to be described in the next section. The hypotheses H_i may form a continuous set (for example, H_i may specify that the mean of a population is some specific quantity that can take any value over a wide range, so that there is an infinite number of hypotheses). In that case the summation in the denominator of (3.3) must be replaced by an integral. But Bayes' theorem always takes the same basic form: prior probabilities are converted to posterior probabilities by multiplication in proportion to likelihoods.

The example provides an indication of the way in which Bayes' theorem may be used as an aid to diagnosis. In practice there are severe problems in estimating the probabilities appropriate for the population of patients under treatment; for example, the distribution of diseases observed in a particular centre is likely to vary with time. The determination of the likelihoods will involve extensive and carefully planned surveys and the definition of the outcome categories may be difficult.

One of the earliest applications of Bayes' theorem to medical diagnosis was that of Warner *et al.* (1961). They examined data from a large number of patients with congenital heart disease. For each of 33 different diagnoses they estimated the prior probability, π_i, and the probabilities $l_{y|i}$ of various combinations of symptoms. Altogether 50 symptoms, signs and other variables were measured on each individual. Even if all these had been dichotomies there would have been 2^{50} possible values of y, and it would clearly be impossible to get reliable estimates of all the $l_{y|i}$. Warner *et al.* overcame this problem by making an assumption which has often been made by later workers in this field, namely that the symptoms and other variables are statistically independent. The probability of any particular combination of symptoms, y, can then be obtained by multiplying together the separate, or *marginal*, probabilities of each. In this study firm diagnoses for certain patients could be made by intensive investigation and these were compared with the diagnoses given by Bayes' theorem and also with those made by experienced cardiologists using the same information. Bayes' theorem seems to emerge well from the comparison. Nevertheless, the assumption of independence of symptoms is potentially dangerous and should not be made without careful thought.

A number of papers illustrating the use of Bayesian methods and related techniques of decision theory to problems in medical diagnosis, prognosis and decision-making are to be found in the journal *Medical Decision Making*. For a review of decision analysis see Glasziou and Schwartz (1991). The aim here is to provide rules for the choice among decisions to be made during the course of medical treatment. These may involve such questions as whether to proceed immediately with an operation or whether to delay the decision while the patient is kept under observation or until the results of laboratory tests become available. Such choices depend not only on assessments of the probabilities of life-threatening diseases, based on the evidence currently available, but also on assessments of the expected gain (or *utility*) to be derived from various outcomes. Bayesian methods are central to the calculation of probabilities, but the assignment of utilities may be difficult and indeed highly subjective.

For further discussion see Bailey (1977, §4.7), Weinstein and Fineberg (1980), Spiegelhalter and Knill-Jones (1984) and Pauker and Kassirer (1992).

Example 3.1

Fraser and Franklin (1974) studied 700 case records of patients with liver disease. The initial set of over 300 symptoms, signs and test results was reduced to 97 variables for purposes of analysis. In particular, groups of symptoms and signs recognized to be clinically interdependent were amalgamated so as to minimize the danger inherent in the independence assumption discussed above. Patients with rare diagnoses (those represented by less than 12 patients) or multiple diagnoses were omitted, as were those with incomplete records. There remained 480 cases. Prior probabilities were estimated from the relative frequencies of the various diagnoses, and likelihoods for particular combinations of symptoms, signs and test results were obtained by multiplication of marginal frequencies.

Application of Bayes' theorem to each of the patient records gave posterior probabilities. For example, the posterior probabilities for one patient were:

Acute infective hepatitis	0·952
Cholestatic infective hepatitis	0·048
All other diagnoses	0·000

In a large number of cases the first or first two diagnoses accounted for a high probability, as in this instance.

This first analysis led to some revisions of the case records, and the exercise was repeated on a reduced set of 419 patients and the predicted diagnoses compared with the true diagnoses. A result was categorized as 'equivocal' if the highest posterior probability was less than three times as great as the second highest. Similar predictions were done on the basis of the likelihoods alone (i.e. ignoring the prior probabilities). The results were:

	Correct	Equivocal	Incorrect
Likelihood	316 (75%)	51 (12%)	52 (12%)
Bayesian	325 (78%)	48 (11%)	46 (11%)

It seems likely that the Bayesian results would have shown a greater improvement over the likelihood results if the rare diseases had not been excluded (because the priors would then have been relatively more important).

There is a danger in validating such a diagnostic procedure on the data set from which the method has been derived, because the estimates of probability are 'best' for this particular set and less appropriate for other sets. Fraser and Franklin therefore checked the method on 70 new cases with diagnoses falling into the group previously considered. The Bayesian method gave 44 (63%) correct, 12 (17%) equivocal and 14 (20%) incorrect results, with the likelihood method again slightly worse.

The following example illustrates the application of Bayes' theorem to genetic counselling.

Example 3.2

From genetic theory it is known that a woman with a haemophiliac brother has a probability of $\frac{1}{2}$ of being a carrier of a haemophiliac gene. A recombinant DNA diagnostic probe test provides information that contributes towards discriminating between carriers and non-carriers of a haemophiliac gene. It has been observed that 90% of women known to be carriers give a positive test result, whilst 20% of non-carriers have a positive result. The woman has the test. What is the probability that she is a carrier if the result is negative?

The probability may be evaluated using (3.3). Let H_1 be the hypothesis that the woman is a carrier and H_2 that she is not. Then $\pi_1 = \pi_2 = 0.5$. If outcome y represents a negative test then $l_{y|1}$, the probability of a negative test result if the woman is a carrier,

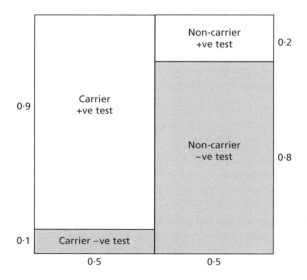

equals $1 - 0.9 = 0.1$, and $l_{y|2}$, the probability of a negative test result if the woman is not a carrier, equals 0.8. Therefore,

$$P(\text{carrier given} -\text{ve test}) = \frac{0.5 \times 0.1}{0.5 \times 0.1 + 0.5 \times 0.8}$$
$$= 0.11.$$

Thus, the posterior probability is less than the prior probability, as would be expected, since the extra information, a negative test, is more probable if the woman is not a carrier.

A diagrammatic representation of the calculation is as follows. A square with sides of length 1 unit is divided vertically according to the prior probabilities of each hypothesis, and then horizontally within each column according to the probabilities of outcome. Then by the multiplication rule (3.2) each of the four rectangles has an area equal to the probability of the corresponding hypothesis and outcome.

Once it is known that the outcome is negative, then only the shaded area is relevant and the probability that the woman is a carrier is the proportion of the shaded area that is in the carrier column, leading to the same numerical answer as direct application of (3.3).

3.4 **Probability distributions**

Table 3.1 provides our first example of a *probability distribution*. That is, it shows how the total probability, equal to 1, is distributed among the different types of family. A variable whose different values follow a probability distribution is known as a *random variable*. In Table 3.1 the number of boys in a family is a random variable. So is the number of girls.

If a random variable can be associated with different points on a scale, the probability distribution can be represented visually by a histogram, just as for frequency distributions. We shall consider first some examples of ungrouped discrete random variables. Here the vertical scale of the histogram measures the probability for each value of the random variable, and each probability is represented by a vertical line.

Example 3.3

In repeated tosses of an unbiased coin, the outcome is a random variable with two values, H and T. Each value has a probability $\frac{1}{2}$. The distribution is shown in Fig. 3.2, where the two outcomes, H and T, are allotted to arbitrary points on the horizontal axis.

Example 3.4

In a genetic experiment we may cross two heterozygotes with genotypes Aa (that is, at a particular gene locus, each parent has one gene of type A and one of type a). The progeny will be homozygotes (aa or AA) or heterozygotes (Aa), with the probabilities shown below.

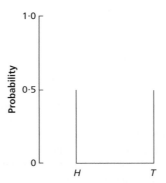

Fig. 3.2 Probability distribution for random variable with two values: the results of tossing a coin with equal probabilities of heads and tails.

Genotype	No. of A genes	Probability
aa	0	$\frac{1}{4}$
Aa	1	$\frac{1}{2}$
AA	2	$\frac{1}{4}$
		$\overline{1}$

The three genotypes may be allotted to points on a scale by using as a random variable the number of A genes in the genotype. This random variable takes the values 0, 1 and 2, and the probability distribution is depicted in Fig. 3.3.

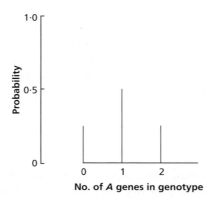

No. of A genes in genotype

Fig. 3.3 Probability distribution for random variable with three values: the number of A genes in the genotype of progeny of an $Aa \times Aa$ cross.

Example 3.5

A third example is provided by the characterization of families of four children by the number of boys. The probabilities, in the particular numerical case considered in §3.2, are given in Table 3.1, and they are depicted in Fig. 3.4.

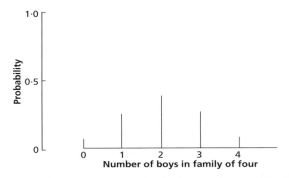

Fig. 3.4 Probability distribution of number of boys in family of four children if male births occur independently with probability 0.51 (Table 3.1).

When the random variable is continuous, it is of little use to refer to the probabilities of particular values of the variable, because these probabilities are in general zero. For example, the probability that the exact height of a male adult is 70 in. is zero, because in the virtually infinite population of exact heights of adult males a negligible proportion will be exactly 70 in. If, however, we consider a small interval centred at 70 in., say $70 - h$ to $70 + h$, where h is very small, there will be a small non-zero probability associated with this interval. Furthermore, the probability will be very nearly proportional to h. Thus, the probability of a height between 69·98 and 70·02 in. will be very nearly double the probability for the interval 69·99 to 70·01. It is therefore a reasonable representation of the situation to suppose that there is a *probability density* characteristic of the value 70 in., which can be denoted by $f(70)$, such that the probability for a small interval $70 - h$ to $70 + h$ is very close to

$$2hf(70).$$

The probability distribution for a continuous random variable, x, can therefore be depicted by a graph of the probability density $f(x)$ against x, as in Fig. 3.5. This is, in fact, the frequency curve discussed in §2.3. The reader familiar with the calculus will recognize $f(x)$ as the derivative with respect to x of the probability $F(x)$ that the random variable assumes a value less than or equal to x. $F(x)$ is called the *distribution function* and is represented by the area underneath the curve in Fig. 3.5 from the left end of the distribution (which may be at minus infinity) up to the value x. The distribution function corresponding to the density function of Fig. 3.5 is shown in Fig. 3.6. Note that the height of the density function is proportional to the slope of the distribution function; in the present example both these quantities are zero at the lower and upper extremes of the variables and attain a maximum at an intermediate point.

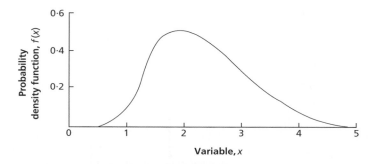

Fig. 3.5 Probability density function for a continuous random variable.

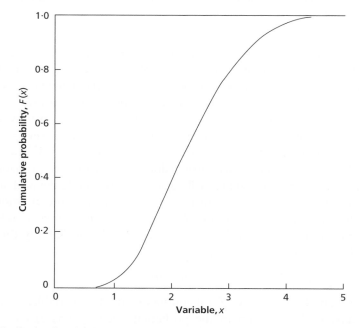

Fig. 3.6 Distribution function corresponding to the density function shown in Fig. 3.5.

The shape of a probability distribution may be characterized by the features already used for frequency distributions. In particular, we may be concerned with the number and position of the modes, the values of the random variable at which the probability, or (for continuous variables) the probability density, reaches a maximum. We may be interested too in the skewness of a probability distribution.

By analogy with §§2.4 and 2.6 we are particularly interested in the mean and standard deviation of a random variable, and these concepts are discussed in the next section.

3.5 **Expectation**

There is some difficulty in deciding what is meant by the phrase 'mean of a random variable'. The mean has been defined earlier only for a finite number, n, of observations. With a probability distribution such as that in Table 3.1 the number of observations must be thought of as infinite. How, then, is the mean to be calculated?

Suppose n is very large—so large that the relative frequencies of the different values of a discrete random variable like that in Table 3.1 can be taken to be very nearly equal to the probabilities. If they were exactly equal to the probabilities, the frequency distribution of the number of boys would be as follows:

x No. of boys	Frequency
0	$0·0576n$
1	$0·2400n$
2	$0·3747n$
3	$0·2600n$
4	$0·0677n$
	n

The mean value of x would be

$$\frac{(0 \times 0·0576n) + (1 \times 0·2400n) + (2 \times 0·3747n) + (3 \times 0·2600n) + (4 \times 0·0677n)}{n}.$$

The factor n may be cancelled from the numerator and denominator of the expression, to give the numerical result $2·04$. The arbitrary sample size, n, does not appear.

If the probabilities of $0, 1, \ldots, 4$ boys are denoted by $P_0, P_1, \ldots, P_4$, the formula for the mean is clearly

$$(0 \times P_0) + (1 \times P_1) + (2 \times P_2) + (3 \times P_3) + (4 \times P_4).$$

In general, if x is a discrete random variable taking values $x_0, x_1, x_2, \ldots$, with probabilities $P_0, P_1, P_2, \ldots$, the mean value of x is calculated as

$$\sum_i x_i P_i. \tag{3.6}$$

The mean value of a random variable, calculated in this way, is often called the *expected value*, the *mathematical expectation* or simply the *expectation* of x, and the operation involved (multiplying each value of x by its probability, and then adding) is denoted by $E(x)$. The expectation of a random variable is often allotted a Greek symbol like μ (lower-case Greek letter 'mu'), to distinguish it from a mean value calculated from a finite number of observations (denoted usually by symbols such as $\bar{x}$ or $\bar{y}$).

As a second example, consider the probability distribution of x, the number of A genes in the genotypes shown in Example 3.4. Here,

$$E(x) = (0 \times 0.25) + (1 \times 0.50) + (2 \times 0.25)$$
$$= 1.$$

If x follows a continuous distribution, the formula given above for $E(x)$ cannot be used. However, one could consider a discrete distribution in which possible values of x differed by a small interval $2h$. To any value X_0 we could allot the probability given by the continuous distribution for values of x between $X_0 - h$ and $X_0 + h$ (which, as we have seen, will be close to $2hf(X_0)$ if h is small enough). The expectation of x in this discrete distribution can be calculated by the general rule. As the interval h gets smaller and smaller, the discrete distribution will approach more and more closely the continuous distribution, and in general the expectation will approach a quantity which formally is given by the expression

$$\mu = \int_{-\infty}^{\infty} xf(x) \, dx.$$

This provides a definition of the expectation of x for a continuous distribution.

The *variance* of a random variable is defined as

$$\text{var}(x) = E(x - \mu)^2;$$

that is, as the expectation of the squared difference from the mean. This is an obvious development from the previous formula $\sum (x_i - \bar{x})^2/n$ for the variance of a finite number, n, of observations, since this quantity is the mean value of the squared difference from the sample mean, $\bar{x}$. The distinction between the divisor of n and that of $n - 1$ becomes of no importance when we are dealing with probability distributions since n is effectively infinite.

The variance of a random variable is customarily given the symbol σ^2 (σ being the lower-case Greek letter 'sigma'). The standard deviation is again defined as σ, the square root of the variance.

By analogy with the short-cut formula (2.3) for the sample variance, we shall find it convenient to use the following relationship:

$$\sigma^2 = E(x^2) - \mu^2. \tag{3.7}$$

The two formulae for the variance may be illustrated by the distribution in Example 3.4, for which we have already obtained $\mu = 1$. With the direct formula, we proceed as follows:

x	P	$x - \mu$	$(x - \mu)^2$
0	0.25	−1	1
1	0.50	0	0
2	0.25	1	1

$$\sigma^2 = E(x - \mu)^2$$
$$= (1 \times 0.25) + (0 \times 0.50) + (1 \times 0.25)$$
$$= 0.5.$$

With the short-cut formula,

x	P	x^2
0	0.25	0
1	0.50	1
2	0.25	4

$$E(x^2) = (0 \times 0.25) + (1 \times 0.50) + (4 \times 0.25)$$
$$= 1.5;$$
$$\sigma^2 = E(x^2) - \mu^2$$
$$= 1.5 - 1^2$$
$$= 0.5,$$

as before.

We have so far discussed probability distributions in rather general terms. In the next three sections we consider three specific forms of distribution which play a very important role in statistical theory and practice.

3.6 **The binomial distribution**

We have already met a particular case of this form of distribution in the example of §3.2 on the sex distribution in families of four.

In general, suppose we have a random sequence in which the outcome of each individual trial is of one of two types, A or B, these outcomes occurring with probabilities π and $1 - \pi$, respectively. (The symbol π, the lower-case Greek letter 'pi', is used merely as a convenient Greek letter and has no connection at all with the mathematical constant $\pi = 3.14159\ldots$) In the previous example, A and B were boys and girls, and π was 0.51.

Consider now a group of n observations from this random sequence (in the example $n = 4$). It will be convenient to refer to each such group as a 'sample' of n observations. What is the probability distribution of the number of As in the sample? This number we shall call r, and clearly r must be one of the numbers $0, 1, 2, \ldots, n - 1, n$. Define also $p = r/n$, the *proportion* of As in the sample, and $q = (n - r)/n = 1 - p$, the proportion of Bs.

As in the example, we argue that the probability of r As and $n - r$ Bs is

$$\pi^r (1 - \pi)^{n-r}$$

multiplied by the number of ways in which one can choose r out of the n sample members to receive a lable 'A'. This multiplying factor is called a *binomial coefficient.* In the example the binomial coefficients were worked out by simple enumeration, but clearly this could be tedious with large values of *n* and *r*. The binomial coefficient is usually denoted by

$$\binom{n}{r}$$

(referred to in speaking as '*n* binomial *r*'), or

$$^{n}C_{r}.$$

Tables of binomial coefficients are provided in most books of mathematical tables. For moderate values of *n* and *r* they can be calculated directly from:

$$\binom{n}{r} = \frac{n(n-1)(n-2)\ldots(n-r+1)}{1\cdot2\cdot3\ldots r} \qquad (3.8)$$

(where the single dots are multiplication signs and the rows of dots mean that all the intervening integers are used). The quantity $1\cdot2\cdot3\ldots r$ is called 'factorial *r*' or '*r* factorial' and is usually written *r*!. Since the expression $n(n-1)\ldots(n-r+1)$, which occurs in the numerator of

$$\binom{n}{r},$$

can be written as

$$\frac{n!}{(n-r)!},$$

it follows that

$$\binom{n}{r} = \frac{n!}{r!(n-r)!} \qquad (3.9)$$

This formula involves unnecessarily heavy multiplication, but it draws attention to the symmetry of the binomial coefficients:

$$\binom{n}{r} = \binom{n}{n-r}. \qquad (3.10)$$

This is, indeed, obvious from the definition. Any selection of *r* objects out of *n* is automatically a selection of the $n-r$ objects which remain.

If we put $r = 0$ in (3.8), both the numerator and the denominator are meaningless. Putting $r = n$ would give

$$\binom{n}{n} = \frac{n!}{n!} = 1,$$

and it would accord with the symmetry result to put

$$\binom{n}{0} = 1. \tag{3.11}$$

This is clearly the correct result, since there is precisely one way of selecting 0 objects out of n to be labelled as As: namely to select all the n objects to be labelled as Bs. Note that (3.11) accords with (3.9) if we agree to call $0! = 1$; this is merely a convention since $0!$ is strictly not covered by our previous definition of the factorial, but it provides a useful extension of the definition which is used generally in mathematics.

The binomial coefficients required in the example of §3.2 could have been obtained from (3.8) as follows:

$$\binom{4}{0} = 1$$

$$\binom{4}{1} = \frac{4}{1} = 4$$

$$\binom{4}{2} = \frac{4 \cdot 3}{1 \cdot 2} = 6$$

$$\binom{4}{3} = \frac{4 \cdot 3 \cdot 2}{1 \cdot 2 \cdot 3} = 4$$

$$\binom{4}{4} = \frac{4 \cdot 3 \cdot 2 \cdot 1}{1 \cdot 2 \cdot 3 \cdot 4} = 1.$$

A useful way to obtain binomial coefficients for small values of n, without any multiplication, is by means of Pascal's triangle:

```
n                    1
1                 1    1
2              1    2    1
3           1    3    3    1
4        1    4    6    4    1
5     1    5   10   10    5    1
etc.                etc.
```

In this triangle of numbers, which can be extended downwards indefinitely, each entry is obtained as the sum of the two adjacent numbers on the line above. Thus, in the fifth row (for $n = 4$),

$$4 = 1 + 3, \quad 6 = 3 + 3, \quad \text{etc.}$$

Along each row are the binomial coefficients

$$\binom{n}{0}, \binom{n}{1}, \dots \quad \text{up to} \binom{n}{n-1}, \binom{n}{n}.$$

The probability that the sample of n individuals contains r As and $n - r$ Bs, then, is

$$\binom{n}{r}\pi^r(1-\pi)^{n-r}. \tag{3.12}$$

If this expression is evaluated for each value of r from 0 to n, the sum of these $n+1$ values will represent the probability of obtaining 0 As or 1 A or 2 As, etc., up to n As. These are the only possible results from the whole sequence and they are mutually exclusive; the sum of the probabilities is, therefore, 1. That this is so follows algebraically from the classical binomial theorem, for

$$\binom{n}{0}\pi^0(1-\pi)^n + \binom{n}{1}\pi^1(1-\pi)^{n-1} + \ldots + \binom{n}{n}\pi^n(1-\pi)^0$$
$$= [\pi + (1-\pi)]^n$$
$$= 1^n$$
$$= 1.$$

This result was verified in the particular example of Table 3.1.

The expectation and variance of r can now be obtained by applying the general formulae (3.6) and (3.7) to the probability distribution (3.12) and using standard algebraic results on the summation of series. Alternative derivations are given in §4.4. The results are:

$$E(r) = n\pi \tag{3.13}$$

and

$$\text{var}(r) = n\pi(1-\pi). \tag{3.14}$$

The formula for the expectation is intuitively acceptable. The mean number of As is equal to the number of observations multiplied by the probability that an individual result is an A. The expectation of the number of boys out of four, in our previous example, was shown in §3.5 to be 2·04. We now see that this result could have been obtained from (3.13):

$$E(r) = 4 \times 0·51 = 2·04.$$

The formula (3.14) for the variance is less obvious. For a given value of n, $\text{var}(r)$ reaches a maximum value when $\pi = 1 - \pi = \frac{1}{2}$ (when $\text{var}(r) = \frac{1}{4}n$), and falls off markedly as π approaches 0 or 1. If π is very small, the factor $1-\pi$ in (3.14) is very close to 1, and $\text{var}(r)$ becomes very close to $n\pi$, the value of $E(r)$.

We shall often be interested in the probability distribution of p, the *proportion* of As in the sample. Now $p = r \times (1/n)$, and the multiplying factor $1/n$ is constant from one sample to another. It follows that

$$E(p) = E(r) \times (1/n) = \pi \tag{3.15}$$

and

$$\text{var}(p) = \text{var}(r) \times (1/n)^2 = \frac{\pi(1-\pi)}{n}. \tag{3.16}$$

The square in the multiplying factor for the variance arises because the units in which the variance is measured are the squares of the units of the random variable.

It will sometimes be convenient to refer to the standard deviations of r or of p. These are the square roots of the corresponding variances:

$$SD(r) = \sqrt{[n\pi(1 - \pi)]}$$

and

$$SD(p) = \sqrt{\left[\frac{\pi(1 - \pi)}{n}\right]}.$$

Some further properties of the binomial distribution are given in §4.4. Binomial probabilities can be evaluated in many statistical packages.

Example 3.6

Table 3.2 is given by Lancaster (1965) from data published by Roberts *et al.* (1939). These authors observed 551 crosses between rats, with one parent heterozygous for each of five factors and the other parent homozygous recessive for each. The distribution is that of the number of dominant genes out of five, for each offspring. The theoretical distribution is the binomial with $n = 5$ and $\pi = \frac{1}{2}$, and the 'expected' frequencies, obtained by multiplying the binomial probabilities by 551, are shown in the table. The agreement between observed and expected frequencies is satisfactory.

The binomial distribution is characterized by the mathematical variables π and n. Variables such as these which partly or wholly characterize a probability distribution are known as *parameters*. They are, of course, entirely distinct from

Table 3.2 Distribution of number of dominant genes at five loci, in crosses between parents heterozygous for each factor and those homozygous recessive for each (Lancaster, 1965).

Number of dominant genes	Number of offspring	
	Observed	Expected
0	17	17·2
1	81	86·1
2	152	172·2
3	180	172·2
4	104	86·1
5	17	17·2
	551	551·0

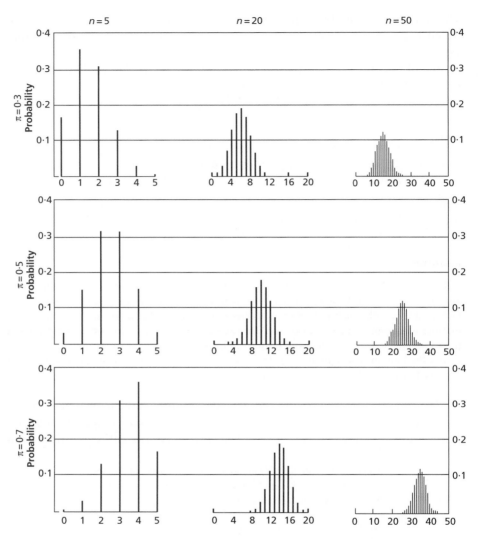

Fig. 3.7 Binomial distribution for various values of π and n. The horizontal scale in each diagram shows values of r.

random variables. Figure 3.7 illustrates the shape of the distribution for various combinations of π and n. Note that, for a particular value of n, the distribution is symmetrical for $\pi = \frac{1}{2}$ and asymmetrical for $\pi < \frac{1}{2}$ or $\pi > \frac{1}{2}$; and that for a particular value of π the asymmetry decreases as n increases.

Statistical methods based on the binomial distribution are described in detail in §§4.4, 4.5 and 8.5.

3.7 **The Poisson distribution**

This distribution is named after S.D. Poisson (1781–1840), a French mathematician. It is sometimes useful as a limiting form of the binomial, but it is important also in its own right as a distribution arising when events of some sort occur randomly in time, or when small particles are distributed randomly in space.

   We shall first consider random events in time. Suppose that a certain type of event occurs repeatedly, with an average rate of λ per unit time but in an entirely random fashion. To make the idea of randomness rather more precise we can postulate that in any very small interval of time of length h (say 1 ms) the probability that an event occurs is approximately proportional to h, say λh. (For example, if h is doubled the very small probability that the interval contains an event is also doubled.) The probability that the interval contains more than one event is supposed to be proportionately smaller and smaller as h gets smaller, and can therefore be ignored. Furthermore, we suppose that what happens in any small interval is independent of what happens in any other small interval which does not overlap the first.

   A very good instance of this probability model is that of the emission of radioactive particles from some radioactive material. The rate of emission, λ, will be constant, but the particles will be emitted in a purely random way, each successive small interval of time being on exactly the same footing, rather than in a regular pattern. The model is the analogy, in continuous time, of the random sequence of independent trials discussed in §3.1, and is called the *Poisson process*.

   Suppose that we observe repeated stretches of time, of length T time units, from a Poisson process with a rate λ. The number, x, of events occurring in an interval of length T will vary from one interval to another. In fact, it is a random variable, the possible values of which are 0, 1, 2, ... What is the probability of a particular value x?

   A natural guess at the value of x would be λT, the rate of occurrence multiplied by the time interval. We shall see later that λT is the mean of the distribution of x, and it will be convenient to denote λT by the single symbol μ.

   Let us split any one interval of length T into a large number n of subintervals each of length T/n (Fig. 3.8). Then, if n is sufficiently large, the number of events in the subinterval will almost always be 0, will occasionally be 1 and will hardly ever be more than 1. The situation is therefore almost exactly the same as a sequence of n binomial trials (a trial being the observation of a subinterval), in each of which there is a probability $\lambda(T/n) = \mu/n$ of there being an event and $1 - \mu/n$ of there being no event. The probability that the whole series of n trials provides exactly x events is, in this approximation, given by the binomial distribution:

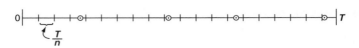

Fig. 3.8 The occurrence of events in a Poisson process, with the time-scale subdivided into small intervals.

$$\frac{n(n-1)\ldots(n-x+1)}{x!}\left(\frac{\mu}{n}\right)^x\left(1-\frac{\mu}{n}\right)^{n-x}. \tag{3.17}$$

Now, this binomial approximation will get better and better as n increases. What happens to (3.17) as n increases indefinitely? We can replace

$$n(n-1)\ldots(n-x+1)$$

by n^x since x will be negligible in comparison with n. Similarly we can replace $(1-\mu/n)^{n-x}$ by $(1-\mu/n)^n$ since $(1-\mu/n)^x$ will approach 1 as n increases. It is a standard mathematical result that, as n increases indefinitely, $(1-\mu/n)^n$ approaches $e^{-\mu}$, where e is the base of natural (or Napierian) logarithms ($e = 2\cdot718\ldots$).

Finally, then, in the limit as n increases indefinitely, the probability of x events approaches

$$P_x = \frac{n^x}{x!}\left(\frac{\mu}{n}\right)^x e^{-\mu} = \frac{\mu^x e^{-\mu}}{x!}. \tag{3.18}$$

The expression (3.18) defines the Poisson probability distribution. The random variable x takes the values $0, 1, 2,\ldots$ with the successive probabilities obtained by putting these values of x in (3.18). Thus,

$$P_0 = e^{-\mu}$$
$$P_1 = \mu e^{-\mu}$$
$$P_2 = \tfrac{1}{2}\mu^2 e^{-\mu}, \text{etc.}$$

Note that, for $x = 0$, we replace $x!$ in (3.18) by the value 1, as was found to be appropriate for the binomial distribution. To verify that the sum of the probabilities is 1,

$$P_0 + P_1 + P_2 + \ldots = e^{-\mu}\left(1 + \mu + \tfrac{1}{2}\mu^2 + \ldots\right)$$
$$= e^{-\mu} \times e^{\mu}$$
$$= 1,$$

the replacement of the infinite series on the right-hand side by e^{μ} being a standard mathematical result.

Before proceeding to further consideration of the properties of the Poisson distribution, we may note that a similar derivation may be applied to the situation in which particles are randomly distributed in space. If the space is one-dimensional (for instance the length of a cotton thread along which flaws may occur with constant probability at all points), the analogy is immediate. With two-dimensional space (for instance a microscopic slide over which bacteria are distributed at random with perfect mixing technique) the total area of size A may be divided into a large number n of subdivisions each of area A/n; the argument then carries through with A replacing T. Similarly, with three-dimensional space (bacteria well mixed in a fluid suspension), the total volume V is divided into n small volumes of size V/n. In all these situations the model envisages particles distributed at random with density λ per unit length (area or volume). The number of particles found in a length (area or volume) of size l (A or V) will follow the Poisson distribution (3.18) where the parameter $\mu = \lambda l$ (λA or λV).

The shapes of the distribution for $\mu = 1$, 4 and 15 are shown in Fig. 3.9. Note that for $\mu = 1$ the distribution is very skew, for $\mu = 4$ the skewness is much less and for $\mu = 15$ it is almost absent.

The distribution (3.18) is determined entirely by the one parameter, μ. It follows that all the features of the distribution in which one might be interested are functions only of μ. In particular the mean and variance must be functions of μ. The mean is

$$E(x) = \sum_{x=0}^{\infty} xP_x$$

$$= \mu,$$

this result following after a little algebraic manipulation.

By similar manipulation we find

$$E(x^2) = \mu^2 + \mu$$

and

$$var(x) = E(x^2) - \mu^2$$

$$= \mu \tag{3.19}$$

Thus, the variance of x, like the mean, is equal to μ. The standard deviation is therefore $\sqrt{\mu}$.

Much use is made of the Poisson distribution in bacteriology. To estimate the density of live organisms in a suspension the bacteriologist may dilute the suspension by a factor of, say, 10^{-5}, take samples of, say, $1\,cm^3$ in a pipette and drop the contents of the pipette on to a plate containing a nutrient medium on which the bacteria grow. After some time each organism dropped on to the plate will have formed a colony and these colonies can be counted. If the original suspension was well mixed, the volumes sampled are accurately determined and

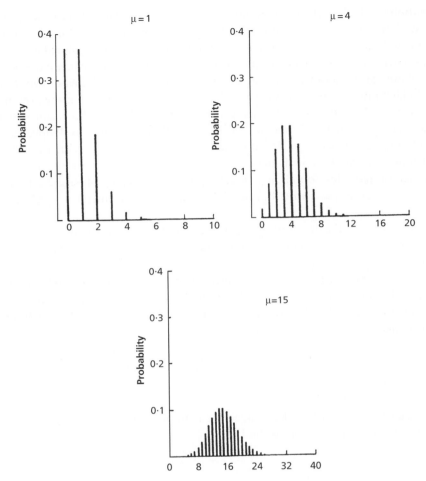

Fig. 3.9 Poisson distribution for various values of μ. The horizontal scale in each diagram shows values of *x*.

the medium is uniformly adequate to sustain growth, the number of colonies in a large series of plates could be expected to follow a Poisson distribution. The mean colony count per plate, $\bar{x}$, is an estimate of the mean number of bacteria per $10^{-5}\,\mathrm{cm}^3$ of the original suspension, and a knowledge of the theoretical properties of the Poisson distribution permits one to measure the precision of this estimate (see §5.2).

Similarly, for total counts of live and dead organisms, repeated samples of constant volume may be examined under the microscope and the organisms counted directly.

Example 3.7

As an example, Table 3.3 shows a distribution observed during a count of the root nodule bacterium (*Rhizobium trifolii*) in a Petroff–Hausser counting chamber. The 'expected' frequencies are obtained by calculating the mean number of organisms per square, $\bar{x}$, from the frequency distribution (giving $\bar{x} = 2 \cdot 50$) and calculating the probabilities P_x of the Poisson distribution with μ replaced by $\bar{x}$. The expected frequencies are then given by $400\,P_x$. The observed and expected frequencies agree quite well. This organism normally produces gum and therefore clumps readily. Under these circumstances one would not expect a Poisson distribution, but the data in Table 3.3 were collected to show the effectiveness of a method of overcoming the clumping.

In the derivation of the Poisson distribution use was made of the fact that the binomial distribution with a large n and small π is an approximation to the Poisson with mean $\mu = n\pi$.

Conversely, when the correct distribution is a binomial with large n and small π, one can approximate this by a Poisson with mean $n\pi$. For example, the number of deaths from a certain disease, in a large population of n individuals subject to a probability of death π, is really binomially distributed but may be taken as approximately a Poisson variable with mean $\mu = n\pi$. Note that the standard deviation on the binomial assumption is $\sqrt{[n\pi(1-\pi)]}$, whereas the Poisson standard deviation is $\sqrt{(n\pi)}$. When π is very small these two expressions are almost equal. Table 3.4 shows the probabilities for the Poisson distribution with $\mu = 5$, and those for various binomial distributions with $n\pi = 5$. The similarity between the binomial and the Poisson improves with increases in n (and corresponding decreases in π).

Table 3.3 Distribution of counts of root nodule bacterium (*Rhizobium trifolii*) in a Petroff–Hausser counting chamber (data from Wilson and Kullman, 1931).

Number of bacteria per square	Number of squares Observed	Expected
0	34	32·8
1	68	82·1
2	112	102·6
3	94	85·5
4	55	53·4
5	21	26·7
6	12	11·1
7–	4	5·7
	400	399·9

Table 3.4 Binomial and Poisson distributions with $\mu = 5$.

r	n	π = 0·5, n = 10	0·10, 50	0·05, 100	Poisson
0		0·0010	0·0052	0·0059	0·0067
1		0·0098	0·0286	0·0312	0·0337
2		0·0439	0·0779	0·0812	0·0842
3		0·1172	0·1386	0·1396	0·1404
4		0·2051	0·1809	0·1781	0·1755
5		0·2461	0·1849	0·1800	0·1755
6		0·2051	0·1541	0·1500	0·1462
7		0·1172	0·1076	0·1060	0·1044
8		0·0439	0·0643	0·0649	0·0653
9		0·0098	0·0333	0·0349	0·0363
10		0·0010	0·0152	0·0167	0·0181
>10		0	0·0094	0·0115	0·0137
		1·0000	1·0000	1·0000	1·0000

Probabilities for the Poisson distribution may be obtained from many statistical packages.

3.8 The normal (or Gaussian) distribution

The binomial and Poisson distributions both relate to a discrete random variable. The most important continuous probability distribution is the *Gaussian* (C.F. Gauss, 1777–1855, German mathematician) or, as it is frequently called, the *normal* distribution. Figures 3.10 and 3.11 show two frequency distributions, of height and of blood pressure, which are similar in shape. They are both approximately symmetrical about the middle and exhibit a shape rather like a bell, with a pronounced peak in the middle and a gradual falling off of the frequency in the two tails. The observed frequencies have been approximated by a smooth curve, which is in each case the probability density of a normal distribution.

Frequency distributions resembling the normal probability distribution in shape are often observed, but this form should not be taken as the norm, as the name 'normal' might lead one to suppose. Many observed distributions are undeniably far from 'normal' in shape and yet cannot be said to be abnormal in the ordinary sense of the word. The importance of the normal distribution lies not so much in any claim to represent a wide range of observed frequency distributions but in the central place it occupies in sampling theory, as we shall see in Chapters 4 and 5. For the purposes of the present discussion we shall regard the normal distribution as one of a number of theoretical forms for a continuous random variable, and proceed to describe some of its properties.

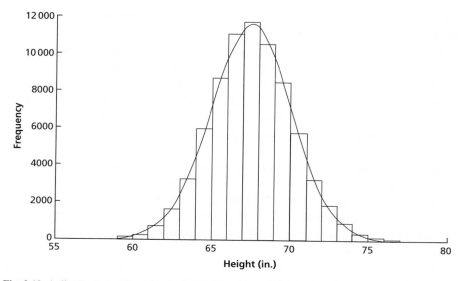

Fig. 3.10 A distribution of heights of young adult males, with an approximating normal distribution (Martin, 1949, Table 17 (Grade 1)).

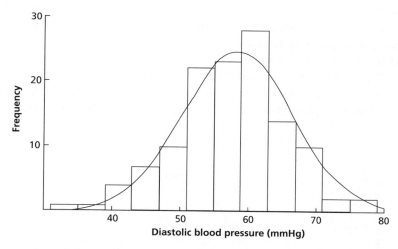

Fig. 3.11 A distribution of diastotic blood pressures of schoolboys with an approximating normal distribution (Rose, 1962, Table 1).

The probability density, $f(x)$, of a normally distributed random variable, x, is given by the expression

$$f(x) = \frac{1}{\sigma\sqrt{(2\pi)}} \exp\left[-\frac{(x-\mu)^2}{2\sigma^2}\right],\tag{3.20}$$

where $\exp(z)$ is a convenient way of writing the exponential function e^z (e being the base of natural logarithms), μ is the expectation or mean value of x and σ is the standard deviation of x. (Note that π is the mathematical constant $3.14159\ldots$, not, as in §3.6, the parameter of a binomial distribution.)

The curve (3.20) is shown in Fig. 3.12, on the horizontal axis of which are marked the positions of the mean, μ, and the values of x which differ from μ by $\pm\sigma$, $\pm 2\sigma$ and $\pm 3\sigma$. The symmetry of the distribution about μ may be inferred from (3.20), since changing the sign but not the magnitude of $x - \mu$ leaves $f(x)$ unchanged.

Figure 3.12 shows that a relatively small proportion of the area under the curve lies outside the pair of values $x = \mu + 2\sigma$ and $x = \mu - 2\sigma$. The area under the curve between two values of x represents the probability that the random variable x takes values within this range (see §3.4). In fact the probability that x lies within $\mu \pm 2\sigma$ is very nearly 0.95, and the probability that x lies outside this range is, correspondingly, 0.05.

It is important for the statistician to be able to find the area under any part of a normal distribution. Now, the density function (3.20) depends on two parameters, μ and σ. It might be thought, therefore, that any relevant probabilities would have to be worked out separately for every pair of values of μ and σ. Fortunately this is not so. In the previous paragraph we made a statement about the probabilities inside and outside the range $\mu \pm 2\sigma$, without any assumption about the particular values taken by μ and σ. In fact the probabilities depend on an expression of the departure of x from μ as a multiple of σ. For example, the points marked on the axis of Fig. 3.12 are characterized by the multiples ± 1, ± 2 and ± 3, as shown on the lower scale. The probabilities under various parts of any normal distribution can therefore be expressed in terms of the *standardized deviate* (or *z-value*)

$$z = \frac{x - \mu}{\sigma}.$$

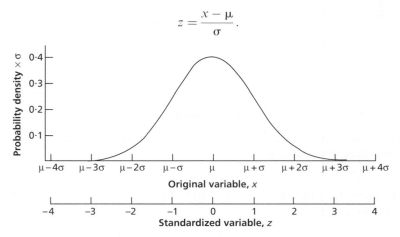

Fig. 3.12 The probability density function of a normal distribution showing the scales of the original variable and the standardized variable.

Table 3.5 Some probabilities associated with the normal distribution.

Standardized deviate $z = (x - \mu)/\sigma$	Probability of greater deviation	
	In either direction	In one direction
0·0	1·000	0·500
1·0	0·317	0·159
2·0	0·046	0·023
3·0	0·0027	0·0013
1·645	0·10	0·05
1·960	0·05	0·025
2·576	0·01	0·005

A few important results, relating values of z to single- or double-tail area probabilities, are shown in Table 3.5. More detailed results are given in Appendix Table A1, and are also readily available from programs in computer packages or on statistical calculators.

It is convenient to denote by $N(\mu, \sigma^2)$ a normal distribution with mean μ and variance σ^2 (i.e. standard deviation σ). With this notation, the standardized deviate z follows the *standard normal distribution*, $N(0, 1)$.

The use of tables of the normal distribution may be illustrated by the next example.

Example 3.8

The heights of a large population of men are found to follow closely a normal distribution with a mean of 172·5 cm and a standard deviation of 6·25 cm. We shall use Table A1 to find the proportions of the population corresponding to various ranges of height.

1 *Above 180 cm.* If $x = 180$, the standardized deviate $z = (180 - 172·5)/6·25 = 1·20$. The required proportion is the probability that z exceeds 1·20, which is found from Table A1 to be 0·115.

2 *Below 170 cm.* $z = (170 - 172·5)/6·25 = -0·40$. The probability that z falls below $-0·40$ is the same as that of exceeding $+0·40$, namely 0·345.

3 *Below 185 cm.* $z = (185 - 172·5)/6·25 = 2·00$. The probability that z falls below 2·00 is one minus the probability of exceeding 2·00, namely $1 - 0·023 = 0·977$.

4 *Between 165 and 175 cm.* For $x = 165$, $z = -1·20$; for $x = 175$, $z = 0·40$. The probability that z falls between $-1·20$ and 0·40 is one minus the probability of (i) falling below $-1·20$ or (ii) exceeding 0·40, namely

$$1 - (0·115 + 0·345) = 1 - 0·460 = 0·540.$$

The normal distribution is often useful as an approximation to the binomial and Poisson distributions. The binomial distribution for any particular value of π

approaches the shape of a normal distribution as the other parameter n increases indefinitely (see Fig. 3.7); the approach to normality is more rapid for values of π near $\frac{1}{2}$ than for values near 0 or 1, since all binomial distributions with $\pi = \frac{1}{2}$ have the advantage of symmetry. Thus, provided n is large enough, a binomial variable r (in the notation of §3.6) may be regarded as approximately normally distributed with mean $n\pi$ and standard deviation $\sqrt{[n\pi(1-\pi)]}$.

The Poisson distribution with mean μ approaches normality as μ increases indefinitely (see Fig. 3.9). A Poisson variable x may, therefore, be regarded as approximately normal with mean μ and standard deviation $\sqrt{\mu}$.

If tables of the normal distribution are to be used to provide approximations to the binomial and Poisson distributions, account must be taken of the fact that these two distributions are discrete whereas the normal distribution is continuous. It is useful to introduce what is known as a *continuity correction*, whereby the exact probability for, say, the binomial variable r (taking integral values) is approximated by the probability of a normal variable between $r - \frac{1}{2}$ and $r + \frac{1}{2}$. Thus, the probability that a binomial variable took values greater than or equal to r when $r > n\pi$ (or less than or equal to r when $r < n\pi$) would be approximated by the normal tail area beyond a standardized normal deviate

$$z = \frac{|r - n\pi| - \frac{1}{2}}{\sqrt{[n\pi(1-\pi)]}},$$

the vertical lines indicating that the 'absolute value', or the numerical value ignoring the sign, is to be used.

Tables 3.6 and 3.7 illustrate the normal approximations to some probabilities for binomial and Poisson variables.

Table 3.6 Examples of the approximation to the binomial distribution by the normal distribution with continuity correction.

π	n	Mean $n\pi$	Standard deviation $\sqrt{[n\pi(1-\pi)]}$	Values of r	Exact probability	Normal approximation with continuity correction	
						z	Probability
0·5	10	5	1·581	≤ 2	0·0547	1·581	0·0579
				≥ 8	0·0547		
0·1	50	5	2·121	≤ 2	0·1117	1·179	0·1192
				≥ 8	0·1221		
0·5	40	20	3·162	≤ 14	0·0403	1·739	0·0410
				≥ 26	0·0403		
0·2	100	20	4·000	≤ 14	0·0804	1·375	0·0846
				≥ 26	0·0875		

Table 3.7 Examples of the approximation to the Poisson distribution by the normal distribution with continuity correction.

Mean μ	Standard deviation $\sqrt{\mu}$	Values of x	Exact probability	Normal approximation with continuity correction $z = \frac{|x-\mu|-\frac{1}{2}}{\sqrt{\mu}}$	Probability
5	2·236	0	0·0067	2·013	0·0221
		≤2	0·1246	1·118	0·1318
		≥8	0·1334	1·118	0·1318
		≥10	0·0318	2·013	0·0221
20	4·472	≤10	0·0108	2·214	0·0168
		≤15	0·1565	1·006	0·1572
		≥25	0·1568	1·006	0·1572
		≥30	0·0218	2·124	0·0168
100	10·000	≤80	0·0226	1·950	0·0256
		≤90	0·1714	0·950	0·1711
		≥110	0·1706	0·950	0·1711
		≥120	0·0282	1·950	0·0256

The importance of the normal distribution extends well beyond its value in modelling certain symmetric frequency distributions or as an approximation to the binomial and Poisson distributions. We shall note in §4.2 a central role in describing the sampling distribution of means of large samples and, more generally, in §5.4, its importance in the large-sample distribution of a wider range of statistics.

The $\chi^2_{(1)}$ distribution

Many probability distributions of importance in statistics are closely related to the normal distribution, and will be introduced later in the book. We note here one especially important distribution, the χ^2 ('chi-square' or 'chi-squared') *distribution on one degree of freedom*, written as $\chi^2_{(1)}$. It is a member of a wider family of χ^2 distributions, to be described more fully in §5.1; at present we consider only this one member of the family.

Suppose z denotes a standardized normal deviate, as defined above. That is, z follows the N(0,1) distribution. The squared deviate, z^2, is also a random variable, the value of which must be non-negative, ranging from 0 to ∞. Its distribution, the $\chi^2_{(1)}$ distribution, is depicted in Fig. 3.13. The percentiles (p.38) of the distribution are tabulated on the first line of Table A2. Thus, the column headed $P = 0.050$ gives the 95th percentile. Two points may be noted at this stage.

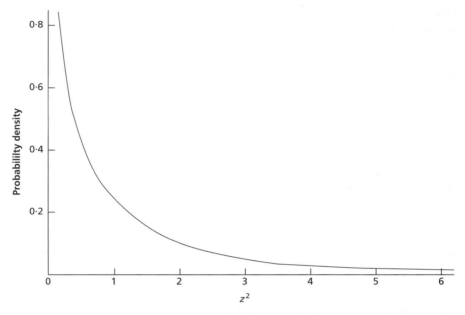

Fig. 3.13 Probability density function for a variate z^2 following a χ^2 distribution on one degree of freedom.

1 $E(z^2) = E(x - \mu)^2/\sigma^2 = \sigma^2/\sigma^2 = 1$. The mean value of the distribution is 1.

2 The percentiles may be obtained from those of the normal distribution. From Table A1 we know, for instance, that there is a probability 0·05 that z exceeds $+1·960$ or falls below $-1·960$. Whenever either of these events happens, z^2 exceeds $(1·960)^2 = 3·84$. Thus, the 0·05 level of the $\chi^2_{(1)}$ distribution is 3·84, as is confirmed by the entry in Table A2. A similar relationship holds for all the other percentiles.

This equivalence between the standard normal distribution, N(0,1), and the $\chi^2_{(1)}$ distribution, means that many statements about normally distributed random variables can be equally well expressed in terms of either distribution. It must be remembered, though, that the use of z^2 removes the information about the *sign* of z, and so if the direction of the deviation from the mean is important the N(0, 1) distribution must be used.

4 Analysing means and proportions

4.1 **Statistical inference: tests and estimation**

Population and sample

We noted in Chapter 1 that statistical investigations invariably involve observations on groups of individuals. Large groups of this type are usually called *populations*, and as we saw earlier the individuals comprising the populations may be human beings, other living organisms or inanimate objects. The statistician may refer also to a population of observations—for example, the population of heights of adult males resident in England at a certain moment, or the population of outcomes (death or survival) for all patients suffering from a particular illness during some period.

To study the properties of some populations we often have recourse to a *sample* drawn from that population. This is a subgroup of the individuals in the population, usually proportionately few in number, selected to be, to some degree, representative of the population. In most situations the sample will not be fully representative. Something is lost by the process of sampling. Any one sample is likely to differ in some respect from any other sample that might have been chosen, and there will be some risk in taking any sample as representing the population. The statistician's task is to measure and to control that risk.

Techniques for the design of sample surveys, and examples of their use in medical research, are discussed in §19.2. In the present chapter we are concerned only with the simplest sort of sampling procedure, *simple random sampling*, which means that every possible sample of a given size from the population has an equal probability of being chosen. A particular sample may, purely by chance, happen to be dissimilar from the population in some serious respect, but the theory of probability enables us to calculate how large these discrepancies are likely to be. Much of statistical analysis is concerned with the estimation of the likely magnitude of these *sampling errors*, and in this and the next chapter we consider some of the most important results.

Statistical inference

In later sections of this chapter we shall enquire about the likely magnitude of sampling errors when samples are drawn from specific populations. The argument will be essentially from population to sample. Given the distribution of a variable in a population we can obtain results about the distribution of various quantities, such as the mean and variance, calculated from the sample observations and therefore varying from sample to sample. Such a quantity is called a *statistic*. The population itself can be characterized by various quantities, such as the mean and variance, and these are called *parameters*. The *sampling distributions* of statistics, given the parameters, are obtained by purely deductive arguments.

In general, though, it is of much more practical interest to argue in the opposite direction, from sample to population—a problem of induction rather than deduction. Having obtained a single sample, a natural step is to try to *estimate* the population parameter by some appropriate statistic from the sample. For example, the population mean of some variable might be estimated by the sample mean, and we shall need to ask whether this is a reasonable procedure. This is a typical example of an argument from sample to population—the form of reasoning called *statistical inference*.

We have assumed so far that the data at our disposal form a random sample from some population. In some sampling enquiries this is known to be true by virtue of the design of the investigation. In other studies a more complex form of sampling may have been used (§19.2). A more serious conceptual difficulty is that in many statistical investigations there is no formal process of sampling from a well-defined population. For instance, the prevalence of a certain disease may be calculated for all the inhabitants of a village and compared with that for another village. A clinical trial may be conducted in a clinic, with the participation of all the patients seen at the clinic during a given period. A doctor may report the duration of symptoms among a consecutive series of 50 patients with a certain form of illness. Individual readings may vary haphazardly, whether they form a random sample or whether they are collected in a less formal way, and it will often be desirable to assess the effect that this basic variability has on any statistical calculations that are performed. How can this be done if there is no well-defined population and no strictly random sample?

It can be done by arguing that the observations are subject to random, unsystematic variation, which makes them appear very much like observations on a random variable. The population formed by the whole distribution is not a real, well-defined entity, but it may be helpful to think of it as a hypothetical population which would be generated if an indefinitely large number of observations, showing the same sort of random variation as those at our disposal, could be made. This concept seems satisfactory when the observations vary in a patternless way. We are putting forward a *model*, or conceptual framework, for the random variation, and propose to make whatever statements we can about the relevant features of this model, just as we wish to make statements about the relevant features of a population in a strict sampling situation. Sometimes, of course, the supposition that the data behave like a simple random sample is blatantly unrealistic. There may, for instance, be a systematic tendency for the earliest observations to be greater in magnitude than those made later. Such trends, and other systematic features, can be allowed for by increasing the complexity of the model. When such modifications have been made, there will still remain some degree of apparently random variation, the underlying probability distribution of which is a legitimate object of study.

The estimation of the population mean by the sample mean is an example of the type of inference known as *point estimation*. It is of limited value unless supplemented by other devices. A single value quoted as an estimate of a population parameter is of little use unless it is accompanied by some indication of its precision. In the following parts of this section we shall describe various ways of enhancing the value of point estimates. However, it will be useful here to summarize some important attributes that may be required for an estimator:

1   A statistic is an *unbiased* estimator of a parameter if, in repeated sampling, its expectation (i.e. mean value) equals the parameter. This is useful, but not essential: it may for instance be more convenient to use an estimator whose median, rather than mean, is the parameter value.

2   An estimator is *consistent* if it gives the value of the parameter when applied to the whole population, i.e. in very large samples. This is a more important criterion than **1**. It would be very undesirable if, in large samples, where the estimator is expected to be very precise, it pointed misleadingly to the wrong answer.

3   The estimator should preferably have as little sampling error as possible. A consistent estimator which has minimum sampling error is called *efficient*.

4   A statistic is *sufficient* if it captures all the information that the sample can provide about a particular parameter. This is an important criterion, but its implications are somewhat outside the scope of this book.

Likelihood

In discussing Bayes' theorem in §3.3, we defined the likelihood of a hypothesis as the probability of observing the given data if the hypothesis were true. In other words, the *likelihood function* for a parameter expresses the probability (or probability density) of the data for different values of the parameter. Consider a simple example. Suppose we make one observation on a random variable, x, which follows a normal distribution with mean μ and variance 1, where μ is

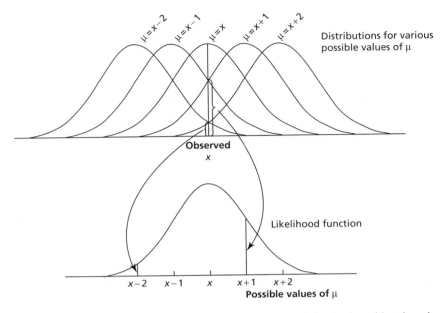

Fig. 4.1 The likelihood function for an observation from a normal distribution with unit variance. The likelihood for a particular value of μ in the lower diagram is equal to the probability density of x in the distribution with mean μ in the upper diagram.

unknown. What can be said about μ on the basis of the single value x? The likelihoods of the possible values of μ are shown in Fig. 4.1. This curve, showing the likelihood function, has exactly the same shape as a normal distribution with mean μ and variance 1, but it should not be thought of as a probability distribution since the ordinate for each value represents a density from a *different* distribution. The likelihood function can be used in various ways to make inferences about the unknown parameter μ, and we shall explore its use further in Chapter 6 in relation to Bayesian methods. At this stage we note its usefulness in providing a point estimate of μ. The peak of the likelihood function in Fig. 4.1 is at the value x, and we say that the *maximum likelihood estimate* (or *estimator*) of μ is x. Of course, in this simple example, the result is entirely unsurprising, but the method of maximum likelihood, advocated and developed by R.A. Fisher, is the most useful general method of point estimation. It has various desirable properties. A maximum likelihood estimator may be biased, but its *bias* (the difference between its expectation and the true parameter value) becomes smaller as the sample size increases, and is rarely important. The estimator is consistent, and in large samples it is efficient. Its sampling distribution in large samples becomes close to a normal distribution, which enables statements of probability to be made by using tables of the normal distribution.

Significance tests

Data are often collected to answer specified questions, such as: (i) do workers in a particular industry have reduced lung function compared with a control group? or (ii) is a new treatment beneficial to those suffering from a certain disease compared with the standard treatment? Such questions may be answered by setting up a hypothesis and then using the data to test this hypothesis. It is generally agreed that some caution should be exercised before claiming that some effect, such as a reduced lung function or an improved cure rate, has been established. The way to proceed is to set up a *null hypothesis*, that there is *no* effect. So, in (ii) above the null hypothesis is that the new treatment and the standard treatment are equally beneficial. Then an effect is claimed only if the data are inconsistent with this null hypothesis; that is, they are unlikely to have arisen if it were true.

The formal way of proceeding is one of the most important methods of statistical inference, and is called a *significance test*. Suppose a series of observations is selected randomly from a population and we are interested in a certain null hypothesis that specifies values for one or more parameters of the population. The question then arises: do the observations in the sample throw any light on the plausibility of the hypothesis? Some samples will have certain features which would be unlikely to arise if the null hypothesis were true; if such a sample were observed, there would be reason to suspect that the null hypothesis was untrue.

A very important question now is how we decide which sample values are 'likely' and which are 'unlikely'. In most situations, *any* set of sample values is peculiar in the sense that precisely the same values are unlikely ever to be chosen again. A random sample of 5 from a normal distribution with mean zero and unit variance might give the values (rounded to one decimal) 0·2, −1·1, 0·7, 0·8, −0·6. There is nothing very unusual about this set of values: its mean happens to be zero, and its sample variance is somewhat less than unity. Yet precisely those values are very unlikely to arise in any subsequent sample. But, if we did not know the population mean, and our null hypothesis specified that it was zero, we should have no reason at all for doubting its truth on the basis of this sample. On the other hand, a sample comprising the values 2·2, 0·9, 2·7, 2·8, 1·4, the mean of which is 2·0, would give strong reason for doubting the null hypothesis. The reason for classifying the first sample as 'likely' and the second as 'unlikely' is that the latter is proportionately very much more likely on an alternative hypothesis that the population mean is greater than zero, and we should like our test to be sensitive to possible departures from the null hypothesis of this form.

The significance test is a rule for deciding whether any particular sample is in the 'likely' or 'unlikely' class, or, more usefully, for assessing the strength of the conflict between what is found in the sample and what is predicted by the null hypothesis. We need first to decide what *sort* of departures from those expected are to be classified as 'unlikely', and this will depend on the sort of alternatives to the null hypothesis to which we wish our test to be sensitive. The dividing line between the 'likely' and 'unlikely' classes is clearly arbitrary but is usually defined in terms of a probability, *P*, which is referred to as the *significance level*. Thus, a result would be declared *significant at the 5% level* if the sample were in the class containing those samples most removed from the null hypothesis, in the direction of the relevant alternatives, and that class contained samples with a total probability of no more than 0·05 on the null hypothesis. An alternative and common way of expressing this is to state that the result was *statistically significant* ($P < 0·05$).

The 5% level and, to a lesser extent, the 1% level have become widely accepted as convenient yardsticks for assessing the significance of departures from a null hypothesis. This is unfortunate in a way, because there should be no rigid distinction between a departure which is just beyond the 5% significance level and one which just fails to reach it. It is perhaps preferable to avoid the dichotomy—'significant' or 'not significant'—by attempting to measure *how* significant the departure is. A convenient way of measuring this is to report the probability, *P*, of obtaining, if the null hypothesis were true, a sample as extreme as, or more extreme than, the sample obtained. One reason for the origin of the use of the dichotomy, significant or not significant, is that significance levels had to be looked up in tables, such as Appendix Tables A2, A3 and A4, and this restricted the evaluation of *P* to a range. Nowadays significance tests are usually carried out by a computer and most statistical computing packages give the calculated *P* value. It is preferable to quote this value and we shall follow this practice. However, when analyses are carried out by hand, or the calculated *P* value is not given in computer output, then a range of values could be quoted. This should be done as precisely as possible, particularly when the result is of borderline significance; thus, '$0·05 < P < 0·1$' is far preferable to 'not significant ($P > 0·05$)'.

Although a 'significant' departure provides some degree of evidence against a null hypothesis, it is important to realize that a 'non-significant' departure does not provide positive evidence in favour of that hypothesis. The situation is rather that we have failed to find strong evidence against the null hypothesis.

It is important also to grasp the distinction between statistical significance and clinical significance or practical importance. The analysis of a large body of data might produce evidence of departure from a null hypothesis which is highly significant, and yet the difference may be of no practical importance—either because the effect is clinically irrelevant or because it is too small. Conversely, another investigation may fail to show a significant effect—perhaps because the study is too small or because of excessive random variation—and yet an effect large enough to be important may be present: the investigation may have been too insensitive to reveal it.

A significance test for the value of a parameter, such as a population mean, is generally *two-sided*, in the sense that sufficiently large departures from the null hypothesis, in either direction, will be judged significant. If, for some reason, we decided that we were interested in possible departures only in one specified direction, say that a new treatment was superior to an old treatment, it would be reasonable to count as significant only those samples that differed sufficiently from the null hypothesis in that direction. Such a test is called *one-sided*. For a one-sided test at, say, the 5% level, sensitive to positive deviations from the null hypothesis (e.g. a population mean higher than the null value), a sample would be significant if it were in the class of samples deviating most from the null hypothesis in the positive direction and this class had a total probability of no more than 0·05.

A one-sided test at level P is therefore equivalent to a two-sided test at level $2P$, except that departures from the null hypothesis are counted in one direction only. In a sense the distinction is semantic. On the other hand, there is a temptation to use one-sided rather than two-sided tests because the probability level is lower and therefore the *apparent* significance is greater. A decision to use a one-sided test should *never* be made after looking at the data and observing the direction of the departure. Before the data are examined, one should decide to use a one-sided test only if it is quite certain that departures in one direction will always be ascribed to chance, and therefore regarded as non-significant however large they are. This situation rarely arises in practice, and it will be safe to assume that significance tests should almost always be two-sided. We shall make this assumption in this book unless otherwise stated.

No null hypothesis is likely to be exactly true. Why, then, should we bother to test it, rather than immediately rejecting it as implausible? There are several rather different situations in which the use of a significance test can be justified:

1 *To test a simplifying hypothesis.* Sometimes the null hypothesis specifies a simple model for a situation which is really likely to be more complex than the model admits. For instance, in studying the relationship between two variables, as in Chapter 7, it will be useful to assume for simplicity that a trend is linear (i.e. follows a straight line) if there is no evidence to the contrary, even though common sense tells us that the true trend is highly unlikely to be precisely linear.

2 *To test a null hypothesis which might be approximately true.* In a clinical trial to test a new drug against a placebo, it may be that the drug will either be very nearly inert or will have a marked effect. The null hypothesis that the drug is completely inert (and therefore has exactly the same effect as a placebo) is then a close approximation to a possible state of affairs.

3   *To test the direction of a difference from a critical value.* Suppose we are interested in whether a certain parameter, θ, has a value greater or less than some value θ_0. We could test the null hypothesis that θ is precisely θ_0. It may be quite clear that this will not be true. Nevertheless we give ourselves the opportunity to assert in which direction the difference lies. If the null hypothesis is significantly contradicted, we shall have good evidence either that $\theta > \theta_0$ or that $\theta < \theta_0$.

Finally, it must be remembered that the investigator's final judgement on any question should not depend *solely* on the results of a significance test. He or she must take into account the initial plausibility of various hypotheses and the evidence provided by other relevant studies. The balancing of different types of evidence will often be a subjective matter not easily formulated in clearly defined procedures. Formal methods based on Bayes' theorem are described in Chapters 6 and 16.

Confidence intervals

We have noted that a point estimate is of limited value without some indication of its precision. This is provided by the *confidence interval* which has a specified probability (the *confidence coefficient* or *coverage probability*) of containing the parameter value. The most commonly used coverage probability is 0·95. The interval is then called the 95% confidence interval, and the ends of this interval the 95% *confidence limits*; less frequently 90% or 99% limits may be used.

Two slightly different ways of interpreting a confidence interval may be useful:

1   The values of the parameter inside the 95% confidence interval are precisely those which would not be contradicted by a two-sided significance test at the 5% level. Values outside the interval, on the other hand, would all be contradicted by such a test.

2   We have said that the confidence interval contains the parameter with probability 0·95. This is not quite the same thing as saying that the parameter has a probability of 0·95 of being within the interval, because the parameter is not a random variable. In any particular case, the parameter either is or is not in the interval. What we are doing is to imagine a series of repeated random samples from a population with a fixed parameter value. In the long run, 95% of the confidence intervals will include the parameter value and the confidence statement will in these cases be true. If, in any particular problem, we calculate a confidence interval, we may happen to be unlucky in that this may be one of the 5% of cases in which the interval does not contain the parameter; but we are applying a procedure that will work 95% of the time.

The first approach is akin to the system of interval estimation used by R.A. Fisher, leading to *fiducial limits*; in most cases these coincide with confidence limits. The second approach was particularly stressed by J. Neyman (1894–1981), who was responsible for the development of confidence intervals in the 1930s. Interval estimation was used widely throughout the nineteenth century, often with precisely the same computed values as would be given nowadays by confidence intervals. The theory was at that time supported by concepts of prior probability, as discussed in Chapters 6 and 16. The approaches of both Fisher and Neyman dispense with the need to consider prior probability,

It follows from **1** above that a confidence interval may be regarded as equivalent to performing a significance test for all values of a parameter, not just the single value corresponding to the null hypothesis. Thus the confidence interval contains more information than a single significance test and, for this reason, it is sometimes argued that significance tests could be dispensed with and all results expressed in terms of a point estimate together with a confidence interval. On the other hand, the null hypothesis often has special importance, and quoting the P value, and not just whether the result is or is not significant at the 5% level, does provide information about the plausibility of the null hypothesis beyond that provided by the 95% confidence interval. In the last decade or two there has been an inceasing tendency to encourage the use of confidence limits in preference to significance tests (Rothman, 1978; Gardner & Altman, 1989). In general we recommend that, where possible, results should be expressed by a confidence interval, and that, when a null hypothesis is particularly relevant, the significance level should be quoted as well.

The use of confidence intervals facilitates the distinction between statistical significance and clinical significance or practical importance. Five possible interpretations of a significance test are illustrated in terms of the confidence interval for a difference between two groups in Fig. 4.2, adapted from Berry (1986, 1988): (a) the difference is significant and certainly large enough to be of practical importance; (b) the difference is significant but it is unclear whether it is large enough to be important; (c) the difference is significant but too small to be important; (d) the difference is not significant but may be large enough to be important; and (e) the difference is not significant and also not large enough to be important. One of the tasks in planning investigations is to ensure that a difference large enough to be important is likely, if it really exists, to be statistically significant and thus to be detected (cf. §4.6), and possibly to ensure that it is clear whether or not the difference is large enough to be important.

Finally, it should be remembered that confidence intervals for a parameter, even for a given coverage such as 95%, are not unique. First, even for the same set of data, the intervals may be based on different statistics. The aim should be to use an efficient statistic; the sample mean, for example, is usually an efficient way of estimating the population mean. Secondly, the same coverage may be achieved by allowing the non-coverage probability to be distributed in different ways between the two tails. A symmetric pair of 95% limits would allow

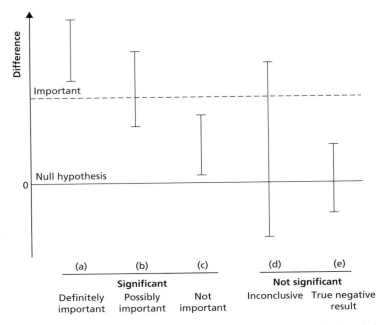

Fig. 4.2 Confidence intervals showing five possible interpretations in terms of statistical significance and practical importance.

non-coverage probabilities of $2\frac{1}{2}\%$ in each direction. Occasionally one might wish to allow 5% in one direction and zero in the other, the latter being achieved by an infinitely long interval in that direction. It is customary to use symmetric intervals unless otherwise stated.

In the following sections, and in Chapter 5, these different strands of statistical inference will be applied to a number of different situations and the detailed methodology set out.

4.2 **Inferences from means**

The sampling error of a mean

We now apply the general principles described in the last section to the making of inferences from mean values. The first task is to enquire about the sampling variation of a mean value of a set of observations.

Suppose that x is a quantitative random variable with mean μ and variance σ^2, and that $\bar{x}$ is the mean of a random sample of n values of x. For example, x may be the systolic blood pressure of men aged 30–34 employed in a certain industrial occupation, and $\bar{x}$ the mean of a random sample of n men from this very large population. We may think of $\bar{x}$ as itself a random variable, for each sample will have its own value of $\bar{x}$, and if the random sampling procedure is repeated indefinitely the values of $\bar{x}$ can be regarded as following a probability distribution (Fig. 4.3). The nature of this distribution of $\bar{x}$ is of considerable importance, for it determines how much uncertainty is conferred upon $\bar{x}$ by the very process of sampling.

Two features of the variability of $\bar{x}$ seem intuitively clear. First, it must depend on σ: the more variable is the blood pressure in the industrial population, the more variable will be the means of different samples of size n. Secondly, the variability of $\bar{x}$ must depend on n: the larger the size of each random sample, the closer together the values of $\bar{x}$ will be expected to lie.

Mathematical theory provides three basic results concerning the distribution of $\bar{x}$, which are of great importance in applied statistics.

1 $E(\bar{x}) = \mu$; that is, the mean of the distribution of the sample mean is the same as the mean of the individual measurements.

2 $\text{var}(\bar{x}) = \sigma^2/n$. The variance of the sample mean is equal to the variance of the individual measurements divided by the sample size. This provides a

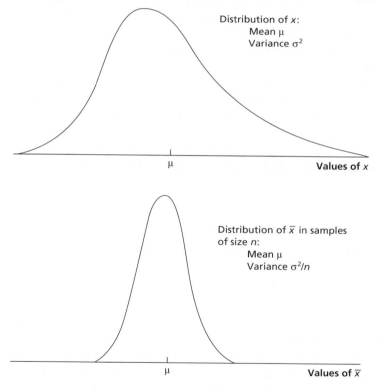

Fig. 4.3 The distribution of a random variable and the sampling distribution of means in random samples of size n.

formal expression of the intuitive feeling, mentioned above, that the variability of $\bar{x}$ should depend on both σ and n; the precise way in which this dependence acts would perhaps not have been easy to guess. The standard deviation of $\bar{x}$ is

$$\sqrt{\left(\frac{\sigma^2}{n}\right)} = \frac{\sigma}{\sqrt{n}}. \tag{4.1}$$

This quantity is often called the *standard error* of the mean and written $\mathrm{SE}(\bar{x})$. It is quite convenient to use this nomenclature as it helps to avoid confusion between the standard deviation of x and the standard deviation of $\bar{x}$, but it should be remembered that a standard error is not really a new concept: it is merely the standard deviation of some quantity calculated from a sample (in this case, the mean) in an indefinitely long series of repeated samplings.

3   If the distribution of x is normal, so will be the distribution of $\bar{x}$. Much more importantly, even if the distribution of x is not normal, that of $\bar{x}$ will become closer and closer to the normal distribution with mean μ and variance σ^2/n as n gets larger. This is a consequence of a mathematical result known as the *central limit theorem*, and it accounts for the central importance of the normal distribution in statistics.

The normal distribution is strictly only the limiting form of the sampling distribution of $\bar{x}$ as n increases to infinity, but it provides a remarkably good approximation to the sampling distribution even when n is small and the distribution of x is far from normal. Table 4.1 shows the results of taking random samples of five digits from tables of random numbers. These tables may be thought of as forming a probability distribution for a discrete random variable x, taking the values $0, 1, 2, \ldots, 9$ with equal probabilities of $0\cdot1$. This is clearly far from normal in shape. The mean and variance may be found by the methods of §3.5:

$$\mu = \mathrm{E}(x) = 0\cdot1(1 + 2 + \ldots + 9) = 4\cdot5,$$
$$\sigma^2 = \mathrm{E}(x^2) - \mu^2$$
$$= 0\cdot1(1^2 + 2^2 + \ldots + 9^2) - (4\cdot5)^2$$
$$= 8\cdot25,$$
$$\sigma = \sqrt{8\cdot25} = 2\cdot87,$$
$$\mathrm{SE}(\bar{x}) = \sqrt{(8\cdot25/5)} = \sqrt{1\cdot65} = 1\cdot28.$$

Two thousand samples of size 5 were taken (actually, by generating the random numbers on a computer rather than reading from printed tables), the mean $\bar{x}$ was calculated for each sample, and the 2000 values of $\bar{x}$ formed into the frequency distribution shown in Table 4.1. The distribution can be seen to be similar in shape to the normal distribution. The closeness of the approximation may be

Table 4.1 Distribution of means of 2000 samples of five random numbers.

Mean, $\bar{x}$	Frequency
0·4–	1
0·8–	4
1·2–	11
1·6–	22
2·0–	43
2·4–	88
2·8–	104
3·2–	178
3·6–	196
4·0–	210
4·4–	272
4·8–	200
5·2–	193
5·6–	154
6·0–	129
6·4–	92
6·8–	52
7·2–	30
7·6–	13
8·0–	7
8·4–	1
	2000

seen from Fig. 4.4, which shows the histogram corresponding to Table 4.1, together with a curve the height of which is proportional to the density of a normal distribution with mean 4·5 and standard deviation 1·28.

The theory outlined above applies strictly to random sampling from an infinite population or for successive independent observations on a random variable. Suppose a sample of size n has to be taken from a population of finite size N. Sampling is usually *without replacement*, which means that if an individual member of the population is selected as one member of a sample it cannot again be chosen in that sample. The expectation of $\bar{x}$ is still equal to μ, the population mean. The formula (4.1) must, however, be modified by a 'finite population correction', to become

$$\text{SE}(\bar{x}) = \frac{\sigma}{\sqrt{n}}\sqrt{(1-f)}, \tag{4.2}$$

where $f = n/N$, the *sampling fraction*. The effect of the finite population correction, $1 - f$, is to reduce the sampling variance substantially as f approaches 1, i.e.

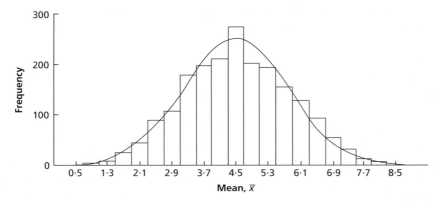

Fig. 4.4 The distribution of means from 2000 samples of five random digits (Table 4.1), with the approximating normal distribution.

as the sample size approaches the population size. Clearly, when $n = N$, $f = 1$ and $\mathrm{SE}(\bar{x}) = 0$, there is only one possible random sample, consisting of all the members of the population, and for this sample $\bar{x} = \mu$.

The sampling error of the sample median has no simple general expression. In random samples from a normal distribution, however, the standard error of the median for large n is approximately $1 \cdot 253\sigma/\sqrt{n}$. The fact that this exceeds $\sigma/\sqrt{n}$ shows that the median is more variable than the sample mean (or, technically, it is less *efficient* as an estimator of μ). This comparison depends on the assumption of normality for the distribution of x, however, and for certain other distributional forms the median provides the more efficient estimator.

Inferences from the sample mean

We consider first the situation in which the population standard deviation, σ, is known; later we consider what to do when σ is unknown.

Known σ

Let us consider in some detail the problem of testing the null hypothesis (which we shall denote by H_0) that the parameters of a normal distribution are $\mu = \mu_0$ and $\sigma = \sigma_0$, using the mean, $\bar{x}$, of a random sample of size n.

If H_0 is true, we know that the probability is only $0 \cdot 05$ that $\bar{x}$ falls outside the interval $\mu_0 - 1 \cdot 96\sigma_0/\sqrt{n}$ to $\mu_0 + 1 \cdot 96\sigma_0/\sqrt{n}$. For a value of $\bar{x}$ outside this range, the standardized normal deviate

$$z = \frac{\bar{x} - \mu_0}{\sigma_0/\sqrt{n}} \tag{4.3}$$

would be less than -1.96 or greater than 1.96. Such a value of $\bar{x}$ could be regarded as sufficiently far from μ_0 to cast doubt on the null hypothesis. Certainly, H_0 *might* be true, but if so an unusually large deviation would have arisen—one of a class that would arise by chance only once in 20 times. On the other hand such a value of $\bar{x}$ would be quite likely to occur if μ had some value other than μ_0, closer, in fact, to the observed $\bar{x}$. The particular critical values adopted here for z, ± 1.96, correspond to the quite arbitrary probability level of 0.05. If z is numerically greater than 1.96 the difference between μ_0 and $\bar{x}$ is said to be *significant at the 5% level*. Similarly, an even more extreme difference yielding a value of z numerically greater than 2.58 is *significant at the 1% level*. Rather than using arbitrary levels, such as 5% or 1%, we might enquire how far into the tails of the expected sampling distribution the observed value of $\bar{x}$ falls. A convenient way of measuring this tendency is to measure the probability, P, of obtaining, if the null hypothesis were true, a value of $\bar{x}$ as extreme as, or more extreme than, the value observed. If $\bar{x}$ is just significant at the 5% level, $z = \pm 1.96$ and $P = 0.05$ (the probability being that in both tails of the distribution). If $\bar{x}$ is beyond the 5% significance level, $z > 1.96$ or < -1.96 and $P < 0.05$. If $\bar{x}$ is not significant at the 5% level, $P > 0.05$ (Fig. 4.5). If the observed value of z were, say, 2.20, one could either give the exact value of P as 0.028 (from Table A1), or, by comparison with the percentage points of the normal distribution, write $0.02 < P < 0.05$.

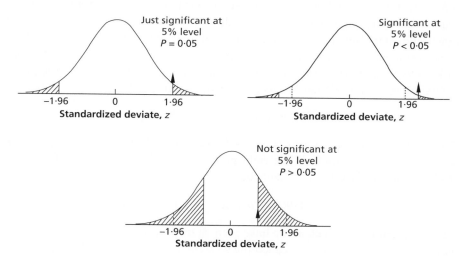

Fig. 4.5 Significance tests at the 5% level based on a standardized normal deviate. The observed deviate is marked by an arrow.

Example 4.1

A large number of patients with cancer at a particular site, and of a particular clinical stage, are found to have a mean survival time from diagnosis of 38·3 months with a standard deviation of 43·3 months. One hundred patients are treated by a new technique and their mean survival time is 46·9 months. Is this apparent increase in mean survival explicable as a random fluctuation?

We test the null hypothesis that the 100 recent results are effectively a random sample from a population with mean $\mu_0 = 38\cdot3$ and standard deviation $\sigma_0 = 43\cdot3$. Note that this distribution must be extremely skew, since a deviation of even one standard deviation below the mean gives a negative value $(38\cdot3 - 43\cdot3 = -5\cdot0)$, and no survival times can be negative. However, 100 is a reasonably large sample size, and it would be safe to use the normal theory for the distribution of the sample mean. Putting $n = 100$ and $\bar{x} = 46\cdot9$, we have a standardized normal deviate

$$\frac{46\cdot9 - 38\cdot3}{(43\cdot3/\sqrt{100})} = \frac{8\cdot6}{4\cdot33} = 1\cdot99.$$

This value just exceeds the 5% value of 1·96, and the difference is therefore just significant at the 5% level $(P < 0\cdot05)$. Referring to Appendix Table A1, the actual value of P is $2 \times 0\cdot0233 = 0\cdot047$.

This significant difference suggests that the increase in mean survival time is rather unlikely to be due to chance. It would not be safe to assume that the new treatment has improved survival, as certain characteristics of the patients may have changed since the earlier data were collected; for example, the disease may be diagnosed earlier. All we can say is that the difference is not very likely to be a chance phenomenon.

Suppose we wish to draw inferences about the population mean, μ, without concentrating on a single possible value μ_0. In a rough sense, μ is more likely to be near $\bar{x}$ than very far from $\bar{x}$. Can this idea be made more precise by asserting something about the probability that μ lies within a given interval around $\bar{x}$? This is the confidence interval approach. Suppose that the distribution of x is normal with known standard deviation, σ. From the general sampling theory, the probability is 0·95 that $\bar{x} - \mu$ lies between $-1\cdot96\sigma/\sqrt{n}$ and $+1\cdot96\sigma/\sqrt{n}$, i.e. that

$$-1\cdot96\sigma/\sqrt{n} < \bar{x} - \mu < 1\cdot96\sigma/\sqrt{n}. \tag{4.4}$$

Rearrangement of the left part of (4.4), namely $-1\cdot96\sigma/\sqrt{n} < \bar{x} - \mu$, gives $\mu < \bar{x} + 1\cdot96\sigma/\sqrt{n}$; similarly the right part gives $\bar{x} - 1\cdot96\sigma/\sqrt{n} < \mu$. Therefore (4.4) is equivalent to the statement that

$$\bar{x} - 1\cdot96\sigma/\sqrt{n} < \mu < \bar{x} + 1\cdot96\sigma/\sqrt{n}. \tag{4.5}$$

The statement (4.5), which as we have seen, is true with probability 0·95, asserts that μ lies in a certain interval called the 95% *confidence interval*. The ends of this interval, which are called the 95% *confidence limits*, are symmetrical about $\bar{x}$ and (since σ and n are known) can be calculated from the sample data. The

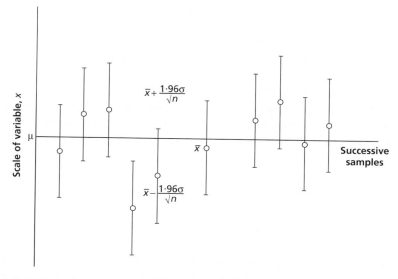

Fig. 4.6 Confidence limits (95%) for the mean of a normal distribution with known standard deviation, from a series of random samples of size n.

confidence interval provides a formal expression of the uncertainty which must be attached to $\bar{x}$ on account of sampling errors alone.

Interpretation **2** of a confidence interval (p. 90) is illustrated in Fig. 4.6. An imaginary series of repeated random samples from a population with a fixed value of μ will give different values of $\bar{x}$ and therefore different confidence intervals but, in the long run, 95% of these intervals will include μ, whilst in 5% $\bar{x}$ will be more than 1·96 standard errors away from μ (as in the fourth sample in Fig. 4.6) and the interval will not include μ.

Example 4.1, continued

In this example, the 95% confidence limits are

$$46 \cdot 9 \pm (1 \cdot 96)(4 \cdot 33)$$
$$= 38 \cdot 4 \text{ and } 55 \cdot 4.$$

The fact that this interval just excludes the possible value 38·3, which was tested previously, corresponds to the fact that this value was just contradicted by a significance test at the 5% level.

The assumption of normality is not crucial if n is reasonably large, because of the near-normality of the distribution of $\bar{x}$ in samples from almost any population.

For a higher degree of confidence than 95% we may use some other percentile of the normal distribution. The 99% limits, for instance, are

$$\bar{x} \pm 2 \cdot 58\sigma/\sqrt{n}.$$

In general, the $1 - \alpha$ confidence limits are

$$\bar{x} \pm z_{\alpha}\sigma/\sqrt{n},$$

where z_{α} is the standardized normal deviate exceeded (in either direction) with probability α. (The notation here is not universally standard: in some usages the subscript α refers to either the *one-tailed* probability, which we write as $\frac{1}{2}\alpha$, or the *distribution function*, $1 - \frac{1}{2}\alpha$.)

Unknown σ: the t distribution

Suppose now that we wish to test a null hypothesis which specifies the mean value of a normal distribution ($\mu = \mu_0$) but does not specify the variance σ^2, and that we have no evidence about σ^2 besides that contained in our sample. The procedure outlined above cannot be followed because the standard error of the mean, $\sigma/\sqrt{n}$, cannot be calculated. It seems reasonable to replace σ by the estimated standard deviation in the sample, s, giving a standardized deviate

$$t = \frac{\bar{x} - \mu_0}{s/\sqrt{n}} \qquad (4.6)$$

instead of the normal deviate z given by (4.3). The statistic t would be expected to follow a sampling distribution close to that of z (i.e. close to a standard normal distribution with mean 0 and variance 1) when n is large, because then s will be a good approximation to σ. When n is small, s may differ considerably from σ, purely by chance, and this will cause t to have substantially greater random variability than z.

In fact, t follows what is known as the *t distribution on $n - 1$ degrees of freedom* (DF). The t distributions form a family, distinguished by an index, the 'degrees of freedom', which in the present application is one less than the sample size. As the degrees of freedom increase, the t distribution tends towards the standard normal distribution (Fig. 4.7). Appendix Table A3 shows the percentiles of t, i.e. the values exceeded with specified probabilities, for different values of the degrees of freedom, v. For $v = \infty$, the tabulated values agree with those of the standard normal distribution. The 5% point, which always exceeds the normal value of 1·960, is nevertheless close to 2·0 for all except quite small values of v. The t distribution was derived by W.S. Gosset (1876–1937) and published under the pseudonym of 'Student' in 1908; the distribution is frequently referred to as Student's t distribution.

The t distribution is strictly valid only if the distribution of x is normal. Nevertheless, it is reasonably *robust* in the sense that it is approximately valid for quite marked departures from normality.

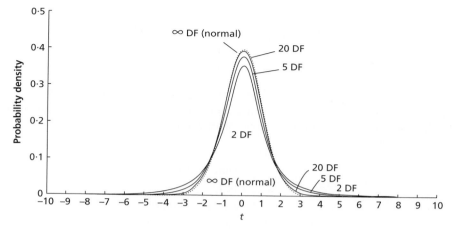

Fig. 4.7 Probability density function for t distributions on 2, 5, 20 and infinite degrees of freedom; the last is the standard normal distribution.

Calculation of the confidence interval proceeds as before, but using the t distribution instead of the normal distribution. If

$$t = \frac{\bar{x} - \mu}{s/\sqrt{n}},$$

the probability is 0·95 that t lies between $\pm t_{\nu,\,0\cdot05}$, the tabulated 5% point of the t distribution on $\nu = n - 1$ degrees of freedom. A little rearrangement gives an equivalent statement: the probability is 0·95 that

$$\bar{x} - t_{\nu,\,0\cdot05}(s/\sqrt{n}) < \mu < \bar{x} + t_{\nu,\,0\cdot05}(s/\sqrt{n}). \qquad (4.7)$$

This is the 95% confidence interval. It differs from (4.5) in the replacement of the percentage point of the normal distribution by that of the t distribution, which as we have seen is a somewhat larger number. The necessity to estimate the standard error from the sample has led to an interval based on a somewhat larger multiple of the standard error.

As in significance tests, normality of the distribution of x is necessary for the strict validity of (4.7), but moderate departures from normality will have little effect on the validity.

Example 4.2

The following data are the uterine weights (in mg) of each of 20 rats drawn at random from a large stock. Is it likely that the mean weight for the whole stock could be 24 mg, a value observed in some previous work?

9	18	21	26
14	18	22	27
15	19	22	29
15	19	24	30
16	20	24	32

Here $n = 20$, $\sum x = 420$ and $\bar{x} = 420/20 = 21 \cdot 0$. For t, we need the estimated standard error of the mean, $s/\sqrt{n}$, which it is convenient to calculate as $\sqrt{(s^2/n)}$, to avoid taking two separate square roots. From the usual short-cut formula,

$$\sum(x - \bar{x})^2 = \sum x^2 - (\sum x)^2/n$$
$$= 9484 - 8820$$
$$= 664,$$
$$s^2 = 664/19 = 34 \cdot 947,$$
$$s^2/n = 34 \cdot 947/20 = 1 \cdot 7474,$$
$$\sqrt{(s^2/n)} = 1 \cdot 3219$$

and

$$t = \frac{21 \cdot 0 - 24 \cdot 0}{1 \cdot 3219} = -2 \cdot 27.$$

The degrees of freedom are $\nu = 20 - 1 = 19$, and Table A3 shows the relevant percentage points as

| P | 0·05 | 0·02 |
| t | 2·093 | 2·539 |

Thus, the observed value is significant at between 2% and 5% ($0 \cdot 02 < P < 0 \cdot 05$). If these calculations had been done on a computer which gave the precise significance level, we should have had $P = 0 \cdot 035$. There is a rather strong suggestion that the mean weight of the stock is different from 24 mg (and, indeed, *less* than this value).

The 95% confidence limits for μ are

$$21 \cdot 00 \pm (2 \cdot 093)(1 \cdot 3219)$$
$$= 18 \cdot 23 \text{ and } 23 \cdot 77.$$

The exclusion of the value 24 corresponds to the significant result of testing this value at the 5% level. The 99% limits are

$$21 \cdot 00 \pm (2 \cdot 861)(1 \cdot 3219)$$
$$= 17 \cdot 22 \text{ and } 24 \cdot 78,$$

now including 24, since this value for μ was not significantly contradicted at the 1% level.

4.3 Comparison of two means

The investigator frequently needs to compare the means from two separate sets of data—for example, the mean weight gains in two groups of animals receiving different diets. These are *independent* samples, because there is no particular connection between a member of one group and a member of the other group.

A different situation arises when there is a connection between paired members of the two groups—for instance, if the observations are systolic blood pressures on the *same* group of men at two different times. These two situations need to be treated in different ways. We start with the *paired* case, which is technically rather simpler.

Paired case

Suppose we have two samples of size n:

$$x_{11}, x_{12}, \ldots, x_{1i}, \ldots, x_{1n}$$

drawn at random from a distribution with mean μ_1 and variance σ_1^2, and

$$x_{21}, x_{22}, \ldots, x_{2i}, \ldots, x_{2n}$$

drawn at random from a distribution with mean μ_2 and variance σ_2^2. If there is some sense in which x_{1i} is paired with x_{2i}, it will usually be true that high values of x_{1i} tend to be associated with high values of x_{2i}, and low with low. For example, x_{1i} and x_{2i} might be blood-pressure readings on the ith individual in a group of n, on each of two occasions. Some individuals would tend to give high values on both occasions, and some would tend to give low values. In such situations,

$$E(x_{1i} - x_{2i}) = \mu_1 - \mu_2.$$

However, the tendency of high or low values on one occasion to be associated with high or low values on the other occasion means that var $(x_{1i} - x_{2i})$ is lower than would be the case in the absence of such an association. Now, $\bar{x}_1 - \bar{x}_2$, the difference between the two means, is the mean of the n individual differences $x_{1i} - x_{2i}$, and these differences are independent of each other. The sampling error of $\bar{x}_1 - \bar{x}_2$ can therefore be obtained by analysing the n individual differences. This automatically ensures that, whatever the nature of the relationship between the paired readings, the appropriate sampling error is calculated. If the differences are normally distributed then the methods of §4.2 can be applied.

Example 4.3

In a small clinical trial to assess the value of a new tranquillizer on psychoneurotic patients, each patient was given a week's treatment with the drug and a week's treatment with a placebo, the order in which the two sets of treatments were given being determined at random. At the end of each week the patient had to complete a questionnaire, on the

Table 4.2 Anxiety scores recorded for 10 patients receiving a new drug and a placebo in random order.

| Patient | Anxiety score | | Difference d_i |
	Drug	Placebo	(drug − placebo)
1	19	22	−3
2	11	18	−7
3	14	17	−3
4	17	19	−2
5	23	22	1
6	11	12	−1
7	15	14	1
8	19	11	8
9	11	19	−8
10	8	7	1
			−13

basis of which he or she was given an 'anxiety score' (with possible values from 0 to 30), high scores corresponding to states of anxiety. The results are shown in Table 4.2.

The last column of Table 4.2 shows the difference, d_i, between the anxiety score for the ith subject on the drug and on the placebo. A t test on the 10 values of d_i gives

$$\sum d_i = -13,$$
$$\sum d_i^2 = 203,$$
$$\sum (d_i - \bar{d})^2 = 186 \cdot 1.$$

Therefore,

$$\bar{d} = -1 \cdot 30.$$
$$s^2 = 186 \cdot 1/9 = 20 \cdot 68,$$
$$\sqrt{(s^2/n)} = \sqrt{(20 \cdot 68/10)} = \sqrt{2 \cdot 068} = 1 \cdot 438,$$

and, to test the null hypothesis that $E(d_i) = 0$,

$$t = \frac{-1 \cdot 30}{1 \cdot 438} = -0 \cdot 90 \text{ on 9DF}.$$

The difference is clearly not significant ($P = 0 \cdot 39$).

The 95% confidence limits for the mean difference are

$$-1 \cdot 30 \pm (2 \cdot 262)(1 \cdot 438)$$
$$= -4 \cdot 55 \text{ and } 1 \cdot 95.$$

To conclude, this trial provided no convincing evidence that the new tranquillizer reduced anxiety when compared with a placebo ($P = 0 \cdot 39$). The 95% confidence interval for the reduction in anxiety was from 4·6 points on a 30-point scale in the tranquilliser's favour to 2.0 units in favour of the placebo.

In Table 4.2, some subjects, like Nos. 6 and 10, tend to give consistently low scores, whereas others, like Nos. 1 and 5, score highly on both treatments. These systematic differences between subjects are irrelevant to the comparison between treatments, and it is therefore appropriate that the method of differencing removes their effect.

Unpaired case: two independent samples

It will be useful to start by considering a rather general situation. Suppose that we have two random variables y_1 and y_2, that y_1 is distributed with mean m_1 and variance v_1, and y_2 with mean m_2 and variance v_2. We take an observation at random on y_1 and an *independent* random observation on y_2. What can be said about the distribution of $y_1 - y_2$ in an indefinite series of repetitions of this procedure?

Two important results are:

$$E(y_1 - y_2) = m_1 - m_2 \tag{4.8}$$

and

$$\text{var}(y_1 - y_2) = v_1 + v_2. \tag{4.9}$$

That is, the mean of the observed difference is the difference between the population means, as might be expected. The variance of the observed difference is the *sum* of the two population variances: the variability of each of the two observations combine to produce a greater variation in the difference.

We now apply the general results (4.8) and (4.9) to the particular case in which $y_1 = \bar{x}_1$, the mean of a random sample of size n_1 from a population with mean μ_1 and variance σ_1^2; and $y_2 = \bar{x}_2$, the mean of an independent random sample of size n_2 from a population with mean μ_2 and variance σ_2^2. Here, from (4.1),

$$m_1 = \mu_1 \text{ and } v_1 = \sigma_1^2/n_1;$$
$$m_2 = \mu_2 \text{ and } v_2 = \sigma_2^2/n_2.$$

Therefore, from (4.8) and (4.9),

$$\left. \begin{aligned} E(\bar{x}_1 - \bar{x}_2) &= \mu_1 - \mu_2 \\[2ex] \text{var}(\bar{x}_1 - \bar{x}_2) &= \frac{\sigma_1^2}{n_1} + \frac{\sigma_2^2}{n_2}. \end{aligned} \right\} \tag{4.10}$$

and

If the distributions of the xs are normal, and σ_1^2 and σ_2^2 are known, (4.10) can be used immediately for inferences about $\mu_1 - \mu_2$. To test the null hypothesis that $\mu_1 - \mu_2$, the standardized normal deviate

$$z = \frac{\bar{x}_1 - \bar{x}_2}{\sqrt{\left(\dfrac{\sigma_1^2}{n_1} + \dfrac{\sigma_2^2}{n_2}\right)}}$$

is used. For confidence limits for $\mu_1 - \mu_2$, the appropriate multiple of the standard error (i.e. of the denominator of z) is measured on either side of $\bar{x}_1 - \bar{x}_2$.

The normality of the xs is not a serious restriction if the sample sizes are not too small, because $\bar{x}_1 - \bar{x}_2$, like $\bar{x}_1$ and $\bar{x}_2$ separately, will be almost normally distributed. The lack of knowledge of σ_1^2 and σ_2^2 is more serious. These variances have to be estimated in some way, and we shall distinguish between two situations, in the first of which σ_1^2 and σ_2^2 are assumed to be equal and a common estimate is used for both parameters, and in the second of which no such assumption is made.

Equal variances: the two-sample t test

There are many instances in which it is reasonable to assume $\sigma_1^2 = \sigma_2^2$.

1   In testing a null hypothesis that the two samples are from distributions with the same mean and variance. For example, if the two samples are observations made on patients treated with a possibly active drug and on other patients treated with a pharmacologically inert placebo, the null hypothesis might specify that the drug was completely inert. In that case equality of variance is as much a part of the null hypothesis as equality of means, although we want a test based on $\bar{x}_1 - x_2$ so that we can hope to detect drugs which particularly affect the mean value of x.

2   It may be known from general experience that the sort of changes which distinguish sample 1 from sample 2 may affect the mean but are not likely to affect the variance appreciably. The sample estimates of variance, s_1^2 and s_2^2, may differ considerably, but in these situations we should, on general grounds, be prepared to regard most of the difference as due to sampling fluctuations in s_1^2 and s_2^2 rather than to a corresponding difference in σ_1^2 and σ_2^2.

If σ_1^2 and σ_2^2 are equal, their common value may be denoted by σ^2 without a subscript. How should σ^2 be estimated? From the first sample we have the estimator

$$s_1^2 = \frac{\sum_{(1)}(x - \bar{x}_1)^2}{n_1 - 1},$$

the subscript (1) after $\sum$ denoting a summation over the first sample. From the second sample, similarly, σ^2 is estimated by

$$s_2^2 = \frac{\sum_{(2)}(x - \bar{x}_2)^2}{n_2 - 1}.$$

A common estimate could be obtained by a straightforward mean of s_1^2 and s_2^2, but it is better to take a weighted mean, giving more weight to the estimate from the larger sample. It can be shown to be appropriate to take

$$s^2 = \frac{(n_1 - 1)s_1^2 + (n_2 - 1)s_2^2}{(n_1 - 1) + (n_2 - 1)}$$

$$= \frac{\sum_{(1)}(x - \bar{x}_1)^2 + \sum_{(2)}(x - \bar{x}_2)^2}{n_1 + n_2 - 2}.$$

This step enables us to use the t distribution on $n_1 + n_2 - 2$ degrees of freedom, as an exact solution to the problem if the xs are exactly normally distributed and as an approximate solution if the distribution of the xs is not grossly non-normal.

The standard error of $\bar{x}_1 - \bar{x}_2$ is now estimated by

$$\text{SE}(\bar{x}_1 - \bar{x}_2) = \sqrt{\left[s^2 \left(\frac{1}{n_1} + \frac{1}{n_2} \right) \right]}.$$

To test the null hypothesis that $\mu_1 = \mu_2$, we take

$$t = \frac{\bar{x}_1 - \bar{x}_2}{\text{SE}(\bar{x}_1 - \bar{x}_2)}$$

as following the t distribution on $n_1 + n_2 - 2$ DF.

Confidence limits are given by

$$\bar{x}_1 - \bar{x}_2 \pm t_{v,\,0.05}\text{SE}(\bar{x}_1 - \bar{x}_2),$$

with $v = n_1 + n_2 - 2$.

Example 4.4

Two groups of female rats were placed on diets with high and low protein content, and the gain in weight between the 28th and 84th days of age was measured for each rat. The results are given in Table 4.3.

The calculations proceed as follows

$$\sum_{(1)} x = 1\,440 \qquad\qquad \sum_{(2)} x = 707$$

$$n_1 = 12 \qquad\qquad n_2 = 7$$

$$\bar{x}_1 = 120 \cdot 0 \qquad\qquad \bar{x}_2 = 101 \cdot 0$$

$$\sum_{(1)} x^2 = 177\,832 \qquad\qquad \sum_{(2)} x^2 = 73\,959$$

$$(\sum_{(1)} x)^2/n_1 = 172\,800 \cdot 00 \qquad\qquad (\sum_{(2)} x)^2/n_2 = 71\,407 \cdot 00$$

$$\sum_{(1)} (x - \bar{x}_1)^2 = 5\,032 \cdot 00 \qquad\qquad \sum_{(2)} (x - \bar{x}_2)^2 = 2\,552 \cdot 00$$

$$s^2 = \frac{5032 + 2552}{17} = 446 \cdot 12.$$

$$
\begin{aligned}
\mathrm{SE}(\bar{x}_1 - \bar{x}_2) &= \sqrt{[(446 \cdot 12)(\tfrac{1}{12} + \tfrac{1}{7})]} \\
&= \sqrt{[(446 \cdot 12)(0 \cdot 22619)]} \\
&= \sqrt{100 \cdot 9} \\
&= 10 \cdot 04.
\end{aligned}
$$

To test the null hypothesis that $\mu_1 = \mu_2$,

$$t = \frac{120 \cdot 0 - 101 \cdot 0}{10 \cdot 04} = \frac{19 \cdot 0}{10 \cdot 04} = 1 \cdot 89 \text{ on 17 DF } (P = 0 \cdot 076).$$

The difference is not quite significant at the 5% level, and would provide merely suggestive evidence for a dietary effect.

Table 4.3 Gain in weight (g) between 28th and 84th days of age of rats receiving diets with high and low protein content.

	High protein	Low protein
	134	70
	146	118
	104	101
	119	85
	124	107
	161	132
	107	94
	83	
	113	
	129	
	97	
	123	
Total	1440	707

The 95% confidence limits for $\mu_1 - \mu_2$ are

$$19\cdot0 \pm (2\cdot110)(10\cdot04)$$
$$= 19\cdot0 \pm 21\cdot2$$
$$= -2\cdot2 \text{ and } 40\cdot2.$$

The range of likely values for $\mu_1 - \mu_2$ is large. If the experimenter feels dissatisfied with this range of uncertainty, the easiest remedy is to repeat the experiment with more observations. Higher values of n_1 and n_2 will tend to decrease the standard error of $\bar{x}_1 - \bar{x}_2$ and hence increase the precision of the comparison.

It might be tempting to apply the unpaired method to paired data. This would be incorrect because systematic differences between pairs would not be eliminated but would form part of the variance used in the denominator of the t statistic. Thus, using the unpaired method for paired data would lead to a less sensitive analysis except in cases where the pairing proved ineffective.

Unequal variances

In other situations it may be either clear that the variances differ considerably or prudent to assume that they may do so. One possible approach, in the first case, is to work with a transformed scale of measurement (§10·8). If the means, as well as the variances, differ, it may be possible to find a transformed scale, such as the logarithm of the original measurement, on which the means differ but the variances are similar. On the other hand, if the original means are not too different, it will usually be difficult to find a transformation that substantially reduces the disparity between the variances.

In these situations the main defect in the methods based on the t distribution is the use of a pooled estimate of variance. It is better to estimate the standard error of the difference between the two means as

$$\mathrm{SE}(\bar{x}_1 - \bar{x}_2) = \sqrt{\left(\frac{s_1^2}{n_1} + \frac{s_2^2}{n_2}\right)}.$$

A significance test of the null hypothesis may be based on the statistic

$$d = \frac{\bar{x}_1 - \bar{x}_2}{\sqrt{\left(\dfrac{s_1^2}{n_1} + \dfrac{s_2^2}{n_2}\right)}},$$

which is approximately a standardized normal deviate if n_1 and n_2 are reasonably large. Similarly, approximate $100(1 - \alpha)\%$ confidence limits are given by

$$\bar{x}_1 - \bar{x}_2 \pm z_\alpha \mathrm{SE}(\bar{x}_1 - \bar{x}_2),$$

where z_α is the appropriate standardized normal deviate corresponding to the two-sided probability α.

However, this method is no more exact for finite values of n_1 and n_2 than would be the use of the normal approximation to the t distribution in the case of equal variances. The appropriate analogue of the t distribution is both more complex than the t distribution and more contentious. One solution, due to B.L. Welch, is to use a distribution for d (tabulated, for example, in Pearson and Hartley, 1966, Table 11). The critical value for any particular probability level depends on s_1^2/s_2^2, n_1 and n_2. Another solution, similarly dependent on s_1^2/s_2^2, n_1 and n_2, is that of W.V. Behrens, tabulated as Table VI in Fisher and Yates (1963). The distinction between these two approaches is due to different approaches to the logic of statistical inference. Underlying Welch's test is an interpretation of probability levels, either in significance tests or confidence intervals, as long-term frequencies in repeated samples from the same populations. The Behrens test was advocated by R.A. Fisher as an example of the use of fiducial inference, and it arises also from the Bayesian approach (§6.2).

A feature of Welch's approach is that the critical value for d may be less than the critical value for a t distribution with $n_1 + n_2 - 2$ DF, and this is unsatisfactory. A simpler approximate solution which does not have this disadvantage is to test d against the t distribution with degrees of freedom, ν, dependent on s_1^2/s_2^2, n_1 and n_2 according to the following formula (Satterthwaite, 1946):

$$\frac{(s_1^2/n_1 + s_2^2/n_2)^2}{\nu} = \frac{(s_1^2/n_1)^2}{n_1 - 1} + \frac{(s_2^2/n_2)^2}{n_2 - 1}. \tag{4.11}$$

Although this test uses the t distribution, it should not be confused with the more usual two-sample t test based on equal variances. This approximate test is included in some statistical software packages.

Example 4.5

A suspension of virus particles is prepared at two dilutions. If the experimental techniques are perfect, preparation B should have 10 times as high a concentration of virus particles as preparation A. Equal volumes from each suspension are inoculated on to the chorioallantoic membrane of chick embryos. After an appropriate incubation period the membranes are removed and the number of pocks on each membrane is counted. The numbers are as follows:

Preparation	A	B
Counts	0	10
	0	13
	1	13
	1	14
	1	19
	1	20
	2	21
	2	26
	3	29

Are these results consistent with the hypothesis that, in a large enough series of counts, the mean for preparation B will be 10 times that for preparation A? If the counts on B are divided by 10 and denoted by x_2, the counts on A being denoted by x_1, an equivalent question is whether the means of x_1 and x_2 differ significantly.

Preparation	A	B
Counts	x_1	x_2
	0	1·0
	0	1·3
	1	1·3
	1	1·4
	1	1·9
	1	2·0
	2	2·1
	2	2·6
	3	2·9
	$n_1 = 9$	$n_2 = 9$
	$\bar{x}_1 = 1·2222$	$\bar{x}_2 = 1·8333$
	$s_1^2 = 0·9444$	$s_2^2 = 0·4100.$

The estimates of variance are perhaps not sufficiently different here to cause great disquiet, but it is known from experience with this type of data that estimates of variance of pock counts, standardized for dilution as we did for x_2, tend to decrease as the original counts increase. The excess of s_1^2 over s_2^2 is therefore probably not due to sampling error. We have

$$d = \frac{1·2222 - 1·8333}{\sqrt{\left(\dfrac{0·9444}{9} + \dfrac{0·4100}{9}\right)}} = \frac{-0·6111}{0·3879} = -1·58.$$

Note that, when, as here, $n_1 = n_2$, d turns out to have exactly the same numerical value as t, because the expression inside the square root can be written either as

$$\frac{s_1^2}{n} + \frac{s_2^2}{n}$$

or as

$$\frac{1}{2}(s_1^2 + s_2^2)\left(\frac{1}{n} + \frac{1}{n}\right).$$

Using Satterthwaite's approximation, the test statistic of 1.58 can be referred to the t distribution with DF given by

$$\nu = \frac{0·1504^2}{0·1049^2/8 + 0·0455^2/8} = 13·8.$$

Using 14 DF the significance level is 0·14. The 95% confidence limits for the difference between the two means are

$$-0 \cdot 6111 \pm 2 \cdot 145 \times 0 \cdot 3879$$
$$= -1 \cdot 4 \text{ and } 0 \cdot 2.$$

In any of these approaches, if the sample means are sufficiently close and the sample sizes are sufficiently large, the confidence interval for the difference in means may be narrow enough to allow one to conclude that the means are effectively equal for all practical purposes. The investigator must, however, be careful not to conclude that the two populations are identical unless there is good reason to believe that the variances are also equal.

4.4 **Inferences from proportions**

The sampling error of a proportion

This has already been fully discussed in §3.6. If individuals in an infinitely large population are classified into two types A and B, with probabilities π and $1 - \pi$, the number r of individuals of type A in a random sample of size n follows a binomial distribution. We shall now apply the results of §4.2 to prove the formulae previously given for the mean and variance of r.

Suppose we define a quantitative variable x, which takes the value 1 for each A individual and 0 for each B. We may think of x as a score attached to each member of the population. The point of doing this is that, in a sample of n consisting of r As and $n - r$ Bs,

$$\sum x = (r \times 1) + [(n - r) \times 0]$$
$$= r$$

and

$$\bar{x} = r/n, \ = p \text{ in the notation of §3.6.}$$

The sample proportion p may therefore be identified with the sample mean of x, and to study the sampling variation of p we can apply the general results established in §4.2. We shall need to know the population mean and standard deviation of x. From first principles these are

$$E(x) = (\pi \times 1) + [(1 - \pi) \times 0] \tag{4.12}$$
$$= \pi,$$

and

$$\mathrm{var}(x) = E(x^2) - [E(x)]^2$$
$$= (\pi \times 1^2) + [(1 - \pi) \times 0^2] - \pi^2$$
$$\pi(1 - \pi).$$

From (4.1),

$$\text{var}(\bar{x}) = \frac{\pi(1 - \pi)}{n}. \tag{4.13}$$

Writing (4.12) and (4.13) in terms of p rather than x and $\bar{x}$, we have

$$E(p) = \pi$$

and

$$\text{var}(p) = \frac{\pi(1 - \pi)}{n},$$

as in (3.15) and (3.16). Since $r = np$,

$$E(r) = n\pi$$

and

$$\text{var}(r) = n\pi(1 - \pi),$$

as in (3.13) and (3.14).

One more result may be taken from §4.2. As n approaches infinity, the distribution of $\bar{x}$ (that is, of p) approaches the normal distribution, with the corresponding mean and variance. The increasing symmetry has already been noted in §3.6.

Inferences from the proportion in a sample

Suppose that, in a large population, individuals drawn at random have an unknown probability π of being of type A. In a random sample of n individuals, a proportion p $(= r/n)$ are of type A. What can be said about π?

Suppose first that we wish to test a null hypothesis specifying that π is equal to some value π_0. On this hypothesis, the number of type A individuals, r, found in repeated random samples of size n would follow a binomial distribution. To express the departure of any observed value, r, from its expected value, $n\pi_0$, we could state the extent to which r falls into either of the tails of its sampling distribution. As in §4.1 this extent could be measured by calculating the probability in the tail area. The situation is a little different here because of the discreteness of the distribution of r. Do we calculate the probability of obtaining a larger deviation than that observed, $r - n\pi_0$, or the probability of a deviation at least as great? Since we are saying something about the degree of surprise elicited by a certain observed result, it seems reasonable to include the probability of this result in the summation. Thus, if $r > n\pi_0$ and the probabilities in the binomial distribution with parameters π_0 and n are $P_0, P_1, \ldots, P_n$, the P value for a one-sided test will be

$$P_+ = P_r + P_{r+1} + \ldots + P_n.$$

For a two-sided test we could add the probabilities of deviations at least as large as that observed, in the other direction. The P value for the other tail is

$$P_- = P_r' + P_{r'-1} + \ldots + P_0,$$

where r' is equal to $2n\pi_0 - r$ if this is an integer, and the highest integer less than this quantity otherwise. The P value for the two-sided test is then $P = P_- + P_+$.
For example, if $r = 8, n = 10$ and $\pi_0 = \frac{1}{2}$,

$$P_+ = P_8 + P_9 + P_{10}$$

and

$$P_- = P_2 + P_1 + P_0.$$

If $r = 17, n = 20$ and $\pi_0 = \frac{1}{3}$,

$$P_+ = P_{17} + P_{18} + P_{19} + P_{20}$$
$$P_- = 0.$$

If $r = 15, n = 20$ and $\pi_0 = 0.42$,

$$P_+ = P_{15} + P_{16} + P_{17} + P_{18} + P_{19} + P_{20}$$
$$P_- = P_1 + P_0.$$

An alternative, and perhaps preferable, approach is to regard a two-sided test at level α as being essentially the combination of two one-sided tests each at level $\frac{1}{2}\alpha$. The two-sided P value is then obtained simply by doubling the one-sided value.

Considerable simplification is achieved by approximating to the binomial distribution by the normal (§3.8). On the null hypothesis

$$\frac{r - n\pi_0}{\sqrt{[n\pi_0(1 - \pi_0)]}}$$

is approximately a standardized normal deviate. Using the continuity correction, (p.80), the tail area required in the significance test is approximated by the area beyond a standardized normal deviate

$$z = \frac{|r - n\pi_0| - \frac{1}{2}}{\sqrt{[n\pi_0(1 - \pi_0)]}}, \tag{4.14}$$

and the result will be significant at, say, the 5% level if this probability is less than 0·05.

Example 4.6

In a clinical trial to compare the effectiveness of two analgesic drugs, X and Y, each of 100 patients receives X for a period of 1 week and Y for another week, the order of administration being determined randomly. Each patient then states a preference for one of the two drugs. Sixty-five patients prefer X and 35 prefer Y. Is this strong evidence for the view that, in the long run, more patients prefer X than Y?

Test the null hypothesis that the preferences form a random series in which the probability of an X preference is $\frac{1}{2}$. This would be true if X and Y were equally effective in all respects affecting the patients' judgements. The standard error of r is

$$\sqrt{(100 \times \tfrac{1}{2} \times \tfrac{1}{2})} = \sqrt{25} = 5.$$

The observed deviation, $r - n\pi_0$, is

$$65 - 50 = 15.$$

With continuity correction, the standardized normal deviate is $(15 - \frac{1}{2})/5 = 2\cdot90$. Without continuity correction, the value would have been $15/5 = 3\cdot00$, a rather trivial difference. In this case the continuity correction could have been ignored. The normal tail area for $z = 2\cdot90$ is $0\cdot0037$; the departure from the null hypothesis is highly significant, and the evidence in favour of X is strong. The exact value of P, from the binomial distribution, is $0\cdot0035$, very close to the normal approximation.

The 95% confidence limits for π are the two values, π_L and π_U, for which the observed value of r is just significant on a one-sided test at the $2\frac{1}{2}\%$ level (Fig. 4.8). These values may be obtained fairly readily from tables of the binomial distribution, and are tabulated in the Geigy Scientific Tables (1982, Vol. 2, pp. 89–102). They may be obtained also from Fisher and Yates (1963, Table VIII1).

The normal approximation may be used in a number of ways.

1 The tail areas could be estimated from (4.14). Thus, for 95% confidence limits, approximations to π_L and π_U are given by the formulae

$$\frac{r - n\pi_L - \frac{1}{2}}{\sqrt{[n\pi_L(1 - \pi_L)]}} = 1\cdot96$$

and

$$\frac{r - n\pi_U + \frac{1}{2}}{\sqrt{[n\pi_U(1 - \pi_U)]}} = -1\cdot96.$$

2 In method **1**, if n is large, the continuity correction of $\frac{1}{2}$ may be omitted.

Method **1** involves the solution of a quadratic equation for each of π_L and π_U; method **2** involves a single quadratic equation. A further simplification is as follows.

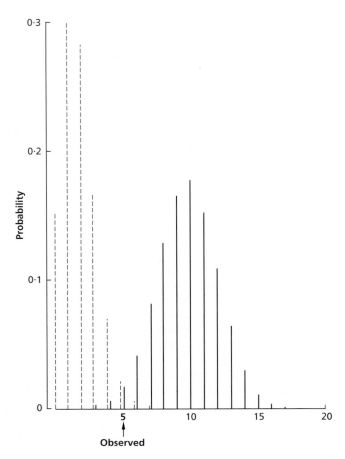

Fig. 4.8 Binomial distributions illustrating the 95% confidence limits for the parameter π based on a sample with five individuals of a certain type out of 20. For $\pi = \pi_L = 0\cdot09$ the probability of 5 or more is $0\cdot025$; for $\pi = \pi_U = 0\cdot49$ the probability of 5 or less is $0\cdot025$. $(- - -)\ \pi_L = 0\cdot09$; $(\underline{\qquad\qquad})$ $\pi_U = 0\cdot49$.

3 Replace $\pi_L(1 - \pi_L)$ and $\pi_U(1 - \pi_U)$ by $p(1 - p)$. This is not too drastic a step, as $p(1 - p)$ changes rather slowly with changes in p, particularly for values of p near $\frac{1}{2}$. Ignoring the continuity correction, as in **2**, we have the most frequently used approximation to the 95% confidence limits:

$$p \pm 1\cdot96\sqrt{(pq/n)},$$

where, as usual, $q = 1 - p$. The simplification here is due to the replacement of the standard error of p, which involves the unknown value π, by the approximate form $\sqrt{(pq/n)}$, which can be calculated entirely from known quantities.

Newcombe (1998a), in an extensive study of various methods, recommends method **2**. Method **3** has a coverage probability well below the nominal 95%, tending to shorten the interval unduly in the direction from p towards $\frac{1}{2}$.

Exact limits require the calculation of tail-area probabilities for the binomial distribution. The lower limit π_L, for instance, is the solution of

$$\sum_{j=r}^{n} \binom{n}{j} \pi_L^j (1 - \pi_L)^{n-j} = 0{\cdot}025. \tag{4.15}$$

The binomial tail areas can be obtained from many statistical packages. Alternatively, they can be obtained from tables of another important distribution: the F distribution. This is described in more detail in §5.1. We note here that the distribution is indexed by two parameters, v_1 and v_2, called *degrees of freedom* (DF). Table A4 shows the value of F exceeded with probability P for various combinations of v_1, v_2 and P, denoted by F_{P, v_1, v_2}.

It can be shown that the left-hand side of (4.15) equals the probability that a variable distributed as F with $2n - 2r + 2$ and $2r$ degrees of freedom exceeds $r(1 - \pi_L)/(n - r + 1)\pi_L$. Therefore

$$\frac{r(1 - \pi_L)}{(n - r + 1)\pi_L} = F_{0{\cdot}025, \, 2n-2r+2, \, 2r}.$$

That is,

$$\left. \begin{array}{c} \pi_L = \dfrac{r}{r + (n - r + 1)F_{0{\cdot}025, \, 2n-2r+2, \, 2r}} \\[4mm] \text{and similarly,} \\[4mm] \pi_U = \dfrac{r + 1}{r + 1 + (n - r)F^{-1}_{0{\cdot}025, \, 2r+2, \, 2n-2r}} \end{array} \right\} \tag{4.16}$$

(Miettinen, 1970).

Example 4.6, continued

With $n = 100$, $p = 0{\cdot}65$, the exact 95% confidence limits are found to be $0{\cdot}548$ and $0{\cdot}743$.

Method **1** will be found to give $0{\cdot}548$ and $0{\cdot}741$, method **2** gives $0{\cdot}552$ and $0{\cdot}736$, and method **3** gives

$$0{\cdot}65 \pm 1{\cdot}96 \sqrt{\left[\frac{(0{\cdot}65)(0{\cdot}35)}{100} \right]}$$
$$= 0{\cdot}65 \pm (1{\cdot}96)(0{\cdot}0477)$$
$$= 0{\cdot}557 \text{ and } 0{\cdot}743$$

In this example method **3** is quite adequate.

Example 4.7

As a contrasting example with small numbers, suppose $n = 20$ and $p = 0.25$. The exact 95% confidence limits are 0.087 and 0.491 (see Fig. 4.8).

Method **1** gives 0.096 and 0.494, method **2** gives 0.112 and 0.469, method **3** gives 0.060 and 0.440. Method **3** is clearly less appropriate here than in Example 4.6. In general, method **3** should be avoided if either np or $n(1 - p)$ is small (say, less than 10). Methods **2** and **3** may also be unreliable when either $n\pi_L$ or $n(1 - \pi_U)$ is less than 5. In this case, $n\pi_L$ is about 2 so it is not surprising that the lower confidence limit is not too well approximated by the normal approximation.

Example 4.8

As an example of finding the exact limits using the F distribution, consider the data of Fig. 4.8, where $r = 5$ and $n = 20$. Then,

$$\pi_L = 5/(5 + 16F_{0.025, 32, 10})$$

and

$$\pi_U = 6/(6 + 15F_{0.025, 12, 30}^{-1}).$$

The value of $F_{0.025, 32, 10}$ can be obtained by interpolation in Table A4 where interpolation is linear in the reciprocal of the degrees of freedom. Thus,

$$F_{0.025, 32, 10} = 3.37 - (3.37 - 3.08) \times \left(\frac{1}{24} - \frac{1}{32}\right) \bigg/ \frac{1}{24}$$

$$= 3.30.$$

Therefore $\pi_L = 0.0865$ and, since $F_{0.025, 12, 30} = 2.41$, $\pi_U = 0.4908$. In this example, interpolation was required for one of the F values and then only in the first of the degrees of freedom, but in general interpolation would be required for both F values and in both the degrees of freedom. This is tedious and can be avoided by using a method based on the normal approximation except when this method gives values such that either $n\pi_L$ or $n(1 - \pi_U)$ is small (say, less than 5).

It was remarked earlier that the discreteness of the distribution of r made inferences from proportions a little different from those based on a variable with a continuous distribution, and we now discuss these differences. For a continuous variable an exact significance test would give the result $P < 0.05$ for exactly 5% of random samples drawn from a population in which the null hypothesis were true, and a 95% confidence interval would contain the population value of the estimated parameter for exactly 95% of random samples. Neither of these properties is generally true for a discrete variable. Consider a binomial variable from a distribution with $n = 10$ and $\pi = 0.5$ (Table 3.4, p. 76). Using the exact test, for the hypothesis that $\pi = 0.5$, significance at the 5% level is found only for $r = 0, 1, 9$ or 10 and the probability of one or other of these values is 0.022.

Therefore, a result significant at the 5% level would be found in only 2·2% of random samples if the null hypothesis were true. This causes no difficulty if the precise level of P is stated. Thus if $r = 1$ we have $P = 0·022$, and a result significant at a level of 0·022 or less would occur in exactly 2·2% of random samples. The normal approximation with continuity correction is then the best approximate test, giving, in this case, $P = 0·027$.

A similar situation arises with the confidence interval. The exact confidence limits for the binomial parameter are conservative in the sense that the probability of including the true value is *at least* as great as the nominal confidence coefficient. This fact arises from the debatable decision to include the observed value in the calculation of tail-area probabilities. The limits are termed 'exact' because they are obtained from exact calculations of the binomial distribution, rather than from an approximation, but not because the confidence coefficient is achieved exactly. This problem cannot be resolved, in the same way as for the significance test, by changing the confidence coefficient. First, this is difficult to do but, secondly and more importantly, whilst for a significance test it is desirable to estimate P as precisely as possible, in the confidence interval approach it is perfectly reasonable to specify the confidence coefficient in advance at some conventional value, such as 95%. The approximate limits using the continuity correction also tend to be conservative. The limits obtained by methods **2** and **3**, however, which ignore the continuity correction, will tend to have a probability of inclusion nearer to the nominal value. This suggests that the neglect of the continuity correction is not a serious matter, and may, indeed, be an advantage.

The problems discussed above, due to the discreteness of the distribution, have caused much controversy in the statistical literature, particularly with the analysis of data collected to compare two proportions, to be discussed in §4.5. One approach, suggested by Lancaster (1952, 1961), is to use *mid-P* values, and this approach has been advocated more widely recently (Williams, 1988; Barnard, 1989; Hirji, 1991; Upton, 1992; Berry & Armitage, 1995; Newcombe, 1998a). The mid-P value for a one-sided test is obtained by including in the tail only one-half of the probability of the observed sample. Thus, for a binomial sample with r observed out of n, where $r > n\pi_0$, the one-sided mid-P value for testing the hypothesis that $\pi = \pi_0$ will be

$$\text{mid-}P_+ = \tfrac{1}{2}P_r + P_{r+1} + \ldots + P_n.$$

It has to be noted that the mid-P value is not the probability of obtaining a significant result by chance when the null hypothesis is true. Again, consider a binomial variable from a distribution with $n = 10$ and $\pi = 0·5$ (Table 3.4, p. 76). For the hypothesis that $\pi = 0·5$, a mid-P value less than 0·05 would be found only for $r = 0, 1, 9$ or 10, since the mid-P value for $r = 2$ is 2[0·0010

$+0{\cdot}0098 + \frac{1}{2}(0{\cdot}0439)] = 0{\cdot}0655$, and the probability of one or other of these values is $0{\cdot}022$.

Barnard (1989) has recommended quoting both the P and the mid-P values, on the basis that the former is a measure of the statistical significance when the data under analysis are judged alone, whereas the latter is the appropriate measure of the strength of evidence against the hypothesis under test to be used in combination with evidence from other studies. This arises because the mid-P value has the desirable feature that, when the null hypothesis is true, its average value is $0{\cdot}5$ and this property makes it particularly suitable as a measure to be used when combining results from several studies in making an overall assessment (meta-analysis; §18.10). Since it is rare that the results of a single study are used without support from other studies, our recommendation is also to give both the P and mid-P values, but to give more emphasis to the latter.

Corresponding to mid-P values are mid-P confidence limits, calculated as those values which, if taken as the null hypothesis value, give a corresponding mid-P value; that is, the 95% limits correspond to one-sided mid-P values of $0{\cdot}025$.

Where a normal approximation is adequate, P values and mid-P values correspond to test statistics calculated with and without the correction for continuity, respectively. Correspondingly, confidence intervals and mid-P confidence intervals can be based on normal approximations, using and ignoring the continuity correction, respectively. Thus, the mid-P confidence limits for a binomial probability would be obtained using method **2** rather than method **1** (p. 115).

Where normal approximations are inadequate, the mid-P values are calculated by summing the appropriate probabilities. The mid-P limits are more tedious to calculate, as they are not included in standard sets of tables and there is no direct formula corresponding to (4.16). The limits may be obtained fairly readily using a personal computer or programmable calculator by setting up the expression to be evaluated using a general argument, and then by trial and error finding the values that give tails of $0{\cdot}025$.

Example 4.7, continued

The mid-P limits are given by

$$P_0 + P_1 + P_2 + P_3 + P_4 + \tfrac{1}{2}P_5 = 0{\cdot}975 \text{ or } 0{\cdot}025,$$

where P_i is the binomial probability (as in (3.12)) for i events with $n = 20$ and $\pi = \pi_L$ or π_U. This expression was set up on a personal computer for general π, and starting with the knowledge that the confidence interval would be slightly narrower than the limits of $0{\cdot}0865$ and $0{\cdot}4908$ found earlier the exact 95% mid-P confidence limits were found as $0{\cdot}098$ and $0{\cdot}470$. Method **2** gives the best approximation to these limits but, as noted earlier, the lower confidence limit is less well approximated by the normal approximation, because $n\pi_L$ is only about 2.

4.5 **Comparison of two proportions**

As in the comparison of two means, considered in §4.3, we can distinguish between two situations according to whether individual members of the two samples are or are not paired.

Paired case

Suppose there are N observations in each sample, forming therefore N pairs of observations. Denoting the samples by 1 and 2, and describing each individual as A or not A, there are clearly four types of pairs:

Type	Sample 1	Sample 2	Number of pairs
1	A	A	k
2	A	Not A	r
3	Not A	A	s
4	Not A	Not A	m

If the number of pairs of the four types are as shown above, another way of exhibiting the same results is in the form of a two-way table:

		Sample 2 A	Sample 2 Not A	
Sample 1	A	k	r	$k + r$
	Not A	s	m	$s + m$
		$k + s$	$r + m$	N

The proportions of A individuals in the two samples are $(k + r)/N$ in sample 1 and $(k + s)/N$ in sample 2. We are interested in the difference between the two proportions, which is clearly $(r - s)/N$.

Consider first a significance test. The null hypothesis is that the expectation of $(r - s)/N$ is zero, or in other words that the expectations of r and s are equal. This can conveniently be tested by restricting our attention to the $r + s$ pairs in which the two members are of different types. Denote $r + s$ by n. On the null hypothesis, given n disparate or 'untied' pairs, the number of pairs of type 2 (or, indeed, of type 3) would follow a binomial distribution with a parameter equal to $\frac{1}{2}$. The test therefore follows precisely the methods of §4.4. A large-sample test is obtained by regarding

$$z = \frac{r - \frac{1}{2}n}{\frac{1}{2}\sqrt{n}} \tag{4.17}$$

as a standardized normal deviate. A continuity correction may be applied by reducing the absolute value of $r - \frac{1}{2}n$ by $\frac{1}{2}$. This test is sometimes known as McNemar's test. An alternative form of (4.17), with continuity correction included, is

$$z^2 = \frac{(|r - s| - 1)^2}{r + s},$$
(4.18)

where z^2 may be regarded as a $\chi^2_{(1)}$ variate (§3.8). This is one of the few statistical calculations that really can be done in one's head; see also (5.8).

McNemar's test is based on the normal approximation to the discrete binomial distribution. The situation is similar to that considered in §4.4 except for the complication of the tied pairs, k and m; with the correction for continuity, (4.17) corresponds to (4.14) with $\pi_0 = \frac{1}{2}$. The significance test (4.18) will be satisfactory except for small values of $r + s$ (less than about 10), and in such cases an exact test may be carried out on the $r + s$ untied pairs. For this purpose the F distribution may be used, as in (19.28).

It should be noted that, although the significance test is based entirely on the two frequencies r and s, the estimated difference between the proportions of positives and therefore also its standard error depend also on N. That is, evidence as to the existence of a difference is provided solely by the united pairs; an assessment of the *magnitude* of that difference must allude to the remainder of the data. The distinction between statistical and clinical significance, referred to in §4.1, must be borne in mind.

The calculation of confidence limits for the difference between the two proportions involves accounting for the variation in the number of united pairs, $r + s$. This may be achieved by deriving the standard error from the properties of the multinomial distribution, which is an extension of the binomial distribution when there are more than two classes. Approximate confidence limits for the difference between the two proportions are then given by taking its standard error to be

$$\frac{1}{N} \sqrt{\left[r + s - \frac{(r - s)^2}{N} \right]}$$
(4.19)

(Fleiss, 1981), and using the usual normal theory. However, this method is unreliable for small frequencies, when the probability that the parameter is included within the interval tends to be considerably less than the nominal confidence coefficient (Newcombe, 1998c). In extreme cases the limits may fall outside the permissible range of [0, 1]. More satisfactory methods, such as Newcombe's recommended Method 10, require extensive computation, and are best implemented by a computer program such as that included in StatsDirect (1999).

There is a potential discrepancy between the test (4.17) and the confidence limits obtained using (4.19). If the test is just significant at the 5% level, with

$z = 1.96$, the lower confidence limit is higher than zero. This arises because of the second term within the square root in (4.19). The discrepancy will be slight except for large differences between r and s.

When data of this type are obtained in a case–control study, emphasis is often directed to the odds ratio (see (4.22)), which can, for paired data, be estimated by the simple ratio r/s (see (19.26)). Tests and confidence limits can be obtained by the standard methods applied to the simple proportion $r/(r+s)$ (see (19.27)).

Example 4.9

Fifty specimens of sputum are each cultured on two different media, A and B, the object being to compare the ability of the two media to detect tubercle bacilli. The results are shown in Table 4.4. The null hypothesis that the media are equally effective is tested by the standardized normal deviate

$$z = \frac{12 - (\frac{1}{2})(14)}{\frac{1}{2}\sqrt{14}} = \frac{5}{1.871} = 2.67 \quad (P = 0.008).$$

There is very little doubt that A is more effective than B. The continuity correction would reduce the normal deviate to $4.5/1.871 = 2.41$, still a significant result ($P = 0.016$).

The exact significance level is given by

$$P = 2 \times \left(\tfrac{1}{2}\right)^{14}[1 + 14 + (14 \times 13/2)] = 0.013.$$

Table 4.4 Distribution of 50 specimens of sputum according to results of culture on two media.

Type	Medium A	B	Number of sputa
1	+	+	20
2	+	−	12
3	−	+	2
4	−	−	16
			50

Alternative layout

		Medium B +	−	Total
Medium A	+	20	12	32
	−	2	16	18
Total		22	28	50

The mid-P value is obtained by taking only one-half of the last term in the above expression and is 0.007, close to the approximate value 0.008 obtained above.

The approximate 95% confidence limits for the difference between the proportions of positive sputum on the two media are, from (4.19),

$$\frac{(12-2)}{50} \pm \frac{1.96\sqrt{(14-10^2/50)}}{50}$$
$$= 0.20 \pm 0.14$$
$$= 0.06 \text{ and } 0.34.$$

More exact limits (Newcombe, 1998c) are 0.06 and 0.33 (StatsDirect, 1999).

Unpaired case: two independent samples

Suppose these are two populations in which the probabilities that an individual shows characteristic A are π_1 and π_2. A random sample of size n_1 from the first population has r_1 members showing the characteristic (and a proportion $p_1 = r_1/n_1$), while the corresponding values for an independent sample from the second population are n_2, r_2, and $p_2 = r_2/n_2$. In the general formulae (4.8) and (4.9),

$$m_1 = \pi_1 \text{ and } v_1 = \pi_1(1-\pi_1)/n_1;$$
$$m_2 = \pi_2 \text{ and } v_2 = \pi_2(1-\pi_2)/n_2.$$

Hence,

$$\left. \begin{aligned} \mathrm{E}(p_1 - p_2) &= \pi_1 - \pi_2 \\[2mm] \text{and} \quad \mathrm{var}(p_1 - p_2) &= \frac{\pi_1(1-\pi_1)}{n_1} + \frac{\pi_2(1-\pi_2)}{n_2} \end{aligned} \right\}. \tag{4.20}$$

For confidence limits, π_1 and π_2 are unknown and may be replaced by p_1 and p_2, respectively, to give

$$\mathrm{var}(p_1 - p_2) = \frac{p_1 q_1}{n_1} + \frac{p_2 q_2}{n_2}, \tag{4.21}$$

where

$$q_1 = 1 - p_1$$

and

$$q_2 = 1 - p_2.$$

Approximate limits then follow by applying the usual normal theory. Newcombe (1998b) shows that this method tends to give confidence intervals with too low a coverage probability. His paper describes another method (Method 10) with more acceptable properties. A more complex method of Miettinen and Nurminen (1985), implemented in StatsDirect (1999), also has satisfactory coverage properties.

Suppose we wish to test the null hypothesis that $\pi_1 = \pi_2$. Call the common value π. Then p_1 and p_2 are both estimates of π, and there is little point in estimating π (as in (4.21)) by two different quantities in two different places in the expression. If the null hypothesis is true, both samples are from effectively the same population, and the best estimate of π will be obtained by pooling the two samples, to give

$$p = \frac{r_1 + r_2}{n_1 + n_2}.$$

This pooled estimate is now substituted for both π_1 and π_2 to give

$$\mathrm{var}(p_1 - p_2) = pq\left(\frac{1}{n_1} + \frac{1}{n_2}\right),$$

writing as usual $q = 1 - p$. The null hypothesis is thus tested approximately by taking

$$z = \frac{p_1 - p_2}{\sqrt{\left[pq\left(\dfrac{1}{n_1} + \dfrac{1}{n_2}\right)\right]}}$$

as a standardized normal deviate.

Example 4.10

In a clinical trial to assess the value of a new method of treatment (A) in comparison with the old method (B), patients were divided at random into two groups. Of 257 patients treated by method A, 41 died; of 244 patients treated by method B, 64 died. Thus, $p_1 = 41/257 = 0.1595$ and $p_2 = 64/244 = 0.2623$.

The difference between the two fatality rates is estimated as $0.1595 - 0.2623 = -0.1028$. For 95% confidence limits we take

$$\mathrm{var}(p_1 - p_2) = \frac{(0.1595)(0.8405)}{257} + \frac{(0.2623)(0.7377)}{244}$$
$$= 0.0005216 + 0.0007930$$
$$= 0.0013146$$

and

$$\mathrm{SE}(p_1 - p_2) = \sqrt{0.0013146} = 0.0363.$$

Thus, 95% confidence limits are

$$-0.1028 \pm (1.96)(0.0363) = -0.0317 \text{ and } -0.1739,$$

the minus sign merely serving to indicate in which direction the difference lies.

For the significance test, we form the pooled proportion

$$p = 105/501 = 0\cdot2096$$

and estimate $\mathrm{SE}(p_1 - p_2)$ as

$$\sqrt{\left[(0\cdot2096)(0\cdot7904)\left(\frac{1}{257} + \frac{1}{244}\right)\right]}$$
$$= 0\cdot0364.$$

Thus, the normal deviate is

$$\frac{-0\cdot1028}{0\cdot0364} = -2\cdot82(P = 0\cdot005).$$

There is strong evidence of a difference in fatality rates, in favour of A.

In this example, the frequencies are sufficiently large to justify the approximate formula for confidence limits. Newcombe's (1998b) Method 10 gives 95% limits as $(-0\cdot0314, -0\cdot1736)$; the method of Miettinen and Nurminen (1985) gives $(-0\cdot0316, -0\cdot1743)$.

Note that, in Example 4.10, the use of p changed the standard error only marginally, from $0\cdot0363$ to $0\cdot0364$. In fact, there is likely to be an appreciable change only when n_1 and n_2 are very unequal and when p_1 and p_2 differ substantially. In other circumstances, either standard error formula may be regarded as a good approximation to the other, and used accordingly.

In epidemiological studies it is often appropriate to measure the difference in two proportions by their ratio, p_1/p_2, rather than their difference. This measure is referred to as the *risk ratio, rate ratio* or *relative risk*, depending on the type of study. In case–control studies the relative risk cannot be evaluated directly but, in many circumstances, the *odds ratio*, defined by

$$OR = \frac{p_1/(1 - p_1)}{p_2/(1 - p_2)} \qquad (4.22)$$

is a good approximation to the relative risk (Chapter 19). From the point of view of significance testing it makes no difference which measure is used and the method above or the extensions given later in this section are appropriate.

The confidence limits for the risk ratio and odds ratio both involve the use of logarithms, and the *natural* or Napierian logarithm must be used. In natural logarithms the base is e $(= 2\cdot7183)$; $\log_e x$ is usually written as $\ln x$, and $\ln x = 2\cdot3026 \log_{10} x$. Most pocket calculators have a key for $\ln x$ and for the antilogarithm, the exponential of x, often written as e^x, so that the conversion formula is not normally required.

Writing R for p_1/p_2, we have

$$R = \frac{r_1/n_1}{r_2/n_2} \tag{4.23}$$

and approximately (using formula (5.19) given later)

$$\text{SE}(\ln R) = \sqrt{\left(\frac{1}{r_1} - \frac{1}{n_1} + \frac{1}{r_2} - \frac{1}{n_2} \right)} \tag{4.24}$$

and the 95% confidence interval for R is

$$\exp[\ln R \pm 1 \cdot 96 \text{SE}(\ln R)].$$

For more exact limits, see Koopman (1984), Miettinen and Nurminen (1985) and Gart and Nam (1988).

For a case–control study (§19.4) we must change the notation since there are no longer samples from the two populations, but instead cases of disease and controls (non-cases) are sampled separately and their exposure to some factor established. Suppose the frequencies are as follows:

		Cases	Controls	
	+	a	c	$a + c$
Factor				
	−	b	d	$b + d$
		$a + b$	$c + d$	n

Then the observed odds ratio is given by

$$OR = \frac{ad}{bc} \tag{4.25}$$

and, approximately,

$$\text{SE}[\ln(OR)] = \sqrt{\left(\frac{1}{a} + \frac{1}{b} + \frac{1}{c} + \frac{1}{d} \right)}. \tag{4.26}$$

Confidence limits based on a normal approximation using (4.26) are sometimes known as *logit limits*; they are illustrated below in Example 4.11. If any of the cell frequencies are small, more complex methods should be used. Exact limits are mentioned later, on p. 137, but an adequate approximation is often given by the method of Cornfield (1956). The expected values of the frequencies used in (4.25) will give a 'true' odds ratio denoted by ψ. The 95% confidence limits are the two values of ψ for which, given the marginal totals, the observed value of a has a one-sided P value of $0 \cdot 025$. That is, the limits are the solutions of

$$\frac{a - A(\psi)}{\sqrt{\text{var}(a; \psi)}} = \pm 1 \cdot 96, \tag{4.27}$$

where $A(\psi)$ is the value of a which, with the observed marginal totals, would give an odds ratio of ψ, and var $(a; \psi)$ is the variance of a for that value of ψ. That is,

$$\frac{A(d - a + A)}{(a + b - A)(a + c - A)} = \psi \tag{4.28}$$

and

$$\mathrm{var}(a; \psi) \simeq \left(\frac{1}{A} + \frac{1}{a + c - A} + \frac{1}{a + b - A} + \frac{1}{d - a + A} \right)^{-1}. \tag{4.29}$$

It is tedious to solve (4.27), but the calculation can readily be set up as a spreadsheet calculation and solved quickly by trial and error. Using a trial value for A, ψ is obtained from (4.28) and var$(a; \psi)$ from (4.29). These are then substituted in the left-hand side of (4.27). The aim is to choose values of A so that (4.27) gives $\pm 1 \cdot 96$. This is achieved by trying different values and iterating. See also Breslow and Day (1980, §4.3) or Fleiss (1981, §5.6).

Example 4.11

Liddell *et al.* (1984) reported on a case–control study investigating the association of bronchial carcinoma and asbestos exposure in the Canadian chrysolite mines and mills. The data were as follows:

Asbestos exposure	Lung cancer	Controls
Exposed	148 (a)	372 (c)
Not exposed	75 (b)	343 (d)

The calculations are:

$$OR = (148 \times 343)/(75 \times 372) = 1 \cdot 82$$
$$\ln OR = 0 \cdot 599$$

$$SE(\ln OR) = \sqrt{\left(\frac{1}{148} + \frac{1}{75} + \frac{1}{372} + \frac{1}{343} \right)} = \sqrt{0 \cdot 02569} = 0 \cdot 160.$$

$$95\% \text{ confidence interval for } \ln OR = 0 \cdot 599 \pm 1 \cdot 96 \times 0 \cdot 160$$
$$= 0 \cdot 285 \text{ to } 0 \cdot 913,$$
$$95\% \text{ confidence interval for } OR = \exp(0 \cdot 285) \text{ to } \exp (0 \cdot 913)$$
$$= 1 \cdot 33 \text{ to } 2 \cdot 49.$$

Cornfield's method, using (4.27)–(4.29), gives the same limits of $1 \cdot 33$ and $2 \cdot 49$.

2×2 tables and χ^2 tests

An alternative way of displaying the data of Example 4.10 is shown in Table 4.5. This is called a *2 × 2*, or sometimes a *fourfold, contingency table*. The total frequency, 501 in this example, is shown in the lower right corner of the table. This total frequency or *grand total* is split into two different dichotomies represented by the two horizontal rows of the table and the two vertical columns. In this example the rows represent the two treatments and the columns represent the two outcomes of treatment. There are thus $2 \times 2 = 4$ combinations of row and column categories, and the corresponding frequencies occupy the four *inner cells* in the body of the table. The total frequencies for the two row categories and those for the two columns are shown at the right and at the foot, and are called *marginal totals*.

We have already used a 2×2 table (Table 4.4) to display the results needed for a comparison of proportions in paired samples, but the purpose was a little different from the present approach, which is concerned solely with the *unpaired* case.

We are concerned, in Table 4.5, with possible differences between the fatality rates for the two treatments. Given the marginal totals in Table 4.5, we can easily calculate what numbers would have had to be observed in the body of the table to make the fatality rates for A and B exactly equal. In the top left cell, for example, this *expected* number is

$$\frac{105 \times 257}{501} = 53 \cdot 862,$$

since the overall fatality rate is 105/501 and there are 257 individuals treated with A. Similar expected numbers can be obtained for each of the four inner cells, and are shown in Table 4.6 (where the observed and expected numbers are distinguished by the letters O and E). The expected numbers are not integers and have been rounded off to 3 decimal places. Clearly one could not possibly observe $53 \cdot 862$ individuals in a particular cell. These expected numbers should be thought of as expectations, or mean values, over a large number of possible tables with the same marginal totals as those observed, when the null hypothesis is true.

Note that the values of E sum, over both rows and columns, to the observed marginal totals. It follows that the *discrepancies*, measured by the differences $O - E$, add to zero along rows and columns; in other words, the four discrepancies are numerically the same (12.862 in this example), two being positive and two negative.

In a rough sense, the greater the discrepancies, the more evidence we have against the null hypothesis. It would therefore seem reasonable to base a significance test somehow on these discrepancies. It also seems reasonable to take account of the absolute size of the frequencies: a discrepancy of 5 is much more important if $E = 5$ than if $E = 100$.

It turns out to be appropriate to calculate the following index:

$$X^2 = \sum \frac{(O - E)^2}{E}, \tag{4.30}$$

Table 4.5 2×2 table showing results of a clinical trial.

Treatment	Death	Survival	Total
	Outcome		
A	41	216	257
B	64	180	244
Total	105	396	501

Table 4.6 Expected frequencies and contributions to X^2 for data in Table 4.5.

Treatment		Death	Survival	Total
		Outcome		
A	O	41	216	257
	E	53·862	203·138	257
	$O - E$	−12·862	12·862	0
	$(O - E)^2$	165·431	165·431	
	$(O - E)^2/E$	3·071	0·814	
B	O	64	180	244
	E	51·138	192·862	244
	$O - E$	12·862	−12·862	0
	$(O - E)^2$	165·431	165·431	
	$(O - E)^2/E$	3·235	0·858	
Total	O	105	396	501
	E	105	396	
	$O - E$	0	0	

the summation being over the four inner cells of the table. The contributions to X^2 from the four cells are shown in Table 4.6. The total is

$$X^2 = 3 \cdot 071 + 0 \cdot 814 + 3 \cdot 235 + 0 \cdot 858$$
$$= 7 \cdot 978.$$

On the null hypothesis, X^2 follows the $\chi^2_{(1)}$ distribution (see §3.8), the approximation improving as the expected numbers get larger. There is one degree of freedom because only one of the values of E is necessary to complete the whole table. Reference to Table A2 shows that the observed value of 7·978 is beyond the 0·01 point of the $\chi^2_{(1)}$ distribution, and the difference between the two fatality rates is therefore significant at the 1% level. The precise significance level may be obtained by taking the square root of 7·978 ($= 2\cdot82$) and referring to Table A1; this gives 0·005.

On p. 126, we derived a standardized normal deviate by calculating the standard error of the difference between the two proportions, obtaining the numerical value of 2·82. This agrees with the value obtained as the square root of X^2. In fact it can be shown algebraically that the X^2 index is always the same as the square of the normal deviate given by the first method. The probability levels given by the two tests are therefore always in agreement.

The X^2 index is often denoted by χ^2, although it seems slightly preferable to reserve the latter for the theoretical distribution, denoting the calculated value by X^2.

There are various alternative formulae for X^2, of which we may note one. Denote the entries in the table as follows:

		Column		
		1	2	
Row	1	a	b	r_1
	2	c	d	r_2
		s_1	s_2	N

Then

$$X^2 = \frac{(ad - bc)^2 N}{r_1 r_2 s_1 s_2}. \tag{4.31}$$

This version is particularly suitable for use with a calculator.

We have, then, two entirely equivalent significance tests. Which the user chooses to use is to some extent a matter of taste and convenience. However, there are two points to be made. First, the standard error method, as we have seen, not only yields a significance test but also leads naturally into the calculation of confidence intervals. This, then, is a strong argument for calculating differences and standard errors, and basing the test on these values rather than on the X^2 index. The main counter-argument is that, as we shall see in §8.5 and §8.6 the X^2 method can be generalized to contingency tables with more than two rows and columns.

It is important to remember that the X^2 index can only be calculated from 2×2 tables in which the entries are frequencies. A common error is to use it for a table in which the entries are mean values of a certain variable; this practice is completely erroneous.

A closely related method of deriving a significance test is to work with one of the frequencies in the 2×2 table. With the notation above, the frequency denoted by a could be regarded as a random variable and its significance assessed against its expectation and standard error calculated conditionally on the marginal totals. This method proceeds as follows, using O, E and V to represent the observed value, expected value and variance of a:

$$\left. \begin{aligned} E &= \frac{(a+b)(a+c)}{N} \\ V &= \frac{(a+b)(c+d)(a+c)(b+d)}{N^2(N-1)} \\ X^2 &= \frac{(O-E)^2}{V} \end{aligned} \right\}. \tag{4.32}$$

Apart from a factor of $(N-1)/N$, (4.32) is equivalent to (4.31). This form is particularly convenient when combining the results of several studies since the values of O, E and V may be summed over studies before calculating the test statistic. Yusuf *et al.* (1985) proposed an approximate method of estimating the odds ratio and its standard error by

$$\left. \begin{aligned} OR &= \exp\left(\frac{O-E}{V}\right) \\ \mathrm{SE}[\ln(OR)] &= \frac{1}{\sqrt{V}} \end{aligned} \right\}. \tag{4.33}$$

This method was introduced for the combination of studies where the effect was small, and is known to be biased when the odds ratio is not small (Greenland & Salvan, 1990).

More details of such methods are given in §15.6 and of their application in overviews or meta-analyses in §18.10.

Example 4.12

Consider the data of Example 4.11. We have

$$O = 148, \quad E = 123 \cdot 62, \quad V = 42 \cdot 038$$

and (4.33) gives

$$OR = \exp(24 \cdot 38 / 42 \cdot 038) = 1 \cdot 79$$
$$\mathrm{SE}[\ln(OR)] = 0 \cdot 154.$$

These values are close to those found in Example 4.11.

Both the standard error test and the χ^2 test are based on approximations which are valid particularly when the frequencies are high. In general, two methods of improvement are widely used: the application of a continuity correction and the calculation of exact probabilities.

Continuity correction for 2 × 2 tables

This method was described by F. Yates and is often called *Yates's correction*. The $\chi^2_{(1)}$ distribution has been used as an approximation to the distribution of X^2 on the null hypothesis and subject to fixed marginal totals. Under the latter constraint only a finite number of tables are possible. For the marginal totals of Table 4.5, for example, all the possible tables can be generated by increasing or decreasing one of the entries by one unit at a time, until either that entry or some other reaches zero. (A fuller discussion follows later in this section.) The position, therefore, is rather like that discussed in §3.8 where a discrete distribution (the binomial) was approximated by a continuous distribution (the normal). In the present case one might base the significance test on the probability of the observed table or one showing a more extreme departure from the null hypothesis. An improvement in the estimation of this probability is achieved by reducing the absolute value of the discrepancy, $O - E$, by $\frac{1}{2}$ before calculating X^2. In Example 4.10, Table 4.6, this would mean taking $|O - E|$ to be 12·362 instead of 12·862, and the corrected value of X^2, denoted by X^2_c, is 7·369, somewhat less than the uncorrected value but still highly significant.

The continuity correction has a relatively greater effect when the expected frequencies are small than when they are large. The use of the continuity correction gives an approximation to the P value in the exact test described below. As in the analogous situations discussed earlier in this chapter (and see also p. 137), we prefer the mid-P value, which corresponds to the *uncorrected* χ^2 test. We therefore recommend that the continuity correction should not routinely be employed.

The continuity-corrected version of (4.31) is

$$X^2_c = \frac{(|ad - bc| - \frac{1}{2}N)^2 N}{r_1 r_2 s_1 s_2}. \tag{4.34}$$

If the continuity correction is applied in the χ^2 test, it should logically be applied in the standard error test. The procedure there is to calculate $p_1 - p_2$ after the frequencies have been moved half a unit nearer their expected values, the standard error remaining unchanged. Thus, in Example 4.10, we should have $p_{1(c)} = 41\cdot5/257 = 0\cdot1615, p_{2(c)} = 63\cdot5/244 = 0\cdot2602$, giving $z_{(c)} = -0\cdot0987/0\cdot0364 = -2\cdot71$. Since $(-2\cdot71)^2 = 7\cdot34$, the result agrees with that for X^2_c apart from rounding errors.

The exact test for 2 × 2 tables

Even with the continuity correction there will be some doubt about the adequacy of the χ^2 approximation when the frequencies are particularly small. An exact test was suggested almost simultaneously in the mid-1930s by R.A. Fisher, J.O. Irwin and F. Yates, and is often called 'Fisher's exact test'. It consists in calculating the exact probabilities of the possible tables described in the previous subsection. The probability of a table with frequencies

$$
\begin{array}{cc|c}
a & b & r_1 \\
c & d & r_2 \\
\hline
s_1 & s_2 & N
\end{array}
$$

is given by the formula

$$
\frac{r_1!\; r_2!\; s_1!\; s_2!}{N!\; a!\; b!\; c!\; d!}. \tag{4.35}
$$

This is, in fact, the probability of the observed cell frequencies *conditional* on the observed marginal totals, under the null hypothesis of no association between the row and column classifications.

Given any observed table, the probabilities of all tables with the same marginal totals can be calculated, and the P value for the significance test calculated by summation. Example 4.13 illustrates the calculations and some of the difficulties of interpretation which may arise.

Example 4.13

The data in Table 4.7, due to M. Hellman, are discussed by Yates (1934).

There are six possible tables with the same marginal totals as those observed, since neither a nor c (in the notation given above) can fall below 0 or exceed 5, the smallest marginal total in the table. The cell frequencies in each of these tables are shown in Table 4.8.

The probability that $a = 0$ is, from (4.35),

$$
P_0 = \frac{20!\; 22!\; 5!\; 37!}{42!\; 0!\; 20!\; 5!\; 17!} = 0 \cdot 03096.
$$

Tables of log factorials (Fisher & Yates, 1963, Table XXX) are often useful for this calculation, and many scientific calculators have a factorial key (although it may only function correctly for integers less than 70). Alternatively the expression for P_0 can be calculated without factorials by repeated multiplication and division after cancelling common factors:

$$
P_0 = \frac{22 \times 21 \times 20 \times 19 \times 18}{42 \times 41 \times 40 \times 39 \times 38} = 0 \cdot 03096.
$$

Table 4.7 Data on malocclusion of teeth in infants (reproduced from Yates (1934) with permission from the author and publishers).

	Infants with		
	Normal teeth	Malocclusion	Total
Breast-fed	4	16	20
Bottle-fed	1	21	22
Total	5	37	42

Table 4.8 Cell frequencies in tables with the same marginal totals as those in Table 4.7.

0	20	20		1	19	20		2	18	20
5	17	22		4	18	22		3	19	22
5	37	42		5	37	42		5	37	42
3	17	20		4	16	20		5	15	20
2	20	22		1	21	22		0	22	22
5	37	42		5	37	42		5	37	42

The probabilities for $a = 1, 2, \ldots, 5$ can be obtained in succession. Thus,

$$P_1 = \frac{5 \times 20}{1 \times 18} \times P_0$$

$$P_2 = \frac{4 \times 19}{2 \times 19} \times P_1, \text{etc.}$$

The results are:

a	Probability
0	0·0310
1	0·1720
2	0·3440
3	0·3096
4	0·1253
5	0·0182
	1·0001

This is the complete *conditional distribution* for the observed marginal totals, and the probabilities sum to unity, as would be expected. Note the importance of carrying enough significant digits in the first probability to be calculated; the above calculations were carried out with more decimal places than recorded by retaining each probability in the calculator for the next stage.

The observed table has a probability of 0·1253. To assess its significance we could measure the extent to which it falls into the tail of the distribution by calculating the probability of that table or of one more extreme. For a one-sided test the procedure clearly gives

$$P = 0·1253 + 0·0182 = 0·1435.$$

The result is not significant at even the 10% level.

For a two-sided test the other tail of the distribution must be taken into account, and here some ambiguity arises. Many authors advocate that the one-tailed P value should be doubled. In the present example, the one-tailed test gave $P = 0·1435$ and the two-tailed test would give $P = 0·2870$. An alternative approach is to calculate P as the total probability of tables, in either tail, which are at least as extreme as that observed in the sense of having a probability at least as small. In the present example we should have

$$P = 0·1253 + 0·0182 + 0·0310 = 0·1745.$$

The first procedure is probably to be preferred on the grounds that a significant result is interpreted as strong evidence for a difference in the *observed direction*, and there is some merit in controlling the chance probability of such a result to no more than half the two-sided significance level. The tables of Finney *et al.* (1963) enable one-sided tests at various significance levels to be made without computation provided the frequencies are not too great.

To calculate the mid-P value only half the probability of the observed table is included and we have

$$\text{mid-}P = \tfrac{1}{2}(0·1253) + 0·0182 = 0·0808$$

as the one-sided value, and the two-sided value may be obtained by doubling this to give 0·1617.

The results of applying the exact test in this example may be compared with those obtained by the χ^2 test with Yates's correction. We find $X^2 = 2·39 (P = 0·12)$ without correction and $X_c^2 = 1·14 (P = 0·29)$ with correction. The probability level of 0·29 for X_c^2 agrees well with the two-sided value 0·29 from the exact test, and the probability level of 0·12 for X^2 is a fair approximation to the exact mid-P value of 0·16.

Cochran (1954) recommends the use of the exact test, in preference to the χ^2 test with continuity correction, (i) if $N < 20$, or (ii) if $20 < N < 40$ and the smallest expected value is less than 5. With modern scientific calculators and statistical software the exact test is much easier to calculate than previously and should be used for any table with an expected value less than 5.

The exact test and therefore the χ^2 test with Yates's correction for continuity have been criticized over the last 50 years on the grounds that they are conservative in the sense that a result significant at, say, the 5% level will be found in less than 5% of hypothetical repeated random samples from a population in which the null hypothesis is true. This feature was discussed in §4.4 and it was remarked that the problem was a consequence of the discrete nature of the data and causes no difficulty if the precise level of P is stated. Another source of criticism has been that the tests are conditional on the observed margins, which frequently would not all be fixed. For example, in Example 4.13 one could imagine repetitions of sampling in which 20 breast-fed infants were compared with 22 bottle-fed infants but in many of these samples the number of infants with normal teeth would differ from 5. The conditional argument is that, whatever inference can be made about the association between breast-feeding and tooth decay, it has to be made within the context that exactly five children had normal teeth. If this number had been different then the inference would have been made in this different context, but that is irrelevant to inferences that can be made when there are five children with normal teeth. Therefore, we do not accept the various arguments that have been put forward for rejecting the exact test based on consideration of possible samples with different totals in one of the margins. The issues were discussed by Yates (1984) and in the ensuing discussion, and by Barnard (1989) and Upton (1992), and we shall not pursue this point further. Nevertheless, the exact test and the corrected χ^2 test have the undesirable feature that the average value of the significance level, when the null hypothesis is true, exceeds 0.5. The mid-P value avoids this problem, and so is more appropriate when combining results from several studies (see §4.4). As for a single proportion, the mid-P value corresponds to an uncorrected χ^2 test, whilst the exact P value corresponds to the corrected χ^2 test.

The probability distribution generated by (4.35), for different values of the cell frequencies, a, b, c and d, is called the *hypergeometric distribution*. When the null hypothesis is not true, the expected frequencies will have an odds ratio, ψ, different from 1. In that case, the probabilities for the various values of a are proportional to the expression (4.35) multiplied by ψ^a and are somewhat awkward to evaluate. Nevertheless, an exact test for the non-null hypothesis that $\psi = \psi_0$ can, in principle, be obtained in a manner similar to that used for the exact test of the null hypothesis. This enables exact confidence limits to be obtained by finding those values of ψ, denoted by ψ_L and ψ_U, that give the appropriate tail-area probabilities in the two directions. Mid-P significance levels will, in large samples, give confidence limits similar to the approximate limits given by (4.26)–(4.29). The inclusion of the observed table in the tail-area calculations will give rather wider limits. In Example 4.11, these wider 95% limits (obtained from an algorithm of Thomas (1971) and implemented in StatsDirect (1999)) are 1·32 and 2·53; Cornfield's (1956) method (4.27)–(4.29), with a continuity correction reducing by $\frac{1}{2}$ the absolute value of the numerator $a - A(\psi)$ in (4.27), gives 1·31 and 2·52.

4.6 **Sample-size determination**

One of the questions most commonly asked about the planning of a statistical study, and one of the most difficult to answer, is: how many observations should be made? Other things being equal, the greater the sample size or the larger the experiment, the more precise will be the estimates of the parameters and their differences. The difficulty lies in deciding what degree of precision to aim for. An increase in the size of a survey or of an experiment costs more money and takes more time. Sometimes a limit is imposed by financial resources or by the time available, and the investigator will wish to make as many observations as the resources permit, allowing in the budget for the time and cost of the processing and analysis of the data. In other situations there will be no obvious limit, and the investigator will have to balance the benefits of increased precision against the cost of increased data collection or experimentation. In some branches of technology the whole problem can be looked at from a purely economic point of view, but this will rarely be possible in medical research since the benefit of experimental or survey information is so difficult to measure financially. The determination of sample size is thus likely to be an adaptive process requiring subjective judgement. The balancing of precision against availability of resources may take place by trial and error, until a solution is found which satisfies both requirements. In many situations there may be a range of acceptable solutions, so that a degree of arbitrariness remains in the choice of sample size.

In any review of these problems at the planning stage it is likely to be important to relate the sample size to a specified degree of precision. We shall consider first the problem of comparing the means of two populations, μ_1 and μ_2, assuming that they have the same known standard deviation, σ, and that two equal random samples of size n are to be taken. If the standard deviations are known to be different, the present results may be thought of as an approximation (taking σ^2 to be the mean of the two variances). If the comparison is of two proportions, π_1 and π_2, σ may be taken approximately to be the pooled value

$$\sqrt{\{\tfrac{1}{2}[\pi_1(1-\pi_1) + \pi_2(1-\pi_2)]\}}.$$

We now consider three ways in which the precision may be specified.
1 *Given standard error.* Suppose it is required that the standard error of the difference between the observed means, $\bar{x}_1 - \bar{x}_2$, is less than ε; equivalently the width of the 95% confidence intervals might be specified to be not wider than $\pm 2\varepsilon$. This implies

$$\sigma\sqrt{(2/n)} < \varepsilon$$

or

$$n > 2\sigma^2/\varepsilon^2. \tag{4.36}$$

If the requirement is that the standard error of the mean of one sample shall be less than ε, the corresponding inequality for n is

$$n > \sigma^2/\varepsilon^2. \tag{4.37}$$

2 *Given difference to be significant.* We might require that, if $\bar{x}_1 - \bar{x}_2$ is greater in absolute value than some value d_1, then it shall be significant at some specified level (say at a two-sided 2α level). Denote by $z_{2\alpha}$ the standardized normal deviate exceeded (in either direction) with probability 2α (for $2\alpha = 0.05, z_{2\alpha} = 1.96$). Then

$$d_1 > z_{2\alpha}\sigma\sqrt{(2/n)}$$

or

$$n > 2\left(\frac{z_{2\alpha}\sigma}{d_1}\right)^2. \tag{4.38}$$

3 *Given power against specified difference.* Criterion **2** is defined in terms of a given *observed* difference, d. The true difference, δ, may be either less or greater than d, and it seems preferable to base the requirement on the value of δ. It might be possible to specify a value of δ, say δ_1, which one did not wish to overlook, in the sense that if $\delta > \delta_1$ one would like to get a significant result at, say, the two-sided 2α level. However, a significant difference cannot be guaranteed. Sampling fluctuations may lead to a value of $|d|$ much less than $|\delta|$ and not significantly different from zero. The probability of this is denoted by β and referred to as the *Type II error rate*, that is the probability of failing to detect a real difference (false negative). The significance level is referred to as the *Type I error rate*, that is the probability of incorrectly rejecting the null hypothesis (false positive). While the Type I error rate is controlled at a low value by choice of significance level during analysis, the Type II error rate can only be controlled at the design stage. One might specify that the Type II error rate be no greater than some low value, or equivalently that the probability of correctly detecting the difference as significant, $1 - \beta$, should be not less than some high value. This value is called the *power* of the study.

The situation is represented in Fig. 4.9. Positive values of d are significant at the stated level if

$$d > z_{2\alpha}\text{SE}(d), \tag{4.39}$$

that is, d is to the right of the point A. For a power $> 1 - \beta$ the point A must be to the left of a point cutting off a one-sided probability of β on the right-hand distribution. That is,

$$z_{2\alpha}\text{SE}(d) < \delta_1 - z_{2\beta}\text{SE}(d)$$

or

$$\delta_1 > (z_{2\alpha} + z_{2\beta})\text{SE}(d). \tag{4.40}$$

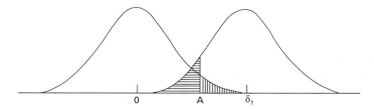

Fig. 4.9 Distributions of d; the left-hand distribution represents the null hypothesis and the right-hand distribution the alternative hypothesis. The vertically shaded area represents the significance level (Type I error rate) and the horizontally shaded area is the Type II error rate.

If d represents the difference, $\bar{x}_1 - \bar{x}_2$, of the means of a continuous variable between two independent groups each of size n then $SE(d) = \sigma \sqrt{(2/n)}$ and (4.40) becomes

$$n > 2 \left[\frac{(z_{2\alpha} + z_{2\beta})\sigma}{\delta_1} \right]^2. \tag{4.41}$$

The distinction between **2** and **3** is important. For instance, if $2\alpha = 0.05$ and $1 - \beta = 0.95$, $z_{2\alpha} = 1.96$ and $z_{2\beta} = 1.64$. If d_1 is put equal to δ_1, the values of n given by (4.41) and (4.38) are thus in the ratio $(1.96 + 1.64)^2 : 1.96^2$ or $3.4 : 1$.

We have assumed, in both **2** and **3**, that the null hypothesis under test specifies a zero value for the true difference, δ. This is usually the case, but there are situations where the null hypothesis specifies a non-zero value, δ_0 for δ, as in equivalence trials (§18.9). The formulae (4.38)–(4.41) still hold, provided that d_1 is interpreted as the difference between $\bar{x}_1 - \bar{x}_2$ and δ_0, and δ_1 is replaced by $\delta_1 - \delta_0$.

Example 4.14

The lung functions of two groups of men are to be compared using the forced expiratory volume (FEV). From previous work the standard deviation of FEV is 0.5 l. A two-sided significance level of 0.05 is to be used and a power of 80% is required against a specified mean difference between the groups of 0.25 l. How many men should there be in each group?

Using (4.41) with $z_{2\alpha} = 1.96$, $z_{2\beta} = 0.842$, $\sigma = 0.5$, and $\delta_1 = 0.25$ gives

$$n > 2 \left[\frac{(1.96 + 0.842)(0.5)}{0.25} \right]^2$$

$$= 62.8.$$

Therefore 63 men should be included in each group.

The formulae given above assume a knowledge of the standard deviation (SD), σ. In practice, σ will rarely be known in advance, although sometimes the investigator will be able to make use of an estimate of σ from previous data which is felt to be reasonably accurate. The approaches outlined above may be modified in two ways. The first way would be to recognize that the required values of n can be specified only in terms of the ratio of a critical interval (ε, d_1 or δ_1) to an estimated or true standard deviation (s or σ). For instance, in **1** we might specify the estimated standard error to be a certain multiple of s; in **2** d_1 might be specified as a certain multiple of s; in **3**, the power might be specified against a given ratio of δ_1 to σ. In **2** and **3**, because the test will use the t distribution rather than the normal, the required values of n will be rather greater than those given by (4.38) or (4.41), but the adjustments will only be important for small samples, that is, those giving 30 or fewer DF for the estimated SD. In this case an adjusted sample size can be given by a second use of (4.41), replacing $z_{2\alpha}$ and $z_{2\beta}$ by the corresponding values from the t distribution, with DF given by the sample size obtained in the initial application of (4.41).

The specification of critical distances as multiples of an unknown standard deviation is not an attractive suggestion. An alternative approach would be to estimate σ by a relatively small pilot investigation and then to use this value in formulae (4.36)–(4.41), to provide an estimate of the total sample size, n. Again, some adjustment is called for because of the uncertainty introduced by estimating σ, but the effect will be small provided that the initial pilot sample is not too small.

The above discussion has been in terms of two independent samples, where the analysis is the two-sample t test (§4.3). If the two groups are paired, the method of analysis would be the paired t test and (4.40) would be used with SE(d) substituted by $\sigma/\sqrt{n}$, where σ is the standard deviation of the differences between paired values and n is the number of pairs. In terms of the methods of analysis of variance, to be introduced in Chapter 8, σ is the 'residual' standard deviation.

The comparison of two independent proportions follows a similar approach. In this case the standard error of the difference depends on the values of the proportions (§4.5). Following approach **3**, specification would be in terms of requiring detection of a difference between true proportions π_1 and π_2, using a test of the null hypothesis that each proportion is equal to the pooled value π. The equation corresponding to (4.41) is

$$n > \left\{ \frac{z_{2\alpha}\sqrt{[2\pi(1-\pi)]} + z_{2\beta}\sqrt{[\pi_1(1-\pi_1) + \pi_2(1-\pi_2)]}}{\pi_1 - \pi_2} \right\}^2 . \qquad (4.42)$$

This equation is slightly more complicated than (4.41) because the standard error of the difference between two observed proportions is different for the null and alternative hypotheses (§4.5). Use of (4.42) gives sample sizes that are appropriate when statistical significance is to be determined using the uncorrected χ^2 test (4.30). Fleiss *et al.* (1980) show that for the continuity-corrected test (4.34), $2/|\pi_1 - \pi_2|$ should be added to the solution given by (4.42).

Casagrande *et al.* (1978) give tables for determining sample sizes that are based on the exact test for 2×2 tables (§4.5), and Fleiss (1981) gives a detailed set of tables based on a formula that gives a good approximation to the exact values. Appendix Table A8 gives the sample size required in each of the two groups, calculated using (4.42) and including the continuity correction for some common situations. Although in general we favour uncorrected tests, Table A8 refers to the corrected version since in those cases where the difference is of practical consequence it would be advisable to aim on the high side.

Example 4.15

A trial of a new treatment is being planned. The success rate of the standard treatment to be used as a control is 0·25. If the new treatment increases the success rate to 0·35, then it is required to detect that there is an improvement with a two-sided 5% significance test and a power of 90%. How many patients should be included in each group?

Using (4.42) with $\pi_1 = 0\cdot25$, $\pi_2 = 0\cdot35$, $\pi = 0\cdot3$, $z_{2\alpha} = 1\cdot96$, and $z_{2\beta} = 1\cdot282$ gives

$$n > \left[\frac{1\cdot96\sqrt{0\cdot42} + 1\cdot282\sqrt{(0\cdot1875 + 0\cdot2275)}}{0\cdot1} \right]^2 .$$
$$= 439\cdot4$$

Including Fleiss *et al.*'s (1980) correction gives

$$n = 439\cdot4 + 2/0\cdot1$$
$$= 459\cdot4$$

From Table A8 the sample size is given as 459 (the same value is given in both Casagrande *et al.*'s (1978) and Fleiss's (1981) tables).

Case–control studies

In a case–control study the measure of association is the odds ratio, or approximate relative risk (§4.5 and §19.5), and this measure is used in determining sample size. For hypothesis testing the data are arranged in a 2×2 table and the significance test is then a comparison of the proportions of individuals in the case and control groups who are exposed to the risk factor. Then the problem of sample size determination can be converted to that of comparing two independent proportions. The controls represent the general population and we need to specify the proportion of controls exposed to the risk factor, p. The first step is to find the proportion of cases, p', that would be exposed for a specified odds ratio, OR_1. This may easily be determined using (4.22). To eliminate this step, and the need to interpolate in tables such as Table A8, tables have been produced that are indexed by the proportion of exposed in the controls and the specified value of the true odds ratio for which it is required to establish statistical significance. Table A9 is a brief table covering commonly required situations. This table is based on (4.22) and (4.42) with the continuity correction. Schlesselman (1982) gives a more extensive set of tables; these tables give smaller sample sizes than Table A9, since Schlesselman did not include Fleiss's addition for the continuity correction.

Example 4.16

A case–control study is being planned to assess the association between a disease and a risk factor. It is estimated that 20% of the general population are exposed to the risk factor. It is required to detect an association if the relative risk is 2 or greater with 80% power at the 5% significance level. How many cases and controls are required?

Using (4.22) with $p = 0.2$ and $OR_1 = 2.0$ gives $p' = 0.3333$. Then, using (4.42), with $\pi_1 = 0.3333$ and $\pi_2 = 0.2$, and using the continuity correction, gives $n = 186.5$. So the study should consist of at least 187 cases and the same number of controls. The above calculations can be avoided by direct use of Appendix Table A9, which gives $n = 187$.

Inverse formulation

The sample-size problem is usually expressed as one of determining *sample size* given the *power* and magnitude of the *specified effect* to be detected. But it could be considered as finding any one of these three items for given values of the other two. This is often a useful approach since the sample size may be limited by other considerations. Then, the relevant questions are: what effect could be detected; or what would the power be? The next example considers the inverse problem of estimating what can be achieved with a given sample size.

Exampe 4.17

Consider the situation of Example 4.14 but suppose that resources are available to include only 50 men in each group.
(a) What would be the power of the study?
    Substituting in (4.41) with $z_{2\beta}$ as unknown gives

$$50 = 2\left[\frac{(1.96 + z_{2\beta})(0.5)}{0.25}\right]^2,$$

and therefore

$$z_{2\beta} = 0\cdot540.$$

From Table A1 this corresponds to a power of

$$1 - 0\cdot2946 = 0\cdot7054 \text{ or } 71\%.$$

(b) What size of mean difference between the groups could be detected with 80% power? Substituting in (4.41) with δ_1 as unknown gives

$$50 = 2\left[\frac{(1\cdot96 + 0\cdot842)(0\cdot5)}{\delta_1}\right]^2,$$

and therefore $\delta_1 = 0\cdot28$. A mean difference of $0\cdot28$ l could be detected.

Note that, if the sample size has already been determined for a specified δ_1, the revised value is quickly obtained by noting that the difference that can be detected is proportional to the reciprocal of the square root of the sample size. Thus, since for $\delta_1 = 0\cdot25$ the sample size was calculated as 62·8, then for a sample size of 50 we have $\delta_1 = 0\cdot25 \times \sqrt{(62\cdot8/50)} = 0\cdot28$.

For the inverse problem of determining the power or the size of effect that could be detected with a given sample size, the formulae (4.41) and (4.42) can be used but the tables are less convenient. Since it is often required to consider what can be achieved with a range of sample sizes, it is convenient to be able to calculate approximate solutions more simply. This can be achieved by noting that, in (4.41), δ_1 is proportional to $1/\sqrt{n}$ and $z_{2\alpha} + z_{2\beta}$ is proportional to $\sqrt{n}$. These relationships apply exactly for a continuous variable but also form a reasonable approximation for comparing proportions.

Example 4.18

In Example 4.15 suppose only 600 patients are available so that $n = 300$.
(a) What size of difference could be detected with 90% power?
Approximately

$$\delta_1 = 0\cdot10 \times \sqrt{(459\cdot4/300)}$$
$$= 0\cdot124.$$

Using (4.42) gives $\delta_t = 0\cdot126$ so the approximation is good. An increase in success rate to about 37·6% could be detected.
(b) What would be the power to detect a difference of $0\cdot1$?
Approximately

$$1\cdot96 + z_{2\beta} = (1\cdot96 + 1\cdot282) \times \sqrt{(300/459\cdot4)}$$
$$= 2\cdot620$$

Therefore $z_{2\beta} = 0\cdot660$ and the revised power is 74.5%.
Using (4.42) gives $z_{2\beta} = 0\cdot626$ and a revised power of 73·4%.

Unequal-sized groups

It is usually optimal when comparing two groups to have equal numbers in each group. But sometimes the number available in one group may be restricted, e.g. for a rare disease in a case–control study (§19.4). In this case the power can be increased to a limited extent by having more in the other group. If one group contains m subjects and the other rm, then the study is approximately equivalent to a study with n in each group where

$$\frac{2}{n} = \frac{1}{m} + \frac{1}{rm}.$$

That is,

$$m = \frac{(r+1)n}{2r}. \tag{4.43}$$

This expression is derived by equating the expressions for the standard error of the difference between two means used in a two-sample t test, and is exact for a continuous variable and approximate for the comparison of two proportions. Fleiss *et al.* (1980) give a formula for the general case of comparing two proportions where the two samples are not of equal size, and their formula is suitable for the inverse problem of estimating power from known sample sizes.

The total number of subjects in the study is

$$\frac{(r+1)^2}{4r} \times 2n,$$

which is a minimum for $r = 1$.

Other considerations

The situations considered in this section are relatively simple—those of comparing two groups without any complicating features. The determination of sample size is often facilitated by the use of tables and, in addition to those mentioned earlier, the book by Lemeshow *et al.* (1990) contains a number of sets of tables. Even in these simple situations it is necessary to have a reasonable idea of the likely form of the data to be collected before sample size can be estimated. For example, when comparing means it is necessary to have an estimate of the standard deviation, or in comparing proportions the approximate size of one of the proportions is required at the planning stage. Such information may be available from earlier studies using the same variables or may be obtained from a pilot study. In more complicated situations more information is required but (4.41) can be used in principle, provided that it is possible to find an expression for σ, the standard deviation relevant to the comparison of interest.

For a comparison of proportions using paired samples, where the significance test is based on the untied pairs (§4.5), it is necessary to have information on the likely effectiveness of the matching, which would determine the proportion of pairs that were tied (Connor, 1987). As such information may be unavailable, the effect of matching is often ignored in the determination of sample size, but this would lead to a larger sample size than necessary if the matching were effective (Parker and Bregman, 1986).

Other more complicated situations are discussed elsewhere in this book. These include Bayesian methods (p. 182), equivalence trials (p. 638), and non-compliance in clinical trials (p. 613). Schlesslman (1982) and Donner (1984) consider sample-size determination in the presence of a confounder (Chapter 19). Tables for sample-size determination in survival analysis (Chapter 17) are given by Lemeshow *et al.* (1990) and Machin *et al.* (1997). For a more detailed review, see Lachin (1998).

Many investigations are concerned with more than one variable measured on the same individual. In a morbidity survey, for example, a wide range of symptoms, as well as the results of certain diagnostic tests, may be recorded for each person. Sample sizes deemed adequate for one purpose may, therefore, be inadequate for others. In many investigations the sample size chosen would be the largest of the separate requirements for the different variables; it would not matter too much that for some variables the sample size was unnecessarily high. In other investigations, in contrast, this may be undesirable, because either the cost or the trouble incurred by taking the extra observations is not negligible. A useful device in these circumstances is *multiphase sampling*. In the first phase certain variables are observed on all the members of the initial sample. In the second phase a subsample of the original sample is then taken, either by simple random sampling or by one of the other methods described in §19.2, and other variables are observed only on the members of the subsample. The process could clearly be extended to more than two phases.

Some population censuses have been effectively multiphase samples in which the first phase is a 100% sample to which some questions are put. In the second phase, a subsample (say, 1 in 10 of the population) is asked certain additional questions. The justification here would be that complete enumeration is necessary for certain basic demographic data, but that for certain more specialized purposes (perhaps information about fertility or occupation) a 1-in-10 sample would provide estimates of adequate precision. Material savings in cost are achieved by restricting these latter questions to a relatively small subsample.

5 Analysing variances, counts and other measures

5.1 Inferences from variances

The sampling error of a variance estimate

Suppose that a quantitative random variable x follows a distribution with mean μ and variance σ^2. In a sample of size n, the estimated variance is

$$s^2 = \frac{\sum(x_i - \bar{x})^2}{n - 1}.$$

In repeated random sampling from the distribution, s^2 will vary from one sample to another; it will itself be a random variable. We now consider the nature of the variation in s^2.

An important result is that the mean value, or expectation, of s^2 is σ^2. That is,

$$\mathrm{E}(s^2) = \sigma^2. \tag{5.1}$$

Another way of stating the result (5.1) is that s^2 is an *unbiased* estimator of σ^2. It is this property which makes s^2, with its divisor of $n - 1$, a satisfactory estimator of the population variance: the statistic (2.1), with a divisor of n, has an expectation $(n - 1)\sigma^2/n$, which is less than σ^2. Note that $\mathrm{E}(s)$ is not equal to σ; it is in fact less than σ. The reason for paying so much attention to $\mathrm{E}(s^2)$ rather than $\mathrm{E}(s)$ will appear in Chapters 8 and 9.

What else can be said about the sampling distribution of s^2? Let us, for the moment, tighten our requirements about the distribution of x by assuming that it is strictly normal. In this particular instance, the distribution of s^2 is closely related to one of a family of distributions called the χ^2 distributions (*chi-square* or *chi-squared*), which are of very great importance in statistical work, and it will be useful to introduce these distributions by a short discussion before returning to the distribution of s^2, which is the main concern of this section.

Denote by X_1 the standardized deviate corresponding to the variable x. That is, $X_1 = (x - \mu)/\sigma$. X_1^2 is a random variable, whose value must be non-negative. As was noted in §3.8, the distribution of X_1^2 is called the χ^2 *distribution on one degree of freedom* (1 DF), and is often called the $\chi^2_{(1)}$ distribution. It is depicted as the first curve in Fig. 5.1. The *percentage points* of the χ^2 distribution are tabulated in Table A2. The values exceeded with probability P are often called the $100(1 - P)$th *percentiles*; thus, the column headed

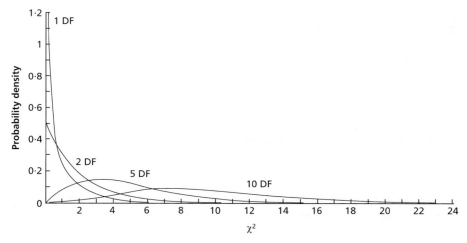

Fig. 5.1 Probability density functions for χ^2 distributions with various numbers of degrees of freedom.

$P = 0\cdot050$ gives the 95th percentile. Two points may be noted at this stage.

1 $E(X_1^2) = E(x - \mu)^2/\sigma^2 = \sigma^2/\sigma^2 = 1$. The mean value of the distribution is 1.

2 The percentiles may be obtained from those of the normal distribution. From Table A1 we know, for instance, that there is a probability 0·05 that $(x - \mu)/\sigma$ exceeds $+1\cdot960$ or falls below $-1\cdot960$. Whenever either of these events happens, $(x - \mu)^2/\sigma^2$ exceeds $(1\cdot960)^2 = 3\cdot84$. Thus, the 0·05 level of the $\chi^2_{(1)}$ distribution is 3·84. A similar relationship holds for all the other percentiles.

Now let x_1 and x_2 be two independent observations on x, and define

$$X_2^2 = \frac{(x_1 - \mu)^2}{\sigma^2} + \frac{(x_2 - \mu)^2}{\sigma^2}.$$

X_2^2 follows what is known as the χ^2 *distribution on two degrees of freedom* $(\chi^2_{(2)})$. The variable X_2^2, like X_1^2, is necessarily non-negative. Its distribution is shown as the second curve in Fig. 5.1, and is tabulated along the second line of Table A2. Note that X_2^2 is the sum of two independent observations on X_1^2. Hence

$$E(X_2^2) = 2E(X_1^2) = 2.$$

Similarly, in a sample of n independent observations x_i, define

$$X_n^2 = \sum_{i=1}^{n} \frac{(x_i - \mu)^2}{\sigma^2} = \frac{\sum(x_i - \mu)^2}{\sigma^2}. \tag{5.2}$$

This follows the χ^2 *distribution on n degrees of freedom* $(\chi^2_{(n)})$, and $E(X_n^2) = n$.

Figure 5.1 and Table A2 show that, as the degrees of freedom increase, the χ^2 distribution becomes more and more symmetric. Indeed, since it is the sum of n independent $\chi^2_{(1)}$ variables, the central limit theorem (which applies to sums as well as to means) shows that $\chi^2_{(n)}$ tends to normality as n increases. The variance of the $\chi^2_{(n)}$ distribution is $2n$.

The result (5.2) enables us to find the distribution of the sum of squared deviations about the population mean μ. In the formula for s^2, we use the sum of squares about the sample mean $\bar{x}$, and it can be shown that

$$\sum(x_i - \bar{x})^2 \le \sum(x_i - \mu)^2.$$

In fact, $\sum(x_i - \bar{x})^2/\sigma^2$ follows the $\chi^2_{(n-1)}$ distribution. The fact that differences are taken from the sample mean rather than the population mean is compensated for by the subtraction of 1 from the degrees of freedom. Now

$$s^2 = \frac{\sum(x_i - \bar{x})^2}{n-1} = \frac{\sigma^2}{n-1} \frac{\sum(x_i - \bar{x})^2}{\sigma^2}$$

$$= \frac{\sigma^2}{n-1} \chi^2_{(n-1)}.$$

That is, s^2 behaves as $\sigma^2/(n-1)$ times a $\chi^2_{(n-1)}$ variable. It follows that

$$E(s^2) = \frac{\sigma^2}{n-1} E(\chi^2_{(n-1)}) = \frac{\sigma^2}{n-1}(n-1) = \sigma^2,$$

as was noted in (5.1), and

$$\text{var}(s^2) = \frac{\sigma^4}{(n-1)^2} \text{var}(\chi^2_{(n-1)}) = \frac{\sigma^4}{(n-1)^2} 2(n-1)$$

$$= \frac{2\sigma^4}{n-1}. \tag{5.3}$$

The formula (5.3) for $\text{var}(s^2)$ is true only for samples from a normal distribution; indeed, the whole sampling theory for s^2 is more sensitive to non-normality than that for the mean.

Inferences from a variance estimate

For normally distributed variables, the methods follow immediately from previous results.

Suppose s^2 is the usual estimate of variance in a random sample of size n from a normal distribution with variance σ^2; the population mean need not be specified. For a test of the null hypothesis that $\sigma^2 = \sigma_0^2$, calculate

$$X^2 = \frac{(n-1)s^2}{\sigma_0^2}, \quad \text{or equivalently} \quad \frac{\sum(x - \bar{x})^2}{\sigma_0^2}, \tag{5.4}$$

and refer this to the $\chi^2_{(n-1)}$ distribution. For a two-sided test at a significance level α, the critical values for X^2 will be those corresponding to tabulated probabilities of $1 - \frac{1}{2}\alpha$ and $\frac{1}{2}\alpha$. For a two-sided 5% level, for example, the entries under the headings 0·975 and 0·025 must be used. We may denote these by $\chi^2_{n-1, 0·975}$ and $\chi^2_{n-1, 0·025}$.

For confidence limits for σ^2 we can argue that the probability is, say, 0·95 that

$$\chi^2_{n-1, 0·975} < \frac{\sum(x - \bar{x})^2}{\sigma^2} < \chi^2_{n-1, 0·025}$$

and hence that

$$\frac{\sum(x - \bar{x})^2}{\chi^2_{n-1, 0·025}} < \sigma^2 < \frac{\sum(x - \bar{x})^2}{\chi^2_{n-1, 0·975}}.$$

These are the required confidence limits.

As already pointed out, the sampling theory for s^2 is particularly sensitive to non-normality, and the results in the present section should be interpreted cautiously if serious departures from normality are present.

Comparison of two variances

Suppose that two independent samples provide observations on a variable x, the first sample of n_1 observations giving an estimated variance s_1^2, and the second sample of n_2 observations giving an estimated variance s_2^2. If each sample is from a normal distribution, the two estimates of variance can be compared by considering the *ratio* of the two variance estimates,

$$F = s_1^2 / s_2^2.$$

If the null hypothesis is true, the distribution of F, in repeated pairs of samples of size n_1 and n_2 from normal distributions, is known exactly. It depends on n_1 and n_2 (or, equivalently, on the degrees of freedom, $v_1 = n_1 - 1$ and $v_2 = n_2 - 1$) but not on the common population variance σ^2. A tabulation of the F distributions as complete as that provided in Table A2 for the χ^2 distributions is impracticable because of the dependence on both v_1 and v_2. The standard books of tables (Fisher & Yates, 1963; Pearson & Hartley, 1966; Geigy Scientific Tables, 1982) provide a table of critical values of F at each of a number of significance levels. An abbreviated version is shown in Appendix Table A4.

For particular values of v_1 and v_2, F can clearly assume values on either side of 1, and significant departures from the null hypothesis may be marked either by very small or by very large values of F. The tabulated critical values are, however, all greater than 1 and refer only to the upper tail of the F distribution. This is not a serious restriction because the labelling of the two samples by the numbers 1 and 2 is arbitrary, and a mere reversal of the labels will convert a ratio less than 1 into a value greater than 1.

To use Table A4 we denote by s_1^2 the *larger* of the two variance estimates; ν_1 is the corresponding number of degrees of freedom (which, of course, is not necessarily the larger of ν_1 and ν_2). For a two-sided test, care should be taken to set P in Table A4 equal to half the two-sided significance level. For a two-sided test at the 5% level, for instance, the entries for $P = 0.025$ are used.

The tables of the F distribution may be used to provide confidence limits for σ_1^2/σ_2^2. The ratio

$$F' = \frac{s_1^2/\sigma_1^2}{s_2^2/\sigma_2^2}$$

follows the F distribution on ν_1 and ν_2 degrees of freedom (on the null hypothesis $\sigma_1^2 = \sigma_2^2$ and $F' = F$). We no longer require $s_1^2 > s_2^2$. Denote by F_{α, ν_1, ν_2} the tabulated critical value of F for ν_1 and ν_2 degrees of freedom and a one-sided significance level α and by F_{α, ν_2, ν_1}, the corresponding entry with ν_1 and ν_2 interchanged. Then the probability is α that

$$F' > F_{\alpha, \nu_1, \nu_2},$$

i.e. that

$$F > F_{\alpha, \nu_1, \nu_2}(\sigma_1^2/\sigma_2^2);$$

and also α that

$$1/F' > F_{\alpha, \nu_2, \nu_1},$$

i.e. that

$$F < (1/F_{\alpha, \nu_2, \nu_1})(\sigma_1^2/\sigma_2^2).$$

Consequently, the probability is $1 - 2\alpha$ that

$$(1/F_{\alpha, \nu_2, \nu_1})(\sigma_1^2/\sigma_2^2) < F < F_{\alpha, \nu_1, \nu_2}(\sigma_1^2/\sigma_2^2)$$

or that

$$F/F_{\alpha, \nu_1, \nu_2} < \sigma_1^2/\sigma_2^2 < F \times F_{\alpha, \nu_2, \nu_1}.$$

For a 95% confidence interval, therefore, the observed value of F must be divided by the tabulated value $F_{0.025, \nu_1, \nu_2}$ and multiplied by the value $F_{0.025, \nu_2, \nu_1}$.

Example 5.1

Two different microscopic methods, A and B, are available for the measurement of very small dimensions. Repeated observations on the same standard object give estimates of variance as follows:

Method	A	B
Number of observations	$n_1 = 10$	$n_2 = 20$
Estimated variance (square micrometres)	$s_1^2 = 1 \cdot 232$	$s_2^2 = 0 \cdot 304$

For a significance test we calculate

$$F = s_1^2/s_2^2 = 4 \cdot 05.$$

The tabulated value for $v_1 = 9$ and $v_2 = 19$ for $P = 0 \cdot 025$ is $2 \cdot 88$ and for $P = 0 \cdot 005$ is $4 \cdot 04$. (Interpolation in Table A4 is needed.) The observed ratio is thus just significant at the two-sided 1% level, that is $P = 0 \cdot 010$.

For 95% confidence limits we need the tabulated values

$$F_{0 \cdot 025, \, 9, \, 19} = 2 \cdot 88$$

and

$$F_{0 \cdot 025, \, 19, \, 9} = 3 \cdot 69$$

(interpolating in the table where necessary). The confidence limits for the ratio of population variances, σ_1^2/σ_2^2, are therefore

$$\frac{4 \cdot 05}{2 \cdot 88} = 1 \cdot 24$$

and

$$(4 \cdot 05)(3 \cdot 69) = 14 \cdot 9.$$

Two connections may be noted between the F distributions and other distributions already met.

1   When $v_1 = 1$, the F distribution is that of the square of a quantity following the t distribution on v_2 DF. For example, for a one-sided significance level $0 \cdot 05$, the tabulated value of F for $v_1 = 1, v_2 = 10$ is $4 \cdot 96$; the two-sided value for t on 10 DF is $2 \cdot 228$; $(2 \cdot 228)^2 = 4 \cdot 96$.

This relationship follows because a t statistic is essentially the ratio of a normal variable with zero mean to an independent estimate of its standard deviation. Squaring the numerator gives a χ^2 variable (equivalent to an estimate of variance on 1 DF), and squaring the denominator similarly gives an estimate of variance on the appropriate number of degrees of freedom. Both the positive and negative tails of the t distribution have to be included because, after squaring, they both give values in the upper tail of the F distribution.

2   When $v_2 = \infty$, the F distribution is the same as that of a $\chi^2_{(v_1)}$ variable divided by v_1. Thus, for $v_1 = 10, v_2 = \infty$, the tabulated F for a one-sided level $0 \cdot 05$ is $1 \cdot 83$; that for $\chi^2_{(10)}$ is $18 \cdot 31$; $18 \cdot 31 \, / \, 10 = 1 \cdot 83$.

The reason here is similar to that advanced above. An estimate of variance s_2^2 on $\nu_2 = \infty$ DF must be exactly equal to the population variance σ^2. Thus, F may be written as $s_1^2/\sigma^2 = \chi_{(\nu_1)}^2/\nu_1$ (see p. 149).

The F test and the associated confidence limits provide an exact treatment of the comparison of two variance estimates from two independent *normal* samples. Unfortunately, the methods are rather sensitive to the assumption of normality—much more so than in the corresponding uses of the t distribution to compare two means. This defect is called a lack of *robustness*.

The methods described in this section are appropriate only for the comparison of two *independent* estimates of variances. Sometimes this condition fails because the observations in the two samples are paired, as in the first situation considered in §4.2. The appropriate method for this case makes use of a technique described in Chapter 7, and is therefore postponed until p. 203.

A different use of the F distribution has already been noted on p. 117.

5.2 **Inferences from counts**

Suppose that x is a count, say, of the number of events occurring during a certain period or a number of small objects observed in a biological specimen, which can be assumed to follow the Poisson distribution with mean μ (§3.7). What can be said about μ?

Suppose first that we wish to test a null hypothesis specifying that μ is equal to some value μ_0. On this hypothesis, x would follow a Poisson distribution with expectation μ_0. The departure of x from its expected value, μ_0, is measured by the extent to which x falls into either of the tails of the hypothesized distribution. The situation is similar to that of the binomial (§3.6). Thus if $x > \mu_0$ and the probabilities in the Poisson distribution are $P_0, P_1, \ldots$, the P value for a one-sided test will be

$$P_+ = P_x + P_{x+1} + P_{x+2} + \ldots$$
$$= 1 - P_0 - P_1 - \ldots - P_{x-1}.$$

The possible methods of constructing a two-sided test follow the same principles as for the binomial in §3.6.

Again considerable simplification is achieved by approximating the Poisson distribution by the normal (§3.8). On the null hypothesis, and including a continuity correction,

$$z = \frac{|x - \mu_0| - \frac{1}{2}}{\sqrt{\mu_0}} \tag{5.5}$$

is approximately a standardized normal deviate. Excluding the continuity correction corresponds to the mid-P value obtained by including only $\frac{1}{2}P_x$ in the summation of Poisson probabilities.

Example 5.2

In a study of asbestos workers a large group was followed over several years and 33 died of lung cancer. Making allowance for age, using national death rates, the expected number of deaths due to lung cancer was 20·0. How strong is this evidence that there is an excess risk of death due to lung cancer?

On the null hypothesis that the national death rates applied, the standard error of x is $\sqrt{20·0} = 4·47$. The observed deviation is $33 - 20·0 = 13·0$. With continuity correction, the standardized normal deviate is $(13·0 - 0·5)/4·47 = 2·80$, giving a one-sided normal tail area of $0·0026$. The exact one-sided value of P, from the Poisson distribution, is $0·0047$, so the normal test exaggerated the significance. Two-sided values may be obtained by doubling these values, and both methods show that the evidence of excess mortality due to lung cancer is strong.

The exact one-sided mid-P value is $0·0037$ and the corresponding standardized normal deviate is $13·0/4·47 = 2·91$, giving a one-sided level of $0·0018$.

The 95% confidence limits for μ are the two values, μ_L and μ_U, for which x is just significant by a one-sided test at the $2\frac{1}{2}\%$ level. These values may be obtained from tables of the Poisson distribution (e.g. Pearson & Hartley, 1966, Table 7) and Bailar and Ederer (1964) give a table of confidence factors. Table VIII1 of Fisher and Yates (1963) may also be used.

The normal approximation may be used in similar ways to the binomial case.
1 The tail areas could be estimated from (5.5). Thus approximations to the 95% limits are given by

$$\frac{x - \mu_L - \frac{1}{2}}{\sqrt{\mu_L}} = 1·96$$

and

$$\frac{x - \mu_U + \frac{1}{2}}{\sqrt{\mu_U}} = -1·96.$$

2 If x is large the continuity correction in method **1** may be omitted.
3 Replace $\sqrt{\mu_L}$ and $\sqrt{\mu_U}$ by $\sqrt{x}$. This is only satisfactory for large values (greater than 100).

The exact limits may be obtained by using tables of the χ^2 distribution. This follows from the mathematical link between the Poisson and the χ^2 distributions (see Liddell, 1984). The limits are

$$\left.\begin{aligned}
\mu_L &= \tfrac{1}{2}\chi^2_{2x,\,0·975} \\[2mm]
\mu_U &= \tfrac{1}{2}\chi^2_{2x+2,\,0·025}
\end{aligned}\right\} . \tag{5.6}$$

and

Example 5.2, continued

With $x = 33$, the exact 95% confidence limits are found to be 22·7 and 46·3. Method **1** gives 23·1 and 46·9, method **2** gives 23·5 and 46·3, and method **3** gives 21·7 and 44·3. In this example methods **1** and **2** are adequate. The 95% confidence limits for the relative death rate due to lung cancer, expressed as the ratio of observed to expected, are 22·7/20·0 and 46·3/20·0 = 1·14 and 2·32. The mid-P limits are obtained from method **2** as 23·5/20·0 and 46·3/20·0 = 132.

Example 5.3

As an example where exact limits should be calculated, suppose that, in a similar situation to Example 5.2, there were two deaths compared with an expectation of 0·5. Then

$$\mu_L = \tfrac{1}{2}\chi^2_{4,\,0.975} = 0\cdot 24$$

and

$$\mu_U = \tfrac{1}{2}\chi^2_{6,\,0.025} = 7\cdot 22.$$

The limits for the ratio of observed to expected deaths are $0\cdot24/0\cdot5$ and $7\cdot22/0\cdot5 = 0\cdot5$ and 14·4. The mid-P limits of μ may be obtained by trial and error on a programmable calculator or personal computer as those values for which $P(x = 0)\ + P(x = 1)+ \tfrac{1}{2}P(x = 2) = 0\cdot975$ or $0\cdot025$. This gives $\mu_L = 0\cdot335$ and $\mu_U = 6\cdot61$ so that the mid-P limits of the ratio of observed to expected deaths are 0·7 and 13·2. The evidence of excess mortality is weak but the data do not exclude the possibility of a large excess.

Suppose that in Example 5.3 there had been no deaths, then there is some ambiguity on the calculation of a 95% confidence interval. The point estimate of μ is zero and, since the lower limit cannot exceed the point estimate and also cannot be negative, its only possible value is zero. There is a probability of zero that the lower limit exceeds the true value of μ instead of the nominal value of $2\tfrac{1}{2}\%$, and a possibility is to calculate the upper limit as $\mu_U = \tfrac{1}{2}\chi^2_{2,\,0.05} = 3\cdot00$, rather than as $\tfrac{1}{2}\chi^2_{2,\,0.025} = 3\cdot69$, so that the probability that the upper limit is less than the true value is approximately 5%, and the interval has approximately 95% coverage. Whilst this is logical and provides the narrowest 95% confidence interval it seems preferable that the upper limit corresponds to $2\tfrac{1}{2}\%$ in the upper tail to give a uniform interpretation. It turns out that the former value, $\mu = 3\cdot00$, is the upper mid-P limit. Whilst it is impossible to find a lower limit with this interpretation, this is clear from the fact that the limit equals the point estimate and that both are at the extreme of possible values. This rationale is similar to that in our recommendation that a two-sided significance level should be double the one-sided level.

Comparison of two counts

Suppose that x_1 is a count which can be assumed to follow a Poisson distribution with mean μ_1. Similarly let x_2 be a count independently following a Poisson distribution with mean μ_2. How might we test the null hypothesis that $\mu_1 = \mu_2$?

One approach would be to use the fact that the variance of $x_1 - x_2$ is $\mu_1 + \mu_2$ (by virtue of (3.19) and (4.9)). The best estimate of $\mu_1 + \mu_2$ on the basis of the available information is $x_1 + x_2$. On the null hypothesis $E(x_1 - x_2) = \mu_1 - \mu_2 = 0$, and $x_1 - x_2$ can be taken to be approximately normally distributed unless μ_1 and μ_2 are very small. Hence,

$$z = \frac{x_1 - x_2}{\sqrt{(x_1 + x_2)}} \tag{5.7}$$

can be taken as approximately a standardized normal deviate.

A second approach has already been indicated in the test for the comparison of proportions in paired samples (§4.5). Of the total frequency $x_1 + x_2$, a portion x_1 is observed in the first sample. Writing $r = x_1$ and $n = x_1 + x_2$ in (4.17) we have

$$z = \frac{x_1 - \frac{1}{2}(x_1 + x_2)}{\frac{1}{2}\sqrt{(x_1 + x_2)}} = \frac{x_1 - x_2}{\sqrt{(x_1 + x_2)}}$$

as in (5.7). The two approaches thus lead to exactly the same test procedure.

A third approach uses a rather different application of the χ^2 test from that described for the 2×2 table in §4.5, the total frequency of $x_1 + x_2$ now being divided into two components rather than four. Corresponding to each observed frequency we can consider the expected frequency, on the null hypothesis, to be $\frac{1}{2}(x_1 + x_2)$:

Observed	x_1	x_2
Expected	$\frac{1}{2}(x_1 + x_2)$	$\frac{1}{2}(x_1 + x_2)$

Applying the usual formula (4.30) for a χ^2 statistic, we have

$$\begin{aligned} X^2 &= \frac{[x_1 - \frac{1}{2}(x_1 + x_2)]^2}{\frac{1}{2}(x_1 + x_2)} + \frac{[x_2 - \frac{1}{2}(x_1 + x_2)]^2}{\frac{1}{2}(x_1 + x_2)} \\ &= \frac{(x_1 - x_2)^2}{x_1 + x_2}. \end{aligned} \tag{5.8}$$

As for (4.30) X^2 follows the $\chi^2_{(1)}$ distribution, which we already know to be the distribution of the square of a standardized normal deviate. It is therefore not surprising that X^2 given by (5.8) is precisely the square of z given by (5.7). The third approach is thus equivalent to the other two, and forms a particularly useful method of computation since no square root is involved in (5.8).

Consider now an estimation problem. What can be said about the ratio μ_1/μ_2? The second approach described above can be generalized, when the null hypothesis is not necessarily true, by saying that x_1 follows a binomial distribution with parameters $x_1 + x_2$ (the n of §3.7) and $\mu_1/(\mu_1 + \mu_2)$ (the π of §3.6). The methods of §4.4 thus provide confidence limits for $\pi = \mu_1/(\mu_1 + \mu_2)$, and hence for μ_1/μ_2 which is merely $\pi/(1 - \pi)$. The method is illustrated in Example 5.4.

The difference $\mu_1 - \mu_2$ is estimated by $x_1 - x_2$, and the usual normal theory can be applied as an approximation, with the standard error of $x_1 - x_2$ estimated as in (5.7) by $\sqrt{(x_1 + x_2)}$.

Example 5.4

Equal volumes of two bacterial cultures are spread on nutrient media and after incubation the numbers of colonies growing on the two plates are 13 and 31. We require confidence limits for the ratio of concentrations of the two cultures.

The estimated ratio is $13/31 = 0.4194$. From the Geigy tables a binomial sample with 13 successes out of 44 provides the following 95% confidence limits for π: 0·1676 and 0·4520. Calculating $\pi/(1 - \pi)$ for each of these limits gives the following 95% confidence limits for μ_1/μ_2:

$$0.1676/0.8324 = 0.2013$$

and

$$0.4520/0.5480 = 0.8248.$$

The mid-P limits for π, calculated exactly as described in §4.4, are 0·1752 and 0·4418, leading to mid-P limits for μ_1/μ_2 of 0·2124 and 0·7915.

The normal approximations described in §4.4 can, of course, be used when the frequencies are not too small.

Example 5.5

Just as the distribution of a proportion, when n is large and π is small, is well approximated by assuming that the number of successes, r, follows a Poisson distribution, so a comparison of two proportions under these conditions can be effected by the methods of this section. Suppose, for example, that, in a group of 1000 men observed during a particular year, 20 incurred a certain disease, whereas, in a second group of 500 men, four cases occurred. Is there a significant difference between these proportions? This question could be answered by the methods of §4.5. As an approximation we could compare the observed proportion of deaths falling into group 2, $p = 4/24$, with the theoretical proportion $\pi = 500/1500 = 0.3333$. The equivalent χ^2 test would run as follows:

	Group 1	Group 2	Total
Observed cases	20	4	24
Expected cases	$\dfrac{1000 \times 24}{1500} = 16$	$\dfrac{500 \times 24}{1500} = 8$	24

With continuity correction

$$X_c^2 = (3\tfrac{1}{2})^2/16 + (3\tfrac{1}{2})^2/8$$
$$= 0.766 + 1.531$$
$$= 2.30 \ (P = 0.13).$$

The difference is not significant. Without the continuity correction, $X^2 = 3.00$ $(P = 0.083)$.

If the full analysis for the 2×2 table is written out it will become clear that this abbreviated analysis differs from the full version in omitting the contributions to X^2 from the non-affected individuals. Since these are much more numerous than the cases, their contributions to X^2 have large denominators and are therefore negligible in comparison with the terms used above. This makes it clear that the short method described here must be used only when the proportions concerned are very small.

Example 5.6

Consider a slightly different version of Example 5.5. Suppose that the first set of 20 cases occurred during the follow-up of a large group of men for a total of 1000 man-years, whilst the second set of four cases occurred amongst another large group followed for 500 man-years. Different men may have different risks of disease, but, under the assumptions that each man has a constant risk during his period of observation and that the lengths of follow-up are unrelated to the individual risks, the number of cases in each group will approximately follow a Poisson distribution. As a test of the null hypothesis that the mean risks per unit time in the two groups are equal, the χ^2 test shown in Example 5.5 may be applied.

Note, though, that a significant difference may be due to failure of the assumptions. One possibility is that the risk varies with time, and that the observations for one group are concentrated more heavily at the times of high risk than is the case for the other group; an example would be the comparison of infant deaths, where one group might be observed for a shorter period after birth, when the risk is high. Another possibility is that lengths of follow-up are related to individual risk. Suppose, for example, that individuals with high risk were observed for longer periods than those with low risk; the effect would be to increase the expected number of cases in that group.

Further methods for analysing follow-up data are described in Chapter 17.

5.3 **Ratios and other functions**

We saw, in §4.2, that inferences about the population mean are conveniently made by using the standard error of the sample mean. In §§4.4 and 5.2, approximate methods for proportions and counts made use of the appropriate standard errors, invoking the normal approximations to the sampling distributions. Similar normal approximations are widely used in other situations, and it is therefore useful to obtain formulae for standard errors (or, equivalently, their squares, the sampling variances) for various other statistics.

Many situations involve functions of one or more simple statistics, such as means or proportions. We have already, in (4.9), given a general formula for the variance of a difference between two independent random variables, and applied it, in §§4.3, 4.5 and 5.2, to comparisons of means, proportions and counts. In the present section we give some other useful formulae for the variances of functions of independent random variables.

Two random variables are said to be *independent* if the distribution of one is unaffected by the value taken by the other. One important consequence of independence is that mean values can be multiplied. That is, if x_1 and x_2 are independent and $y = x_1 x_2$, then

$$E(y) = E(x_1)E(x_2). \tag{5.9}$$

Linear function

Suppose $x_1, x_2, \ldots, x_k$ are independent random variables, and

$$y = a_1 x_1 + a_2 x_2 + \ldots + a_k x_k,$$

the *a*s being constants. Then,

$$\mathrm{var}(y) = a_1^2 \mathrm{var}(x_1) + a_2^2 \mathrm{var}(x_2) + \ldots + a_k^2 \mathrm{var}(x_k). \tag{5.10}$$

The result (4.9) is a particular case of (5.10) when $k = 2, a_1 = 1$ and $a_2 = -1$.

The independence condition is important. If the *x*s are not independent, there must be added to the right-hand side of (5.10) a series of terms like

$$2a_i a_j \mathrm{cov}(x_i, x_j), \tag{5.11}$$

where 'cov' stands for the *covariance* of x_i and x_j, which is defined by

$$\mathrm{cov}(x_i, x_j) = E\{[x_i - E(x_i)] \, [x_j - E(x_j)]\}.$$

The covariance is the expectation of the product of deviations of two random variables from their means. When the variables are independent, the covariance is zero. When all k variables are independent, all the covariance terms vanish and we are left with (5.10).

Ratio

In §5.1, we discussed the ratio of two variance estimates and (at least for normally distributed data) were able to use specific methods based on the F distribution. In §5.2, we noted that the ratio of two counts could be treated by using results established for the binomial distribution. In general, though, exact methods for ratios are not available, and recourse has to be made to normal approximations.

Let $y = x_1/x_2$, where again x_1 and x_2 are independent. No general formula can be given for the variance of y. Indeed, it may be infinite. However, if x_2 has a small coefficient of variation, the distribution of y will be rather similar to a distribution with a variance given by the following formula:

$$\text{var}(y) = \frac{\text{var}(x_1)}{[\text{E}(x_2)]^2} + \frac{[\text{E}(x_1)]^2}{[\text{E}(x_2)]^4}\text{var}(x_2). \tag{5.12}$$

Note that if x_2 has no variability at all, (5.12) reduces to

$$\text{var}(y) = \frac{\text{var}(x_1)}{x_2^2},$$

which is an exact result when x_2 is a constant.

Approximate confidence limits for a ratio may be obtained from (5.12), with the usual multiplying factors for $\text{SE}(y)$ $[= \sqrt{\text{var}(y)}]$ based on the normal distribution. However, if x_1 and x_2 are normally distributed, an exact expression for confidence limits is given by *Fieller's theorem* (Fieller, 1940). This covers a rather more general situation, in which x_1 and x_2 are dependent, with a non-zero covariance. We suppose that x_1 and x_2 are normally distributed with variances and a covariance which are known multiples of some unknown parameter σ^2, and that σ^2 is estimated by a statistic s^2 on f DF. Define $\text{E}(x_1) = m_1$, $\text{E}(x_2) = m_2$, $\text{var}(x_1) = v_{11}\sigma^2$, $\text{var}(x_2) = v_{22}\sigma^2$ and $\text{cov}(x_1, x_2) = v_{12}\sigma^2$. Denote the unknown ratio m_1/m_2 by ρ, so that $m_1 = \rho m_2$. It then follows that the quantity $z = x_1 - \rho x_2$ is distributed as $\text{N}[0, (v_{11} - 2\rho v_{12} + \rho^2 v_{22})\sigma^2]$, and so the ratio

$$T = \frac{x_1 - \rho x_2}{s\sqrt{(v_{11} - 2\rho v_{12} + \rho^2 v_{22})}} \tag{5.13}$$

follows a t distribution on f DF. Hence, the probability is $1 - \alpha$ that

$$-t_{f,\alpha} < T < t_{f,\alpha},$$

or, equivalently,

$$T^2 < t_{f,\alpha}^2. \tag{5.14}$$

Substitution of (5.13) in (5.14) gives a quadratic inequality for ρ, leading to $100(1 - \alpha)\%$ confidence limits for ρ given by

$$\rho_L, \rho_U = \frac{y - \dfrac{gv_{12}}{v_{22}} \pm t_{f,\alpha}\dfrac{s}{x_2}\left[v_{11} - 2yv_{12} + y^2v_{22} - g\left(v_{11} - \dfrac{v_{12}^2}{v_{22}}\right)\right]^{\frac{1}{2}}}{1 - g}, \tag{5.15}$$

where

$$g = \frac{t_{f,\alpha}^2 s^2 v_{22}}{x_2^2} \tag{5.16}$$

and $[\ \ ]^{\frac{1}{2}}$ indicates a square root.

If g is greater than 1, x_2 is not significantly different from zero at the α level, and the data are consistent with a zero value for m_2 and hence an infinite value for ρ. The confidence set will then either be the two intervals $(-\infty, \rho_L)$ and (ρ_U, ∞), excluding the observed value y, or the whole set of values $(-\infty, \infty)$.

Otherwise, the interval (ρ_L, ρ_U) will include y, and when g is very small the limits will be close to those given by the normal approximation using (5.12). This may be seen by setting $g = 0$ in (5.15), when the limits become

$$y \pm t_{f,\alpha} \left[\frac{\operatorname{var}(x_1)}{x_2^2} - \frac{2x_1}{x_2^3} \operatorname{cov}(x_1, x_2) + \frac{x_1^2}{x_2^4} \operatorname{var}(x_2) \right]^{\frac{1}{2}}. \tag{5.17}$$

Equation (5.17) agrees with (5.12), with the replacement of expectations of x_1 and x_2 by their observed values, and the inclusion of the covariance term.

The validity of (5.15) depends on the assumption of normality for x_1 and x_2. Important use is made of Fieller's theorem in biological assay (§20.2) where the normality assumption is known to be a good approximation.

A situation commonly encountered is the comparison of two independent samples when the quantity of interest is the ratio of the location parameters rather than their difference. The formulae above may be useful, taking x_1 and x_2 to be the sample means, and using standard formulae for their variances. The use of Fieller's theorem will be problematic if (as is usually the case) the variances are not estimated as multiples of the same s^2, although approximations may be used. An alternative approach is to work with the logarithms of the individual readings, and make inferences about the difference in the means of the logarithms (which is the logarithm of their ratio), using the standard procedures of §4.3.

Product

Let $y = x_1 x_2$, where x_1 and x_2 are independent. Denote the means of x_1 and x_2 by μ_1 and μ_2, and their variances by σ_1^2 and σ_2^2. Then

$$\operatorname{var}(y) = \mu_1^2 \sigma_2^2 + \mu_2^2 \sigma_1^2 + \sigma_1^2 \sigma_2^2. \tag{5.18}$$

The assumption of independence is crucial.

General function

Suppose we know the mean and variance of the random variable x. Can we calculate the mean and variance of any general function of x such as $3x^3$ or

$\sqrt{(\log x)}$? There is no simple formula, but again a useful approximation is available when the coefficient of variation of x is small. We have to assume some knowledge of calculus at this point. Denote the function of x by y. Then

$$\text{var}(y) \simeq \left(\frac{dy}{dx}\right)^2_{x=E(x)} \text{var}(x), \qquad (5.19)$$

the symbol $\simeq$ standing for 'approximately equal to'. In (5.19), dy/dx is the differential coefficient (or derivative) of y with respect to x, evaluated at the mean value of x.

If y is a function of two variables, x_1 and x_2,

$$\text{var}(y) \simeq \left(\frac{\partial y}{\partial x_1}\right)^2 \text{var}(x_1) + 2\left(\frac{\partial y}{\partial x_1}\right)\left(\frac{\partial y}{\partial x_2}\right) \text{cov}(x_1, x_2) + \left(\frac{\partial y}{\partial x_2}\right)^2 \text{var}(x_2), \quad (5.20)$$

where $\partial y/\partial x_1$ and $\partial y/\partial x_2$ are the *partial* derivatives of y with respect to x_1 and x_2, and these are again evaluated at the mean values. The reader with some knowledge of calculus will be able to derive (4.9) as a particular case of (5.20) when $\text{cov}(x_1, x_2) = 0$. An obvious extension of (5.20) to k variables gives (5.10) as a special case. Equations (5.12) and (5.18) are special cases of (5.20), when $\text{cov}(x_1, x_2) = 0$. In (5.18), the last term becomes negligible if the coefficients of variation of x_1 and x_2 are very small; the first two terms agree with (5.20).

The method of approximation by (5.19) and (5.20) is known as the *delta method*.

5.4 Maximum likelihood estimation

In §4.1 we noted several desirable properties of point estimators, and remarked that many of these were achieved by the method of maximum likelihood. In Chapter 4 and the earlier sections of the present chapter, we considered the sampling distributions of various statistics chosen on rather intuitive grounds, such as the mean of a sample from a normal distribution. Most of these turn out to be maximum likelihood estimators, and it is useful to reconsider their properties in the light of this very general approach.

In §3.6 we derived the binomial distribution and in §4.4 we used this result to obtain inferences from a sample proportion. The probability distribution here is a two-point distribution with probabilities π and $1 - \pi$ for the two types of individual. There is thus one parameter, π, and a maximum likelihood (ML) estimator is obtained by finding the value that maximizes the probability shown in (3.12). The answer is p, the sample proportion, which was, of course, the statistic chosen intuitively. We shall express this result by writing

$$\hat{\pi} = p,$$

the 'hat' symbol indicating the ML estimator.

Two of the properties already noted in §3.6 follow from general properties of ML estimators: first, in large samples (i.e. for large values of n), the distribution of p tends to become closer and closer to a normal distribution; and, secondly, p is a *consistent* estimator of π because its variance decreases as n increases, and so p fluctuates more and more closely around its mean, π.

A third property of ML estimators is their *efficiency*: no other estimator would have a smaller variance than p in large samples. One other property of p is its *unbiasedness*, in that its mean value is π. This can be regarded as a bonus, as not all ML estimators are unbiased, although in large samples any bias must become proportionately small in comparison with the standard error, because of the consistency property.

Since the Poisson distribution is closely linked with the binomial, as explained in §3.7, it is not surprising that similar properties hold. There is again one parameter, μ, and the ML estimator from a sample of n counts is the observed mean count:

$$\hat{\mu} = \bar{x}.$$

An equivalent statement is that the ML estimator of $n\mu$ is $n\bar{x}$, which is the total count $\sum x$. The large-sample normality of ML estimators implies a tendency towards normality of the Poisson distribution with a large mean ($n\mu$ here), confirming the decreased skewness noted in connection with Fig. 3.9. The consistency of $\bar{x}$ is illustrated by the fact that

$$\mathrm{var}(\bar{x}) = \mathrm{var}(x)/n = \mu/n,$$

so, as n increases, the distribution of $\bar{x}$ becomes more tightly concentrated around its mean μ. Again, the unbiasedness is a bonus.

In Fig. 4.1, the concept of maximum likelihood estimation was illustrated by reference to a single observation from a normal distribution $N(\mu, 1)$. The ML estimator of μ is clearly x. In a sample of size n from the same distribution, the situation would be essentially the same, except that the distributions of $\bar{x}$ for different values of μ would now have a variance of $1/n$ rather than 1. The ML estimator would clearly be $\bar{x}$, which has the usual properties of consistency and efficiency and, as a bonus, unbiasedness.

In practice, if we are fitting a normal distribution to a set of n observations, we shall not usually know the population variance, and the distribution we fit, $N(\mu, \sigma^2)$, will have *two* unknown parameters. The likelihood now has to be maximized simultaneously over all possible values of μ and σ^2. The resulting ML estimators are:

$$\hat{\mu} = \bar{x},$$

as expected, and

$$\hat{\sigma}^2 = \frac{\sum (x_i - \bar{x})^2}{n}.$$

This is the *biased* estimator of the variance, (2.1), with divisor n, rather than the *unbiased* estimator s^2 given by (2.2). As we noted in §2.6, the bias of (2.1) becomes proportionately unimportant as n gets large, and the estimator is consistent, as we should expect.

Proofs that the ML estimators noted here do maximize the likelihood are easily obtained by use of the differential calculus. That is, in fact, the general approach for maximum likelihood solutions to more complex problems, many of which we shall encounter later in the book. In some of these more complex models, such as logistic regression (§14.2), the solution is obtained by a computer program, acting iteratively, so that each round of the calculation gets closer and closer to the final value.

Two points may be noted finally:

1 The ML solution depends on the model put forward for the random variation. Choice of an inappropriate model may lead to inefficient or misleading estimates. For certain non-normal distributions, for instance, the ML estimator of the location parameter may not be (as with the normal distribution) the sample mean $\bar{x}$. This corresponds to the point made in §§2.4 and 2.5 that for skew distributions the median or geometric mean may be a more satisfactory measure than the arithmetic mean.

2 There are some alternative approaches to estimation, other than maximum likelihood, that also provide large-sample normality, consistency and efficiency. Some of these, such as generalized estimating equations (§12.6), will be met later in the book.

6 Bayesian methods

6.1 Subjective and objective probability

Our approach to the interpretation of probability, and its application in statistical inference, has hitherto been *frequentist*. That is, we have regarded the probability of a random event as being the long-run proportion of occasions on which it occurs, conditional on some specified hypothesis. Similarly, in methods of inference, a P value is defined as the proportion of trials in which some observed result would have been observed on the null hypothesis; and a confidence interval is characterized by the probability of inclusion of the true value of a parameter in repeated samples.

Bayes' theorem (§3.3) allowed us to specify prior probabilities for hypotheses, and hence to calculate posterior probabilities after data had been observed, but the prior probabilities were, at that stage, justified as representing the long-run frequencies with which these hypotheses were true. In medical diagnosis, for example, we could speak of the probabilities of data (symptoms, etc.) on certain hypotheses (diagnoses), and attribute (at least approximately) probabilities to the diagnoses according to the relative frequencies seen in past records of similar patients.

It would be attractive if one could allot probabilities to hypotheses like the following: 'The use of tetanus antitoxin in cases of clinical tetanus reduces the fatality of the disease by more than 20%,' for which no frequency interpretation is possible. Such an approach becomes possible only if we interpret the probability of a hypothesis as a measure of our degree of belief in its truth. A probability of zero would correspond to complete disbelief, a value of one representing complete certainty. These numerical values could be manipulated by Bayes' theorem, measures of prior belief being modified in the light of observations on random variables by multiplication by likelihoods, resulting in measures of posterior belief.

It is often argued that this is a more 'natural' interpretation of probability than the frequency approach, and that non-specialist users of statistical methods often erroneously interpret the results of significance tests or confidence intervals in this subjective way. That is, a non-significant result may be wrongly interpreted as showing that the null hypothesis has low probability, and a parameter may be claimed to have a 95% probability of lying inside a confidence interval.

This argument should not be used to justify an incorrect interpretation, but it does lend force to attempts to develop a coherent approach in terms of degrees of belief.

Such an approach to probability and statistical inference was, in fact, conventional in the late eighteenth century and most of the nineteenth century, following the work of T. Bayes and P.-S. Laplace (1749–1827), the 'degrees of belief' interpretation being termed 'inverse probability' in contrast to the frequentist 'direct probability'. As we shall see, there are close parallels between many results obtained by the two approaches, and the distinction became blurred during the nineteenth century. The frequentist approach dominated during the early part of the twentieth century, especially through the influence of R.A. Fisher (1890–1962), but many writers (Good, 1950; Savage, 1954; Jeffreys, 1961; Lindley, 1965) have advocated the inverse approach (now normally called 'Bayesian') as the basis for statistical inference, and it is at present very influential.

The main problem is how to determine prior probabilities in situations where frequency interpretations are meaningless, but where values in between the two extremes of complete disbelief and complete certainty are needed. One approach is to ask oneself what odds one would be prepared to accept for a bet on the truth or falsehood of a particular proposition. If the acceptable odds were judged to be 4 to 1 against, the proposition could be regarded as having a probability of 1/5 or 0·2. However, the contemplation of hypothetical gambles on outcomes that may never be realized, is an unattractive prospect, and seems inappropriate for the large number of probability assessments that would be needed in any realistic scientific study. It is therefore more convenient to use some more flexible approach to capture the main features of a prior assessment of the plausibility of different hypotheses.

Most applications of statistics involve inference about parameters in models. It is often possible to postulate a family of probability distributions for the parameter, the various members of which allow sufficient flexibility to meet the needs of most situations. At one extreme are distributions with a very wide dispersion, to represent situations where the user has little prior knowledge or belief. At the other extreme are distributions with very low dispersion, for situations where the user is confident that the parameter lies within a small range. We shall see later that there are particular mathematical distributions, called *conjugate priors*, that present such flexibility and are especially appropriate for particular forms of distribution for the data, in that they combine naturally with the likelihoods in Bayes' theorem.

The first extreme mentioned above, leading to a prior with wide dispersion, is of particular interest, because there are many situations in which the investigator has very little basis for an informed guess, especially when a scientific study is being done for the first time. It is then tempting to suggest that a prior distribution should give equal probabilities, or probability densities, to all the possible values of the parameter. However, that approach is ambiguous, because a uniform distribution of probability across all values of a parameter would lead to a non-uniform distribution on a transformed scale of measurement that might be just as attractive as the original. For example, for a parameter θ representing a proportion of successes in an experiment, a uniform distribution of θ between 0 and 1 would not lead to a uniform distribution of the logit of θ ((14.5), p. 488) between $-\infty$ and ∞. This problem was one of the main objections to Bayesian methods raised throughout the nineteenth century.

A convenient way out of the difficulty is to use the family of conjugate priors appropriate for the situation under consideration, and to choose the extreme member of that family to represent ignorance. This is called a *non-informative* or *vague* prior. A further consideration is that the precise form of the prior distribution is important only for small quantities of data. When the data are extensive, the likelihood function is tightly concentrated around the maximum likelihood value, and the only feature of the prior that has much influence in Bayes' theorem is its behaviour in that same neighbourhood. Any prior distribution will be rather flat in that region unless it is is very concentrated there or elsewhere. Such a prior will lead to a posterior distribution very nearly proportional to the likelihood, and thus almost independent of the prior. In other words, as might be expected, large data sets almost completely determine the posterior distribution unless the user has very strong prior evidence.

The main body of statistical methods described in this book was built on the frequency view of probability, and we adhere mainly to this approach. Bayesian methods based on suitable choices of non-informative priors (Lindley, 1965) often correspond precisely to the more traditional methods, when appropriate changes of wording are made. We shall indicate many of these points of correspondence in the later sections of this chapter. Nevertheless, there are points at which conflicts between the viewpoints necessarily arise, and it is wrong to suggest that they are merely different ways of saying the same thing.

In our view both Bayesian and non-Bayesian methods have their proper place in statistical methodology. If the purpose of an analysis is to express the way in which a set of initial beliefs is modified by the evidence provided by the data, then Bayesian methods are clearly appropriate. Formal introspection of this sort is somewhat alien to the working practices of most scientists, but the informal synthesis of prior beliefs and the assessment of evidence from data is certainly commonplace. Any sensible use of statistical information must take some account of prior knowledge and of prior assessments about the plausibility of various hypotheses. In a card-guessing experiment to investigate extrasensory perception, for example, a score in excess of chance expectation which was just significant at the 1% level would be regarded by most people with some scepticism: many would prefer to think that the excess had arisen by chance (to say nothing of the possibility of experimental laxity) rather than by the intervention of telepathy or clairvoyance. On the other hand, in a clinical trial to compare an active drug with a placebo, a similarly significant result would be widely accepted as evidence for a drug effect because such findings are commonly made. The question, then, is not whether prior beliefs should be taken into account, but rather whether this should be done formally, through a Bayesian analysis, or informally, using frequentist methods for data analysis.

The formal approach is particularly appropriate when decisions need to be taken, for instance about whether a pharmaceutical company should proceed with the development of a new product. Here, the evidence, subjective and objective, for the ultimate effectiveness of the product, needs to be assessed together with the financial and other costs of taking alternative courses of action.

Another argument in favour of Bayesian methods has emerged in recent decades as a result of research into new models for complex data structures. In general, Bayesian methods lead to a simplification of computing procedures in that the calculations require the likelihood function based on the observed data, whereas frequentist methods using tail-area probabilities require that results should be integrated over sets of data not actually observed. Nevertheless, Bayesian calculations for complex problems involve formidable computing resources, and these are now becoming available in general computer packages (Goldstein, 1998) as well as in specialist packages such as BUGS (Thomas *et al.*, 1992; Spiegelhalter *et al.*, 2000; available from http://www.mrc-bsu.cam.ac.uk/bugs/); see Chapter 16.

With more straightforward data sets arising in the general run of medical research, the investigator may have no strong prior beliefs to incorporate into the analysis, and the emphasis will be on the evidence provided by the data. The statistician then has two options: either to use frequentist methods such as those described in this book, or to keep within the Bayesian framework by calculating likelihoods. The latter can be presented directly, as summarizing the evidence from the data, enabling the investigator or other workers to incorporate whatever priors they might wish to use. It may sometimes be useful to report a 'sensitivity analysis' in which the effects of different prior assumptions can be explored.

Bayesian methods for some simple situations are explained in the following sections, and Bayesian approaches to more complex situations are described in Chapter 16. Fuller accounts are to be found in books such as Lee (1997), Carlin and Louis (2000) and, at a rather more advanced level, Box and Tiao (1973).

6.2 **Bayesian inference for a mean**

The frequentist methods of inference for a mean, described in §4.2, made use of the fact that, for large sample sizes, the sample mean tends to be normally distributed. The methods developed for samples from a normal distribution therefore provide a reliable approximation for samples from non-normal distributions, unless the departure from normality is severe or the sample size is very small. The same is true in Bayesian inference, and we shall concentrate here on methods appropriate for samples from normal distributions.

Figure 4.1 describes the likelihood function for a single observation x from a normal distribution with unit variance, $N(\mu, 1)$. It is a function of μ which takes the shape of a normal curve with mean x and unit variance. This result can immediately be extended to give the likelihood from a sample mean. Suppose that $\bar{x}$ is the mean of a sample of size n from a normal distribution $N(\mu, \sigma^2)$. From §4.2, we know that $\bar{x}$ is distributed as $N(\mu, \sigma^2/n)$, and the likelihood function is therefore a normal curve $N(\bar{x}, \sigma^2/n)$.

Suppose now that μ follows a normal prior distribution $N(\mu_0, \sigma_0^2)$. Then, application of Bayes' theorem shows that the posterior distribution of μ is

$$N\left(\frac{\bar{x} + \mu_0\sigma^2/n\sigma_0^2}{1 + \sigma^2/n\sigma_0^2}, \frac{\sigma^2/n}{1 + \sigma^2/n\sigma_0^2}\right). \tag{6.1}$$

The mean of this distribution can be written in the form

$$\frac{\bar{x}\left(\dfrac{n}{\sigma^2}\right) + \mu_0\left(\dfrac{1}{\sigma_0^2}\right)}{\dfrac{n}{\sigma^2} + \dfrac{1}{\sigma_0^2}}, \tag{6.2}$$

which is a weighted mean of the observed mean $\bar{x}$ and the prior mean μ_0, the weights being inversely proportional to the two variances of these quantities (the sampling variance of $\bar{x}$, σ^2/n, and the prior variance of μ, σ_0^2). Thus, the observed data and the prior information contribute to the posterior mean in proportion to their precision. The fact that the posterior estimate of μ is shifted from the sample mean $\bar{x}$, in the direction of the prior mean μ_0, is an example of the phenomenon known as *shrinkage*, to be discussed further in §6.4.

The variance of the posterior distribution (6.1) may be written in the form

$$\frac{(\sigma^2/n)\sigma_0^2}{(\sigma^2/n) + \sigma_0^2}, \tag{6.3}$$

which is less than either of the two separate variances, σ^2/n and σ_0^2. In this sense, precision has been gained by combining the information from the data and the prior information.

These results illustrate various points made in §6.1. First, the family chosen for the prior distributions, the normal, constitutes the conjugate family for the normal likelihood. When the prior is chosen from a conjugate family, the posterior distribution is always another member of the same family, but with parameters altered by the incorporation of the likelihood. Although this is mathematically very convenient, it does not follow that the prior should necessarily be chosen in this way. For example, in the present problem, the user might believe that the mean lies in the neighbourhood of either of two values, θ_0 or θ_1. It might then be appropriate to use a bimodal prior distribution with peaks at these two values. In that case, the simplicity afforded by the conjugate family would be lost, and the posterior distribution would no longer take the normal form (6.1).

Secondly, if either n is very large (when the evidence from the data overwhelms the prior information) or if σ_0^2 is very large (when the prior evidence is very weak and the prior distribution is *non-informative*), the posterior distribution (6.1) tends towards the likelihood $N(\bar{x}, \sigma^2/n)$.

In principle, once the formulations for the prior and likelihood have been accepted as appropriate, the posterior distribution provides all we need for inference about μ. In practice, as in frequentist inference, it will be useful to consider ways of answering specific questions about the possible value of μ. In particular, what are the Bayesian analogues of the two principal modes of inference discussed in §4.1: significance tests and confidence intervals?

Bayesian significance tests

Suppose that, in the formulation leading up to (6.1), we wanted to ask whether there was strong evidence that $\mu < 0$ or $\mu > 0$. In frequentist inference we should test the hypothesis that $\mu = 0$, and see whether it was strongly contradicted by a significant result in either direction. In the present Bayesian formulation there is no point in considering the probability that μ is exactly 0, since that probability is zero (although $\mu = 0$ has a non-zero *density*). However, we can state directly the probability that, say $\mu < 0$ by calculating the tail area to the left of zero in the normal distribution (6.1).

It is instructive to note what happens in the limiting case considered above, when the sample size is large or the prior is non-informative and the posterior distribution is $N(\bar{x}, \sigma^2/n)$. The posterior probability that $\mu < 0$ is the probability of a standardized normal deviate less than

$$\frac{0 - \bar{x}}{\sigma/\sqrt{n}} = \frac{-\bar{x}\sqrt{n}}{\sigma},$$

and this is precisely the same as the one-sided P value obtained in a frequentist test of the null hypothesis that $\mu = 0$. The posterior tail area and the one-sided P value are thus numerically the same, although of course their strict interpretations are quite different.

Example 6.1

Example 4.1 described a frequentist significance test based on a sample of $n = 100$ survival times of patients with a form of cancer. The observed mean was $\bar{x} = 46{\cdot}9$ months, and the hypothesis tested was that the population mean was (in the notation of the present section) $\mu = 38\cdot3$ months, the assumed standard deviation being $\sigma = 43\cdot3$ months. (The subscript 0 used in that example is dropped here, since it will be needed for the parameters of the prior distribution.) Although, as noted in Example 4.1, the individual survival times x must be positive, and the large value of σ indicates a highly skew distribution, the normal theory will provide a reasonable approximation for the distribution of the sample mean.

Table 6.1 shows the results of applying (6.1) with various assumptions about the prior distribution $N(\mu_0, \sigma_0^2)$. Since μ must be positive, a normal distribution is strictly inappropriate, and a distributional form allowing positive values only would be preferable. However, if (as in Table 6.1) σ_0/μ_0 is small, the normal distribution will assign very little probability to the range $\mu < 0$, and the model provides a reasonable approach.

Case A represents a vague prior centred around the hypothesized value. The usual assumption for a non-informative prior, that $\sigma_0 = \infty$, is inappropriate here, as it would assign too much probability to negative values of μ; the value chosen for σ_0 would allow a wide range of positive values, and would be suitable if the investigator had very little preconception of what might occur. The final inference is largely determined by the likelihood from the data. The probability of $\mu < 38\cdot3$ is small, and close to the one-sided P value of $0\cdot023$ (which is half the two-sided value quoted in Example 4.1).

Cases B, C and D represent beliefs that the new treatment might have a moderate effect in improving or worsening survival, in comparison with the previous mean of $38\cdot3$, with respectively scepticism, agnosticism and enthusiasm. The final inferences reflect these different prior judgements, with modest evidence for an improvement in C and strong evidence, boosted by the prior belief, in D. In B, the evidence from the data in favour of the new treatment is unable to counteract the gloomy view presented by the prior.

Case E represents a strong belief that the new treatment is better than the old, with a predicted mean survival between about 38 and 42 months. This prior belief is supported by the data, although the observed mean of $46\cdot9$ is somewhat above the presumed range. The evidence for an improvement is now strong.

Note that in each of these cases the posterior standard deviation is less than the standard error of the mean, $4\cdot33$, indicating the additional precision conferred by the prior assumptions.

Table 6.1 Various prior distributions for Example 4.1.

	Prior distribution		Posterior distribution		
	μ_0	σ_0	Mean	SD	$P(\mu < 38\cdot3)$
A	38·3	10	45·54	3·97	0·034
B	30	5	39·66	3·27	0·34
C	40	5	43·94	3·27	0·043
D	50	5	48·23	3·27	0·001
E	40	1	40·35	0·97	0·017

In some situations it may be appropriate to assign a non-zero probability to a null hypothesis such as $\mu = 0$. For example, in a clinical trial to study the efficacy of a drug, it might be held that there is a non-negligible probability ϕ_0 that the drug is ineffective, whilst the rest of the prior probability, $1 - \phi_0$, is spread over a range of values. This model departs from the previous one in not using a normal (and hence conjugate) prior distribution, and various possibilities may be considered. For instance, the remaining part of the distribution may be assumed to be normal over an infinite range, or it may be distributed in some other way, perhaps over a finite range. We shall not examine possible models in any detail here, but one or two features should be noted. First, if the observed mean $\bar{x}$ is sufficiently close to zero, the posterior odds in favour of the null hypothesis, say $\phi_1/(1 - \phi_1)$, will tend to be greater than the prior odds $\phi_0/(1 - \phi_0)$. That is, the observed mean tends to confirm the null hypothesis. Conversely, an observed mean sufficiently far from zero will tend to refute the null hypothesis, and the posterior odds will be less than the prior odds. However, the close relationship with frequentist methods breaks down. A value of $\bar{x}$ which is just significantly different from zero at some level α may, in sufficiently large samples, confirm the null hypothesis by producing posterior odds greater than the prior odds. Moreover, the proportionate increase in odds increases with the sample size.

This result, often called Lindley's paradox, has been much discussed (Lindley, 1957; Cox & Hinkley, 1974, §10.5; Shafer, 1982; Senn, 1997, pp. 179–184). It arises because, for large samples, the prior distribution need be considered only in a small neighbourhood of the maximum likelihood estimate $\bar{x}$, and with a diffuse distribution of the non-null part of the prior the contribution from this neighbourhood is very small and leads to a low posterior probability against the null hypothesis. Lindley's paradox is often used as an argument against the use of frequentist methods, or at least to assert that large samples require very extreme significance levels (i.e. small values of α) before they become convincing. However, it can equally well be argued that, with a sample mean near, but significantly different from, the null value in large samples, the initial choice of a diffuse prior for the non-null hypothesis was inappropriate. A more concentrated distribution around the null value would have removed the difficulty.

This example illustrates the dilemma facing the Bayesian analyst if the evidence from the data is in some way inconsistent with the prior assumptions. A purist approach would suggest that the prior distribution represents prior opinion and should not be changed by hindsight. A more pragmatic approach would be to recognize that the initial choice was ill-informed, and to consider analyses using alternative formulations.

Unknown mean and variance

We have assumed so far in this section that, in inferences about the mean μ, the variance σ^2 is known. In practice, as noted in §4.2, the variance is usually unknown, and this is taken into account in the frequentist approach by use of the *t* distribution.

The Bayesian approach requires a prior distribution for σ^2 as well as for μ, and in the absence of strong contraindications it is useful to introduce the conjugate family for the distribution of variance. This turns out to be an *inverse gamma* distribution, which means that some multiple of the reciprocal of σ^2 is assumed to have a χ^2 distribution on some appropriate degrees of freedom (see §5.1). There are two arbitrary constants here—the multiplying factor and the degrees of freedom—so the model presents a wide range of possible priors.

The full development is rather complicated, but simplification is achieved by the use of non-informative priors for the mean and variance, and the further assumption that these are independent. We assume as before that σ_0^2, the prior variance for μ, is infinite; and a non-informative version of the inverse gamma distribution for σ^2 (with zero mean and zero 'degrees of freedom') is chosen. The posterior distribution of μ is then centred around $\bar{x}$, the variation around this mean taking the form of $t_{(n-1)}$ times the usual standard error, $s/\sqrt{n}$, where $t_{(n-1)}$ is a variate following the t distribution on $n - 1$ DF. There is thus an analogy with frequentist methods similar to that noted for the case with known variance. In particular, the posterior probability that $\mu < 0$ is numerically the same as the one-sided P value in a frequentist t test of the null hypothesis that $\mu = 0$.

The comparison of the means of two independent samples, for which frequentist methods were described in §4.3, requires further assumptions about the prior distributions for the two pairs of means and variances. If these are all assumed to be non-informative, as in the one-sample case, and independent, the posterior distribution of the difference between the two means, $\mu_1 - \mu_2$, involves the Fisher–Behrens distribution referred to in §4.3.

Bayesian estimation

The posterior distribution provides all the information needed for Bayesian estimation, but, as with frequentist methods, more compact forms of description will usually be sought.

Point estimation

As noted in §4.1, a single-valued point estimator, without any indication of its variability, is of limited value. Nevertheless, estimates of important parameters such as means are often used, for instance in tabulations. A natural suggestion is that a parameter should be estimated by a measure of location of the posterior distribution, such as the mean, median or mode. Decision theory suggests that the choice between these should be based on the *loss function*—the way in which the adverse consequences of making an incorrect estimate depend on the difference between the true and estimated values. The mean is an appropriate choice if the loss is proportional to the square of this difference; and the median is appropriate if the loss is proportional to the absolute value of the difference. These are rather abstruse considerations in the context of simple data analysis, and it may be wise to choose the mean as being the most straightforward, unless the distribution has extreme outlying values which affect the mean, in which case the median might be preferable. The mode is less easy to justify, being appropriate for a loss function which is constant for all incorrect values.

If the posterior distribution is normal, as in the discussion leading up to Example 6.1, the three measures of location coincide, and there is no ambiguity. We should emphasize, though, that a Bayesian point estimate will, as in Example 6.1, be influenced by the prior distribution, and may be misleading for many purposes where the reader is expecting a simple descriptive statement about the data rather than a summary incorporating the investigator's preconceptions.

Finally, note that for a non-informative prior, when the posterior distribution is proportional to the likelihood, the mode of the posterior distribution coincides with the maximum likelihood estimator. In Example 6.1, case A, the prior is almost non-informative, and the posterior mean (coinciding here with the mode and median) is close to the sample mean of 46·9, the maximum likelihood value.

Interval estimation

A natural approach is to select an interval containing a specified high proportion, say $1 - \alpha$, of the posterior probability. The resulting interval may be termed a *Bayesian confidence interval*, although it is important to realize that the interpretation is quite different from that of the frequentist confidence interval presented in §4.1. Alternative phrases such as *credibility interval* or *Bayesian probability interval* are preferable.

The choice of a $1 - \alpha$ credibility interval is not unique, as any portion of the posterior distribution covering the required probability of $1 - \alpha$ could be selected. (A similar feature of frequentist confidence intervals was noted in §4.1.) The simplest, and most natural, approach is to choose the interval with equal tail areas of $\frac{1}{2}\alpha$. In the situation described at the beginning of this section, with a normal sampling distribution with known variance, and a non-informative normal prior, the $1 - \alpha$ credibility interval coincides with the usual symmetric $1 - \alpha$ confidence interval centred around the sample mean. When the variance is unknown, the non-informative assumptions described earlier lead to the use of the t distribution, and again the credibility interval coincides with the usual confidence interval. In other situations, and with more specific prior assumptions, the Bayesian credibility interval will not coincide with that obtained from a frequentist approach.

6.3 **Bayesian inference for proportions and counts**

The model described in §6.2, involving a normal likelihood and a normal prior, will serve as a useful approximation in many situations where these conditions are not completely satisfied, as in Example 6.1. In particular, it may be adequate for analyses involving proportions and counts, provided that the normal approximations to the sampling distributions, described in §3.8, are valid, and that a normal distribution reasonably represents the prior information.

However, for these two situations, more exact methods are available, based on the binomial distribution for proportions (§3.6) and the Poisson distribution for counts (§3.7).

Bayesian inference for a proportion

Consider the estimation of a population proportion π from a random sample of size n in which r individuals are affected in some way. The sampling results, involving the binomial distribution, were discussed in §3.6 and §4.4. In the Bayesian approach we need a prior distribution for π. A normal distribution can clearly provide only a rough approximation, since π must lie between 0 and 1. The most convenient and flexible family of distributions for this purpose, which happens also to be the conjugate family, is that of the *beta distributions*. The density of a beta distribution takes the form

$$f(\pi) = \frac{\pi^{a-1}(1-\pi)^{b-1}}{\mathrm{B}(a,b)},\tag{6.4}$$

where the two parameters a and b must both be positive. The denominator $\mathrm{B}(a, b)$ in (6.4), which is needed to ensure that the total probability is 1, is known as the *beta function*. When a and b are both integers, it can be expressed in terms of factorials (see §3.6), as follows:

$$\mathrm{B}(a,b) = \frac{(a-1)!\,(b-1)!}{(a+b-2)!}.\tag{6.5}$$

We shall refer to (6.4) as the Beta (a, b) distribution. The mean and variance of π are, respectively,

$$\mathrm{E}(\pi) = \pi_0 = a/(a+b), \quad \text{and} \quad \mathrm{var}(\pi) = ab/(a+b)^2(a+b+1).$$

The mean is $<, =$ or $> \frac{1}{2}$ according to whether $a <, =$ or $> b$. The variance decreases as $a + b$ increases, so strong prior evidence is represented by high values of $a + b$.

The shape of the beta distribution is determined by the values of a and b. If $a = b = 1$, $f(\pi)$ is constant, and the distribution of π is *uniform*, all values between 0 and 1 having the same density. If a and b are both greater than 1, the distribution of π is unimodal with a mode at $\pi = (a-1)/(a+b-2)$. If a and b are both less than 1, the distribution is U-shaped, with modes at 0 and 1. If $a > 1$ and $b < 1$, the distribution is J-shaped, with a mode at 1, and the reverse conditions for a and b give a reversed J-shape, with a mode at 0.

With (6.4) as the prior distribution, and the binomial sampling distribution for the observed value r, application of Bayes' theorem shows that the posterior distribution of π is again a beta distribution, Beta $(r+a, n-r+b)$. The posterior mean is thus

$$\tilde{\pi} = \frac{r+a}{n+a+b}, \tag{6.6}$$

which lies between the observed proportion of affected individuals, $p = r/n$, and the prior mean π_0. The estimate of the population proportion is thus shrunk from the sample estimate towards the prior mean. For very weak prior evidence and a large sample ($a+b$ small, n large), the posterior estimate will be close to the sample proportion p. For strong prior evidence and a small sample ($a+b$ large, n small) the estimate will be close to the prior mean π_0.

As a representation of prior ignorance, it might seem natural to choose the uniform distribution, which is the member of the conjugate family of beta distributions with $a = b = 1$. Note, however, from (6.6) that this gives $\tilde{\pi} = (r+1)/(n+2)$, a slightly surprising result. The more expected result with $\tilde{\pi} = p$, the sample proportion, would be obtained only with $a = b = 0$, which is strictly not an allowable combination of parameters for a beta distribution. Theoretical reasons have been advanced for choosing, instead, $a = b = \frac{1}{2}$, although this choice is not normally adopted. The dilemma is of little practical importance, however. The change of parameters in the beta function, in moving from the prior to the posterior, is effectively to add a hypothetical number of a affected individuals to the r observed, and b non-affected to the $n-r$ observed, and unless r or $n-r$ is very small none of the choices mentioned above will have much effect on the posterior distribution.

Statements of the posterior probability for various possible ranges of values of π require calculations of the area under the curve (i.e. the integral) for specified portions of the beta distribution. These involve the *incomplete beta function*, and can be obtained from suitable tables (e.g. Pearson & Hartley, 1966, Tables 16 and 17 and §8) or from tabulations of the F distribution included in some computer packages. Using the latter approach, the probability that $\pi < \pi'$ in the Beta (a, b) distribution is equal to the probability that $F > F'$ in the F distribution with $2b$ and $2a$ degrees of freedom, where

$$F' = \frac{a(1-\pi')}{b\pi'}.$$

We illustrate some of the points discussed above by reference in §6.2 to the data analysed earlier by frequentist methods in Example 4.6.

Example 6.2

In the clinical trial described in Example 4.6, 100 patients receive two drugs, X and Y, in random order; 65 prefer X and 35 prefer Y. Denote by π the probability that a patient prefers X. Example 4.6 described a frequentist significance test of the null hypothesis that $\pi = \frac{1}{2}$ and, in the continuation on p. 117, provided 95% confidence limits for π.

Table 6.2 shows the results of Bayesian analyses with various prior beta distributions for π.

In case A, the uniform distribution, Beta (1, 1), represents vague prior knowledge as indicated earlier, and the posterior distribution is determined almost entirely by the data. The central 95% posterior probability region is very similar to the 95% confidence range given in Example 4.6 (continued on p. 117), method **2**. The probability that $\pi < 0.5$ agrees (to four decimal places) with the one-sided mid-P significance level in a test of the null hypothesis that $\pi = 0.5$.

The tighter prior distribution used in case B suggests that the observed proportion $p = 0.65$ is an overestimate of the true probability π. The posterior mean is shrunk towards 0.5, but the probability that $\pi < 0.5$ is still very low.

In case C, the prior distribution is even more tightly packed around 0.5 and the posterior mean is shrunk further. The lower limit of the central 95% posterior probability region barely exceeds 0.5, and $P(\pi < 0.5)$ is correspondingly only a little short of 0.025. With such strong prior belief the highly significant difference between p and 0.5 (as judged by a frequentist test) is heavily diluted, although still providing a moderate degree of evidence for a verdict in favour of drug X.

Bayesian comparison of two proportions

In the comparison of two proportions, discussed from a frequentist standpoint in §4.5, a fully Bayesian approach would require a formulation for the prior distributions of the two parameters π_1 and π_2, allowing for the possibility that their random variation is associated in some way. In most situations, however, progress can be made by concentration on a single measure of the contrast between the two parameters.

For the paired case, treated earlier on p. 121, the analysis may be reduced to that of a single proportion by consideration of the relative proportions of the two types of untied pairs, for which the observed frequencies (p. 121) are r and s.

Table 6.2 Various prior distributions for Example 6.2.

	Prior distribution				Posterior distribution				
	a	b	Mean	Central 95% probability region	a	b	Mean	Central 95% probability region	$P(\pi < 0.5)$
A	1	1	0.5	(0.025, 0.975)	66	36	0.650	(0.552, 0.736)	0.0013
B	30	30	0.5	(0.375, 0.625)	95	65	0.595	(0.517, 0.668)	0.0085
C	60	60	0.5	(0.411, 0.589)	125	95	0.569	(0.502, 0.633)	0.0212

In the unpaired case (p. 124), one possible simplification is to express the contrast between π_1 and π_2 in terms of the log of the odds ratio,

$$\log \Psi = \log \frac{\pi_1(1-\pi_2)}{(1-\pi_1)\pi_2}. \tag{6.7}$$

In the notation used in (4.25), $\log \Psi$ may be estimated by the log of the observed odds ratio ad/bc, the variance of which is given approximately by the square of the standard error (4.26) divided by $(2 \cdot 3026)^2 = 5 \cdot 3019$ (to convert from natural to common logs). Unless some of the frequencies are very small, this statistic may be assumed to be approximately normally distributed. The normal theory for the Bayesian estimate of a mean may then be applied. The prior distribution of the parameter (6.7) may also be assumed to be approximately normal, with a mean and variance reflecting prior opinion. The normal theory outlined in §6.2 may then be applied. Note that the formulation in terms of the log of the odds ratio, rather than the odds ratio itself, makes the normal model more plausible, since the parameter and its estimate both have an unlimited range in each direction.

Bayesian inference for a count

Frequentist methods of inference from a count x, following a Poisson distribution with mean μ, were described in §5.2. The Bayesian approach requires the formulation of a prior distribution for μ, which can take positive values between 0 and ∞. The conjugate family here is that of the *gamma distributions*, the density of which is

$$f(\mu) = \frac{\mu^{\alpha-1}e^{-\mu/\beta}}{\Gamma(\alpha)\beta^{\alpha}}, \tag{6.8}$$

where α and β are two adjustable parameters taking positive values. The expression $\Gamma(\alpha)$ indicates the *gamma function*; for integral values of α, $\Gamma(\alpha) = (\alpha-1)!$.

We shall refer to (6.8) as the Gamma (α, β) distribution. The mean and variance of π are, respectively, $\alpha\beta$ and $\alpha\beta^2$. By variation of the two parameters a flexible range of possible prior distributions may be obtained. Essentially, α determines the shape, and β the scale, of the distribution. When $\alpha \leq 1$, the distribution has a reversed J-shape, with a peak at zero; otherwise the distribution is double-tailed. The family of gamma distributions is related closely to the family of chi-square (χ^2) distributions: $2\mu/\beta$ has a χ^2 distribution on 2α degrees of freedom.

For an observed count x, and (6.8) as the prior distribution for μ, the posterior distribution is Gamma $(x + \alpha, \beta/(1+\beta))$. A suitable choice of parameters for a non-informative prior is $\alpha = \frac{1}{2}, \beta = \infty$, which has an infinitely dispersed reversed J-shape. With that assumption, the posterior distribution becomes Gamma $(x + \frac{1}{2}, 1)$, and 2μ has a χ^2 distribution on $2x + 1$ DF.

Example 6.3

Example 5.2 described a study in which $x = 33$ workers died of lung cancer. The number expected at national death rates was 20·0.

The Bayesian model described above, with a non-informative prior, gives the posterior distribution Gamma (33·5, 1), and 2μ has a χ^2 distribution on 67 DF. From computer tabulations of this distribution we find that P ($\mu < 20\cdot0$) is 0·0036, very close to the frequentist one-sided mid-P significance level of 0·0037 quoted in Example 5.2.

If, on the other hand, it was believed that local death rates varied around the national rate by relatively small increments, a prior might be chosen to have a mean count of 20 and a small standard deviation of, say, 2. Setting the mean of the prior to be $\alpha\beta = 20$ and its variance to be $\alpha\beta^2 = 4$, gives $\alpha = 100$ and $\beta = 0\cdot2$, and the posterior distribution is Gamma (133, 0·1667). Thus, 12μ has a χ^2 distribution on 266 DF, and computer tabulations show that P($\mu < 20\cdot0$) is 0·128. There is now considerably less evidence that the local death rate is excessive. The posterior estimate of the expected number of deaths is (133) (0·1667) = 22·17. Note, however, that the observed count is somewhat incompatible with the prior assumptions. The difference between x and the prior mean is $33 - 20 = 13$. Its variance might be estimated as $33 + 4 = 37$ and its standard error as $\sqrt{37} = 6\cdot083$. The difference is thus over twice its standard error, and the investigator might be well advised to reconsider prior assumptions.

Analyses involving the ratio of two counts can proceed from the approach described in §5.2 and illustrated in Examples 5.2 and 5.3. If two counts, x_1 and x_2, follow independent Poisson distributions with means μ_1 and μ_2, respectively, then, given the total count $x_1 + x_2$, the observed count x_1 is binomially distributed with mean $(x_1 + x_2)\mu_1/(\mu_2 + \mu_2)$. The methods described earlier in this section for the Bayesian analysis of proportions may thus be applied also to this problem.

6.4 **Further comments on Bayesian methods**

Shrinkage

The phenomenon of shrinkage was introduced in §6.2 and illustrated in several of the situations described in that section and in §6.3. It is a common feature of parameter estimation in Bayesian analyses. The posterior distribution is determined by the prior distribution and the likelihood based on the data, and its measures of location will tend to lie between those of the prior distribution and the central features of the likelihood function. The relative weights of these two determinants will depend on the variability of the prior and the tightness of the likelihood function, the latter being a function of the amount of data.

The examples discussed in §6.2 and §6.3 involved the means of the prior and posterior distributions and the mean of the sampling distribution giving rise to the likelihood. For unimodal distributions shrinkage will normally also be observed for other measures of location, such as the median or mode. However, if the prior had two or more well-separated modes, as might be the case for some genetic traits, the tendency would be to shrink towards the nearest major mode, and that might be in the opposite direction to the overall prior mean. An example, for normally distributed observations with a prior distribution concentrated at just two points, in given by Carlin and Louis (2000, §4.1.1), who refer to the phenomenon as *stretching*.

We discuss here two aspects of shrinkage that relate to concepts of linear regression, a topic dealt with in more detail in Chapter 7. We shall anticipate some results described in Chapter 7, and the reader unfamiliar with the principles of linear regression may wish to postpone a reading of this subsection.

First, we take another approach to the normal model described at the start of §6.2. We could imagine taking random observations, simultaneously, of the two variables μ and $\bar{x}$. Here, μ is chosen randomly from the distribution $N(\mu_0, \sigma_0^2)$. Then, given this value of μ, $\bar{x}$ is chosen randomly from the conditional distribution $N(\mu, \sigma^2/n)$. If this process is repeated, a series of random pairs $(\mu, \bar{x})$ is generated. These paired observations form a *bivariate normal distribution* (§7.4, Fig. 7.6). In this distribution, $\text{var}(\mu) = \sigma_0^2$, $\text{var}(\bar{x}) = \sigma_0^2 + \sigma^2/n$ (incorporating both the variation of μ and that of $\bar{x}$ given μ), and the correlation (§7.3) between μ and $\bar{x}$ is

$$\rho_0 = \frac{\sigma_0}{\sqrt{(\sigma_0^2 + \sigma^2/n)}}.$$

The regression equation of $\bar{x}$ on μ is

$$E(\bar{x} \mid \mu) = \mu,$$

so the regression coefficient $\beta_{\bar{x} \cdot \mu}$ is 1. From the relationship between the regression coefficients and the correlation coefficient, shown below (7.11), the other regression coefficient is

$$\beta_{\mu \cdot \bar{x}} = \frac{\rho_0^2}{\beta_{\bar{x} \cdot \mu}} = \rho_0^2 = \frac{\sigma_0^2}{\sigma_0^2 + \sigma^2/n}.$$

This result is confirmed by the mean of the distribution (6.1), which can be written as

$$E(\mu \mid \bar{x}) = \mu_0 + \left(\frac{\sigma_0^2}{\sigma_0^2 + \sigma^2/n} \right)(\bar{x} - \mu_0).$$

The fact that $\beta_{\mu \cdot \bar{x}} (= \rho_0^2)$ is less than 1 reflects the shrinkage in the posterior mean. The proportionate shrinkage is

$$1 - \rho_0^2 = \frac{\sigma^2/n}{\sigma_0^2 + \sigma^2/n},$$

which depends on the ratio of the sampling variance, σ^2/n, and the variance of the prior distribution, σ_0^2.

The phenomenon of shrinkage is closely related to that of *regression to the mean*, familiar to epidemiologists and other scientists for many decades. This will be discussed in the context of regression in §7.5.

Prediction

Sometimes the main object of an analysis may be to predict future observations, or at least their distribution, on the assumption that the structure of the random variation remains the same as in the set of data already analysed. If serial observations on a physiological variable have been made for a particular patient, it might be useful to state plausible limits for future observations. The assumption that the relevant distributions remain constant is obviously crucial, and there is the further question whether serial observations in time can be regarded as independent random observations (a topic discussed in more detail in Chapter 12).

Bayesian prediction may also be useful in situations where investigators are uncertain whether to take further observations, and wish to predict the likely range of variation in such observations. For a description of Bayesian predictive methods in clinical trials, see §18.7.

Consider the problem of predicting the mean of a future random sample from the same population as that from which the current sample was drawn. We shall assume the same model and notation as at the start of §6.2, with a normal prior distribution and normal likelihood based on a sample of size n. Suppose that the future sample is to be of size n_1, and denote the unknown mean of this sample by $\bar{x}_1$. If we knew the value of μ, the distribution of $\bar{x}_1$ would be $N(\mu, \sigma^2/n_1)$. In fact, μ is unknown, but its posterior distribution is given by (6.1). The overall distribution of $\bar{x}_1$ is obtained by generating the sampling distribution, with variance σ^2/n_1, for each value of μ in the posterior distribution, and pooling these distributions with weights proportional to the posterior density of μ. The result is a normal distribution with the same mean as in (6.1), but with a variance increased from that in (6.1) by an amount σ^2/n_1. In the simple situation of very weak prior evidence or a very large initial sample (either σ_0^2 or n very large), the predictive distribution for $\bar{x}_1$ becomes

$$N\left[\bar{x}, \sigma^2\left(\frac{1}{n} + \frac{1}{n_1}\right)\right]. \tag{6.9}$$

This effectively expresses the facts that, in the absence of prior knowledge: (i) the best guess at $\bar{x}_1$ is $\bar{x}$; (ii) the variation of $\bar{x}_1$ about $\bar{x}$ is essentially that of the difference between the two estimates; and (iii) the variance of this difference is the sum of the two separate variances, as in (4.9) and (4.10).

In other, more complex, situations, especially those with informative prior distributions, the predictive distributions of future observations will not be as simple as (6.9), and the solutions may be obtainable only by computation. Nevertheless, the simple normal model leading to (6.9) will often provide an adequate approximation.

Sample-size determination

Frequentist methods for sample-size determination were described in some detail in §4.6. In approach **3** of that section, which underlie most of the results described there, the sample size was required to give a specified power (one minus the Type II error rate) against a specified value δ_1 for the unknown parameter δ, in a significance test at level 2α of the null hypothesis that $\delta = 0$. Here, the non-null value δ_1 should not be regarded as a *guess* at the value of δ, but rather as defining the required sensitivity of the study: if δ were as far from zero as δ_1, then we should want to detect the departure by claiming a significant difference.

Although there is no explicit reference in this argument to prior beliefs, the choice of δ_1 is likely to have involved some such considerations. If we believed that $|\delta|$ would be much greater than δ_1, then we have planned a much larger study than was really necessary. Conversely, if we believed that $|\delta|$ was very unlikely to be as large as δ_1, then the study was unlikely to detect any effect and should have been either enlarged or abandoned.

A Bayesian approach to this problem might be to specify a prior distribution for δ, leading to a predictive distribution for the test statistic, and to use this to determine the sample size. For instance, if the prior distribution for δ is $N(\delta_0, \sigma_0^2)$, and the sampling distribution of the test statistic $\bar{x}$ is $N(\delta, \sigma^2/n)$, then the predictive distribution of $\bar{x}$ is $N(\delta_0, \sigma_0^2 + \sigma^2/n)$. By an argument similar to that leading to (4.41), the minimum sample size n for a Type I error rate 2α and a predictive power $1 - \beta$, satisfies the equation

$$z_{2\alpha}\frac{\sigma}{\sqrt{n}} + z_{2\beta}\sqrt{(\sigma_0^2 + \tfrac{\sigma^2}{n})} = \delta_0. \tag{6.10}$$

If $\delta_0 = \delta_1$ and $\sigma_0 = 0$, representing certainty that the true mean is δ_1, then (6.10) gives

$$n = \left[\frac{(z_{2\alpha} + z_{2\beta})\sigma}{\delta_1}\right]^2,$$

which is essentially the same as (4.41), the multiplier 2 in (4.41) arising because the discussion there concerned the difference between *two* means.

This approach has been used in connection with clinical trials by Spiegelhalter and Freedman (1986) and Spiegelhalter *et al.* (1994).

The control of Type I and Type II error rates is somewhat alien to the Bayesian approach, and a more natural Bayesian objective is to choose the sample size in such a way as to achieve a sufficiently compact posterior distribution. The compactness can be measured in various ways, such as the probability contained in an interval of specified length, the length of an interval covering a specified probability, or the variance of the posterior distribution. A useful review by Adcock (1997) appeared in a special issue of *The Statistician* containing other relevant papers.

Lindley (1997) describes a formal approach based on Bayesian decision theory. Here the object is to maximize the expected utility (or negative cost) of any strategy for taking decisions, including, in this case, the decision about the sample size. The utilities to be considered include the benefits deriving from a compact posterior distribution and the countervailing cost of additional sampling. In practice, these costs are very difficult to evaluate, especially in a medical investigation, and the simpler approaches outlined above are likely to be more attractive.

6.5 **Empirical Bayesian methods**

In §3.3, Bayes' theorem was introduced from a frequentist viewpoint: the prior distribution for a parameter was supposed to be determined precisely from previous observations, as in Example 3.1, or by theoretical considerations, as in the use of Mendelian theory in Example 3.2. In the earlier sections of this chapter we have assumed that prior distributions represented personal beliefs, which are unlikely to be supported in any very direct way by objective evidence.

We return now to the earlier scenario, where prior distributions are clearly determined by objective data. The earlier discussion in §3.3 needs to be amplified, because such data are likely to be influenced by random variation, and they will not immediately provide a description of the underlying probability distributions unless this superimposed random variation is allowed for.

There are many situations where statistics are available for each of a number of groups that share some common feature. The results may differ from group to group, but the common features suggest that the information from the whole data set is to some extent relevant to inferences about any one group, as a supplement to the specific statistics for that group. Some examples are as follows:

1 Biochemical test measurements on patients with a specific diagnosis, where repeated measurements on any one patient may fluctuate and their mean is therefore subject to sampling error, but the results for the whole data throw some light on the mean level for that patient. The between-patient

variation may be regarded as the prior distribution, but this is not directly observed. The observed data (mean values for different patients) form a sample from a distribution that is derived from the prior distribution by superimposing on it the random errors derived from the within-patient variation.

2   Biological screening tests done on each of a large number of substances to detect possible pharmacological activity. Test results for any one substance are subject to random error, but again the whole data set provides evidence about the underlying distribution of true mean activity levels.

3   Mortality or morbidity rates for a large number of small areas, each of which is subject to random error. Again, some information relevant to a specific area is provided by the distribution of rates for the whole data set, or at least for a subset of adjacent areas.

In studies of this type it seems reasonable to regard the results for the specific group (patient, substance or area, in the above examples) as being drawn from the same prior distribution as all the other groups unless there are distinguishing features that make this assumption unreasonable (such as a special form of disease in **1**, or an important chemical property in **2**). The likelihood to be used in Bayes' theorem will depend on the particular form of data observed for a particular group, and will often follow immediately from standard results for means, proportions, counts, etc. The prior distribution causes more difficulty because it relates to the 'true' values of the parameters for different groups, and these can only be estimated. In **3**, for instance, the 'true' mortality rate for any area can only be estimated from the observed rate. The variability of the observed rates will always be greater than that of the true rates, because of the additional sampling errors that affect the former. The purpose of empirical Bayes methods is to estimate the prior distribution from the observed data, by adjusting for the sampling errors, and then to use Bayes' theorem to estimate the relevant parameter for any individual group.

We remark here that a strictly Bayesian approach to this problem would proceed rather differently. If the prior distribution is unknown, it would be possible to define it in terms of some parameters (for instance, the parameters a and b in the beta prior in §6.3), and to allow these to be estimated by having their own prior distribution. This is turn might have one or more parameters, which again might have their own prior. This sort of model is called *hierarchical*. It is unusual to involve more than two or three levels of the hierarchy, and at the final stage a prior must be specified, even if (as is likely) it is non-informative. The empirical Bayes approach circumvents the complexity of this procedure, by making an estimate of the first-level prior directly from the data, by frequentist methods.

Consider the normal model described at the start of §6.2. With a slight change of notation, suppose we have k sample means, each of n observations, where the

ith mean, $\bar{x}_i$, is distributed as $N(\mu_i, \sigma^2/n)$ and μ_i has the prior distribution $N(\mu_0, \sigma_0^2)$, the parameters μ_0 and σ_0 being unknown.

As noted in §6.4, the overall variance of the $\bar{x}_i$ is $\sigma_0^2 + \sigma^2/n$, and this can be estimated by the observed variance of the k sample means,

$$s^2 = \frac{\sum (\bar{x}_i - \bar{x}.)^2}{k}, \tag{6.11}$$

where $\bar{x}. = \sum \bar{x}_i/k$, the overall mean value. In (6.11), there are technical reasons for preferring the divisor k to the more usual $k-1$. Hence, an estimate of σ_0^2 is provided by

$$\hat{\sigma}_0^2 = \begin{cases} s^2 - \sigma^2/n & \text{if } s^2 > \sigma^2/n \\ 0 & \text{otherwise.} \end{cases} \tag{6.12}$$

The second condition in (6.12) is needed to avoid a negative estimate of variance.

The prior mean is estimated as $\hat{\mu}_0 = \bar{x}.$, and the usual Bayesian methods proceed, as in §6.2, to provide posterior distributions for each group, and the corresponding shrinkage estimates of the means μ_i. Note that, if $s^2 < \sigma^2/n$, as in the second condition of (6.12), the posterior means of all the groups are shrunk to the same value $\bar{x}.$.

The above account provides an example of *parametric* empirical Bayes. Other approaches are possible. One could postulate a prior distribution of very general form, and estimate this by some efficient method. Such *non-parametric* empirical Bayes analyses tend to produce estimates of the prior distribution in which the probability is concentrated in 'spikes' determined by the values of the observations. Although a prior distribution of this form is wholly implausible, the resulting values of, for instance, the posterior means may be acceptable.

Yet another approach (Efron & Morris, 1975) is to avoid any explicit form of prior distribution, and to obtain shrinkage estimates in terms merely of estimates of the prior variance and the overall variance of the observations (equivalent to $\hat{\sigma}_0^2$ and s^2 in the above account).

Example 6.4

Martuzzi and Elliott (1996) describe a study of the prevalence of respiratory symptoms in schoolchildren aged 7–9 years in 71 school catchment areas in Huddersfield. The sample sizes varied from 1 to 73, with prevalences varying from 14% to 46%, apart from outlying values in areas with fewer than 10 children. A preliminary test of homogeneity showed clear evidence of real variation in prevalence rates. The analysis used variance estimates, as in the last paragraph, but allowing for the variation in sample size. The same estimates would have been obtained from a parametric model assuming a beta prior distribution for the prevalences, as in §3.3.2 of Carlin and Louis (2000).

The resulting shrinkage estimates show much less variability than the crude prevalences, varying between 22% and 39%. A small area with one child who was not a case has a posterior prevalence of 30%, close to the overall mean. A larger area, with 112 children of whom 52 were cases, has a posterior prevalence of 39%, reduced from the crude rate of 46%. A preliminary analysis had shown no evidence of spatial clustering in the prevalence rates, and an alternative empirical Bayes analysis, using as a prior for each area the pooled data for adjacent areas, gave shrinkage estimates very close to those from the global analysis.

In many small area studies of disease prevalence, like that described in Example 6.4, the prevalences are small and the numbers of cases can safely be assumed to have Poisson rather than binomial variation. Some examples are described by Clayton and Kaldor (1987) and, with application to disease mapping, Marshall (1991).

Breslow (1990) gives a useful survey of empirical Bayes and other Bayesian methods in various medical applications.

7 Regression and correlation

7.1 **Association**

In earlier chapters we have been concerned with the statistical analysis of observations on a single variable. In some problems data were divided into two groups, and the dichotomy could, admittedly, have been regarded as defining a second variable. These two-sample problems are, however, rather artificial examples of the relationship between two variables.

In this chapter we examine more generally the association between two quantitative variables. We shall concentrate on situations in which the general trend is linear; that is, as one variable changes the other variable follows *on the average* a trend which can be represented approximately by a straight line. More complex situations will be discussed in Chapters 11 and 12.

The basic graphical technique for the two-variable situation is the *scatter diagram*, and it is good practice to plot the data in this form before attempting any numerical analysis. An example is shown in Fig. 7.1. In general the data refer to a number of *individuals*, each of which provides observations on two variables. In the scatter diagram each variable is allotted one of the two coordinate axes, and each individual thus defines a point, of which the coordinates are the observed values of the two variables. In Fig. 7.1 the individuals are towns and the two variables are the infant mortality rate and a certain index of overcrowding.

The scatter diagram gives a compact illustration of the distribution of each variable and of the relationship between the two variables. Further statistical analysis serves a number of purposes. It provides, first, numerical measures of some of the basic features of the relationship, rather as the mean and standard deviation provide concise measures of the most important features of the distribution of a single variable. Secondly, the investigator may wish to make a prediction of the value of one variable when the value of the other variable is known. It will normally be impossible to predict with complete certainty, but we may hope to say something about the mean value and the variability of the predicted variable. From Fig. 7.1, for instance, it appears roughly that a town with 0·6 persons per room was in 1961 likely to have an infant mortality rate of about 20 per 1000 live births on average, with a likely range of about 14–26. A proper analysis might be expected to give more reliable figures than these rough guesses.

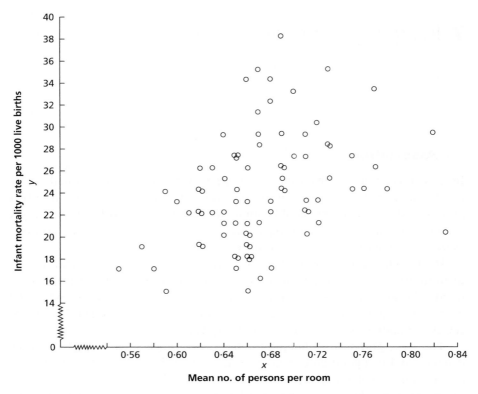

Fig. 7.1 Scatter diagram showing the mean number of persons per room and the infant mortality per 1000 live births for the 83 county boroughs in England and Wales in 1961.

   Thirdly, the investigator may wish to assess the significance of the direction of an apparent trend. From the data of Fig. 7.1, for instance, could it safely be asserted that infant mortality increases on the average as the overcrowding index increases, or could the apparent trend in this direction have arisen easily by chance?

   Yet another aim may be to correct the measurements of one variable for the effect of another variable. In a study of the forced expiratory volume (FEV) of workers in the cadmium industry who had been exposed for more than a certain number of years to cadmium fumes, a comparison was made with the FEV of other workers who had not been exposed. The mean FEV of the first group was lower than that of the second. However, the men in the first group tended to be older than those in the second, and FEV tends to decrease with age. The question therefore arises whether the difference in mean FEV could be explained purely by the age difference. To answer this question the relationship between FEV and age must be studied in some detail. The method is described in §11.5.

We must be careful to distinguish between *association* and *causation*. Two variables are associated if the distribution of one is affected by a knowledge of the value of the other. This does not mean that one variable *causes* the other. There is a strong association between the number of divorces made absolute in the United Kingdom during the first half of this century and the amount of tobacco imported (the 'individuals' in the scatter diagram here being the individual years). It does not follow either that tobacco is a serious cause of marital discontent, or that those whose marriages have broken down turn to tobacco for solace. Association does not imply causation.

A further distinction is between situations in which both variables can be thought of as random variables, the individuals being selected randomly or at least without reference to the values of either variable, and situations in which the values of one variable are deliberately selected by the investigator. An example of the first situation would be a study of the relationship between the height and the blood pressure of schoolchildren, the individuals being restricted to one sex and one age group. Here, the sample may not have been chosen strictly at random, but it can be thought of as roughly representative of a population of children of this age and sex from the same area and type of school. An example of the second situation would arise in a study of the growth of children between certain ages. The nature of the relationship between height and age, as illustrated by a scatter diagram, would depend very much on the age range chosen and the distribution of ages within this range. We return to this point in §7.3.

7.2 **Linear regression**

Suppose that observations are made on variables x and y for each of a large number of individuals, and that we are interested in the way in which y changes on the average as x assumes different values. If it is appropriate to think of y as a random variable for any given value of x, we can enquire how the expectation of y changes with x. The probability distribution of y when x is known is referred to as a *conditional* distribution, and the conditional expectation is denoted by $E(y|x)$. We make no assumption at this stage as to whether x is a random variable or not. In a study of heights and blood pressures of randomly chosen individuals both variables would be random; if x and y were respectively the age and height of children selected according to age, then only y would be random.

The conditional expectation, $E(y|x)$, depends in general on x. It is called the *regression function* of y on x. If $E(y|x)$ is drawn as a function of x it forms the *regression curve*. Two examples are shown in Fig. 7.2. First, the regression in Fig. 7.2(b) differs in two ways from that in Fig. 7.2(a). The curve in Fig. 7.2(b) is a straight line—the *regression line* of y on x. Secondly, the variation of y for fixed x is constant in Fig. 7.2(b), whereas in Fig. 7.2(a) the variation changes as x

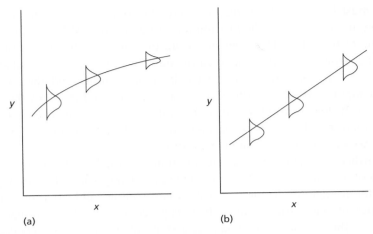

Fig. 7.2 Two regression curves of y on x: (a) non-linear and heteroscedastic; (b) linear and homoscedastic. The distributions shown are those of values of y at certain values of x.

increases. The regression in (b) is called *homoscedastic*, that in (a) being *heteroscedastic*.

The situation represented by Fig. 7.2(b) is important not only because of its simplicity, but also because regressions which are approximately linear and homoscedastic occur frequently in scientific work. In the present discussion we shall make one further simplifying assumption—that the distribution of y for given x is normal.

The model may, then, be described by saying that, for a given x, y follows a normal distribution with mean

$$E(y \mid x) = \alpha + \beta x$$

(the general equation of a straight line) and variance σ^2 (a constant). A set of data consists of n pairs of observations, denoted by $(x_1, y_1), (x_2, y_2), \ldots, (x_n, y_n)$, each y_i being an independent observation from the distribution $N(\alpha + \beta x_i, \sigma^2)$. How can we estimate the parameters α, β and σ^2, which characterize the model?

An intuitively attractive proposal is to draw the regression line through the n points on the scatter diagram so as to minimize the sum of squares of the distances, $y_i - Y_i$, of the points from the line, these distances being measured from the y-axis (Fig. 7.3). This proposal is in accord with theoretical arguments leading to the *least squares* estimators of α and β, a and b, namely the values which minimize the *residual* sum of squares, $\sum(y_i - Y_i)^2$, where Y_i is given by the estimated regression equation

$$Y_i = a + bx_i. \tag{7.1}$$

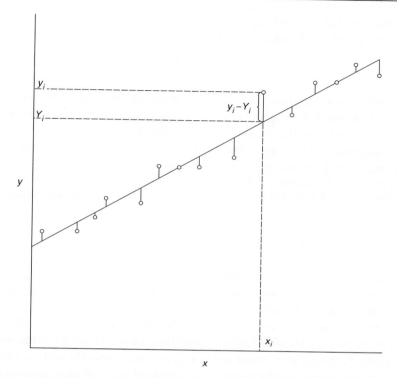

Fig. 7.3 A linear regression line fitted by least squares showing a typical deviation between an observed value y_i and the value Y_i given by the regression line.

The least squares estimators of α and β are also the maximum likelihood estimators (§4.1) and have the smallest standard errors (SE) of all unbiased estimators.

It can be shown by calculus that a and b are given by the formulae

$$a = \bar{y} - b\bar{x}, \tag{7.2}$$

$$b = \frac{\sum(x_i - \bar{x})(y_i - \bar{y})}{\sum(x_i - \bar{x})^2}. \tag{7.3}$$

The regression line can thus be written

$$Y_i = \bar{y} + b(x_i - \bar{x}), \tag{7.4}$$

so that it follows that the line goes through the point $(\bar{x}, \bar{y})$.

The residual sum of squares is

$$S = \sum[y_i - \bar{y} - b(x_i - \bar{x})]^2$$

$$= \sum(y - \bar{y})^2 - \frac{[\sum(x - \bar{x})(y - \bar{y})]^2}{\sum(x - \bar{x})^2}, \tag{7.5}$$

on substituting for b from (7.3).

Finally, it can be shown that an unbiased estimator of σ^2 is

$$s_0^2 = \frac{\sum (y - Y)^2}{n - 2}, \tag{7.6}$$

the residual sum of squares, $\sum (y - Y)^2$, being obtainable from (7.5). The divisor $n - 2$ is often referred to as the residual degrees of freedom, s_0^2 as the *residual mean square*, and s_0 as the *standard deviation about regression*.

The quantities a and b are called the *regression coefficients*; the term is often used particularly for b, the slope of the regression line.

The expression in the numerator of (7.3) is the sum of products of deviations of x and y about their means. A short-cut formula analogous to (2.3) is useful for computational work:

$$\sum (x_i - \bar{x})(y_i - \bar{y}) = \sum x_i y_i - \frac{(\sum x_i)(\sum y_i)}{n}. \tag{7.7}$$

Note that, whereas a sum of squares about the mean must be positive or zero, a sum of products of deviations about the mean may be negative, in which case, from (7.3), b will also be negative.

The above theory is illustrated in the following example, which will also be used later in the chapter after further points have been considered. Although the calculations necessary in a simple linear regression are feasible using a scientific calculator, one would usually use either a statistical package on a computer or a calculator with keys for fitting a regression, and the actual calculations would not be a concern.

Example 7.1

Table 7.1 gives the values for 32 babies of x, the birth weight, and y, the increase in weight between the 70th and 100th day of life expressed as a percentage of the birth weight. A scatter diagram is shown in Fig. 7.4 which suggests an association between the two variables in a negative direction. This seems quite plausible: when the birth weight is low the subsequent rate of growth, *relative to the birth weight*, would be expected to be high, and vice versa. The trend seems reasonably linear.

From Table 7.1 we proceed as follows:

$$n = 32 \quad \sum x = 3576 \qquad \sum y = 2281$$
$$\bar{x} = 3576/32 \qquad \bar{y} = 2281/32$$
$$= 111 \cdot 75. \qquad = 71 \cdot 28.$$

$$\sum x^2 = 409\ 880 \qquad \sum xy = 246\ 032 \qquad \sum y^2 = 179\ 761$$
$$\left(\sum x\right)^2 / n = 399\ 618 \cdot 00 \quad \left(\sum x\right)\left(\sum y\right) / n = 254\ 901 \cdot 75 \quad \left(\sum y\right)^2 / n = 162\ 592 \cdot 53$$
$$\sum (x - \bar{x})^2 = 10\ 262 \cdot 00 \quad \sum (x - \bar{x})(y - \bar{y}) = -8869 \cdot 75 \quad \sum (y - \bar{y})^2 = 17\ 168 \cdot 47.$$

Table 7.1 Birth weights of 32 babies and their increases in weight between 70 and 100 days after birth, expressed as percentages of birth weights.

x, Birth weight (oz)	y, Increase in weight, 70–100 days, as % of x
72	68
112	63
111	66
107	72
119	52
92	75
126	76
80	118
81	120
84	114
115	29
118	42
128	48
128	50
123	69
116	59
125	27
126	60
122	71
126	88
127	63
86	88
142	53
132	50
87	111
123	59
133	76
106	72
103	90
118	68
114	93
94	91

To predict the weight increase from the birth weight, the regression of y on x is needed.

$$b = -\frac{8\ 869 \cdot 75}{10\ 262 \cdot 00}$$
$$= -0 \cdot 8643.$$

The equation of the regression line is, from (7.4),

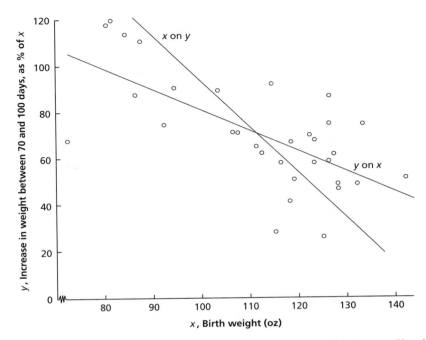

Fig. 7.4 Scatter diagram showing the birth weight, x, and the increase of weight between 70 and 100 days as a percentage of x, for 32 babies, with the two regression lines (Table 7.1).

$$Y = 71 \cdot 28 - 0 \cdot 8643(x - 111 \cdot 75)$$
$$= 167 \cdot 87 - 0 \cdot 8643x.$$

To draw the line, the coordinates of two points suffice, but it is a safeguard to calculate three. Choosing $x = 80$, 100 and 140 as convenient round numbers falling within the range of x used in Fig. 7.4, we find

x	Y
80	98·73
100	81·44
140	46·87

The regression line is now drawn through the three points with these coordinates and is shown in Fig. 7.4.

Note that as x changes from 80 to 120 (i.e. by a factor of $\frac{3}{2}$), y changes on the average from about 100 to 65 (i.e. by a factor of about $\frac{2}{3}$). From the definition of y this implies that *absolute* weight gains are largely independent of x.

For further analyses of these data, see Example 16.1.

In situations in which x, as well as y, is a random variable it may be useful to consider the regression of x on y. This shows how the mean value of x, for a given y, changes with the value of y.

The regression line of x on y may be calculated by formulae analogous to those already used, with x and y interchanged. To avoid confusion between the two lines it will be useful to write the equation of the regression of y on x as

$$Y = \bar{y} + b_{y.x}(x - \bar{x}),$$

with $b_{y.x}$ given by (7.3). The regression equation of x on y is then

$$X = \bar{x} + b_{x.y}(y - \bar{y}),$$

with

$$b_{x.y} = \frac{\sum(x - \bar{x})(y - \bar{y})}{\sum(y - \bar{y})^2}.$$

That the two lines are in general different may be seen from Fig. 7.4. Both lines go through the point $(\bar{x}, \bar{y})$, which is therefore their point of intersection. In Example 7.1 we should probably be interested primarily in the regression of y on x, since it would be natural to study the way in which changes in weight vary with birth weight and to investigate the distribution of change in weight for a particular value of birth weight, rather than to enquire about the distribution of birth weights for a given weight change. In some circumstances both regressions may be of interest.

7.3 **Correlation**

When both x and y are random variables it may be useful to have a measure of the extent to which the relationship between the two variables approaches the extreme situation in which every point on the scatter diagram falls exactly on a straight line. Such an index is provided by the *product–moment correlation coefficient* (or simply *correlation coefficient*), defined by

$$r = \frac{\sum(x - \bar{x})(y - \bar{y})}{\sqrt{\left[\sum(x - \bar{x})^2 \sum(y - \bar{y})^2\right]}}. \tag{7.8}$$

It can be shown that, for any set of data, r falls within the range -1 to $+1$. Figure 7.5 shows five sets of data in which the variation in x and that in y remain approximately constant from one set to another. The marked differences between the five scatter diagrams are summarized by the values of r. Figures 7.5(a) and (e) are examples of perfect correlation, in which the value of y is exactly determined as a linear function of x. The points lie exactly on a straight line; if both variables increase together, as in (a), $r = +1$, while if one variable decreases as the other increases, as in (e), $r = -1$. In each of these cases the two regression lines coincide. Figure 7.5(c) is a very different situation, in which $r = 0$. The two regression coefficients $b_{y.x}$ and $b_{x.y}$ are also zero and the

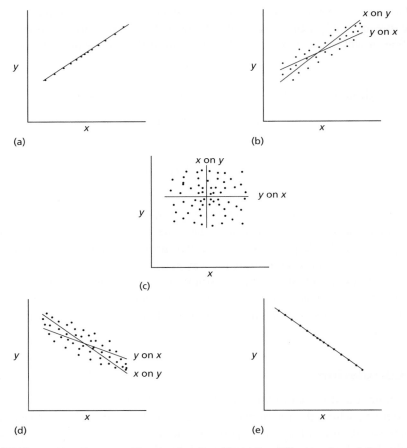

Fig. 7.5 Five scatter diagrams with regression lines illustrating different values of the correlation coefficient. In (a) $r = 1$; (b) $0 < r < 1$; (c) $r = 0$; (d) $-1 < r < 0$; (e) $r = -1$.

regression lines are perpendicular. Intermediate situations are shown in (b), where $0 < r < 1$, and (d), where $-1 < r < 0$. Here, the two regression lines are set at an angle, but point in the same direction.

From the short-cut formulae for sums of squares and products an alternative formula for the correlation coefficient, more convenient for computation, is

$$r = \frac{\sum xy - (\sum x)(\sum y)/n}{\sqrt{\left\{\left[\sum x^2 - (\sum x)^2/n\right]\left[\sum y^2 - (\sum y)^2/n\right]\right\}}}. \qquad (7.9)$$

From (7.5) the sum of squares of y about the regression line of y on x is

$$\sum(y - \bar{y})^2 \left\{ 1 - \frac{\left[\sum(x - \bar{x})(y - \bar{y})\right]^2}{\sum(x - \bar{x})^2 \sum(y - \bar{y})^2} \right\} = \sum(y - \bar{y})^2 \times (1 - r^2). \qquad (7.10)$$

This provides a useful interpretation of the numerical value of r. The squared correlation coefficient is the fraction by which the sum of squares of y is reduced to give the sum of squares of deviations from its regression on x. The same result is true if x and y are interchanged in (7.10). In Figs 7.5(a) and (e), $r^2 = 1$, and (7.10) becomes zero. In (c), $r^2 = 0$ and the sum of squares of either variable is unaffected by regression on the other. In (b) and (d) some reductions take place since $0 < r^2 < 1$.

Two other formulae are easily derived from those for the regression and correlation coefficients:

and

$$\left. \begin{aligned} b_{y.x} &= r\frac{s_y}{s_x} \\[2ex] b_{x.y} &= r\frac{s_x}{s_y} \end{aligned} \right\},$$

$$(7.11)$$

where s_x and s_y are the sample standard deviations of x and y. It follows that

$$b_{y.x}b_{x.y} = r^2.$$

The correlation coefficient has played an important part in the history of statistical methods. It is now of considerably less value than the regression coefficients. If two variables are correlated it is usually much more useful to study the positions of one or both of the regression lines, which permit the prediction of one variable in terms of the other, than to summarize the degree of correlation in a single index.

The restriction of validity of the correlation coefficient to situations in which both variables are observed on a random selection of individuals is particularly important. If, from a large population of individuals, a selection is made by restricting the values of one variable, say x, to a limited range, the correlation coefficient will tend to decrease in absolute value. In the data of Fig. 7.4, for instance, the correlation coefficients calculated on subsets of the data obtained by restricting the range of x values are as follows:

| | Range of x | | Number of observations | Correlation coefficient |
	Lower limit	Upper limit		
All data	70	150	32	-0.668
Subsets	85	135	27	-0.565
	100	120	11	-0.578
	105	115	6	-0.325

Conversely, if the study is restricted to individuals with extreme values of x (including both high and low values), then the correlation coefficient will tend to increase in absolute magnitude. For example, restricting attention to individuals whose birth weight was less than 100 oz or greater than 125 oz gives a correlation coefficient of -0.735.

The interpretation of the numerical value of a correlation coefficient calculated from data selected by values of one variable is thus very difficult.

7.4 **Sampling errors in regression and correlation**

In the regression model of §7.2, suppose that repeated sets of data are generated, each with the same n values of x but with randomly varying values of y. The statistics $\bar{y}$, a and b will vary from one set of data to another. Their sampling variances are obtained as follows:

$$\text{var}(\bar{y}) = \sigma^2/n. \tag{7.12}$$

Note that here σ^2 is the variance of y *for fixed* x, not, as in (4.1), the overall variance of y.

$$\text{var}(b) = \text{var}\left[\frac{\sum y(x - \bar{x})}{\sum(x - \bar{x})^2}\right]$$

(using the fact that $\sum(x - \bar{x})(y - \bar{y}) = \sum(x - \bar{x})y$, the remaining terms vanishing),

$$= \frac{1}{[\sum(x - \bar{x})^2]^2}\sum(x - \bar{x})^2 \,\text{var}(y)$$

$$= \frac{\sigma^2}{\sum(x - \bar{x})^2}. \tag{7.13}$$

$$\text{var}(a) = \text{var}(\bar{y} - b\bar{x})$$
$$= \text{var}(\bar{y}) + \bar{x}^2 \,\text{var}(b)$$

(since it can be shown that b and $\bar{y}$ have zero covariance)

$$= \sigma^2\left[\frac{1}{n} + \frac{\bar{x}^2}{\sum(x - \bar{x})^2}\right]. \tag{7.14}$$

Formulae (7.12), (7.13) and (7.14) all involve the parameter σ^2. If inferences are to be made from one set of n pairs of observations on x and y, σ^2 will be unknown. It can, however, be estimated by the residual mean square, s_0^2 (7.6). Estimated variances are, therefore,

$$\text{var}(\bar{y}) = s_0^2/n, \tag{7.15}$$

$$\text{var}(b) = s_0^2 / \sum(x - \bar{x})^2 \tag{7.16}$$

and

$$\text{var}(a) = s_0^2 \left[\frac{1}{n} + \frac{\bar{x}^2}{\sum(x - \bar{x})^2} \right], \tag{7.17}$$

and hypotheses about $\bar{y}$, a or b can be tested using the t distribution on $n - 2$ degrees of freedom (DF). For example, to test the null hypothesis that $\beta = 0$, i.e. that in the whole population the mean value of y does not change with x, the statistic

$$t = \frac{b}{\text{SE}(b)} \tag{7.18}$$

can be referred to the t distribution on $n - 2$ DF, SE(b) being the square root of (7.16). Similarly, confidence limits for β at, say, the 95% level can be obtained as

$$b \pm t_{n-2, \, 0.05} \text{SE}(b).$$

An important point about the t statistic (7.18) is seen by writing b as $b_{y \cdot x}$ and using (7.3), (7.5), (7.6) and (7.8). We find

$$t = r \sqrt{\left(\frac{n - 2}{1 - r^2} \right)}. \tag{7.19}$$

Since r is symmetric with respect to x and y, it follows that, if, for any set of n paired observations, we calculate the t statistics from $b_{y \cdot x}$ and (by interchanging x and y in the formulae) from $b_{x \cdot y}$, both values of t will be equal to (7.19). In performing the significance test of zero regression and correlation, therefore, it is immaterial whether one tests $b_{y \cdot x}$, $b_{x \cdot y}$ or r. However, we must remember that in some problems only one of the regressions may have a sensible interpretation and it will then be natural to express the test in terms of that regression.

Example 7.1, continued from §7.2

The sum of squares of deviations of y from the regression line is, from (7.5),

$$17 \; 168 \cdot 47 - \frac{(-8869 \cdot 75)^2}{10 \; 262 \cdot 00}$$
$$= 17 \; 168 \cdot 47 - 7666 \cdot 39$$
$$= 9502 \cdot 08.$$

The residual mean square is, from (7.6),

$$s_0^2 = 9502 \cdot 08 / (32 - 2)$$
$$= 316 \cdot 74.$$

From (7.16),

$$\text{var}(b) = 316 \cdot 74 / 10\ 262 \cdot 00$$
$$= 0 \cdot 030\ 865,$$
$$\text{SE}(b) = \sqrt{0 \cdot 030\ 865}$$
$$= 0 \cdot 1757.$$

From (7.18),

$$t = -0 \cdot 8643 / 0 \cdot 1757$$
$$= -4 \cdot 92 \text{ on } 30 \text{ DF } (P < 0 \cdot 001).$$

Alternatively, we could calculate the correlation coefficient

$$r = \frac{-8869 \cdot 75}{\sqrt{[(10\ 262 \cdot 00)(17\ 168 \cdot 47)]}}$$
$$= -\frac{8869 \cdot 75}{13\ 273 \cdot 39}$$
$$= -0 \cdot 668,$$

and, from (7.19),

$$t = -0 \cdot 668 \sqrt{\left(\frac{30}{0 \cdot 554}\right)}$$
$$= -4 \cdot 92,$$

as before.

The sampling error of a correlation coefficient was introduced above in connection with a test of the null hypothesis that its population value is zero. This is the context in which the question usually arises. More rarely we may wish to give confidence limits for the population value in situations in which the individuals providing paired observations can be regarded as randomly drawn from some population. A need arises here to define the nature of the two-dimensional distribution of x and y. A convenient form is the *bivariate normal distribution*, a rough sketch of which is shown in Fig. 7.6. This is a generalization of the familiar univariate normal distribution in which the distribution of y for given x is normal with constant variance, the distribution of x for given y is also normal with constant variance, and both regressions are linear. In large samples from such a distribution the standard error of the correlation coefficient, r, is approximately $(1 - r^2)/\sqrt{n}$, a result which enables approximate confidence limits to be calculated. More refined methods are available for small samples (Geigy Scientific Tables, 1982, Vol. 2, chapter on 'Statistical Methods', §19A; Draper & Smith, 1998, §1.6).

The utility of these results is limited by the importance of the assumption of bivariate normality, and also by the difficulty, referred to earlier, of interpreting the numerical value of a correlation coefficient.

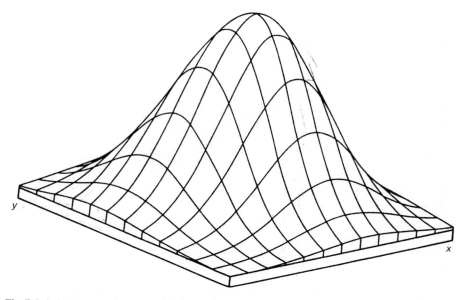

Fig. 7.6 A three-dimensional representation of a bivariate normal distribution, the vertical dimension representing probability density (reprinted from Yule and Kendall, 1950, by permission of the authors and publishers).

Errors of prediction

The best estimate of the mean value of y at a given value of x, say x_0, is given by the regression equation

$$Y = a + bx_0 = \bar{y} + b(x_0 - \bar{x}). \tag{7.20}$$

The sampling variance of Y is

$$\operatorname{var}(Y) = \operatorname{var}(\bar{y}) + (x_0 - \bar{x})^2 \operatorname{var}(b)$$

$$= \sigma^2 \left[\frac{1}{n} + \frac{(x_0 - \bar{x})^2}{\sum(x - \bar{x})^2} \right],$$

which may be estimated by

$$\operatorname{var}(Y) = s_0^2 \left[\frac{1}{n} + \frac{(x_0 - \bar{x})^2}{\sum(x - \bar{x})^2} \right].$$

Again the t distribution on $n - 2$ DF is required. For instance, 95% confidence limits for the predicted mean are

$$Y \pm t_{n-2,\,0.05} s_0 \sqrt{\left[\frac{1}{n} + \frac{(x_0 - \bar{x})^2}{\sum(x - \bar{x})^2} \right]}. \tag{7.21}$$

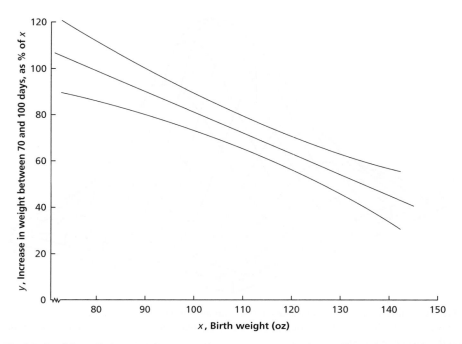

Fig. 7.7 Confidence limits (95%) for the predicted mean value of y for specified values, x_0, of x (data as in Fig. 7.4).

In (7.21) the width of the confidence interval increases with $(x_0 - \bar{x})^2$, and is therefore a minimum when $x_0 = \bar{x}$. Figure 7.7 shows the limits for various values of x_0 in Example 7.1. The reason for the increase in the width of the interval is that slight sampling errors in b will have a greater effect for values of x_0 distant from $\bar{x}$ than for those near $\bar{x}$. The regression line can be thought of as a rod which is free to move up and down (corresponding to the error in $\bar{y}$) and to pivot about a central point (corresponding to the error in b). Points near the ends of the rod will then be subject to greater oscillations than those near the centre.

A different prediction problem is that of estimating an individual value y_0 of y corresponding to a given x_0. The best single estimate is again the value given by the regression equation, but the limits of error are different from those in the previous case. Two slightly different problems can be distinguished.

1   A single prediction is required. The appropriate limits are not strictly confidence limits because the quantity to be estimated is a value taken by a random variable, not a parameter of a distribution. However, writing

$$y_0 = Y + \varepsilon,$$

where ε is the deviation of y_0 from the predicted value Y, we have

$$\text{var}(y_0) = \text{var}(Y) + \text{var}(\varepsilon)$$

$$= \sigma^2 \left[1 + \frac{1}{n} + \frac{(x_0 - \bar{x})^2}{\sum (x - \bar{x})^2} \right], \tag{7.22}$$

and the limits

$$Y \pm t_{n-2,\,0\cdot05} s_0 \sqrt{\left[1 + \frac{1}{n} + \frac{(x_0 - \bar{x})^2}{\sum (x - \bar{x})^2} \right]} \tag{7.23}$$

will include y_0 95% of the time.

2 The object may be to estimate limits within which a certain percentage (say 95%) of the values of y lie when $x = x_0$. Such an interval may be required when a regression has been used to define 'normal' or reference values which are to be used in the assessment of future patients. These limits are

$$\alpha + \beta x_0 \pm 1\cdot96\sigma$$

and are estimated by

$$a + bx_0 \pm 1\cdot96 s_0 = Y \pm 1\cdot96 s_0. \tag{7.24}$$

These limits are a fixed distance from the regression line and lie wholly within the limits of (7.23). When n is very large, $t_{n-2,\,0\cdot05}$ is close to $1\cdot96$, and the second and third terms inside the square root in (7.23) are very small; (7.23) and (7.24) are then almost the same.

Finally, it should be remembered that prediction from a regression formula may be subject to errors other than those of sampling. The linear model may be an inadequate description of the relationship between the two variables. A visual examination of the scatter diagram will provide a partial check, and analytic methods are described in §11.1. Non-linearity may, of course, exist and remain unsuspected because the data at hand provide no indication of it. The danger of using the wrong model is particularly severe if an attempt is made to extrapolate beyond the range of values observed. In Fig. 7.1, for instance, it would be very dangerous to use the regression of y on x to predict the infant mortality in towns with an overcrowding index of $0\cdot4$ or $1\cdot0$.

Comparison of variances in two paired samples

We now return to the comparison of two variances, treated in §5.1 in the case of independent samples. Suppose the two samples are of equal size, n, and there is a natural relationship between a particular value x_{1i} of one sample and the corresponding member x_{2i} of the second sample. Define $X_i = x_{1i} + x_{2i}$ and $Y_i = x_{1i} - x_{2i}$, the sum and difference of paired observations. Thus, we have

Pair	Values of x_1	Values of x_2	Sum	Difference
1	x_{11}	x_{21}	X_1	Y_1
2	x_{12}	x_{22}	X_2	Y_2
.	.	.	.	.
.	.	.	.	.
.	.	.	.	.
n	x_{1n}	x_{2n}	X_n	Y_n

Denoting by x'_{ij} the deviation of x_{ij} from its expectation,

$$\begin{aligned}
\mathrm{cov}(X_i, Y_i) &= \mathrm{E}[(x'_{1i} + x'_{2i})(x'_{1i} - x'_{2i})] \\
&= \mathrm{E}[(x'_{1i})^2 - (x'_{2i})^2] \\
&= \mathrm{var}(x_{1i}) - \mathrm{var}(x_{2i}).
\end{aligned} \tag{7.25}$$

A test of the equality of $\mathrm{var}(x_{1i})$ and $\mathrm{var}(x_{2i})$ is, therefore, the same as a test of the hypothesis that the covariance of X_i and Y_i is zero, which means that the correlation coefficient must also be zero. The test of equality of variances may, therefore, be effected by any of the equivalent tests described above for the hypothesis of zero association between X_i and Y_i. This test is due to E.J.G. Pitman. Its adaptation for purposes of estimation is described by Snedecor and Cochran (1989, §10.8).

7.5 Regression to the mean

The term 'regression' was introduced by Sir Francis Galton (1822–1911) to express the fact that for many inherited characteristics, such as height, the measurements on sons are on average closer to the population mean than the corresponding values for their fathers. The regression coefficient of son's height on father's height is less than 1. The regression of father's height on son's height is also less than 1, so that whether one looks forwards or backwards in generations there is a *regression to the mean*.

Similar phenomena are widely observed in various branches of medicine. Suppose, for instance, that a person's systolic blood pressure is determined by the average of five readings to be 162 mmHg. This is somewhat above the likely population mean of, say, 140 mmHg. If a further reading is taken from the same subject, it will *on average* tend to be less than 162 mmHg. Conversely, a subject with a sample mean less than the population mean will tend to show an increase when retested.

The explanation is closely related to the discussion on shrinkage in §6.4, and anticipates a relevant description of *components of variance* in §8.3. Suppose that repeated blood pressure readings on the ith subject follow a distribution with mean μ_i and variance σ^2, and that the values of μ_i vary from one subject to another with a mean μ_0 and variance σ_0^2. (As noted in §8.3, σ^2 and σ_0^2 are 'components of variance' within and between subjects, respectively.) In terms of the discussion of §6.2, the variation between subjects may be thought of as a prior distribution for μ_i, and the distribution of repeated readings on one subject as providing the likelihood. It follows from the discussion in §§6.2 and 6.4 that, for a subject with a mean blood pressure of $\bar{x}_i$ based on n observations, the estimate of the true mean μ_i will tend to be shrunk from $\bar{x}_i$ towards the population mean μ_0, as will the mean value of a future set of replicate readings.

Suppose that for each subject two independent samples of size n are taken, with means $\bar{x}_{i1}$ and $\bar{x}_{i2}$ for the ith subject. The correlation coefficient between $\bar{x}_{i1}$ and $\bar{x}_{i2}$ is

$$\rho = \frac{\sigma_0^2}{\sigma_0^2 + \sigma^2/n}. \tag{7.26}$$

If the distributions between and within subjects are normal, the joint distribution of $\bar{x}_1$ and $\bar{x}_2$ will be bivariate normal, as in Fig. 7.6, and (7.26) will also measure the regression coefficient of either of the means on the other one. If there were no within-subject variation ($\sigma^2 = 0$), this regression coefficient would be unity. The regression towards the mean is therefore measured by $1 - \rho$, so the smaller ρ is, the greater is the regression towards the mean. Small values of ρ will occur when σ_0^2 is small in relation to the sampling error of the means, e.g. when there is very little real heterogeneity between subjects. High values of ρ will occur when the sampling error is small relative to variance between individuals, and this may be achieved by increasing n.

In some studies of medical interventions, subjects are selected by preliminary screening tests as having high values of a relevant test measurement. For example, in studies of cholesterol-lowering agents, subjects may be selected as having serum cholesterol levels above some critical value, either on a single or on the mean of repeated determinations. On average, even with no effect of the agent under test, subsequent readings on the same subjects would tend to regress toward the mean. A significant reduction below the pretreatment values thus provides no convincing evidence of a treatment effect.

Nevertheless, if precise estimates of the components of variance, and hence of ρ, are available, the extent of regression to the mean can be calculated and allowed for. Gardner and Heady (1973) studied this effect, in relation to cholesterol, blood pressure and daily calorie intake, and gave formulae for the regression effects for various levels of the initial screening cut-off point. As noted above, the effect is reduced by increasing the number of observations made at the initial screen. Johnson and George (1991) extended this work by distinguishing between two sources of within-subject variation: measurement error and physiological fluctuations. The latter type of variation may result in fluctuations that are not independent, showing perhaps cyclical or other trends, a topic discussed in §12.7. In that case, increasing the initial sample size may have a smaller effect on the phenomenon of regression to the mean than would otherwise be so.

Regression to the mean is not a problem when comparing treatments in a randomized controlled trial since both treatment groups will be influenced equally so that the difference will be unbiased, even though the mean improvements of both treatments will include a regression to the mean effect. Another approach is that after selecting patients by a screening test, a second pretreatment value is obtained on admission into the study. This second value, and not the screening value, is used as the initial value in the analysis (McDonald *et al.*, 1983). The extent to which this approach will be successful in eliminating regression to the mean is dependent on the extent to which the second baseline value is independent of the screening value (Senn, 1988).

Newell and Simpson (1990) and Beach and Baron (1998) summarize the phenomenon of regression to the mean and provide additional references.

Example 7.2

Irwig *et al.* (1991) examined the effects of regression to the mean on the screening of individuals to detect those with high levels of blood cholesterol. They considered three hypothetical populations with the following mean values (all values quoted here and below being in units of mmol/l): A, 5·2; B, 5·8; C, 6·4. These values are based on survey data, as being characteristic of men under 35 years and women under 45 (A); men aged 35–74 and women aged 45–64 (B); and women aged 65 and older (C). The calculations are based on the model described above, but with the assumption (again confirmed by observations) that the log of the cholesterol level, rather than the level itself, is normally distributed between and within subjects, with constant within-subject variance.

Standard guidelines would classify levels less than 5·2 as 'desirable', levels between 5·2 and 6·1 as 'borderline high', and those above 6·1 as 'high'. Irwig *et al.* illustrate the effects of regression to the mean in various ways. For instance, an individual in group B with a single screening measurement of 9·0 would have an estimated true mean of 8·4 with 80% confidence limits of 7·7 and 9·2. If the value of 9·0 was based on three measurements, the estimated true level would be 8·8 (limits 8·3, 9·3)—a less pronounced regression effect than for single measurements.

An important concern is that individuals might be classified on the wrong side of a threshold. For instance, an individual in group A with a screening measurement of 4·9 would have a probability of 0·26 of having a true mean above the threshold of 5·2. For a screening measurement of 5·8 there is a probability of 0·10 that the true level is below 5·2.

Other calculations are concerned with the assessment of an intervention intended to lower blood cholesterol. Suppose that an intervention produces a mean reduction of 13% (this figure being based on the results of a particular study). For an individual in group B with three measurements before and one after the intervention, and a pre-intervention mean of 7·8, an observed decrease of 25% corresponds to an estimated true decrease of 19%, while an observed decrease of 0% (no apparent change) corresponds to an estimated true decrease of 5%. In each case there is a shift towards the population mean change of 13%.

The authors conclude that the monitoring of changes in cholesterol levels should play only a limited role in patient management, and that interpretation of such changes should take account of regression to the mean. They argue also that the recommended threshold of 5·2 mmol/l is too low since it is likely to be exceeded by the population mean. Many individuals with single measurements below the threshold, who may for that reason receive reassuring advice, may nevertheless have true values above the threshold.

8 Comparison of several groups

8.1 One-way analysis of variance

The body of techniques called the *analysis of variance* forms a powerful method of analysing the way in which the mean value of a variable is affected by classifications of the data of various sorts. This apparent paradox of nomenclature—that the techniques should be concerned with comparisons of means rather than variances—will be clarified when we come to study the method in detail.

We have already, in §4.3, used the t distribution for the comparison of the means of two groups of data, distinguishing between the paired and unpaired cases. The *one-way analysis of variance*, the subject of the present section, is a generalization of the unpaired t test, appropriate for any number of groups. As we shall see, it is entirely equivalent to the unpaired t test when there are just two groups. The analogous extension of the paired t test will be described in §9.2.

Some examples of a one-way classification of data into several groups are:

1 the reduction in blood sugar recorded for groups of rabbits given different doses of insulin;
2 the value of a certain lung-function test recorded for men of the same age group in a number of different occupational categories;
3 the volumes of liquid taken up by an experimenter using various pipettes to measure a standard quantity, the repeated measurements on any one pipette being grouped together.

In each of these examples a similar question might be asked: What can be said about the variation in blood-sugar reduction from one dose group to another, in lung-function test from one occupational category to another, or in volume of liquid from one pipette to another? There are, however, important differences in the nature of the classification into groups in these three examples. In **1** the groups are defined by dose of insulin and fall into a natural order; in **2** the groups may not fall into a unique order, but some very reasonable classifications of the groups may be suggested—for instance, according to physical effort, intellectual demand, etc.; in **3** the groups of data will almost certainly fall into no natural order. In the present section we are concerned with situations in which no account is taken of any logical ordering of the groups, either because, as in **3**, there is none, or because a consideration of ordering is deferred until a later stage of the analysis.

Suppose there are k groups of observations on a variable y, and that the ith group contains n_i observations. The numbering of the groups from 1 to k will be quite arbitrary, although if there is a simple ordering of the groups it will be natural to use this in the numbering. Further notation is as follows:

Group	1	2 ... i ... k	All groups combined
Number of observations	n_1	n_2 ... n_i ... n_k	$N = \sum_{i=1}^{k} n_i$
Mean of y	$\bar{y}_1$	$\bar{y}_2$ ... $\bar{y}_i$ ... $\bar{y}_k$	$\bar{y} = T/N$
Sum of y	T_1	T_2 ... T_i ... T_k	$T = \sum_{i=1}^{k} T_i$
Sum of y^2	S_1	S_2 ... S_i ... S_k	$S = \sum_{i=1}^{k} S_i$

Note that the entries N, T and S in the final column are the sums along the corresponding rows, but $\bar{y}$ is not the sum of the $\bar{y}_i$ ($\bar{y}$ will be the *mean* of the $\bar{y}_i$ if all the n_i are equal; otherwise $\bar{y}$ is the *weighted mean* of the $\bar{y}_i$, $\sum n_i \bar{y}_i / \sum n_i$). Let the observations within each group be numbered in some arbitrary way, and denote the jth observation in the ith group by y_{ij}.

When a summation is taken over all the N observations, each contributing once to the summation, we shall use the summation sign

$$\sum_{i,j}$$

or, in the text, $\sum_{i,j}$. When the summation is taken over the k groups, each group contributing once, we shall use the sign

$$\sum_{i}$$

or $\sum_i$, whilst summation over the members of a particular group will be denoted by

$$\sum_{j}$$

or $\sum_j$.

The deviation of any observation from the *grand mean*, $\bar{y}$, may be split into two parts, as follows:

$$y_{ij} - \bar{y} = (y_{ij} - \bar{y}_i) + (\bar{y}_i - \bar{y}). \tag{8.1}$$

The first term on the right of (8.1) is the deviation of y_{ij} from its *group mean*, $\bar{y}_i$, and the second term is the deviation of the group mean from the grand mean. If both sides of this equation are squared and summed over all N observations, a similar result holds:

$$\sum_{i,j}(y_{ij} - \bar{y})^2 = \sum_{i,j}(y_{ij} - \bar{y}_i)^2 + \sum_{i,j}(\bar{y}_i - \bar{y})^2, \tag{8.2}$$

since the cross-product term on the right-hand side is zero. This remarkable result means that the 'total' sum of squares about the mean of all N values of y can be partitioned into two parts: (i) the sum of squares of each reading about its own group mean; and (ii) the sum of squares of the deviations of each group mean about the grand mean (these being counted once for every observation). We shall write this result as

Total SSq = Within-Groups SSq + Between-Groups SSq,

'SSq' standing for 'sum of squares'. Note that the Between-Groups SSq may be written

$$\sum_{i,j}(\bar{y}_i - \bar{y})^2 = \sum_{i} n_i(\bar{y}_i - \bar{y})^2,$$

since the contribution $(\bar{y}_i - \bar{y})^2$ is the same for all the n_i observations in the ith group.

Now if there are very large differences between the group means, as compared with the within-group variation, the Between-Groups SSq is likely to be larger than the Within-Groups SSq. If, on the other hand, all the $\bar{y}_i$ are nearly equal and yet there is considerable variation within groups, the reverse is likely to be true. The relative sizes of the Between- and Within-Groups SSq should, therefore, provide an opportunity to assess the variation between group means in comparison with that within groups.

The partitioning of the total sum of squares is most conveniently done by the use of computing formulae analogous to the short-cut formula (2.3) for the sum of squares about the mean of a single sample. These are obtained as follows.

1 *Total SSq.*

$$\sum_{i,j}(y_{ij} - \bar{y})^2 = S - \frac{T^2}{N}, \tag{8.3}$$

by direct application of (2.3).

2 *Within-Groups SSq.*

For the ith group,

$$\sum_{j}(y_{ij} - \bar{y}_i)^2 = S_i - \frac{T_i^2}{n_i}.$$

Summing over the k groups, therefore,

$$\sum_{i,j} (y_{ij} - \bar{y}_i)^2 = \left(S_1 - \frac{T_1^2}{n_1} \right) + \ldots + \left(S_k - \frac{T_k^2}{n_k} \right)$$

$$= \sum_i S_i - \sum_i (T_i^2/n_i)$$

$$= S - \sum_i (T_i^2/n_i). \tag{8.4}$$

3 *Between-Groups SSq.*
  By subtraction, from (8.2),

$$\sum_{i,j} (\bar{y}_i - \bar{y})^2 = \text{Total SSq} - \text{Within-Groups SSq}$$

$$= S - (T^2/N) - \left[S - \sum_i (T_i^2/n_i) \right]$$

$$= \sum_i (T_i^2/n_i) - T^2/N. \tag{8.5}$$

Note that, from (8.5), the Between-Groups SSq is expressible entirely in terms of the group totals, T_i, and the numbers in each group, n_i (and hence in terms of the $\bar{y}_i$ and n_i since $T_i = n_i \bar{y}_i$). This shows clearly that it represents the variation between the group means and not in any way the variation within groups.

Summarizing these results, we have the following formulae for partitioning the total sum of squares:

$$
\left.
\begin{array}{lc}
\text{Between groups} & \sum_i (T_i^2/n_i) - T^2/N \\[2ex]
\text{Within groups} & S - \sum_i (T_i^2/n_i) \\[1ex]
& \rule{3cm}{0.4pt} \\
\text{Total} & S - T^2/N
\end{array}
\right\}. \tag{8.6}
$$

Consider now the problem of testing for evidence of real differences between the groups. Suppose that the n_i observations in the ith group form a random sample from a population with mean μ_i and variance σ^2. As in the two-sample t test, we assume for the moment that σ^2 is the same for all groups. To examine the evidence for differences between the μ_i we shall test the null hypothesis that the μ_i do not vary, being equal to some common unknown value μ. Three ways of estimating σ^2 suggest themselves, as follows.

1 *From the Total SSq.* The whole collection of N observations may be regarded as a random sample of size N, and consequently

$$s_T^2 = \frac{\text{Total SSq}}{N-1}$$

is an unbiased estimate of σ^2.

2   *From the Within-Groups SSq.* Separate unbiased estimates may be got from each group in turn:

$$\frac{S_1 - T_1^2/n_1}{n_1 - 1}, \frac{S_2 - T_2^2/n_2}{n_2 - 1}, \ldots, \frac{S_k - T_k^2/n_k}{n_k - 1}.$$

A combined estimate based purely on variation within groups may be derived (by an extension of the procedure used in the two-sample t test) by adding the numerators and denominators of these ratios, to give the *Within-Groups mean square* (or *MSq*),

$$s_W^2 = \frac{\text{Within-Groups SSq}}{\sum_i (n_i - 1)} = \frac{\text{Within-Groups SSq}}{N-k}.$$

3   *From the Between-Groups SSq.* Since both s_T^2 and s_W^2 are unbiased,

$$\text{E}(s_T^2) = \sigma^2; \text{hence E(Total SSq)} = (N-1)\sigma^2. \tag{8.7}$$

$$\text{E}(s_W^2) = \sigma^2; \text{hence E(Within-Groups SSq)} = (N-k)\sigma^2. \tag{8.8}$$

Subtracting (8.8) from (8.7),

$$\text{E (Between-Groups SSq)} = (N-1)\sigma^2 - (N-k)\sigma^2$$
$$= (k-1)\sigma^2.$$

Hence, a third unbiased estimate is given by the *Between-Groups MSq*,

$$s_B^2 = \frac{\text{Between-Groups SSq}}{k-1}.$$

The divisor $k-1$ is reasonable, being one less than the number of groups, just as the divisor for s_T^2 is one less than the number of observations.

These results hold if the null hypothesis is true. Suppose, however, that the μ_i are not all equal. The Within-Groups MSq is still an unbiased estimate of σ^2, since it is based purely on the variation within groups. The Between-Groups MSq, being based on the variation between group means, will tend to increase. In fact, in general, when the μ_i differ

$$\text{E}(s_B^2) = \sigma^2 + \frac{\sum_i n_i (\mu_i - \bar{\mu})^2}{k-1}, \tag{8.9}$$

where $\bar{\mu}$ is the weighted mean of the μ_i, $\sum_i n_i \mu_i / N$. Some indication of whether the μ_i differ can therefore be obtained from a comparison of s_B^2 and s_W^2. On the null hypothesis these two mean squares estimate the same quantity and therefore should not usually be too different; if the null hypothesis is not true s_B^2 is, from (8.9), on average greater than σ^2 and will tend to be greater than s_W^2.

An appropriate test of the null hypothesis, therefore, may be based on the *variance ratio* (VR) s_B^2/s_W^2, which will be denoted by F. The distribution of F depends on the nature of the distributions of the y_{ij} about their mean $\bar{y}_i$. If the further assumption is made that these distributions are normal, it can be shown that s_B^2 and s_W^2 behave like two *independent* estimates of variance, on $k-1$ and $N-k$ degrees of freedom (DF), respectively. The relevant distribution, the F distribution, has been discussed in §5.1. Departures from the null hypothesis will tend to give values of F greater than unity. A significance test for the null hypothesis should, therefore, count as significant only those values of F which are sufficiently large; that is, a one-sided test is required. As observed in §5.1, the critical levels of F are tabulated in terms of single-tail probabilities, so the tabulated values (Table A4) apply directly to the present situation (the single-tail form of tabulation in fact arose to serve the needs of the analysis of variance).

If $k=2$, the situation considered above is precisely that for which the unpaired (or two-sample) t test was introduced in §4.3. The variance ratio, F, will have 1 and $N-2$ degrees of freedom and t will have $n_1 + n_2 - 2$, i.e. $N-2$ degrees of freedom. The two solutions are, in fact, equivalent in the sense that (i) the value of F is equal to the square of the value of t; (ii) the distribution of F on 1 and $N-2$ degrees of freedom is precisely the same as the distribution of the square of a variable following the t distribution on $N-2$ degrees of freedom. The former statement may be proved algebraically in a few lines. The second has already been noted in §5.1.

If $k=2$ and $n_1 = n_2 = \frac{1}{2}N$ (i.e. there are two groups of equal size), a useful result is that the Between-Groups SSq (8.5) may be written in the alternative form

$$\frac{(T_1 - T_2)^2}{N}. \tag{8.10}$$

If $k>2$, we may wish to examine the difference between a particular pair of means, chosen because the contrast between these particular groups is of logical interest. The standard error (SE) of the difference between two means, say $\bar{y}_g$ and $\bar{y}_h$, may be estimated by

$$\text{SE}(\bar{y}_g - \bar{y}_h) = \sqrt{\left[s_W^2 \left(\frac{1}{n_g} + \frac{1}{n_h}\right)\right]}, \tag{8.11}$$

and the difference $\bar{y}_g - \bar{y}_h$ tested by referring

$$t = \frac{\bar{y}_g - \bar{y}_h}{\text{SE}(\bar{y}_g - \bar{y}_h)}$$

to the t distribution on $N - k$ degrees of freedom (since this is the number of DF associated with the estimate of variance s^2). Confidence limits for the difference in means may be set in the usual way, using tabulated percentiles of t on $N - k$ DF. The only function of the analysis of variance in this particular comparison has been to replace the estimate of variance on $n_g + n_h - 2$ DF (which would be used in the two-sample t test) by the pooled Within-Groups MSq on $N - k$ DF. This may be a considerable advantage if n_g and n_h are small. It has been gained, however, by invoking an assumption that all the groups are subject to the same within-groups variance and if there is doubt about the near-validity of this assumption it will be safer to rely on the data from the two groups alone.

If there are no contrasts between groups which have an a priori claim on our attention, further scrutiny of the differences between means could be made to depend largely on the F test in the analysis of variance. If the variance ratio is not significant, or even suggestively large, there will be little point in examining differences between pairs of means. If F is significant, there is reasonable evidence that real differences exist and are large enough to reveal themselves above the random variation. It then seems natural to see what can safely be said about the direction and magnitude of these differences. This topic will be taken up again in §8.4.

Example 8.1

During each of four experiments on the use of carbon tetrachloride as a worm killer, 10 rats were infested with larvae. Eight days later, five rats were treated with carbon tetrachloride, the other five being kept as controls. After two more days the rats were killed and the number of adult worms counted. It was thought useful to examine the significance of the differences between the means for the four control groups. If significant differences could be established they might be related to definable changes in experimental conditions, thus leading to a reduction of variation in future work. The results and the details of the calculations are shown in Table 8.1. The value of F is 2·27, and comparison with the F table for $v_1 = 3$ and $v_2 = 16$ shows the result to be non-significant at $P = 0.05$. (Actually $P = 0.12$.)

The standard error of the difference between two means is $\sqrt{[2(3997)/5]} = 40.0$. Note that the difference between $\bar{y}_3$ and $\bar{y}_4$ is more than twice its standard error, but since the F value is not significant we should not pay much attention to this particular comparison unless it presents some prior interest (see also §8.4).

Two important assumptions underlying the F test in the one-way analysis of variance are: (i) the normality of the distribution of the y_{ij} about their mean μ_i; and (ii) the equality of the variances in the various groups. The F test is not unduly sensitive to moderate departures from normality, but it will often be worth considering whether some form of transformation (§10.8) will improve matters. The assumption about equality of variances is more serious. It has already been suggested that, for comparisons of two means, where there is

Table 8.1 One-way analysis of variance: differences between four groups of control rats in counts of adult worms.

	Experiment				
	1	2	3	4	All groups
	279	378	172	381	
	338	275	335	346	
	334	412	335	340	
	198	265	282	471	
	303	286	250	318	
T_i	1452	1616	1374	1856	$T = 6298$
n_i	5	5	5	5	$N = 20$
$\bar{y}_i$	290·4	323·2	274·8	371·2	
S_i	434654	540274	396058	703442	$S = 2074428$
T_i^2/n_i	421661	522291	377575	688947	

Between-Groups SSq $= 421\,661 + \ldots + 688\,947 - (6298)^2/20$

$\qquad\qquad\qquad = 2\,010\,474 - 1\,983\,240$

$\qquad\qquad\qquad = 27\,234$

Total SSq $\qquad = 2\,074\,428 - 1\,983\,240$

$\qquad\qquad\qquad = 91\,188$

Within-Groups SSq $= 91\,188 - 27\,234$

$\qquad\qquad\qquad = 63\,954$

Analysis of variance

	SSq	DF	MSq	VR
Between groups	27 234	3	9078	2·27
Within groups	63 954	16	3997	
Total	91 188	19		

doubt about the validity of a pooled within-group estimate of variance, it may be advisable to estimate the variance from the two groups alone. A transformation of the scale of measurement may bring about near-equality of variances. If it fails to do so, an approximate test for differences of means may be obtained by a method described in §8.2.

8.2 The method of weighting

In the one-way analysis of variance we are interested in a series of k means, $\bar{y}_i$, which may have different variances because the group sizes n_i may differ. We ask whether the $\bar{y}_i$ could be regarded as *homogeneous*, in the sense that they could easily differ by sampling variation from some common value, or whether they should be regarded as *heterogeneous*, in the sense that sampling variation is unlikely to explain the differences among them.

We now consider a method of wide generality for tackling other problems of this sort. It depends on certain assumptions, which may or may not be precisely true in any particular application, but it is nevertheless very useful in providing approximate solutions to many problems. The general situation is that data are available in k groups, each providing an estimate of some parameter. We wish first to test whether there is evidence of heterogeneity between the estimates, and then in the absence of heterogeneity to obtain a single estimate of the parameter from the whole data set.

Suppose we observe k quantities, $Y_1, Y_2, \ldots, Y_k$, and we know that Y_i is $N(\mu_i, V_i)$, where the means μ_i are unknown but the variances V_i are known. To test the hypothesis that all the μ_i are equal to some specified value μ, we could calculate a *weighted* sum of squares

$$G_0 = \sum_i [(Y_i - \mu)^2 / V_i] = \sum_i w_i (Y_i - \mu)^2, \qquad (8.12)$$

where $w_i = 1/V_i$. The quantity G_0 is the sum of squares of k standardized normal deviates and, from (5.2), it follows the $\chi^2_{(k)}$ distribution.

However, to test the hypothesis of homogeneity we do not usually wish to specify the value μ. Let us replace μ by the *weighted* mean

$$\overline{Y} = \frac{\sum_i w_i Y_i}{\sum_i w_i}, \qquad (8.13)$$

and calculate

$$G = \sum_i w_i (Y_i - \overline{Y})^2. \qquad (8.14)$$

The quantity w_i is called a *weight*: note that it is the reciprocal of the variance V_i, so if, for example, Y_1 is more precise than Y_2, then $V_1 < V_2$ and $w_1 > w_2$ and Y_1 will be given the higher weight.

A little algebra gives the alternative formula:

$$G = \sum_i w_i Y_i^2 - (\sum_i w_i Y_i)^2 / \sum_i w_i. \qquad (8.15)$$

Note that if all the $w_i = 1$, (8.14) is the usual sum of squares about the mean, $\overline{Y}$ becomes the usual unweighted mean and (8.15) becomes the usual short-cut formula (2.3).

It can be shown that, on the null hypothesis of homogeneity, G is distributed as $\chi^2_{(k-1)}$. Replacing μ by $\overline{Y}$ has resulted in the loss of one degree of freedom. High values of G indicate evidence against homogeneity.

If there is a variable x_i associated with each Y_i then a linear relationship between Y_i and x_i is tested by

$$G_L = \frac{\sum w_i x_i Y_i - \dfrac{\sum w_i x_i \sum w_i Y_i^2}{\sum w_i}}{\sum w_i x_i^2 - \dfrac{(\sum w_i x_i)^2}{\sum w_i}}. \tag{8.16}$$

This follows from the form of the SSq due to regression in Table 11.1 and the method of weighted analysis (see p. 216). On the null hypothesis that Y_i is unassociated with x_i, G_L is distributed as $\chi^2_{(1)}$, whilst high values of G_L indicate evidence against homogeneity in favour of a linear relationship.

If homogeneity is accepted, it will often be reasonable to estimate μ, the common value of the μ_i. The best estimate (in the sense of having the lowest variance) is the weighted mean $\overline{Y}$, defined earlier. Moreover, if the null hypothesis of homogeneity is true, $\mathrm{var}(\overline{Y}) = 1/\sum_i w_i$, and confidence limits for μ may be obtained by using the percentiles of the normal distribution. Thus, 95% limits are

$$\overline{Y} \pm 1\cdot 96\sqrt{(1/\textstyle\sum_i w_i)}.$$

Let us see how this general theory might be applied to the problem of comparing k independent means, using the notation of §8.1. Write $Y_i = \bar{y}_i$ and $V_i = \sigma^2/n_i$. Then

$$\overline{Y} = \sum_i n_i \bar{y}_i / \sum_i n_i = \bar{y},$$

the overall mean; and

$$G = \frac{\sum_i n_i (\bar{y}_i - \bar{y})^2}{\sigma^2} = \frac{\text{Between-Groups SSq}}{\sigma^2}.$$

If σ^2 were known, G could be tested from the $\chi^2_{(k-1)}$ distribution. In practice, we estimate σ^2 by the Within-Groups MSq, s_W^2, and replace G by

$$G' = \frac{\text{Between-Groups SSq}}{s_W^2} = \frac{(k-1)s_B^2}{s_W^2}.$$

This is $k - 1$ times the variance ratio, which we have already seen follows the F distribution on $k - 1$ and $N - k$ DF. For these degrees of freedom the distributions of $(k - 1)F$ and $\chi^2_{(k-1)}$ are exactly equivalent when $N = \infty$ (see §5.1). For reasonably large N the two methods will give closely similar results.

Consider now the possibility mentioned at the end of §8.1, that the groups have different variances σ_i^2. Write $Y_i = \bar{y}_i$ and $V_i = \sigma_i^2/n_i$. Again, the σ_i^2 are unknown, but they may be estimated by

$$s_i^2 = [S_i - (T_i^2/n_i)]/(n_i - 1),$$

and an approximate or *empirical* weight calculated as

$$w_i' = n_i/s_i^2.$$

We calculate the weighted sum of squares (8.15) as

$$G'' = \sum_i w_i' \bar{y}_i^2 - \left(\sum_i w_i' \bar{y}_i\right)^2 / \sum_i w_i'.$$

On the null hypothesis of homogeneity of the μ_i, G'' is distributed approximately as $\chi^2_{(k-1)}$, high values indicating excessive disparity between the $\bar{y}_i$. The approximation is increasingly inaccurate for smaller values of the n_i (say, below about 10), and a refinement is given by James (1951) and Welch (1951). For an application of this method in a comparison of sets of pock counts, see Armitage (1957, p. 579).

8.3 **Components of variance**

In some studies which lead to a one-way analysis of variance, the groups may be of no great interest individually, but may nevertheless represent an interesting source of variation. The result of a pipetting operation, for example, may vary from one pipette to another. A comparison between a particular pair of pipettes would be of little interest; furthermore, a test of the null hypothesis that the different pipettes give identical results on average may be pointless because there may quite clearly be a systematic difference between instruments. A more relevant question here will be: how great is the variation between pipettes as compared with that of repeated readings on the same pipette?

A useful framework is to regard the k groups as being randomly selected from a population of such groups. This will not usually be strictly true, but it serves as an indication that the groups are of interest only as representing a certain type of variation. This framework is often called *Model II*, or the *random-effects model*, as distinct from *Model I*, or the *fixed-effects model*, considered in §8.1.

Suppose, in the first instance, that each group contains the same number, n, of observations. (In the notation of §8.1, all the n_i are equal to n.) Let μ_i be the 'true' mean for the ith group and suppose that in the population of groups μ_i is distributed with mean μ and variance σ_B^2. Readings within the ith group have mean μ_i and variance σ^2. The quantities σ^2 and σ_B^2 are called *components of variance* within and between groups respectively. The situation is illustrated in Fig. 8.1. The data at our disposal consist of a random sample of size n from each of k randomly selected groups.

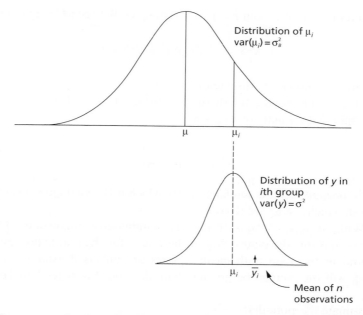

Fig. 8.1 Components of variance between and within groups, with normal distributions for each component of random variation.

Consider first the variance of a single group mean, $\bar{y}_i$. We have

$$\bar{y}_i - \mu = (\mu_i - \mu) + (\bar{y}_i - \mu_i),$$

and the two terms in parentheses represent independent sources of variation—that of μ_i about μ and that of $\bar{y}_i$ about μ_i. Therefore, using (5.10),

$$\text{var}(\bar{y}_i) = \text{var}(\mu_i) + \text{var}(\bar{y}_i, \text{given } \mu_i)$$
$$= \sigma_B^2 + (\sigma^2/n). \tag{8.17}$$

Now, the analysis of variance will have the following structure:

	DF	MSq
Between groups	$k - 1$	s_B^2
Within groups	$k(n - 1)$	s_W^2
Total	$nk - 1 \ (= N - 1)$	

The Between-Groups SSq is (with notation for T_i and T as in §8.1)

$$\frac{\sum T_i^2}{n} - \frac{T^2}{N}$$
$$= n\left[\sum \bar{y}_i^2 - (\sum \bar{y}_i)^2/k\right],$$

summations running from $i = 1$ to k. Thus, the Between-Groups MSq, s_B^2,

$$= n\left[\sum \bar{y}_i^2 - (\sum \bar{y}_i)^2/k\right]/(k-1)$$

$= n$ times an unbiased estimate of $\mathrm{var}(\bar{y}_i)$
$= n$ times an unbiased estimate of $\sigma_B^2 + (\sigma^2/n)$, from (8.17),
$=$ an unbiased estimate of $n\sigma_B^2 + \sigma^2$.
That is,

$$\mathrm{E}\left(s_B^2\right) = \sigma^2 + n\sigma_B^2. \tag{8.18}$$

This important result is similar to (8.9), which is the analogous result for the situation in which the μ_i are fixed.

The Within-Groups MSq is (from §8.1) an unbiased estimate of σ^2. The result (8.18) thus confirms the plausibility of the F test, for the null hypothesis is that $\sigma_B^2 = 0$ and in this case both mean squares are unbiased estimates of σ^2. If $\sigma_B^2 > 0, s_B^2$ will on average be greater than s_W^2, and F will tend to be greater than 1.

To estimate σ_B^2, note that

$$\mathrm{E}(s_B^2 - s_W^2) = \mathrm{E}(s_B^2) - \mathrm{E}(s_W^2)$$
$$= (\sigma^2 + n\sigma_B^2) - \sigma^2$$
$$= n\sigma_B^2.$$

Hence, an unbiased estimate of σ_B^2 is given by

$$\hat{\sigma}_B^2 = \frac{s_B^2 - s_W^2}{n}. \tag{8.19}$$

If $s_B^2 < s_W^2$ (as will often be the case if σ_B^2 is zero or near zero), $\hat{\sigma}_B^2$ is negative. There is a case for replacing $\hat{\sigma}_B^2$ by 0 when this happens, but it should be noted that the unbiased property of (8.19) is then lost.

Example 8.2

Bacharach *et al.* (1940) carried out an experiment on 'diffusing factor', a substance which, when present in an inoculation into the skin of rabbits, spreads the blister caused by the inoculation. They gave inoculations of the same dose at six sites on the back of each of six animals. Their experimental design permitted a study of the influence of the particular site and the order of administration, but there was no evidence that these factors had any effect and we shall regard the data as forming a one-way classification: between and within animals. The variable analysed is the area of the blister (square centimetres).

An analysis of variance was as follows:

	SSq	DF	MSq	VR
Between animals	12·8333	5	2·5667	4·39
Within animals	17·5266	30	0·5842	
Total	30·3599	35		

We have

$$\hat{\sigma}_B^2 = (2 \cdot 5667 - 0 \cdot 5842)/6$$
$$= 0 \cdot 3304.$$

The two components of variance are then estimated as follows, where each is expressed as a percentage of the total:

Between animals	$\hat{\sigma}_B^2$	0·3304	36%
Within animals	s_W^2	0·5842	64%
Total	$\hat{\sigma}_B^2 + s_W^2$	0·9146	100%

The sum of the two components is the estimated variance of a single reading from a randomly chosen rabbit, and the analysis shows that of this total variance 36% is estimated to be attributable to systematic differences between rabbits. (For further analysis of these data, see below; see also Example 9.4, p. 260.)

Confidence limits for σ^2 are obtained from the Within-Groups SSq by use of the χ^2 distribution, as in §5.1. Confidence limits for σ_B^2 are rather more troublesome. An approximate solution is recommended by Boardman (1974). For $100(1 - \alpha)\%$ confidence limits we need various entries in the F table corresponding to a tabulated one-sided level of $\frac{1}{2}\alpha$. Thus, for 95% confidence limits we need entries corresponding to $P = 0 \cdot 025$. Denoting the entry for degrees of freedom ν_1 and ν_2 as F_{ν_1, ν_2}, and putting $f_1 = k - 1$, $f_2 = k(n - 1)$, we need

$$F_1 = F_{f_1, f_2}$$
$$F_2 = F_{f_1, \infty}$$
$$F_3 = F_{f_2, f_1}$$
$$F_4 = F_{\infty, f_1}$$
$$F = \text{observed value}, s_B^2/s_W^2.$$

Then the upper limit for σ_B^2 is

$$\hat{\sigma}_{BU}^2 = F_4 \left(F - \frac{1}{F_3} \right) \left(\frac{s_W^2}{n} \right) \qquad (8.20)$$

and the lower limit is

$$\hat{\sigma}_{BL}^2 = \left(\frac{F - F_1}{F_2} \right) \left(\frac{s_W^2}{n} \right). \qquad (8.21)$$

Note that the lower limit is zero if $F = F_1$, i.e. if F is just significant by the usual test. If $F < F_1$, the lower limit will be negative and in some instances the upper limit may also be negative. For a discussion of this apparent anomaly, see Scheffé (1959, §7.2). The validity of these limits will depend rather heavily on the assumption of normality, particularly for the between-groups variation.

Example 8.2, continued

The 95% confidence limits for σ^2 are (from §5.1)

$$\frac{17 \cdot 5266}{46 \cdot 98}$$

and

$$\frac{17 \cdot 5266}{16 \cdot 79},$$

i.e.

$$0 \cdot 373 \text{ and } 1 \cdot 044,$$

the divisors being the appropriate percentiles of the $\chi^2_{(30)}$ distribution.

For confidence limits for σ^2_B we need the following tabulated values of F, writing $f_1 = 5$, $f_2 = 30$:

$$F_1 = 3 \cdot 03, F_2 = 2 \cdot 57, F_3 = 6 \cdot 23, F_4 = 6 \cdot 02,$$

and the observed F is 4·39. Thus, from (8.20) and (8.21),

$$\hat{\sigma}^2_{BU} = (6 \cdot 02) \left(4 \cdot 39 - \frac{1}{6 \cdot 23} \right) (0 \cdot 0974) = 2 \cdot 48$$

and

$$\hat{\sigma}^2_{BL} = \left(\frac{4 \cdot 39 - 3 \cdot 03}{2 \cdot 57} \right) (0 \cdot 0974) = 0 \cdot 052.$$

The wide ranges of error associated with these estimates makes it clear that the percentage contributions of 36% and 64% are very imprecise estimates indeed.

If the numbers of observations from the groups are unequal, with n_i from the ith group, (8.19) must be modified as follows:

$$\hat{\sigma}^2_B = \frac{s^2_B - s^2_W}{n_0}, \tag{8.22}$$

where

$$n_0 = \frac{1}{(k-1)} \left[N - \frac{\sum n^2_i}{N} \right].$$

A further difficulty is that (8.22) is not necessarily the best way of estimating σ_B^2. The choice of method depends, however, on the unknown ratio of the variance components which are being estimated, and (8.22) will usually be a sensible method if the n_i are not too different. See Searle (1987, §13.3) and Robinson (1998) for a fuller discussion of the issues involved. The situation corresponds to a multilevel model, methods for analysing which are given in §12.5.

8.4 **Multiple comparisons**

We return now to the fixed-effects model of §8.1. In the analysis of data in this form it will usually be important not to rely solely on the analysis of variance table and its F test, but to examine the differences between groups more closely to see what patterns emerge. It is, in fact, good practice habitually to report the mean values $\bar{y}_i$ and their standard errors, calculated as $s_W/\sqrt{n_i}$, in terms of the Within-Groups MSq s_W^2 unless the assumption of constant variance is clearly inappropriate.

The standard error of the difference between two means is given by (8.11), and the t distribution may be used to provide a significance test or to assign confidence limits, as indicated in §8.1. If all the n_i are equal (to n, say), it is sometimes useful to calculate the *least significant difference* (LSD) at a certain significance level. For the 5% level, for instance, this is

$$t_{f_2,\,0.05}\,s_W\,\sqrt{(2/n)},$$

where $f_2 = k(n-1)$, the degrees of freedom within groups. Differences between pairs of means which are significant at this level can then be picked out by eye.

Sometimes interest is focused on comparisons between the group means other than simple differences. These will usually be measurable by a *linear contrast* of the form

$$L = \sum \lambda_i \bar{y}_i, \tag{8.23}$$

where $\sum \lambda_i = 0$. From (5.10),

$$\operatorname{var}(L) = \sum \lambda_i^2 \operatorname{var}(\bar{y}_i),$$

and the standard error of L is thus estimated as

$$\operatorname{SE}(L) = s_W \sqrt{(\sum \lambda_i^2/n)}, \tag{8.24}$$

and the usual t test or confidence limits may be applied.

Some examples of linear contrasts are as follows.

1 *A contrast of one group with the mean of several other groups.* One group may have a special identity, perhaps as a control group, and there may be some reason for pooling a set of q other groups (e.g. if related treatments have been applied to these groups). The relevant comparison will then be

$$\bar{y}_c - \left(\sum_{i=1}^{q} \bar{y}_i\right) \Big/ q,$$

which, when multiplied by q becomes

$$L_1 = q\bar{y}_c - \sum_{i=1}^{q} \bar{y}_i,$$

a particular case of (8.23) with $\lambda_c = q, \lambda_i = -1$ for all i in the set of q groups and $\lambda_i = 0$ otherwise. Note that $\sum \lambda_i = 0$.

2 *A linear regression coefficient.* Suppose that a set of q groups is associated with a variable x_i (for example, the dose of some substance). It might be of interest to ask whether the regression of y on x is significant. Using the result quoted in the derivation of (7.13),

$$L_2 = \sum(x_i - \bar{x})\bar{y}_i,$$

which again is a particular case of (8.23) with $\lambda_i = x_i - \bar{x}$, and again $\sum \lambda_i = 0$.

3 *A difference between two means.* The difference between $\bar{y}_g$ and $\bar{y}_h$ is another case of (8.23) with $\lambda_g = 1, \lambda_h = -1$ and all other $\lambda_i = 0$.

Corresponding to any linear contrast, L, the t statistic, on $k(n-1)$ DF, is from (8.24),

$$t = \frac{L}{\text{SE}(L)} = \frac{L}{s_W \sqrt{\left(\sum \lambda_i^2/n\right)}}.$$

As we have seen, the square of t follows the F distribution on 1 and $k(n-1)$ DF. Thus,

$$F = t^2 = \frac{L^2}{s_W^2 \sum \lambda_i^2/n} = \frac{s_1^2}{s_W^2},$$

where $s_1^2 = L^2/(\sum \lambda_i^2/n)$. In fact, s_1^2 can be regarded as an MSq on 1 DF, derived from an SSq also equal to s_1^2, which can be shown to be part of the SSq between groups of the analysis of variance. The analysis thus takes the following form:

	SSq	DF	MSq	VR
Between groups				
Due to L	$L^2/(\sum \lambda_i^2/n)$	1	s_1^2	$F_1 = s_1^2/s_W^2$
Other contrasts	$\sum T_i^2/n - T^2/n - L^2/(\sum \lambda_i^2/n)$	$k-2$	s_R^2	$F_2 = s_R^2/s_W^2$
Within groups	$S - \sum T_i^2/n$	$k(n-1)$	s_W^2	
Total	$S - T^2/nk$	$nk - 1$		

Separate significance tests are now provided: (i) by F_1 on 1 and $k(n-1)$ DF for the contrast L; as we have seen, this is equivalent to the t test for L; and (ii) by F_2 on $k-2$ and $k(n-1)$ DF for differences between group means other than those measured by L.

Suppose there are two or more linear contrasts of interest:

$$L_1 = \sum \lambda_{1i}\bar{y}_i, \ L_2 = \sum \lambda_{2i}\bar{y}_i, \text{ etc.}$$

Can the single degrees of freedom for these contrasts all be incorporated in the same analysis of variance? They can, provided the Ls are uncorrelated when the null hypothesis is true, and the condition for this is that for any two contrasts (L_p and L_q, say) the sum of products of the coefficients is zero:

$$\sum_{i=1}^{k} \lambda_{pi}\lambda_{qi} = 0.$$

In this case L_p and L_q are said to be *orthogonal*. If there are k' such orthogonal contrasts ($k' < k$), the analysis of variance is extended to include a separate row for each L_i, each with 1 DF, and the SSq for other contrasts, with $k - k' - 1$ DF, is again obtained by subtraction.

The straightforward use of the t or F tests is appropriate for any differences between means or for more general linear contrasts which arise naturally out of the structure of the investigation. However, a difficulty must be recognized. If there are k groups, there are $\frac{1}{2}k(k-1)$ pairs of means which might conceivably be compared and there is no limit to the number of linear contrasts which might be formed. These comparisons are not all independent, but it is fairly clear that, even when the null hypothesis is true, in any set of data *some* of these contrasts are likely to be significant. A sufficiently assiduous search will often reveal some remarkable contrasts which have arisen purely by chance. This may not matter if scrutiny is restricted to those comparisons on which the study was designed to throw light. If, on the other hand, the data are subjected to what is sometimes called a *dredging* procedure—a search for significant contrasts which would not have been thought of initially—there is a real danger that a number of comparisons will be reported as significant, but that they will almost all have arisen by chance.

A number of procedures have been devised to reduce the chance of this happening. They are referred to as methods of making *multiple comparisons* or *simultaneous inference*, and are described in detail by Miller (1981) and Hsu (1996). We mention briefly two methods, one for differences between means and the other for more general linear contrasts.

The first method, based on the distribution of the *studentized range*, is due to Newman (1939) and Keuls (1952). Given a set of p means, each based on n observations, the studentized range, Q, is the range of the $\bar{y}_i$ divided by the estimated standard error. In an obvious notation,

$$Q = \frac{\bar{y}_{\max} - \bar{y}_{\min}}{s/\sqrt{n}}. \tag{8.25}$$

The distribution of Q, on the null hypothesis that all the μ_i are equal, has been studied and some upper 5% and 1% points are given in Appendix Table A5. They depend on the number of groups, p, and the within-groups degrees of freedom, f_2, and are written $Q_{p,0.05}$ and $Q_{p,0.01}$. The procedure is to rank the $\bar{y}_i$ in order of magnitude and to test the Studentized range for all pairs of adjacent means (when it actually reduces to the usual t test), for all adjacent triads, all groups of four adjacent means, and so on. Two means are regarded as differing significantly only if all tests for sets of means, including these two, give a significant result. The procedure is most readily performed in the opposite order to that described, starting with all k, following by the two sets of $k - 1$ adjacent means, and so on. The reason for this is that, if at any stage a non-significant Q is found, that set of means need not be used for any further tests. The procedure will, for example, stop after the first stage if Q for all k means is non-significant.

The following example is taken from Miller (1981, §6.1). Five means, arranged in order, are 16·1, 17·0, 20·7, 21·1 and 26·5; $n = 5$, $f_2 = 20$, and the standard error $s/\sqrt{5} = 1·2$. The values of $Q_{p,0.05}$ for $p = 2$, 3, 4 and 5 are, respectively, 2·95, 3·58, 3·96 and 4·23. Tests are done successively for $p = 5$, 4, 3 and 2, and the results are as follows, where non-significant groupings are indicated by underlining.

A	B	C	D	E
16·1	17·0	20·7	21·1	26·5

The interpretation is that E differs from $\{A, B, C, D\}$, and that within the latter group A differs from C and D, with B occupying an ambiguous position.

In Example 8.1, where we noted that $\bar{y}_3$ and $\bar{y}_4$ differed by more than twice the standard error of the difference, Q calculated for all four groups is

$$(371·2 - 274·8)/\sqrt{(3997/5)} = 96·4/28·3 = 3·41,$$

and from Table A5 $Q_{4,0.05}$ is 4·05, so the test shows no significant difference, as might have been expected in view of the non-significant F test.

The Newman–Keuls procedure has the property that, for a set of groups with equal μ_i, the probability of asserting a significant difference between any of them is at most equal to the specified significance level (0·05 in the above examples). If the null hypothesis is untrue, however, the method has the property that the probability of making at least one incorrect assertion on the pattern of differences between the means may exceed the significance level (Hsu, 1996). A modification to ensure that, whatever the pattern of differences between means, the probability of making at least one incorrect assertion will not exceed the significance level was suggested by Einot and Gabriel (1975). The first step of this modified method is exactly as for the Newman–Keuls method but in subsequent steps the critical values exceed those given in Table A5.

If linear contrasts other than differences are being 'dredged', the infinite number of possible choices suggests that a very conservative procedure should be used, that is, one which indicates significance much less readily than the t test. A method proposed by Scheffé (1959) is as follows. A linear contrast, L, is declared significant at, say, the 5% level if the absolute value of $L/\text{SE}(L)$ exceeds

$$\sqrt{[(k-1)F_{0.05}]}, \tag{8.26}$$

where $F_{0.05}$ is the tabulated 5% point of the F distribution with $k-1$ and $k(n-1)$ DF. When $k = 2$, this rule is equivalent to the use of the t test. For $k > 2$ it is noticeably conservative in comparison with a t test, in that the numerical value of (8.26) may considerably exceed the 5% level of t on $k(n-1)$ degrees of freedom. Scheffé's method has the property that, if the null hypothesis that all μ_i are equal is true, only in 5% of cases will it be possible to find any linear contrast which is significant by this test. Any contrast significant by this test, even if discovered by an exhaustive process of data dredging, may therefore be regarded with a reasonable degree of confidence. In Example 8.1 the contrast between the means for experiments 3 and 4 gives $L/\text{SE}(L) = (371.2 - 274.8)/40.0 = 2.41$; by Scheffé's test the 5% value would be $\sqrt{[3(3.24)]} = 3.12$, and the observed contrast should not be regarded as significant.

It should again be emphasized that the Newman–Keuls and Scheffé procedures, and other multiple-comparison methods, are deliberately conservative in order to reduce the probability of too many significant differences arising by chance in any one study. They are appropriate only when means are being compared in an exploratory way to see what might 'turn up'. When comparisons are made which flow naturally from the plan of the experiment or survey, the usual t test is appropriate.

8.5 Comparison of several proportions: the $2 \times k$ contingency table

In §4.5 the comparison of two proportions was considered from two points of view—the sampling error of the difference between the proportions and the χ^2 significance test applied to the 2×2 table. We saw that these two approaches led to equivalent significance tests of the null hypothesis.

Where more than two proportions are to be compared the calculation of standard errors between pairs of proportions raises points similar to those discussed in §8.4: many comparisons are possible and an undue number of significance differences may arise by chance. However, an overall significance test, analogous to the F test in the analysis of variance, is provided by a straightforward extension of the χ^2 test.

Suppose there are k groups of observations and that in the ith group n_i individuals have been observed, of whom r_i show a certain characteristic (say, being 'positive'). The proportion of positives, r_i/n_i, is denoted by p_i. The data may be displayed as follows:

	1	2	...	i	...	k	All groups combined
Group	1	2	...	i	...	k	combined
Positive	r_1	r_2	...	r_i	...	r_k	R
Negative	$n_1 - r_1$	$n_2 - r_2$	...	$n_i - r_i$	...	$n_k - r_k$	$N - R$
Total	n_1	n_2	...	n_i	...	n_k	N
Proportion positive	p_1	p_2	...	p_i	...	p_k	$P = R/N$

The frequencies form a $2 \times k$ contingency table (there being two rows and k columns, excluding the marginal totals). The χ^2 test follows the same lines as for the 2×2 table (§4.5). For each of the observed frequencies, O, an expected frequency is calculated by the formula

$$E = \frac{\text{Row total} \times \text{Column total}}{N}. \tag{8.27}$$

The quantity $(O - E)^2/E$ is calculated, and, finally

$$X^2 = \sum \frac{(O - E)^2}{E} \tag{8.28}$$

the summation being over the $2k$ cells in the table.

On the null hypothesis that all k samples are drawn randomly from populations with the same proportion of positives, X^2 is distributed approximately as $\chi^2_{(k-1)}$, the approximation improving as the expected frequencies increase in size. An indication of the extent to which the $\chi^2_{(k-1)}$ distribution is valid for small frequencies is given in §8.6. No continuity correction is required, because unless the observed frequencies are very small the number of tables which may be formed with the same marginal totals as those observed is very large, and the distribution of X^2 is consequently more nearly continuous than is the case for 2×2 tables.

An alternative formula for X^2 is of some value. The value of $O - E$ for an entry in the first row of the table (the positives for group i, for instance) is

$$r_i - Pn_i,$$

and this is easily seen to differ only in sign from the entry for the negatives for group i:

$$(n_i - r_i) - (1 - P)n_i = -(r_i - Pn_i).$$

The contribution to X^2 from these two cells is, therefore,

$$(r_i - Pn_i)^2 \left(\frac{1}{Pn_i} + \frac{1}{Qn_i} \right),$$

where $Q = 1 - P$. The expression in the second set of parentheses simplifies to give the following expression for X^2:

$$X^2 = \frac{\sum n_i(p_i - P)^2}{PQ}, \tag{8.29}$$

the summation now being over the k groups. A little manipulation with the summation in (8.29) gives two equivalent expressions,

$$X^2 = \frac{\sum n_i p_i^2 - NP^2}{PQ}$$

and

$$X^2 = \frac{\sum (r_i^2/n_i) - R^2/N}{PQ}. \tag{8.30}$$

The last two expressions are more convenient as computing formulae than (8.29).

The expression (8.29) and the results of §8.2 provide an indication of the reason why X^2 follows the $\chi^2_{(k-1)}$ distribution. In the general formulation of §8.2, we can replace Y_i by p_i, V_i by PQ/n_i and w_i by n_i/PQ. The weighted mean $\bar{Y}$ then becomes

$$\frac{\sum(n_i p_i/PQ)}{\sum(n_i/PQ)} = \frac{\sum n_i p_i}{\sum n_i} = \frac{R}{N} = P,$$

and, from (8.14), the test statistic G, distributed as $\chi^2_{(k-1)}$, becomes

$$X^2 = \sum_i \frac{n_i(p_i - P)^2}{PQ}$$

in agreement with (8.29). We have departed from the assumptions underlying (8.14) in two respects: the variation in p_i is binomial, not normal, and the true variance σ_i^2 has been replaced by the estimated variance PQ/n_i. Both these approximations decrease in importance as the expected frequencies increase in size.

Example 8.3

Table 8.2 shows the numbers of individuals in various age groups who were found in a survey to be positive and negative for *Schistosoma mansoni* eggs in the stool.

Table 8.2 Presence or absence of *S. mansoni* eggs in the stool.

Age (years)	0–	10–	20–	30–	40–	Total
Positive	14	16	14	7	6	57
Negative	87	33	66	34	11	231
Total	101	49	80	41	17	288

The expected number of positives for the age group 0– is

$$(57)(101)/288 = 19\cdot99.$$

The set of expected numbers for the 10 cells in the table is

					Total
19·99	9·70	15·83	8·11	3·36	57
81·01	39·30	64·17	32·89	13·64	231
Total 101	49	80	41	17	288

The fact that the expected numbers add to the same marginal totals as those observed is a useful check.

The contribution to X^2 from the first cell is

$$(14 - 19\cdot99)^2/19\cdot99 = 1\cdot79,$$

and the set of contributions for the 10 cells is

1·79	4·09	0·21	0·15	2·07
0·44	1·01	0·05	0·04	0·51

giving a total of

$$X^2 = 10\cdot36.$$

The degrees of freedom are $k - 1 = 4$, for which the 5% point is 9·49. The departures from the null hypothesis are thus significant at the 5% level ($P = 0\cdot035$).

In this example the column classification is based on a continuous variable, age, and it would be natural to ask whether the proportions of positives exhibit any smooth trend with age. The estimated proportions, with their standard errors calculated as $\sqrt{(p_i q_i/n_i)}$, are

0·14	0·33	0·18	0·17	0·35,
± 0·03	± 0·07	± 0·04	± 0·06	± 0·12

the last being based on particularly small numbers. No clear trend emerges (a method for testing for a trend is given in §15.2). About half the contribution to X^2 comes from the second age group (10–19 years) and there is some suggestion that the proportion of positives in this group is higher than in the neighbouring age groups.

To illustrate the use of (8.30), call the numbers of positives r_i. Then

$$X^2 = (14^2/101 + \ldots + 6^2/17 - 57^2/288)/(0\cdot1979)(0\cdot8021),$$

where $P = 57/288 = 0 \cdot 1979$. This gives

$$X^2 = 10 \cdot 37$$

as before, the discrepancy being due to rounding errors. Note that, if the *negatives* rather than the positives had been denoted by r_i, each of the terms in the numerator of (8.30) would have been different, but the result would have been the same.

8.6 General contingency tables

The form of table considered in the last section can be generalized by allowing more than two rows. Suppose that a total frequency, N, is subdivided by r row categories and c column categories. The null hypothesis, corresponding to that tested in the simpler situations, is that the probabilities of falling into the various columns are independent of the rows; or, equivalently, that the probabilities for the various rows are the same for each column.

The χ^2 test follows closely that applied in the simpler cases. For each cell in the body of the table an expected frequency, E, is calculated by (8.27) and the X^2 index obtained from (8.28) by summation over the rc cells. Various alternative formulae are available, but none is as simple as (8.29) or (8.30) and it is probably most convenient to use the basic formula (8.28). On the null hypothesis, X^2 follows the $\chi^2_{(f)}$ distribution with $f = (r-1)(c-1)$. This number of degrees of freedom may be thought of as the number of arbitrary choices of the frequencies in the body of the table, with the constraint that they should add to the same margins as those observed and thus give the same values of E. (If the entries in $r-1$ rows and $c-1$ columns are arbitrarily specified, those in the other row and column are determined by the marginal totals.)

Again, the χ^2 distribution is an approximation, increasingly valid for large expected frequencies. A rough rule (Cochran, 1954) is that the approximation is safe provided that relatively few expected frequencies are less than 5 (say in 1 cell out of 5 or more, or 2 cells out of 10 or more), and that no expected frequency is less than 1. In tables with smaller expected frequencies the result of the significance test should be regarded with caution. If the result is not obviously either significant or non-significant, it may be wise to pool some of the rows and/or columns in which the small expected frequencies occur and recalculate X^2 (with, of course, a reduced number of degrees of freedom). See also the suggestions made by Cochran (1954, p. 420).

Example 8.4

Table 8.3 shows results obtained in a trial to compare the effects of para-amino-salicylic acid (PAS) and streptomycin in the treatment of pulmonary tuberculosis. In each cell of the table are shown the observed frequencies, O, the expected frequencies, E, and the

Table 8.3 Degrees of positivity of sputa from patients with pulmonary tuberculosis treated with PAS, streptomycin or a combination of both drugs (Medical Research Council, 1950).

Treatment		Positive smear	Negative smear, positive culture	Negative smear, negative culture	Total
		Sputum			
PAS	O	56	30	13	99
	E	50·41	23·93	24·66	
	$O - E$	5·59	6·07	−11·66	
Streptomycin		46	18	20	84
		42·77	20·31	20·92	
		3·23	−2·31	−0·92	
Streptomycin and PAS		37	18	35	90
		45·82	21·76	22·42	
		−8·82	−3·76	12·58	
Total		139	66	68	273

discrepancies, $O - E$. For example, for the first cell, $E = (99)(139)/273 = 50·41$. Note that the values of $O - E$ add to zero along each row and down each column, a useful check on the arithmetic.

$$X^2 = (5·59)^2/50·41 + \ldots + (12·58)^2/22·42$$
$$= 17·64.$$

The degrees of freedom for the χ^2 distribution are $(3 - 1)(3 - 1) = 4$, and from Table A2 the 1% point is 13·28. The relationship between treatment and type of sputum is thus significant at the 1% level ($P = 0·0014$). The magnitudes and signs of the discrepancies, $O - E$, show clearly that the main difference is between PAS (tending to give more positive results) and the combined treatment (more negative results).

Fisher's exact test (§4.5) may be extended to a general $r \times c$ table (Mehta & Patel, 1983). The exact probability level is equal to the sum of all probabilities less than or equal to the observed table, where the probabilities are calculated under the null hypothesis that there is no association and all the marginal totals are fixed. This corresponds to a two-tailed test, using the alternative method of calculating the other tail in a 2×2 table (p. 136), but as the test is of general association there are no defined tails. The calculation is available as 'EXACT' in the SAS program PROC FREQ, and is feasible when $n < 5(r - 1)(c - 1)$, and in StatXact.

8.7 **Comparison of several variances**

The one-way analysis of variance (§8.1) is a generalization of the two-sample t test (§4.3). Occasionally one requires a generalization of the F test (used, as in §5.1, for the comparison of two variances) to the situation where more than two estimates of variance are to be compared. In a one-way analysis of variance, for example, the primary purpose is to compare means, but one might wish to test the significance of differences between variances, both for the intrinsic interest of this comparison and also because the analysis of variance involves an assumption that the group variances are equal.

Suppose there are k estimates of variance, s_i^2, having possibly different degrees of freedom, v_i. (If the ith group contains n_i observations, $v_i = n_i - 1$.) On the assumption that the observations are randomly selected from normal distributions, an approximate significance test due to Bartlett (1937) consists in calculating

$$\bar{s}^2 = \sum v_i s_i^2 / \sum v_i$$
$$M = (\sum v_i)\ln \bar{s}^2 - \sum v_i \ln s_i^2$$

and

$$C = 1 + \frac{1}{3(k-1)}\left[\sum\left(\frac{1}{v_i}\right) - \frac{1}{\sum v_i}\right]$$

and referring M/C to the $\chi^2_{(k-1)}$ distribution. Here 'ln' refers to the *natural* logarithm (see p. 126). The quantity C is likely to be near 1 and need be calculated only in marginal cases. Worked examples are given by Snedecor and Cochran (1989, §13.10).

Bartlett's test is perhaps less useful than might be thought, for two reasons. First, like the F test, it is rather sensitive to non-normality. Secondly, with samples of moderate size, the true variances σ_i^2 have to differ very considerably before there is a reasonable chance of obtaining a significant test result. To put this point another way, even if M/C is non-significant, the estimated s_i^2 may differ substantially, and so may the true σ_i^2. If possible inequality in the σ_i^2 is important, it may therefore be wise to assume it even if the test result is non-significant. In some situations moderate inequality in the σ_i^2 will not matter very much, so again the significance test is not relevant.

An alternative test which is less influenced by non-normality is due to Levene (1960). In this test the deviations of each value from its group mean, or median, are calculated and negative deviations changed to positive, that is, the absolute deviations are used. Then a test of the equality of the mean values of the absolute deviations over the groups using a one-way analysis of variance (§8.1) is carried out. Since the mean value of the absolute deviation is proportional to the standard deviation, then if the variances differ between groups so also will the mean absolute deviations. Thus the variance ratio test for the equality of group means is a test of the homogeneity of variances. Carroll & Schneider (1985) showed that it is preferable to measure the deviations from the group medians to cope with asymmetric distributions.

8.8 Comparison of several counts: the Poisson heterogeneity test

Suppose that k counts, denoted by $x_1, x_2, \ldots, x_i, \ldots, x_k$ are available. It may be interesting to test whether they could reasonably have been drawn at random from Poisson distributions with the same (unknown) mean μ. In many microbiological experiments, as we saw in §3.7, successive counts may be expected to follow a Poisson distribution if the experimental technique is perfect. With imperfect technical methods the counts will follow Poisson distributions with *different* means. In bacteriological counting, for example, the suspension may be inadequately mixed, so that clustering of the organisms occurs; the volumes of the suspension inoculated for the different counts may not be equal; the culture media may not invariably be able to sustain growth. In each of these circumstances heterogeneity of the expected counts is present and is likely to manifest itself by excessive variability of the observed counts. It seems reasonable, therefore, to base a test on the sum of squares about the mean of the x_i. An appropriate test statistic is given by

$$X^2 = \frac{\sum (x - \bar{x})^2}{\bar{x}}, \tag{8.31}$$

which, on the null hypothesis of constant μ, is approximately distributed as $\chi^2_{(k-1)}$. The method is variously called the Poisson *heterogeneity* or *dispersion* test.

The formula (8.31) may be justified from two different points of view. First, it is closely related to the test statistic (5.4) used for testing the variance of a normal distribution. On the present null hypothesis the distribution is Poisson, which we know is similar to a normal distribution if μ is not too small; furthermore, $\sigma^2 = \mu$, which can best be estimated from the data by the sample mean $\bar{x}$. Replacing σ^2_0 by $\bar{x}$ in (5.4) gives (8.31). Secondly, we could argue that, given the total count $\sum x$, the frequency 'expected' at the ith count on the null hypothesis is $\sum x / k = \bar{x}$. Applying the usual formula for a χ^2 index, $\sum [(O - E)^2 / E]$, immediately gives (8.31). In fact, just as the Poisson distribution can be regarded as a limiting form of the binomial for large n and small p, so the present test can be regarded as a limiting form of the χ^2 test for the $2 \times k$ table (§8.5) when R/N is very small and all the n_i are equal; under these circumstances it is not difficult to see that (8.29) becomes equivalent to (8.31).

Example 8.5

The following data were given by 'Student' (1907), who first emphasized the role of the Poisson distribution in microbiology.

Twenty counts of yeast cells in squares of a haemocytometer were as follows:

2	4	4	8
3	3	5	6
7	7	2	7
4	8	5	4
4	1	5	7

Here

$$
\begin{aligned}
k &= 20 \\
\sum x &= 96 \\
\bar{x} &= 4 \cdot 8 \\
\sum x^2 &= 542 \\
(\sum x)^2 / k &= 460 \cdot 8 \\
\sum (x - \bar{x})^2 &= 81 \cdot 2 \\
X^2 &= 81 \cdot 2 / 4 \cdot 8 = 16 \cdot 92 \text{ on 19 DF} \quad (P = 0 \cdot 60).
\end{aligned}
$$

There is no suggestion of variability in excess of that expected from the Poisson distribution.

In referring X^2 to the $\chi^2_{(k-1)}$ distribution we should normally do a one-sided test since heterogeneity tends to give high values of X^2. Occasionally, though, departures from the Poisson distribution will lead to reduced variability. In microbiological counting this might be caused by omission of counts differing widely from the average; Lancaster (1950) has shown that unskilled technicians counting blood cells (which under ideal circumstances provide another example of the Poisson theory) tend to omit extreme values or take repeat observations, presumably because they underestimate the extent of random variation. Other causes of reduced variability are an inability to record accurately high counts (for instance, because of overlapping of bacterial colonies), or physical interference between particles which prevents large numbers from settling close together. The latter phenomenon has been noted by Lancaster (1950) in the counting of red blood cells.

The use of the $\chi^2_{(k-1)}$ distribution in the heterogeneity test is an approximation, but is quite safe provided $\bar{x}$ is greater than about 5, and is safe even for much smaller values of $\bar{x}$ (as low as 2, say) provided k is not too small (> 15, say). For very small values of $\bar{x}$, Fisher (1950, 1964) has shown how to obtain an exact test; the method is illustrated by Oldham (1968, §5.15).

Finally, note that, for $k = 2$, (8.31) is equivalent to $(x_1 - x_2)^2 / (x_1 + x_2)$, which was used as a $\chi^2_{(1)}$ variate in §5.2.

9 Experimental design

9.1 **General remarks**

Notwithstanding the importance of observational studies, such as those to be discussed in Chapter 19, experiments are as fundamental to the advancement of medicine as they are in other branches of science. Experiments are performed to compare the effects of various treatments on some type of experimental unit; the investigator must decide which treatment to allocate to which unit. The following are examples.

1   A comparison of the effects of inoculating animals with different doses of a chemical substance. The units here will be the animals.
2   A prophylactic trial to compare the effectiveness for children of different vaccines against measles. Each child will receive one of the vaccines and may be regarded as the experimental unit.
3   A comparison in one patient suffering recurrent attacks of a chronic disease of different methods of alleviating discomfort. The successive occasions on which attacks occur are now the units for which the choice of treatment is to be made.
4   A study of the relative merits of different programmes of community health education. Each programme would be applied in a different area, and these areas would form the experimental units.

In the last three examples the experiments involve people and this poses special problems. A fuller discussion of this type of experiment and its associated problems is given in Chapter 18. In the present chapter some of the devices of classical experimental design are described. Many of these designs have their basis in agricultural applications and do not adequately address the special problems that arise when the experimental units are people. Nevertheless, aspects of classical design can be useful in this context and these are discussed as they arise in Chapter 18. It should also be noted that the analyses which accompany the designs discussed in this chapter can be useful even when the data have not arisen from a designed experiment.

In **1–4** above a crucial question is how the treatments are to be allotted to the available units. One would clearly wish to avoid any serious disparity between the characteristics of units receiving different treatments. In **2**, for instance, it would be dangerous to give one vaccine to all the children in one school and another vaccine to all the children in a second school, for the exposure of the two groups of children to measles contacts might be quite different. It would then be difficult to decide whether a difference in the incidence of measles was due to different protective powers of the vaccines or to the different degrees of exposure to infection.

It would be possible to arrange that the groups of experimental units to which different treatments were to be applied were made alike in various relevant respects. For example, in **1**, groups of animals with approximately the same mean weight could be formed; in **2**, children from different schools and of different age groups could be represented equally in each treatment group. But, however careful the investigator is to balance factors which seem important, one can never be sure that the treatment groups do not differ markedly in some factor which is also important but which has been ignored in the allocation.

The accepted solution to this dilemma is that advocated by Fisher in the 1920s and 1930s: the allocation should incorporate an element of *randomization*. In its simplest form this means that the choice of treatment for each unit should be made by an independent act of randomization such as the toss of a coin or the use of random-number tables. This would lead to some uncertainty in the numbers of units finally allotted to each treatment, and if these are fixed in advance the groups may be formed by choosing random samples of the appropriate sizes from the total pool of experimental units.

Sometimes a form of *systematic allocation*, analogous to systematic sampling (p. 650), is used as an alternative to random allocation. The units are arranged in a certain order and are then allotted systematically to the treatment groups. This method has much the same advantages and disadvantages as systematic sampling. It is likely to be seriously misleading only if the initial ordering of the units presents some systematic variation of a cyclic type which happens to run in phase with the allocation cycle. However, prior knowledge of which treatment a unit is going to receive can lead to bias (see §18.4), so alternation and other forms of systematic allocation are best avoided in favour of strictly random methods.

A second important principle of experimental design is that of *replication*, the use of more than one experimental unit for each treatment. Various purposes are served by replication. First, an appropriate amount of replication ensures that the comparisons between treatments are sufficiently precise; the sampling error of the difference between two means, for instance, decreases as the amount of replication in each group increases. Secondly, the effect of sampling variation can be estimated only if there is an adequate degree of replication. In the comparison of the means of two groups, for instance, if both sample sizes were as low as two, the degrees of freedom in the t test would only be two (§4.3); the percentage points of t on two degrees of freedom are very high and the test therefore loses a great deal in effectiveness merely because of the inadequacy of the estimate of within-groups variance. Thirdly, replication may be useful in enabling observations to be spread over a wide variety of experimental conditions. In the comparison of two surgical procedures, for instance, it might be useful to organize a cooperative trial in which the methods were compared in each of a number of hospitals, so that the effects of variations in medical and surgical practice and perhaps in the precise type of disease could be studied.

A third basic principle concerns the reduction in random variability between experimental units. The formula for the standard error of a mean, $\sigma/\sqrt{n}$, shows that the effect of random error can be reduced, either by increasing n (more replication) or by decreasing σ. This suggests that experimental units should be as homogeneous as possible in their response to treatment. However, too strenuous an effort to remove heterogeneity will tend to counteract the third reason given above for replication—the desire to cover a wide range of extraneous conditions. In a clinical trial, for example, it may be that a precise comparison could be effected by restricting the age, sex, clinical condition and other features of the patients, but these restrictions may make it too difficult to generalize from the results. A useful solution to this dilemma is to subdivide the units into relatively homogeneous subgroups, called *blocks*. Treatments can then be allocated randomly within blocks so that each block provides a small experiment. The precision of the overall comparisons between treatments is then determined by the random variability *within* blocks rather than that *between* different blocks. This is called a *randomized block* design and is discussed in §9.2. More complex designs, allowing simultaneously for more than one source of extraneous variation, are discussed in §§9.4 and 9.5. Other extensions dealt with in this chapter are designs for the simultaneous comparison of more than one set of treatments; those appropriate for situations similar to that of multistage sampling, in which some units are subdivisions of others; and designs which allow in various ways for the natural restrictions imposed by the experimental material.

9.2 **Two-way analysis of variance: randomized blocks**

In contrast to the data discussed in §§8.1–8.4, outcomes from a randomized block design are classified in two ways, by the block and the treatment. If there are r blocks and c treatments, each block containing c experimental units to which treatments are randomly allocated, there will be a total of $N = rc$ observations on any variable, simultaneously divided into r blocks with c observations in each and c treatment groups with r observations in each.

The analysis of randomized blocks can readily be viewed as a method for the analysis of data that are classified more generally in two ways, say, by the rows and columns of a table. In some experimental situations both the rows and columns of the two-way table may represent forms of treatment. In a blood-clotting experiment, for instance, clotting times may be measured for each combination of r periods of storage of plasma and c concentrations of adrenaline mixed with the plasma. This is a simple example of a *factorial experiment*, to be discussed more generally in §9.3. The distinction between this situation and the randomized block experiment is that in the latter the 'block' classification is introduced mainly to provide extra precision for treatment comparisons; differences between blocks are usually of no intrinsic interest.

Two-way classifications may arise also in non-experimental work, either by classifying in this way data already collected in a survey, or by arranging the data collection to fit a two-way classification.

We consider first the situation in which there is just one observation at each combination of a row and a column; for the ith row and jth column the observation is y_{ij}. To represent the possible effect of the row and column classifications on the mean value of y_{ij}, let us consider an 'additive model' by which

$$E(y_{ij}) = \mu + \alpha_i + \beta_j \qquad (9.1)$$

where α_i and β_j are constants characterizing the rows and columns. By suitable choice of μ we can arrange that

$$\sum_{i=1}^{r} \alpha_i = 0$$

and

$$\sum_{j=1}^{c} \beta_j = 0.$$

According to (9.1) the effect of being in one row rather than another is to change the mean value by adding or subtracting a constant quantity, irrespective of which column the observation is made in. Changing from one column to another has a similar additive or subtractive effect. Any observed value y_{ij} will, in general, vary randomly round its expectation given by (9.1). We suppose that

$$y_{ij} = E(y_{ij}) + \varepsilon_{ij} \qquad (9.2)$$

where the ε_{ij} are independently and normally distributed with a constant variance σ^2. The assumptions are, of course, not necessarily true, and we shall consider later some ways of testing their truth and of overcoming difficulties due to departures from the model.

Denote the total and mean for the ith row by R_i and $\bar{y}_{i.}$, those for the jth column by C_j and $\bar{y}_{.j}$, and those for the whole group of $N = rc$ observations by T and $\bar{y}$ (see Table 9.1). As in the one-way analysis of variance, the total sum of squares (SSq), $\sum(y_{ij} - \bar{y})^2$, will be subdivided into various parts. For any one of these deviations from the mean, $y_{ij} - \bar{y}$, the following is true:

Table 9.1 Notation for two-way analysis of variance data.

		Column				Total	Mean, R_i/c
		1	2...	j...	c		
Row	1	y_{11}	y_{12}...	y_{1j} ...	y_{1c}	R_1	$\bar{y}_{1.}$
	2	y_{21}	y_{22} ...	y_{2j} ...	y_{2c}	R_2	$\bar{y}_{2.}$
	.	.	.	.	.	.	.
	.	.	.	.	.	.	.
	.	.	.	.	.	.	.
	i	y_{i1}	y_{i2} ...	y_{ij} ...	y_{ic}	R_i	$\bar{y}_{i.}$
	.	.	.	.	.	.	.
	.	.	.	.	.	.	.
	.	.	.	.	.	.	.
	r	y_{r1}	y_{r2} ...	y_{rj} ...	y_{rc}	R_r	$\bar{y}_{r.}$
Total		$C1$	C_2 ...	C_j ...	C_c	T	
Mean	C_j/r	$\bar{y}_{.1}$	$\bar{y}_{.2}$ ...	$\bar{y}_{.j}$ ...	$\bar{y}_{.c}$		$(\bar{y} = T/N)$

$$y_{ij} - \bar{y} = (\bar{y}_{i.} - \bar{y}) + (\bar{y}_{.j} - \bar{y}) + (y_{ij} - \bar{y}_{i.} - \bar{y}_{.j} + \bar{y}) \tag{9.3}$$

The three terms on the right-hand side reflect the fact that y_{ij} differs from $\bar{y}$ partly on account of a difference characteristic of the ith row, partly because of a difference characteristic of the jth column and partly by an amount which is not explicable by either row or column differences. If (9.3) is squared and summed over all N observations, we find (the suffixes i, j being implied below each summation sign):

$$\sum(y_{ij} - \bar{y})^2 = \sum(\bar{y}_{i.} - \bar{y})^2 + \sum(\bar{y}_{.j} - \bar{y})^2 + \sum(y_{ij} - \bar{y}_{i.} - \bar{y}_{.j} + \bar{y})^2. \tag{9.4}$$

To show (9.4) we have to prove that all the product terms which arise from squaring the right-hand side of (9.3) are zero. For example,

$$\sum(\bar{y}_{i.} - \bar{y})(y_{ij} - \bar{y}_{i.} - \bar{y}_{.j} + \bar{y}) = 0.$$

These results can be proved by fairly simple algebra.

The three terms on the right-hand side of (9.4) are called the Between-Rows SSq, the Between-Columns SSq and the Residual SSq. The first two are of exactly the same form as the Between-Groups SSq in the one-way analysis, and the usual short-cut method of calculation may be used (see (8.5)).

Between rows:
$$\sum(\bar{y}_{i.} - \bar{y})^2 = \sum_{i=1}^{r} R_i^2/c - T^2/N.$$

Between columns :
$$\sum(\bar{y}_{.j} - \bar{y})^2 = \sum_{j=1}^{c} C_j^2/r - T^2/N.$$

The Total SSq is similarly calculated as

$$\sum(y_{ij} - \bar{y})^2 = \sum y_{ij}^2 - T^2/N,$$

and the Residual SSq may be obtained by subtraction:

Residual SSq = Total SSq − Between-Rows SSq − Between-Columns SSq.

$$(9.5)$$

The analysis so far is purely a consequence of algebraic identities. The relationships given above are true irrespective of the validity of the model. We now complete the analysis of variance by some steps which depend for their validity on that of the model. First, the degrees of freedom (DF) are allotted as shown in Table 9.2. Those for rows and columns follow from the one-way analysis; if the only classification had been into rows, for example, the first line of Table 9.2 would have been shown as Between groups and the SSq shown in Table 9.2 as Between columns and Residual would have added to form the Within-Groups SSq. With $r - 1$ and $c - 1$ as degrees of freedom for rows and columns, respectively, and $N - 1$ for the Total SSq, the DF for Residual SSq follow by subtraction:

$$(rc - 1) - (r - 1) - (c - 1) = rc - r - c + 1 = (r - 1)(c - 1).$$

The mean squares (MSq) for rows, columns and residual are obtained in each case by the formula MSq = SSq/DF, and those for rows and columns may each be tested against the Residual MSq, s^2, as shown in Table 9.2. The test for rows, for instance, has the following justification. On the null hypothesis (which we shall call H_R) that all the row constants α_i in (9.1) are equal (and therefore equal to zero, since $\sum \alpha_i = 0$), both s_R^2 and s^2 are unbiased estimates of σ^2. If H_R is not true, so that the α_i differ, s_R^2 has expectation greater than σ^2 whereas s^2 is still an unbiased estimate of σ^2. Hence F_R tends to be greater than 1, and sufficiently high values indicate a significant departure from H_R. This test is valid whatever values the β_j take, since adding a constant on to all the readings in a particular column has no effect on either s_R^2 or s^2.

Table 9.2 Two-way analysis of variance table.

	SSq	DF	MSq	VR
Between rows	$\sum_i R_i^2/c - T^2/N$	$r - 1$	s_R^2	$F_R = s_R^2/s^2$
Between columns	$\sum_j C_j^2/r - T^2/N$	$c - 1$	s_C^2	$F_C = s_C^2/s^2$
Residual	By subtraction	$(r - 1)(c - 1)$	s^2	
Total	$\sum_{i,j} y_{ij}^2 - T^2/N$	$rc - 1(= N - 1)$		

Similarly, F_C provides a test of the null hypothesis H_C, that all the $\beta_j = 0$, irrespective of the values of the α_i.

If the additive model (9.1) is not true, the Residual SSq will be inflated by discrepancies between $E(y_{ij})$ and the approximations given by the best-fitting additive model, and the Residual MSq will thus be an unbiased estimate of a quantity greater than the random variance. How do we know whether this has happened? There are two main approaches, the first of which is to examine *residuals*. These are the individual expressions $y_{ij} - \bar{y}_{i.} - \bar{y}_{.j} + \bar{y}$. Their sum of squares was obtained, from (9.4), by subtraction, but it could have been obtained by direct evaluation of all the N residuals and by summing their squares. These residuals add to zero along each row and down each column, like the discrepancies between observed and expected frequencies in a contingency table (§8.6), and (as for contingency tables) the number of DF, $(r-1)(c-1)$, is the number of values of residuals which may be independently chosen (the others being then automatically determined). Because of this lack of independence the residuals are not quite the same as the random error terms ε_{ij} of (9.2), but they have much the same distributional properties. In particular, they should not exhibit any striking patterns. Sometimes the residuals in certain parts of the two-way table seem to have predominantly the same sign; provided the ordering of the rows or columns has any meaning, this will suggest that the row-effect constants are not the same for all columns. There may be a correlation between the size of the residual and the 'expected' value* $\bar{y}_{i.} + \bar{y}_{.j} - \bar{y}$: this will suggest that a change of scale would provide better agreement with the additive model.

A second approach is to provide replication of observations, and this is discussed in more detail after Example 9.1.

Example 9.1

Table 9.3 shows the results of a randomized block experiment to compare the effects on the clotting time of plasma of four different methods of treatment of the plasma. Samples of plasma from eight subjects (the 'blocks') were assigned in random order to the four treatments.

The correction term, T^2/N, denoted here by CT, is needed for three items in the SSq column, and it is useful to calculate this at the outset. The analysis is straightforward, and the F tests show that differences between subjects and treatments are both highly significant. Differences between subjects do not interest us greatly as the main purpose of the experiment was to study differences between treatments. The standard error of the difference between two treatment means is $\sqrt{[2(0\cdot6559)/8]} = 0\cdot405$. Clearly, treatments 1, 2 and 3 do not differ significantly among themselves, but treatment 4 gives a significantly higher mean clotting time than the others.

---

*This is the value expected on the basis of the average row and column effects, as may be seen from the equivalent expression $\bar{y} + (\bar{y}_{i.} - \bar{y}) + (\bar{y}_{.j} - \bar{y})$

Table 9.3 Clotting times (min) of plasma from eight subjects, treated by four methods.

Subject	Treatment				Total	Mean
	1	2	3	4		
1	8·4	9·4	9·8	12·2	39·8	9·95
2	12·8	15·2	12·9	14·4	55·3	13·82
3	9·6	9·1	11·2	9·8	39·7	9·92
4	9·8	8·8	9·9	12·0	40·5	10·12
5	8·4	8·2	8·5	8·5	33·6	8·40
6	8·6	9·9	9·8	10·9	39·2	9·80
7	8·9	9·0	9·2	10·4	37·5	9·38
8	7·9	8·1	8·2	10·0	34·2	8·55
Total	74·4	77·7	79·5	88·2	319·8	
Mean	9·30	9·71	9·94	11·02		(9·99)

Correction term, $CT = (319\cdot8)^2/32$ = 3 196·0013

Between-Subjects SSq $= [(39\cdot8)^2 + \ldots + (34\cdot2)^2]/4 - CT$ =   78·9888

Between-Treatments SSq $= [(74\cdot4)^2 + \ldots + (88\cdot2)^2]/8 - CT$ =   13·0163

Total SSq $= (8\cdot4)^2 + \ldots + (10\cdot0)^2 - CT$ =   105·7788

Residual SSq $= 105\cdot7788 - 78\cdot9888 - 13\cdot0163$ =   13·7737

Analysis of variance

	SSq	DF	MSq	VR	
Subjects	78·9888	7	11·2841	17·20	$(P < 0\cdot001)$
Treatments	13·0163	3	4·3388	6·62	$(P = 0\cdot003)$
Residual	13·7737	21	0·6559	1·00	
Total	105·7788	31			

For purposes of illustration the residuals are shown below:

Subject	Treatment				Total
	1	2	3	4	
1	−0·86	−0·27	−0·10	1·22	−0·01
2	−0·33	1·66	−0·87	−0·45	0·01
3	0·37	−0·54	1·33	−1·15	0·01
4	0·37	−1·04	−0·17	0·85	0·01
5	0·69	0·08	0·15	−0·93	−0·01
6	−0·51	0·38	0·05	0·07	−0·01
7	0·21	−0·10	−0·13	−0·01	−0·03
8	0·04	−0·17	−0·30	0·42	−0·01
Total	−0·02	0·00	−0·04	0·02	−0·04

The sum of squares of the 32 residuals in the body of the table is $13 \cdot 7744$, in agreement with the value found by subtraction in Table 9.3 apart from rounding errors. (These errors also account for the fact that the residuals as shown do not add exactly to zero along the rows and columns.) No particular pattern emerges from the table of residuals, nor does the distribution appear to be grossly non-normal. There are 16 negative values and 16 positive values; the highest three in absolute value are positive ($1 \cdot 66$, $1 \cdot 33$ and $1 \cdot 22$), which suggests mildly that the random error distribution may have slight positive skewness.

If the linear model (9.1) is wrong, there is said to be an *interaction* between the row and column effects. In the absence of an interaction the expected differences between observations in different columns are the same for all rows (and the statement is true if we interchange the words 'columns' and 'rows'). If there is an interaction, the expected column differences vary from row to row (and, similarly, expected row differences vary from column to column). With one observation in each row/column cell, the effect of an interaction is inextricably mixed with the residual variation. Suppose, however, that we have more than one observation per cell. The variation between observations *within the same cell* provides direct evidence about the random variance σ^2, and may therefore be used as a basis of comparison for the between-cells residual. This is illustrated in the next example.

Example 9.2

In Table 9.4 we show some hypothetical data related to the data of Table 9.3. There are three subjects and three treatments, and for each subject–treatment combination three replicate observations are made. The mean of each group of three replicates will be seen to agree with the value shown in Table 9.3 for the same subject and treatment. Under each group of replicates is shown the total T_{ij} and the sum of squares, S_{ij} (as indicated for T_{11} and S_{11}).

The Subjects and Treatments SSq are obtained straightforwardly, using the divisor 9 for the sums of squares of row (or column) totals, since there are nine observations in each row (or column), and using a divisor 27 in the correction term. The Interaction SSq is obtained in a similar way to the Residual in Table 9.3, but using the totals T_{ij} as the basis of calculation. Thus,

Interaction SSq = SSq for differences between the nine subject/treatment cells
– Subjects SSq – Treatment SSq,

and the degrees of freedom are, correspondingly, $8 - 2 - 2 = 4$. The Total SSq is obtained in the usual way and the Residual SSq follows by subtraction. The Residual SSq could have been obtained directly as the sum over the nine cells of the sum of squares about the mean of each triplet, i.e. as

$$(S_{11} - T_{11}^2/3) + (S_{12} - T_{12}^2/3) + \ldots + (S_{33} - T_{33}^2/3).$$

The F tests show the effects of subjects and treatments to be highly significant. The interaction term is not significant at the 5% level, but the variance ratio (VR) is nevertheless rather high. It is due mainly to the mean value for subject 8 and treatment 4 being higher than expected.

Table 9.4 Clotting time (min) of plasma from three subjects, three methods of treatment and three replications of each subject–treatment combination.

Subject	Treatment			Total	
	2	3	4		
6	9·8	9·9	11·3		
	10·1	9·5	10·7		
	9·8	10·0	10·7		
	T_{11} 29·7	29·4	32·7	R_1 91·8	
	S_{11} 294·09	288·26	356·67		
7	9·2	9·1	10·3		
	8·6	9·1	10·7		
	9·2	9·4	10·2		
	27·0	27·6	31·2	R_2 85·8	
	243·24	253·98	324·62		
8	8·4	8·6	9·8		
	7·9	8·0	10·1		
	8·0	8·0	10·1		
	24·3	24·6	30·0	R_3 78·9	
	196·97	201·96	300·06		
Total	C_1 81·0	C_2 81·6	C_3 93·9	T 256·5	$\sum y^2$ 2459·85

$$CT = T^2/27 = 2436·75$$

Subjects SSq $= [(91·8)^2 + \ldots + (78·9)^2]/9 - CT$ $= 9·2600$
Treatments SSq $= [(81·0)^2 + \ldots + (93·9)^2]/9 - CT$ $= 11·7800$
Interaction SSq $= [(29·7)^2 + \ldots + (30·0)^2]/3 - CT - \text{Subj. SSq} - \text{Treat.SSq}$ $= 0·7400$
Total SSq $= (9·8)^2 + \ldots + (10·1)^2 - CT = 2459·85 - CT$ $= 23·1000$
Residual SSq $= \text{Total} - \text{Subjects} - \text{Treatments} - \text{Interaction}$ $= 1·3200$

Analysis of variance

	SSq	DF	MSq	VR	
Subjects	9·2600	2	4·6300	63·1	
Treatments	11·7800	2	5·8900	80·3	
Interaction	0·7400	4	0·1850	2·52	$(P = 0·077)$
Residual	1·3200	18	0·0733	1·00	
Total	23·1000	26			

The interpretation of significant interactions and the interpretation of the tests for the 'main effects' (subjects and treatments in Examples 9.1 and 9.2) when interactions are present will be discussed in the next section.

If, in a two-way classification without replication, $c = 2$, the situation is the same as that for which the paired t test was used in §4.3. There is a close analogy here with the relationship between the one-way analysis of variance and the two-sample t test noted in §8.1. In the two-way case the F test provided by the analysis of variance is equivalent to the paired t test in that: (i) F is numerically equal to t^2; (ii) the F statistic has 1 and $r - 1$ DF while t has $r - 1$ DF, and, as noted in §5.1, the distributions of t^2 and F are identical. The Residual MSq in the analysis of variance is half the corresponding s^2 in the t test, since the latter is an estimate of the variance of the difference between the two readings.

In Example 9.2 the number of replications at each row–column combination was constant. This is not a necessary requirement. The number of observations at the ith row and jth column, n_{ij}, may vary, but the method of analysis indicated in Example 9.2 is valid only if the n_{ij} are proportional to the total row and column frequencies; that is, denoting the latter by $n_{i.}$ and $n_{.j}$,

$$n_{ij} = \frac{n_{i.}n_{.j}}{N}. \tag{9.6}$$

In Example 9.2 all the $n_{i.}$ and $n_{.j}$ were equal to 9, N was 27, and $n_{ij} = 81/27 = 3$, for all i and j. If (9.6) is not true, an attempt to follow the standard method of analysis may lead to negative sums of squares for the interaction or residual, which is, of course, an impossible situation.

Condition (9.6) raises a more general issue, namely that many of the relatively straightforward forms of analysis, not only for the two-way layout but also for many of the other arrangements in this chapter, are only possible if the numbers of outcomes in different parts of the experiment satisfy certain quite strict conditions, such as (9.6). Data which fail to satisfy such conditions are said to lack *balance*. In medical applications difficulties with recruitment or withdrawal will readily lead to unbalanced data. In these cases it may be necessary to use more general methods of analysis, such as those discussed in Chapters 11 and 12. If the data are unbalanced because of the absence of just a very small proportion of the data, then one approach is to impute the missing values on the basis of the available data and the fitted model. Details can be found in Cochran and Cox (1957). However, when addressing problems of missing data the issues of why the data are missing can be more important than how to cope with the resulting imbalance: see §12.6.

9.3 **Factorial designs**

In §9.2 an example was described of a design for a factorial experiment in which the variable to be analysed was blood-clotting time and the effects of two factors were to be measured: r periods of storage and c concentrations of adrenaline. Observations were made at each combination of storage periods and adrenaline concentrations. There are two factors here, one at r levels and the other at c levels, and the design is called an $r \times c$ *factorial*.

This design contravenes what used to be regarded as a good principle of experimentation, namely that only one factor should be changed at a time. The advantages of factorial experimentation over the one-factor-at-a-time approach were pointed out by Fisher. If we make one observation at each of the rc combinations, we can make comparisons of the mean effects of different periods of storage on the basis of c observations at each period. To get the same precision with a non-factorial design we would have to choose one particular concentration of adrenaline and make c observations for each storage period: rc in all. This would give us no information about the effect of varying the concentration of adrenaline. An experiment to throw light on this factor with the same precision as the factorial design would need a further rc observations, all with the same storage period. Twice as many observations as in the factorial design would therefore be needed. Moreover, the factorial design permits a comparison of the effect of one factor at different levels of the other: it permits the detection of an interaction between the two factors. This cannot be done without the factorial approach.

The two-factor design considered in §9.2 can clearly be generalized to allow the simultaneous study of three or more factors. Strictly, the term 'factorial design' should be reserved for situations in which the factors are all controllable experimental treatments and in which all the combinations of levels are randomly allocated to the experimental units. The analysis is, however, essentially the same in the slightly different situation in which one or more of the factors represents a form of blocking—a source of known or suspected variation which can usefully be eliminated in comparing the real treatments. We shall therefore include this extended form of factorial design in the present discussion.

Notation becomes troublesome if we aim at complete generality, so we shall discuss in detail a three-factor design. The directions of generalization should be clear. Suppose there are three factors: A at I levels, B at J levels and C at K levels. As in §9.2, we consider a linear model whereby the mean response at the ith level of A, the jth level of B and the kth level of C is

$$E(y_{ijk}) = \mu + \alpha_i + \beta_j + \gamma_k + (\alpha\beta)_{ij} + (\alpha\gamma)_{ik} + (\beta\gamma)_{jk} + (\alpha\beta\gamma)_{ijk}, \qquad (9.7)$$

with

$$\sum_i \alpha_i = \ldots = \sum_i (\alpha\beta)_{ij} = \ldots \sum_i (\alpha\beta\gamma)_{ijk} = 0, \text{etc.}$$

Here, the terms like $(\alpha\beta)_{ij}$ are to be read as single constants, the notation being chosen to indicate the interpretation of each term as an interaction between two or more factors. The constants α_i measure the effects of the different levels of factor A averaged over the various levels of the other factors; these are called the *main effects* of A. The constant $(\alpha\beta)_{ij}$ indicates the extent to which the mean

Table 9.5 Structure of analysis of three-factor design with replication.

	SSq	DF	MSq	VR ($= \text{MSq}/s^2$)
Main effects				
A	S_A	$I - 1$	s_A^2	F_A
B	S_B	$J - 1$	s_B^2	F_B
C	S_C	$K - 1$	s_C^2	F_C
Two-factor interactions				
AB	S_{AB}	$(I-1)(J-1)$	s_{AB}^2	F_{AB}
AC	S_{AC}	$(I-1)(K-1)$	s_{AC}^2	F_{AC}
BC	S_{BC}	$(J-1)(K-1)$	s_{BC}^2	F_{BC}
Three-factor interaction				
ABC	S_{ABC}	$(I-1)(J-1)(K-1)$	s_{ABC}^2	F_{ABC}
Residual	S_R	$IJK(n-1)$	s^2	1
Total	S	$N - 1$		

response at level i of A and level j of B, averaged over all levels of C, is not determined purely by α_i and β_j, and it thus measures one aspect of the interaction of A and B. It is called a *first-order interaction term* or *two-factor interaction term*. Similarly, the constant $(\alpha\beta\gamma)_{ijk}$ indicates how the mean response at the triple combination of A, B and C is not determined purely by main effects and first-order interaction terms. It is called a *second-order* or *three-factor interaction term*.

To complete the model, suppose that y_{ijk} is distributed about $\mathrm{E}(y_{ijk})$ with a constant variance σ^2.

Suppose now that we make n observations at each combination of A, B and C. The total number of observations is $nIJK = N$, say. The structure of the analysis of variance is shown in Table 9.5. The DF for the main effects and two-factor interactions follow directly from the results for two-way analyses. That for the three-factor interaction is a natural extension. The residual DF are $IJK(n-1)$ because there are $n-1$ DF between replicates at each of the IJK factor combinations. The SSq terms are calculated as follows.

1 *Main effects.* As for a one-way analysis, remembering that the divisor for the square of a group total is the total number of observations in that group. Thus, if the total for ith level of A is $T_{i..}$, and the grand total is T, the SSq for A is

$$S_A = \sum_i T_{i..}^2 / nJK - T^2 / N. \tag{9.8}$$

2 *Two-factor interactions.* Form a two-way table of totals, calculate the appropriate corrected sum of squares between these totals and subtract the SSq for the two relevant main effects. For AB, for instance, suppose $T_{ij.}$ is the total for levels i of A and j of B. Then

$$S_{AB} = (\sum_{i,j} T_{ij.}^2/nK - T^2/N) - S_A - S_B. \tag{9.9}$$

3 *Three-factor interaction.* Form a three-way table of totals, calculate the appropriate corrected sum of squares and subtract the SSq for all relevant two-factor interactions and main effects. If T_{ijk} is the total for the three-factor combination at levels i, j, k of A, B, C, respectively,

$$S_{ABC} = (\sum_{i,j,k} T_{ijk}^2/n - T^2/N) - S_{AB} - S_{AC} - S_{BC} - S_A - S_B - S_C. \tag{9.10}$$

4 *Total.* As usual by

$$\sum_{i,j,k} y_{ijkr}^2 - T^2/N,$$

where the suffix r (from 1 to n) denotes one of the replicate observations at each factor combination.

5 *Residual.* By subtraction. It could also have been obtained by adding, over all three factor combinations, the sum of squares between replicates:

$$\sum_{i,j,k} (\sum_{r=1}^{n} y_{ijkr}^2 - T_{ijk}^2/n). \tag{9.11}$$

This alternative formulation unfortunately does not provide an independent check on the arithmetic, as it follows immediately from the other expressions.

The MSq terms are obtained as usual from SSq/DF. Each of these divided by the Residual MSq, s^2, provides an F test for the appropriate null hypothesis about the main effects or interactions. For example, F_A (tested on $I - 1$ and $IJK(n - 1)$ degrees of freedom) provides a test of the null hypothesis that all the α_i, are zero—that is, that the mean responses at different levels of A, averaged over all levels of the other factors, are all equal. Some problems of interpretation of this rather complex set of tests are discussed at the end of this section.

Suppose $n = 1$, so that there is no replication. The DF for the residual become zero, since $n - 1 = 0$. So does the SSq, since all the contributions in parentheses in (9.11) are zero, being sums of squares about the mean of a single observation. The 'residual' line therefore does not appear in the analysis. The position is exactly the same as in the two-way analysis with one observation per cell. The usual practice is to take the highest-order interaction (in this case ABC) as the residual term, and to calculate F ratios using this MSq as the denominator. As in the two-way analysis, this will be satisfactory if the highest-order interaction terms in the *model* (in our case $(\alpha\beta\gamma)_{ijk}$) are zero or near zero. If these terms are substantial, the makeshift Residual MSq, S^2_{ABC}, will tend to be higher than σ^2 and the tests will be correspondingly insensitive.

Table 9.6 Relative weights of right adrenals in mice.

Mother's strain	1 ♀	1 ♂	2 ♀	2 ♂	3 ♀	3 ♂	4 ♀	4 ♂	Totals ♀	Totals ♂	♀+♂
1	0·93	0·69	1·76	0·67	1·46	0·88	1·45	0·95	12·57	6·57	19·14
	1·70	0·83	1·58	0·73	1·89	0·96	1·80	0·86			
2	1·42	0·50	1·85	0·72	2·14	1·00	1·94	0·63	15·25	6·08	21·33
	1·96	0·74	1·69	0·66	2·17	0·96	2·08	0·87			
3	2·22	0·86	1·96	1·04	1·62	0·82	1·51	0·82	15·32	6·69	22·01
	2·33	0·98	2·09	0·96	1·63	0·57	1·96	0·64			
4	1·25	0·56	1·56	1·08	1·88	1·00	1·85	0·43	13·39	6·32	19·71
	1·76	0·75	1·90	0·80	1·81	1·11	1·38	0·59			
Total	13·57	5·91	14·39	6·66	14·60	7·30	13·97	5·79	56·53	25·66	
	19·48		21·05		21·90		19·76				82·19

CT = 105·5499

Analysis of variance

	DF	SSq	MSq	VR	
Mother's strain, M	3	0·3396	0·1132	2·87	
Father's strain, F	3	0·2401	0·0800	2·03	
Sex of animal, S	1	14·8900	14·8900	376·96	($P < 0.001$)
MF	9	1·2988	0·1443	3·65	($P = 0.003$)
MS	3	0·3945	0·1315	3·33	($P = 0.032$)
FS	3	0·0245	0·0082	0·21	
MFS	9	0·2612	0·0290	0·73	
Residual	32	1·2647	0·0395	1·00	
Total	63	18·7134			

Differences ♀ − ♂

Mother's strain	Father's strain 1	2	3	4	Total
1	1·11	1·94	1·51	1·44	6·00
2	2·14	2·16	2·35	2·52	9·17
3	2·71	2·05	1·86	2·01	8·63
4	1·70	1·58	1·58	2·21	7·07
Total	7·66	7·73	7·30	8·18	30·87

Example 9.3

Table 9.6* shows the relative weights of right adrenals (expressed as a fraction of body weight, $\times 10^4$) in mice obtained by crossing parents of four strains. For each of the 16 combinations of parental strains, four mice (two of each sex) were used.

This is a three-factor design. The factors—mother's strain, father's strain and sex—are not, of course, experimental treatments imposed by random allocation. Nevertheless, they represent potential sources of variation whose main effects and interactions may be studied. The DF are shown in the table. The SSq for main effects follow straightforwardly from the subtotals. That for the mother's strain, for example, is

$$[(19{\cdot}14)^2 + \ldots + (19{\cdot}71)^2]/16 - CT,$$

where the correction term, CT, is $(82{\cdot}19)^2/64 = 105{\cdot}5499$. The two-factor interaction, MF, is obtained as

$$[(4{\cdot}15)^2 + \ldots + (4{\cdot}25)^2]/4 - CT - S_M - S_F,$$

where $4{\cdot}15$ is the sum of the responses in the first cell $(0{\cdot}93 + 1{\cdot}70 + 0{\cdot}69 + 0{\cdot}83)$, and S_M and S_F are the SSq for the two main effects. Similarly, the three-factor interaction is obtained as

$$[(2{\cdot}63)^2 + (1{\cdot}52)^2 + \ldots + (3{\cdot}23)^2 + (1{\cdot}02)^2]/2 - CT$$
$$- S_M - S_F - S_S - S_{MF} - S_{MS} - S_{FS}.$$

Here the quantities $2{\cdot}63$, etc. are subtotals of pairs of responses $(2{\cdot}63 = 0{\cdot}93 + 1{\cdot}70)$. The Residual SSq may be obtained by subtraction, once the Total SSq has been obtained.

The F tests show the main effects M and F to be non-significant, although each variance ratio is greater than 1. The interaction MF is highly significant. The main effect of sex is highly significant, and also its interaction with M. To elucidate the strain effects, it is useful to tabulate the sums of observations for the 16 crosses:

Mother's strain	Father's strain				
	1	2	3	4	Total
1	4·15	4·74	5·19	5·06	19·14
2	4·62	4·92	6·27	5·52	21·33
3	6·39	6·05	4·64	4·93	22·01
4	4·32	5·34	5·80	4·25	19·71
Total	19·48	21·05	21·90	19·76	82·19

Strains 2 and 3 give relatively high readings for M and F, suggesting a systematic effect which has not achieved significance for either parent separately. The interaction is due partly to the high reading for (M3, F1).

Each of the 16-cell totals is the sum of four readings, and the difference between any two has a standard error $\sqrt{[(2)(4)(0{\cdot}0395)]} = 0{\cdot}56$. For M3 the difference between F1 and F3 is significantly positive, whereas for each of the other maternal strains the F1 − F3

*The data were kindly provided by Drs R.L. Collins and R.J. Meckler. In their paper (Collins & Meckler, 1965) results from both adrenals are analysed.

difference is negative, significantly so for M2 and M4. A similar reversal is provided by the four entries for M2 and M3, F2 and F3.

The MS interaction may be studied from the previous table of sex contrasts. Each of the row totals has a standard error $\sqrt{[16(0\cdot0395)]} = 0\cdot80$. Maternal strains 2 and 3 show significantly higher sex differences than M1, and M2 is significantly higher also than M4. The point may be seen from the right-hand margin of Table 9.6, where the high responses for M2 and M3 are shown strongly in the female offspring, but not in the males.

This type of experiment, in which parents of each sex from a number of strains are crossed, is called a *diallel cross*. Special methods of analysis are available which allow for the general effect of each strain, exhibited by both males and females, and the specific effects of particular crosses (Bulmer, 1980).

The 2^p factorial design

An interaction term in the analysis of a factorial design will, in general, have many degrees of freedom, and will represent departures of various types from an additive model. The interpretation of a significant interaction may therefore require careful thought. If, however, all the factors are at two levels, each of the main effects and each of the interactions will have only one degree of freedom, and consequently represent linear contrasts which can be interpreted relatively simply. If there are, say, four factors each at two levels, the design is referred to as a $2 \times 2 \times 2 \times 2$, or 2^4, design, and in general for p factors each at two levels, the design is called 2^p. The analysis of 2^p designs can be simplified by direct calculation of each linear contrast. We shall illustrate the procedure for a 2^3 design.

Suppose there are n observations at each of the 8 ($= 2^3$) factor combinations. Since each factor is at two levels we can, by suitable conventions, regard each factor as being positive or negative—say, by the presence or absence of some feature. Denoting the factors by A, B and C, we can identify each factor combination by writing in lower-case letters those factors which are positive. Thus, (ab) indicates the combination with A and B positive and C negative, while (c) indicates the combination with only C positive; the combination with all factors negative will be written as (1). In formulae these symbols can be taken to mean the totals of the n observations at the different factor combinations.

The main effect of A may be estimated by the difference between the mean response at all combinations with A positive and that for A negative. This is a linear contrast,

$$\frac{(a) + (ab) + (ac) + (abc)}{4n} - \left[\frac{(1) + (b) + (c) + (bc)}{4n}\right] = [A]/4n, \qquad (9.12)$$

where

$$[A] = -(1) + (a) - (b) + (ab) - (c) + (ac) - (bc) + (abc), \qquad (9.13)$$

the terms being rearranged here so that the factors are introduced in order. The main effects of B and C are defined in a similar way.

The two-factor interaction between A and B represents the difference between the estimated effect of A when B is positive, and that when B is negative. This is

$$\frac{(ab) + (abc) - (b) - (bc)}{2n} - \left[\frac{(a) + (ac) - (1) - (c)}{2n}\right] = [AB]/2n, \qquad (9.14)$$

where

$$[AB] = (1) - (a) - (b) + (ab) + (c) - (ac) - (bc) + (abc). \qquad (9.15)$$

To avoid the awkwardness of the divisor $2n$ in (9.14) when $4n$ appears in (9.12), it is useful to redefine the interaction as $[AB]/4n$, that is as half the difference referred to above. Note that the terms in (9.15) have a positive sign when A and B are either both positive or both negative, and a negative sign otherwise. Note also that $[AB]/4n$ can be written as

$$\frac{(ab) + (abc) - (a) - (ac)}{4n} - \left[\frac{(b) + (bc) - (1) - (c)}{4n}\right]$$

which is half the difference between the estimated effect of B when A is positive and that when A is negative. This emphasizes the symmetric nature of $[AB]$.

The three-factor interaction $[ABC]$ can similarly be interpreted in a number of equivalent ways. It represents, for instance, the difference between the estimated $[AB]$ interaction when C is positive and when C is negative. Apart from the divisor, this difference is measured by

$$\begin{aligned}[ABC] &= [(c) - (ac) - (bc) + (abc)] - [(1) - (a) - (b) + (ab)]\\ &= -(1) + (a) + (b) - (ab) + (c) - (ac) - (bc) + (abc),\end{aligned} \qquad (9.16)$$

and it is again convenient to redefine the interaction as $[ABC]/4n$.

The results are summarized in Table 9.7. Note that the positive and negative signs for the two-factor interactions are easily obtained by multiplying together the coefficients for the corresponding main effects; and those for the three-factor interaction by multiplying the coefficients for $[A]$ and $[BC]$, $[B]$ and $[AC]$, or $[C]$ and $[AB]$.

The final column of Table 9.7 shows the formula for the SSq and (since each has 1 DF) for the MSq for each term in the analysis. Each term like $[A]$, $[AB]$, etc., has a variance $8n\sigma^2$ on the appropriate null hypothesis (since each of the totals (1), (a), etc., has a variance $n\sigma^2$). Hence $[A]^2/8n$ is an estimate of σ^2. In general, for a 2^p factorial, the divisors for the linear contrasts are $2^{p-1}n$, and those for the SSq are $2^p n$.

The significance of the main effects and of interactions may equivalently be tested by t tests. The residual mean square, s^2, has $8(n - 1)$ DF, and the variance of each of the contrasts $[A]$, $[AB]$, etc., is estimated as $8ns^2$, to give a t test with $8(n - 1)$ DF.

Table 9.7 Calculation of main effects and interactions for a 2^3 factorial design.

Effect		(1)	(a)	(b)	(ab)	(c)	(ac)	(bc)	(abc)	Divisor for contrast	Contributions to SSq
		\multicolumn{8}{c}{Multiplier for total}		
Main effects	A	−1	1	−1	1	−1	1	−1	1	$4n$	$[A]^2/8n$
	B	−1	−1	1	1	−1	−1	1	1	$4n$	$[B]^2/8n$
	C	−1	−1	−1	−1	1	1	1	1	$4n$	$[C]^2/8n$
Two-factor interactions	AB	1	−1	−1	1	1	−1	−1	1	$4n$	$[AB]^2/8n$
	AC	1	−1	1	−1	−1	1	−1	1	$4n$	$[AC]^2/8n$
	BC	1	1	−1	−1	−1	−1	1	1	$4n$	$[BC]^2/8n$
Three-factor interaction	ABC	−1	1	1	−1	1	−1	−1	1	$4n$	$[ABC]^2/8n$

Interpretation of factorial experiments with significant interactions

The analysis of a large-scale factorial experiment provides an opportunity to test simultaneously a number of main effects and interactions. The complexity of this situation sometimes gives rise to ambiguities of interpretation. The following points may be helpful.

1 Whether or not two or more factors interact may depend on the scale of measurement of the variable under analysis. Sometimes a simpler interpretation of the data may be obtained by reanalysing the data after a logarithmic or other transformation (see §10.8). For instance, if we ignore random error, the responses shown in (a) below present an interaction between A and B. Those shown in (b) present no interaction. The responses in (b) are the square roots of those in (a).

	\multicolumn{2}{c}{B}		\multicolumn{2}{c}{B}	
A	Low	High	Low	High
Low	9	16	3	4
High	16	25	4	5
	\multicolumn{2}{c}{(a)}		\multicolumn{2}{c}{(b)}	

The search for a scale of measurement on which interactions are small or non-significant is particularly worth trying if the main effects of one factor, as measured at different levels of the other(s), are related closely to the mean responses at these levels. If the estimated main effects of any one factor are in *opposite directions* for different levels of the other(s), transformations are not likely to be useful. This type of effect is called a *qualitative* interaction, and is likely to be more important than a *quantitative* interaction, in which the effect of one variable is changed in magnitude but not direction by the levels of other variables.

2 In a multifactor experiment many interactions are independently subjected to test; it will not be too surprising if one of these is mildly significant purely by chance. Interactions that are not regarded as inherently plausible should therefore be viewed with some caution unless they are highly significant (i.e. significant at a small probability level such as 1%). Another useful device is the 'half-normal plot' (§11.9).

3 If several high-order interactions are non-significant, their SSq are often pooled with the Residual SSq to provide an increased number of DF and hence more sensitive tests of the main effects or low-order interactions.

There remain some further points of interpretation which are most usefully discussed separately, according as the factors concerned are thought of as having fixed effects or random effects (§8.3).

Fixed effects

If certain interactions are present they can often best be displayed by quoting the mean values of the variable at each of the factor combinations concerned. For instance, in an experiment with A, B and C at two, three and four levels, respectively, if the only significant interaction were BC, the mean values would be quoted at each of the 12 combinations of levels of B and C. These could be accompanied by a statement of the standard error of the difference between two of these means. The reader would then be able to see quickly the essential features of the interaction. Consider the following table of means:

| Level of B | Level of C | | | |
	1	2	3	4
1	2·17	2·25	2·19	2·24
2	1·96	2·01	1·89	1·86
3	2·62	2·67	2·83	2·87

Standard error of difference between two means = 0·05.

Clearly the effect of C is not detectable at level 1 of B; at level 2 of B the two higher levels of C show a decrease in the mean; at level 3 of B the two higher levels of C show an increase.

In situations like this the main effects of B and C are of no great interest. If the effect of C varies with the level of B, the main effect measures the average effect of C over the levels of B; since it depends on the choice of levels of B it will usually be a rather artificial quantity and therefore hardly worth considering. Similarly, if a three-factor interaction is significant and deemed to exist, the interactions between any two of the factors concerned are rather artificial concepts.

Random effects

If, in the previous example, A and C were fixed-effect factors and B was a random-effect factor, the presence of an interaction between B and C would not preclude an interest in the main effect of C—regarded not as an average over the particular levels of B chosen in the experiment, but as an average over the whole population of potential B levels. Under certain conditions (discussed below) the null hypothesis for the main effect of C is tested by comparing the MSq for C against the MSq for the interaction BC. If C has more than two levels, it may be more informative to concentrate on a particular contrast between the levels of C (say, a comparison of level 1 with level 4), and obtain the interaction of this contrast with the factor B.

If one of the factors in a multifactor design is a blocking system, it will usually be natural to regard this as a random-effect factor. Suppose the other factors are controlled treatments (say, A, B and C). Then each of the main effects and interactions of A, B and C may be compared with the appropriate interaction with blocks. Frequently the various interactions involving blocks differ by no more than might be expected by random variation, and the SSq may be pooled to provide extra DF.

The situations referred to in the previous paragraphs are examples in which a *mixed model* is appropriate—some of the factors having fixed effects and some having random effects. If there is just one random factor (as with blocks in the example in the last paragraph), any main effect or interaction of the other factors may be tested against the appropriate interaction with the random factor; for example, if D is the random factor, A could be tested against AD, AB against ABD. The justification for this follows by interpreting the interaction terms involving D in the model like (9.7) as independent observations on random variables with zero mean. The concept of a random interaction is reasonable; if, for example, D is a blocking system, any linear contrast representing part of a main effect or interaction of the other factors can be regarded as varying randomly from block to block. What is more arguable, though, is the assumption that all the components in (9.7) for a particular interaction, say, AD, have the same distribution and are independent of each other. Hence the suggestion, made above, that attention should preferably be focused on particular linear contrasts. Any such contrast, L, could be measured separately in each block and its mean value tested by a t test.

When there are more than two random factors, further problems arise because there may be no exact tests for some of the main effects and interactions. For further discussion, see Snedecor and Cochran (1989, §16.14).

9.4 **Latin squares**

Suppose we wish to compare the effects of a treatments in an experiment in which there are two other known sources of variation, each at a levels. A complete factorial design, with only one observation at each factor combination, would require a^3 observations. Consider the following design, in which $a = 4$. The principal treatments are denoted by A, B, C and D, and the two secondary factors are represented by the rows and columns of the table.

	Column			
Row	1	2	3	4
1	D	B	C	A
2	C	D	A	B
3	A	C	B	D
4	B	A	D	C

Only $a^2 (= 16)$ observations are made, since at each combination of a row and a column only one of the four treatments is used. The design is cunningly balanced, however, in the sense that each treatment occurs precisely once in each row and precisely once in each column. If the effect of making an observation in row 1 rather than row 2 is to add a constant amount on to the measurement observed, the differences between the means for the four treatments are unaffected by the size of this constant. In this sense systematic variation between rows, or similarly between columns, does not affect the treatment comparisons and can be said to have been eliminated by the choice of design.

These designs, called *Latin squares*, were first used in agricultural experiments in which the rows and columns represented strips in two perpendicular directions across a field. Some analogous examples arise in medical research when treatments are to be applied to a two-dimensional array of experimental units. For instance, various substances may be inoculated subcutaneously over a two-dimensional grid of points on the skin of a human subject or an animal. In a plate diffusion assay various dilutions of an antibiotic preparation may be inserted in hollows in an agar plate which is seeded with bacteria and incubated, the inhibition zone formed by diffusion of antibiotic round each hollow being related to the dilution used.

In other experiments the rows and columns may represent two identifiable sources of variation which are, however, not geographically meaningful. The Latin square is being used here as a straightforward generalization of a randomized block design, the rows and columns representing two different systems of blocking. An example would be an animal experiment in which rows represent litters and columns represent different days on which the experiment is performed: the individual animals receive different treatments. An important area of application is when patients correspond to rows and treatment periods to columns. Such designs are referred to as extended crossover designs and are briefly discussed in §18.9.

Latin squares are sometimes used in situations where either the rows or columns or both represent forms of treatment under the experimenter's control. They are then performing some of the functions of factorial designs, with the important proviso that some of the factor combinations are missing. This has important consequences, which we shall note later.

In a randomized block design, treatments are allocated at random within each block. How can randomization be applied in a Latin square, which is clearly a highly systematic arrangement? For any value of a many possible squares can be written down. The safeguards of randomization are introduced by making a random choice from these possible squares. Full details of the procedure are given in Fisher and Yates (1963) and in most books on experimental design. The reader will not go far wrong in constructing a Latin square of the right size by shifting treatments cyclically by one place in successive rows:

$$
\begin{array}{cccc}
A & B & C & D \\
D & A & B & C \\
C & D & A & B \\
B & C & D & A \\
\end{array}
$$

and then permuting the rows and the columns randomly.

As an additive model for the analysis of the Latin square, suppose that the response, y_{ijk}, for the ith row, jth column and kth treatment is given by

$$ y_{ijk} = \mu + \alpha_i + \beta_j + \gamma_k + \varepsilon_{ijk}, \tag{9.17} $$

where μ represents the general mean, $\alpha_i, \beta_j, \gamma_k$ are constants characteristic of the particular row, column and treatment concerned, and ε_{ijk} is a random observation from a normal distribution with zero mean and variance σ^2. The model is, in fact, that of a three-factor experiment without interactions.

The notation for the observations is shown in Table 9.8. The analysis, shown at the foot of Table 9.8, follows familiar lines. The SSq for rows, columns and treatments are obtained by the usual formula in terms of the subtotals, the Total SSq is also obtained as usual, and the residual term is obtained by subtraction:

Residual SSq = Total SSq − (Rows SSq + Columns SSq + Treatments SSq).

The degrees of freedom for the three factors are clearly $a - 1$; the residual DF are found by subtraction to be $a^2 - 3a + 2 = (a - 1)(a - 2)$.

Table 9.8 Notation for Latin square experiment.

Row	Column 1	2 ... j ... a	Total	Mean	Treatment	Total	Mean
1			R_1	$\bar{y}_{1..}$	1	T_1	$\bar{y}_{..1}$
2			R_2	$\bar{y}_{2..}$	2	T_2	$\bar{y}_{..2}$
.			.	.	.	.	.
.			.	.	.	.	.
.			.	.	.	.	.
i		y_{ijk}	R_i	$\bar{y}_{i..}$	k	T_k	$\bar{y}_{..k}$
.			.	.	.	.	.
.			.	.	.	.	.
.			.	.	.	.	.
a			R_a	$\bar{y}_{a..}$	a	T_a	$\bar{y}_{..a}$
Total	C_1	C_2 ... C_j ... C_a	T			T	
Mean	$\bar{y}_{.1.}$	$\bar{y}_{.2.}$ $\bar{y}_{.j.}$ $\bar{y}_{.a.}$		$\bar{y}$			

Analysis of variance

	SSq	DF	MSq	VR
Rows	$\sum R_i^2/a - T^2/a^2$	$a-1$	s_R^2	$F_R = s_R^2/s^2$
Columns	$\sum C_j^2/a - T^2/a^2$	$a-1$	s_C^2	$F_C = s_C^2/s^2$
Treatments	$\sum T_k^2/a - T^2/a^2$	$a-1$	s_T^2	$F_T = s_T^2/s^2$
Residual	By subtraction	$(a-1)(a-2)$	s^2	
Total	$y_{ijk}^2 - T^2/a^2$	$a^2 - 1$		

The basis of the division of the Total SSq is the following identity:

$$y_{ijk} - \bar{y} = (\bar{y}_{i..} - \bar{y}) + (\bar{y}_{.j.} - \bar{y}) + (\bar{y}_{..k} - \bar{y}) + (y_{ijk} - \bar{y}_{i..} - \bar{y}_{.j.} - \bar{y}_{..k} + 2\bar{y}).$$

$$(9.18)$$

When each term is squared and a summation is taken over all the a^2 observations, the four sums of squares are obtained. The product terms such as $\sum(\bar{y}_{.j.} - \bar{y}) \times (\bar{y}_{..k} - \bar{y})$ are all zero, as in the two-way analysis of §9.2.

If the additive model (9.17) is correct, the three null hypotheses about equality of the αs, βs, and γs can all be tested by the appropriate F tests. Confidence limits for differences between pairs of constants (say, between two rows) or for other linear contrasts can be formed in a straightforward way, the standard errors being estimated in terms of s^2. However, the additive model may be incorrect. If the rows and columns are blocking factors, the effect of non-additivity will be to increase the estimate of residual variance. Tests for differences between rows or between columns are of no great interest in this case, and randomization ensures the validity of the tests and estimates for treatment differences; the extra imprecision is automatically accounted for in the increased value of s^2. If, on the other hand, the rows and the columns are treatments, non-additivity means that some interactions exist. The trouble now is that the interactions cannot be measured independently of the main effects, and serious errors may result. In both sets of circumstances, therefore, additivity of responses is a desirable feature, although its absence is more regrettable in the second case than in the first.

Example 9.4

The experiment of Bacharach *et al.* (1940), discussed in Example 8.2, was designed as a Latin square. The design and the measurements are given in Table 9.9. The object of the experiment was to study the possible effects of order of administration in a series of inoculations on the same animal (the 'treatment' factor, represented here by roman numerals), and the choice among six positions on the animal's skin (the row factor), and also to assess the variation between animals (the column factor) in comparison with that within animals.

The Total SSq is obtained as usual as

$$1984 \cdot 0000 - 1953 \cdot 6401 = 30 \cdot 3599.$$

The SSq for animal differences is calculated as

$$[(42 \cdot 4)^2 + (51 \cdot 7)^2 + \cdots + (45 \cdot 1)^2]/6 - 1953 \cdot 6401 = 12 \cdot 8333,$$

the other two main effects follow similarly, and the Residual SSq is obtained by subtraction. The VR for order is less than 1 and need not be referred to the F table. That for positions is certainly not significant. The only significant effect is that for animal differences, and further examination of the between-animals component of variance has already been carried out in Example 8.2.

Replication of Latin squares

An important restriction of the Latin square is, of course, the requirement that the numbers of rows, columns and treatments must all be equal. The nature of the experimental material and the purpose of the experiment often demand that the size of the square should be small. On the other hand, treatment comparisons estimated from a single Latin square are likely to be rather imprecise. Some form of replication is therefore often desirable.

Replication in an experiment like that of Example 9.4 may take various forms, for instance: (i) if the six animals in Table 9.9 were from the same litter, the experiment could be repeated with several litters, a new randomization being used for each litter; (ii) if there were no classification by litters, a single design such as that in Table 9.9 could be used with several animals for each column; (iii)

Table 9.9 Measurements of area of blister (square centimetres) following inoculation of diffusing factor into skin of rabbits in positions a–f on animals' backs, order of administration being denoted by i–vi (Bacharach *et al.*, 1940).

Positions	Animals						Total	Mean
	1	2	3	4	5	6		
a	iii	v	iv	i	vi	ii		
	7·9	8·7	7·4	7·4	7·1	8·2	46·7	7·783
b	iv	ii	vi	v	iii	i		
	6·1	8·2	7·7	7·1	8·1	5·9	43·1	7·183
c	i	iii	v	vi	ii	iv		
	7·5	8·1	6·0	6·4	6·2	7·5	41·7	6·950
d	vi	i	iii	ii	iv	v		
	6·9	8·5	6·8	7·7	8·5	8·5	46·9	7·817
e	ii	iv	i	iii	v	vi		
	6·7	9·9	7·3	6·4	6·4	7·3	44·0	7·333
f	v	vi	ii	iv	i	iii		
	7·3	8·3	7·3	5·8	6·4	7·7	42·8	7·133
Total	42·4	51·7	42·5	40·8	42·7	45·1	265·2	
Mean	7·067	8·617	7·083	6·800	7·117	7·517		7·367

Order	i	ii	iii	iv	v	vi
Total	43·0	44·3	45·0	45·2	44·0	43·7
Mean	7·167	7·383	7·500	7·533	7·333	7·283

$$\sum y_{ijk}^2 = 1984\cdot0000$$
$$T^2/36 = 1953\cdot6401$$

Analysis of variance

	SSq	DF	MSq	VR	
Rows (Positions)	3·8332	5	0·7667	1·17	
Columns (Animals)	12·8333	5	2·5667	3·91	$(P = 0\cdot012)$
Treatments (Order)	0·5632	5	0·1126	<1	
Residual	13·1302	20	0·6565	1·00	
Total	30·3599	35			

if the experiment were repeated with the *same six animals*, on several occasions, again a new randomization should be used for each occasion. In replicated designs of this sort, care needs to be taken to specify the effects to be tested and the correct assignment of degrees of freedom.

9.5 **Other incomplete designs**

The Latin square may be regarded either as a design which allows simultaneously for two extraneous sources of variation—the rows and columns—or as an incomplete factorial design permitting the estimation of three main effects—

rows, columns and treatments—from observations at only a fraction of the possible combinations of factor levels.

Many other types of incomplete design are known. This section contains a very brief survey of some of these designs, with details of construction and analysis omitted. Cox (1958, Chapters 11 and 12) gives a much fuller account of the characteristics and purposes of the various designs, and Cochran and Cox (1957) should be consulted for details of statistical analysis. Most of the designs described in this section have found little use in medical research, examples of their application being drawn usually from industrial and agricultural research. This contrast is perhaps partly due to inadequate appreciation of the less familiar designs by medical research workers, but it is likely also that the organizational problems of experimentation are more severe in medical research than in many other fields, a feature which would tend to favour the use of simple designs.

Graeco-Latin squares

The Latin square generalizes the randomized block design by controlling variation due to two blocking factors. The Graeco-Latin square extends this idea by superimposing on a Latin square a further system of classification which is balanced with respect to the rows, columns and treatments. This is conventionally represented by letters of the Greek alphabet. For example, the following design could be used for an experiment similar to that described in Example 9.4:

Aα	Bβ	Cγ	Dδ	Eε
Bδ	Cε	Dα	Eβ	Aγ
Cβ	Dγ	Eδ	Aε	Bα
Dε	Eα	Aβ	Bγ	Cδ
Eγ	Aδ	Bε	Cα	Dβ

Note that both the 'Latin' (i.e. Roman) letters and the Greek letters form Latin squares with the rows and columns, and also that each Latin letter occurs precisely once with each Greek letter. Suppose that the experimenter wished to compare the effects of five different doses of diffusing factor, allowing simultaneously for the order of administration, differences between animals and differences between positions on the animals' backs. The design shown above could be used, with random allocation of columns to five different animals, rows to five positions, Greek letters to the five places in the order of administration, and Latin letters to the five dilutions.

A general point to remember with Graeco-Latin squares is that the number of DF for the residual mean square is invariably low. Unless, therefore, an estimate of error variance can reliably be obtained from extraneous data, it will often be desirable to introduce sufficient replication to provide an adequately precise estimate of random variation.

Incomplete block designs

In many situations in which a natural blocking system exists, a randomized block design may be ruled out because the number of treatments is greater than the number of experimental units which can conveniently be formed within a block. This limitation may be due to physical restrictions: in an experiment with intradermal inoculations into animals, with an individual animal forming a block, there may be a limit to the number of inoculation sites on an animal. The limitation may be one of convenience; if repeated clinical measurements are made on each of a number of patients, it may be undesirable to subject any one patient to more than a few such observations. There may be a time limit; for example, a block may consist of observations made on a single day. Sometimes when an adequate number of units can be formed within each block this may be undesirable because it leads to an excessively high degree of within-blocks variation.

A possible solution to these difficulties lies in the use of an *incomplete block design*, in which only a selection of the treatments is used in any one block. In general, this will lead to designs lacking the attractive symmetry of a randomized block design. However, certain designs, called *balanced incomplete block designs*, retain a considerable degree of symmetry by ensuring that each treatment occurs the same number of times and each pair of treatments occurs together in a block the same number of times.

There are various categories of balanced incomplete block designs, details of which may be found in books on experimental design. The incompleteness of the design introduces some complexity into the analysis. To compare mean effects of different treatments, for example, it is unsatisfactory merely to compare the observed means for all units receiving these treatments, for these means will be affected by differences between blocks. The observed means are therefore adjusted in a certain way to allow for systematic differences between blocks. This is equivalent to obtaining contrasts between treatments solely from within-blocks differences. For details, see Cochran and Cox (1957, §9.3).

A further class of designs, *Youden squares* or *incomplete Latin squares*, are similar to balanced incomplete block designs, but have the further feature that a second source of extraneous variation is controlled by the introduction of a column classification. They bear the same relation to balanced incomplete block designs as do Latin squares to randomized block designs.

In a Youden square the row and column classifications enter into the design in different ways. The number of rows (blocks) is equal to the number of treatments, so each column contains all the treatments; the number of columns is less than the number of treatments; so only a selection of treatments is used in each row. Sometimes designs are needed for two-way control of variability, in situations in which both classifications must be treated in an incomplete way. A type of design called a *set of balanced lattice squares* may be useful here. For a brief description, see Cox (1958, §11.3(iii)); for details, see Cochran and Cox (1957, Chapter 12).

In a balanced incomplete block design all treatments are handled in a symmetric way. All contrasts between pairs of treatments are, for example, estimated with equal precision. Some other incomplete block designs retain some, but not all, of the symmetry of the balanced designs. They may be adopted because of a deliberate wish to estimate some contrasts more precisely than others. Or it may be that physical restrictions on the size of the experiment do not permit any of the balanced designs to be used. *Lattice designs* (not to be confused with lattice squares), in particular, are useful when a large number of treatments are to be compared and where the smallest balanced design is likely to be too large for practical use.

Sometimes it may be necessary to use incomplete block designs which have no degree of symmetry. For some worked examples, see Pearce (1965, 1983).

Fractional replication and confounding

If the rows and columns of a Latin square represent different treatment factors and the Latin letters represent a third treatment factor, we have an incomplete factorial design. As we have seen in discussing the analysis of the Latin square, one consequence is that the main effects of the factors can be studied only if the interactions are assumed to be absent. There are many other incomplete or *fractional* factorial designs in which only a fraction of all the possible combinations of factor levels are used, with the consequence that not all the main effects or interactions can be separately investigated.

Such designs may be very useful for experiments with a large number of factors in which the number of observations required for a complete factorial experiment is greater than can conveniently be used, or where the main effects can be estimated sufficiently precisely with less than the complete number of observations. If by the use of a fractional factorial design we have to sacrifice the ability to estimate some of the main effects or interactions, it will usually be convenient if we can arrange to lose information about the higher-order interactions rather than the main effects or lower-order interactions, because the former are unlikely to be large without the latter also appearing large, whereas the converse is not true. A further point to remember is that SSq for high-order interactions are often pooled in the analysis of variance to give an estimate of residual variance. The sacrifice of information about some of these will reduce the residual DF, and if this is done too drastically there will be an inadequately precise estimate of error unless an estimate is available from other data.

Fractional factorial designs have been much used in industrial and agricultural work where the simultaneous effects of large numbers of factors have to be studied and where attention very often focuses on the main effects and low-order interactions.

A further way in which a full factorial design can be reduced, in a block experiment, is to arrange that each block contains only a selection of the possible factor combinations. The design is chosen to ensure that some effects, typically main effects and low-order interactions, can be estimated from contrasts *within blocks*, whereas others (of less interest) are estimated from contrasts *between blocks*. The latter are said to be *confounded with blocks*, and are, of course, estimated with lower precision than the unconfounded effects.

9.6 **Split-unit designs**

In a factorial design in which confounding with blocks takes place, as outlined at the end of §9.5, two types of random variation are important: the variation between experimental units within a block, and that between blocks. In some simple factorial designs it is convenient to recognize two such forms of experimental unit, one of which is a subdivision of the other, and to arrange that the levels of some factors are spread across the larger units, while levels of other factors are spread across the smaller units within the larger ones.

This principle was first exploited in agricultural experiments, where the designs are called *split-plot designs*. In some field experiments it is convenient to divide the field into 'main plots' and to compare the levels of one factor—say, the addition of different soil organisms—by allocating them at random to the main plots. At the same time each main plot is divided into a number of 'subplots', and the levels of some other factor—say, different fertilizers—are allocated at random to subplots within a main plot, exactly as in a randomized block experiment. The comparison of fertilizers would be subject to the random variation between subplots, which would be likely to be less than the variation between main plots, which affects organism comparisons. The organisms are thus compared less precisely than the fertilizers. This inequality of precision is likely to be accepted because of the convenience of being able to spread organisms over relatively large areas of ground.

Similar situations arise in medical and other types of biological experimentation. In general the experimental units are not referred to as 'plots', and the design is therefore more appropriately called a *split-unit design*. Another term is *nested design*. If the subunits are serial measurements on the main units then a split-unit analysis is sometimes called a *repeated measures analysis of variance*: for a discussion of some special considerations that apply in this case, see §12.6.

Some examples of the distinction between main units and subunits are as follows:

Main unit	Subunit
Individual human subject or animal	Different occasions with the same subject or animal
Litter	Animals within a litter
Day	Periods during a day

In the first of these instances a split-unit design might be employed to compare the long-term effects of drugs A_1, A_2 and A_3, and simultaneously the short-term effects of drugs B_1, B_2 and B_3. Suppose there are 12 subjects, each of whom must receive one of A_1, A_2 and A_3; and each subject is observed for three periods during which B_1, B_2 and B_3 are to be given in a random order. The design, determine by randomly allocating the As to the different subjects and the Bs to the period within subjects, might be as follows.

Patient	'A' drug throughout	'B' drug during period		
		1	2	3
1	A_3	B_1	B_3	B_2
2	A_1	B_1	B_2	B_3
3	A_1	B_3	B_1	B_2
4	A_2	B_3	B_2	B_1
5	A_3	B_2	B_3	B_1
6	A_2	B_2	B_1	B_3
7	A_1	B_1	B_2	B_3
8	A_3	B_3	B_1	B_2
9	A_3	B_1	B_3	B_2
10	A_2	B_2	B_1	B_3
11	A_1	B_2	B_1	B_3
12	A_2	B_2	B_1	B_3

The analysis of such designs is illustrated in Example 9.5, using data from a survey rather than an experiment.

Example 9.5

The data in Table 9.10 are taken from a survey on the prevalence of upper respiratory tract infection. The variable to be analysed is the number of swabs positive for *Pneumococcus* during a certain period. Observations were made on 18 families, each consisting of a father, a mother and three children, the youngest of whom was always a preschool child. The children are numbered 1, 2 and 3 in descending order of age. Six families were a random selection of such families living in 'overcrowded' conditions, six were in 'crowded' conditions and six were in 'uncrowded' conditions.

The first point to notice is that two types of random variation are relevant: that between families (the main units in this example) and that between people within families (the subunits). Comparisons between degrees of crowding must be made *between families*, comparisons of family status are made *within families*. With designs of any complexity it is a good idea to start the analysis by subdividing the degrees of freedom. The result is shown in the DF column of Table 9.11. The total DF are 89, since there are 90 observations. These are split (as in a one-way analysis of variance) into 17 $(= 18 - 1)$ between families and 72 $(= 18 \times 4)$ within families. The between-families DF are split (again as in a one-way analysis) into 2 $(= 3 - 1)$ for degrees of crowding and 15 $(= 3 \times 5)$ for residual variation within crowding categories. The within-families DF are split into 4 $(= 5 - 1)$ for

Table 9.10 Numbers of swabs positive for *Pneumococcus* during fixed periods.

Crowding category	Family serial number	Father	Mother	Child 1	2	3	Total
Overcrowded	1	5	7	6	25	19	62
	2	11	8	11	33	35	98
	3	3	12	19	6	21	61
	4	3	19	12	17	17	68
	5	10	9	15	11	17	62
	6	9	0	6	9	5	29
		41	55	69	101	114	380
Crowded	7	11	7	7	15	13	53
	8	10	5	8	13	17	53
	9	5	4	3	18	10	40
	10	1	9	4	16	8	38
	11	5	5	10	16	20	56
	12	7	3	13	17	18	58
		39	33	45	95	86	298
Uncrowded	13	6	3	5	7	3	24
	14	9	6	6	14	10	45
	15	2	2	6	15	8	33
	16	0	2	10	16	21	49
	17	3	2	0	3	14	22
	18	6	2	4	7	20	39
		26	17	31	62	76	212
Total		106	105	145	258	276	890

categories of family status, 8 ($= 4 \times 2$) for the interaction between the two main effects, and 60 for within-families residual variation. The latter number can be obtained by subtraction ($60 = 72 - 4 - 8$) or by regarding this source of variation as an interaction between the between-families residual variation and the status factor ($60 = 15 \times 4$). It may be wondered why the interaction between status and crowding is designated as within families when one main effect is between and the other is within families. The reason is that this interaction measures the extent to which the status differences, which are within families, vary from one degree of crowding to another; it is therefore based entirely on within-families contrasts.

Table 9.11 Analysis of variance for data in Table 9.10.

	SSq		DF	MSq	VR against: a	b
Between families	1146·09		17			
Crowding		470·49	2	235·24		5·22*
Residual		675·60	15	45·04[b]	1·78	1·00
Within families	3122·80		72			
Status		1533·67	4	383·42	15·17**	
Status × crowding		72·40	8	9·05	0·36	
Residual		1516·73	60	25·28[a]	1·00	
Total	4268·89		89			

*$P = 0.019$.
**$P < 0.001$.

The calculation of sums of squares follows familiar lines. Thus,

Correction Term CT $= (890)^2/90$	$= 8801 \cdot 11$
Total SSq $= 5^2 + 7^2 + \ldots + 20^2 -$ CT	$= 4268 \cdot 89$
Between-Families SSq $= (62^2 + \ldots + 39^2)/5 -$ CT	$= 1146 \cdot 09$
Within-Families SSq $=$ Total SSq $-$ Between Families SSq	$= 3122 \cdot 80$

Subdividing the Between-Families SSq,

Crowding SSq $= (380^2 + 298^2 + 212^2)/30 -$ CT	$= 470 \cdot 49$
Residual $=$ Between-Families SSq $-$ Crowding SSq	$= 675 \cdot 60$

Subdividing the Within-Families SSq,

Status SSq $= (106^2 + \ldots + 276^2)/18 -$ CT	$= 1533 \cdot 67$
S × C SSq $= (41^2 + \ldots + 76^2)/6 -$ CT$-$ Status SSq $-$	
Crowding SSq	$= 72 \cdot 40$
Residual $=$ Within-Families SSq $-$ Status SSq $-$ S ×C SSq	$= 1516 \cdot 73$

The variance ratios against the Within-Families Residual MSq show that differences due to status are highly significant: we return to these below. The interaction is not significant; there is therefore no evidence that the relative effects of family status vary from one crowding group to another. The variance ratio of 1·78 between the two residuals is just on the borderline of significance at the 5% level. But we should expect a priori that the between-families residual variance would be greater than that within families, and we must certainly test the main effect for crowding against the between-families residual. The variance ratio, 5·22, is significant.

The means for the different members of the family are:

		Child		
F	M	1	2	3
5·6	5·8	8·1	14·3	15·3

The standard error of the difference between two means is $\sqrt{[2(25·28)/18]} = 1·68$. There are clearly no significant differences between the father, mother and eldest child, but the two youngest children have significantly higher means than the other members of the family.

The means for the different levels of crowding are:

Overcrowded	Crowded	Uncrowded
12·7	9·9	7·1

The standard error of the difference between two means is now $\sqrt{[2(45·04)/30]} = 1·73$. There is some evidence of a difference between overcrowded and uncrowded families. However, there seems to be a trend and it might be useful to divide the two degrees of freedom for crowding into one for a linear trend and one for the remaining variation (see §8.4).

Split-unit designs more elaborate than the design described above may be useful. For example, the structure imposed on the main units (which in Example 9.5 was a simple one-way classification) could be a randomized block design or something more complex. The subunit section of the analysis would then be correspondingly enlarged by isolation of the appropriate interactions. Similarly, the subunit structure could be elaborated. Another direction of generalization is in the provision of more than two levels in the hierarchy of nested units. In a study similar to that of Example 9.5, for instance, there might have been several periods of observation for each individual, during which different treatments were administered. There would then be a third section in the analysis, within individuals, with its corresponding residual mean square.

The split-unit design, with its two levels of residual variation, can be regarded as the prototype for multilevel models, a flexible and widely used class of models which will be discussed in §12.5.

The following example illustrates a case in which there are two levels of nested units, but in which the design is very simple. There are no structural factors, the purpose of the analysis being merely to estimate the components of random variation.

Example 9.6

Table 9.12 gives counts of particle emission during periods of 1000 s, for 30 aliquots of equal size of certain radioactive material. Each aliquot is placed twice in the counter. There are three sources of random variation, each with its component of variance, as follows.

1   Variation between aliquots, with a variance component σ_2^2. This may be due to slight variations in size or in radioactivity, or to differences in technique between the 30 occasions on which the different aliquots were examined.

2   Systematic variation between replicate counts causing changes in the expected level of the count, with a variance component σ_1^2. This may be due to systematic biases in counting which affect different counts in different ways, or to inconsistency in the apparatus, due perhaps to variation in the way the material is placed in the counter.

3   Random variation from one time period to another, all other conditions remaining constant: variance component σ_0^2. There is no replication of counts under constant conditions, but we know that this form of variation follows the Poisson distribution (§3.7), in which the variance equals the mean. The mean will vary a little over the whole experiment, but to a close approximation we could estimate σ_0^2 by the observed mean for the whole data, 303·6.

Table 9.12   Radioactivity counts during periods of 1000s.

Aliquot	Counts		Aliquot	Counts	
1	281	291	16	325	267
2	309	347	17	284	296
3	316	356	18	255	281
4	289	277	19	347	285
5	322	292	20	326	302
6	287	321	21	347	307
7	338	320	22	292	344
8	333	275	23	322	308
9	319	311	24	294	272
10	258	302	25	307	303
11	338	294	26	281	331
12	319	281	27	284	322
13	307	247	28	287	305
14	279	259	29	318	352
15	326	272	30	307	301

The analysis of variance is that for a simple one-way classification and is as follows:

	SSq	DF	MSq	Expected value of MSq
Between aliquots	19 898	29	686·1	$\sigma_0^2 + \sigma_1^2 + 2\sigma_2^2$
Within aliquots	20 196	30	673·2	$\sigma_0^2 + \sigma_1^2$
Total	40 094	59		
Poisson			303·6	σ_0^2

The expected values of the mean squares follow from §8.3, if we note that the within-aliquots variance component is $\sigma_0^2 + \sigma_1^2$ (since differences between replicate counts are affected by variation of both type **2** and type **3**), and that the between-aliquots component is σ_2^2.

The estimates of the variance components are now obtained:

$$\sigma_2^2 = (686 \cdot 1 - 673 \cdot 2)/2 = \quad 6 \cdot 4$$
$$\sigma_1^2 = 673 \cdot 2 - 303 \cdot 6 \quad = 369 \cdot 6$$
$$\sigma_0^2 = 303 \cdot 6$$

These estimates are, of course, subject to sampling error, but there is clearly no evidence of any large component, σ_2^2, due to aliquot differences. Replicate counts vary, however, by substantially more than can be explained by the Poisson distribution.

10 Analysing non-normal data

10.1 **Distribution-free methods**

Some of the statistical methods described in §§4.4 and 4.5 for the analysis of proportions have involved rather simple assumptions: for example, χ^2 methods often test simple hypotheses about the probabilities for various categories—that they are equal, or that they are proportional to certain marginal probabilities. The methods used for quantitative data, in contrast, have relied on relatively complex assumptions about distributional forms—that the random variation is normal, Poisson, etc. These assumptions are often likely to be clearly untrue; to overcome this problem we sometimes argue that methods are *robust*—that is, not very sensitive to non-normality. At other times we may use transformations to make the assumptions more plausible.

Clearly, there would be something to be said for methods which avoided unnecessary distributional assumptions. Such methods, called *distribution-free methods*, exist and are widely used by some statisticians. Standard statistical methods frequently use statistics which in a fairly obvious way estimate certain population parameters; the sample estimate of variance s^2, for example, estimates the population parameter σ^2. In distribution-free methods there is little emphasis on population parameters, since the whole object is to avoid a particular functional form for a population distribution. The hypotheses to be tested usually relate to the nature of the distribution as a whole rather than to the values assumed by some of its parameters. For this reason they are often called *non-parametric hypotheses* and the appropriate techniques are often called *non-parametric tests* or *methods*.

The justification for the use of distribution-free methods will usually be along one of the following lines.
1 There may be obvious non-normality.
2 There may be possible non-normality, perhaps to a very marked extent, but the sample sizes may be too small to establish whether or not this is so.
3 One may seek a rapid statistical technique, perhaps involving little or simple calculation. Many distribution-free methods have this property: J.W. Tukey's epithet 'quick and dirty methods' is often used to describe them.

4   A measurement to be analysed may consist of a number of ordered categories, such as $--$, $-$, 0, $+$ and $++$ for degrees of clinical improvement; or a number of observations may form a rank order—for example, patients may be asked to classify six pharmaceutical formulations in order of palatability. In such cases the investigator may be unwilling to allot a numerical scale, but would wish to use methods which took account of the rank order of the observations. Many distribution-free methods are of this type. The first type of data referred to here, namely ordered categorical data, will be discussed at some length in §14.3. There is, in fact, a close relation between some of the methods described there and those to be discussed in the present chapter.

The methods described in the following sections are merely a few of the most useful distribution-free techniques. These methods have been developed primarily as significance tests and are not always easily adapted for purposes of estimation. Nevertheless, the statistics used in the tests can often be said to estimate something, even though the parameter estimated may be of limited interest. Some estimation procedures are therefore described briefly, although the emphasis will be on significance tests. In recent years there have been important advances in so-called *computationally intensive methods*, both for conducting hypothesis tests and for estimation, and these are discussed. Distribution-free methods are frequently used when data do not, at first, appear to conform to the requirements of a method that assumes a given distribution (usually the normal distribution). However, transforming the data so that it has the necessary form is often preferable. Although transformations are not distribution-free methods—indeed, they are a way of avoiding them—they are of sufficient importance in this area to warrant discussion in this chapter.

Fuller accounts of distribution-free methods are given by Siegel and Castellan (1988), who concentrate on significance tests, and by Lehmann (1975), Sprent and Smeeton (2001) and Conover (1999).

10.2 **One-sample tests for location**

In this section we consider tests of the null hypothesis that the distribution of a random variable x is symmetric about zero. If, in some problem, the natural hypothesis to test is that of symmetry about some other value, μ, all that need be done is to subtract μ from each observation; the test for symmetry about zero can then be used. The need to test for symmetry about zero commonly arises with paired comparisons of two treatments, when the variable x is the difference between two paired readings.

The normal-theory test for this hypothesis is, of course, the one-sample t test, and we shall illustrate the present methods by reference to Table 4.2, the data of which were analysed by a paired t test in Example 4.3.

The sign test

Suppose the observations in a sample of size n are $x_1, x_2, \ldots, x_n$, and that of these r are positive and s negative. Some values of x may be exactly zero, and these would not be counted with either the positives or the negatives. The sum $r + s$ may therefore be less than n, and will be denoted by n'.

On the null hypothesis, positive and negative values of x are equally likely. Both r and s therefore follow a binomial distribution with parameters n' (instead of the n of §3.6) and $\frac{1}{2}$ (for the parameter π of §3.6). Excessively high or low values of r (or, equivalently, of s) can be tested exactly from tables of the binomial distribution. For large enough samples, any of the normal approximations (4.17), (4.18), (5.7) or (5.8) may be used (with r and s replacing x_1 and x_2 in (5.7) and (5.8)).

Example 10.1

Consider the differences in the final column of Table 4.2. Here $n' = n = 10$ (since there are no zero values), $r = 4$ and $s = 6$. For a two-sided significance test the probability level is twice the probability of $r \leq 4$, which from tables of the binomial distribution is 0·75. The normal approximation, with continuity correction, would give, for a $\chi^2_{(1)}$ test,

$$X^2 = \frac{(|6 - 4| - 1)^2}{6 + 4} = 0 \cdot 10 \quad (P = 0 \cdot 75).$$

The verdict agrees with that of the t test in Example 4.3: there is no evidence that differences in anxiety score tend to be positive more (or less) often than they are negative. The mid-P value (see §4.4) from the binomial distribution is 0·55, and this corresponds to the uncorrected $\chi^2_{(1)}$ value of 0·40 ($P = 0·53$). Note that these mid-P values approximate more closely to the result of the t test in Example 4.3, where, with $t = -0·90$ on 9 degrees of freedom (DF), $P = 0·39$.

The signed rank sum test

The sign test clearly loses something by ignoring all information about the numerical magnitudes of the observations other than their sign. If a high proportion of the numerically large observations were positive, this would strengthen the evidence that the distribution was asymmetric about zero, and it seems reasonable to try to take this evidence into account. Wilcoxon's (1945) signed rank sum test works as follows. The observations are put in ascending order of magnitude, ignoring the sign, and given the ranks 1 to n' (zero values being ignored as in the sign test). Let T_+ be the sum of the ranks of the positive values and T_- that of the negative. On the null hypothesis T_+ and T_- would not be expected to differ greatly; their sum $T_+ + T_-$ is $\frac{1}{2}n'(n' + 1)$, so an appropriate test would consist in evaluating the probability of a value of, say, T_+ equal to or more extreme than that observed. Table A6 gives critical values for the *smaller* of T_+ and T_-, for two-sided tests at the 5% and 1% levels, for n' up to 25. The distribution is tabulated fully for n' up to 20 by Lehmann (1975, Table H), and other percentiles are given in the Geigy Scientific Tables (1982, p. 163). For larger values of n', T_+ and T_- are approximately normally distributed with variance $n'(n'+1)(2n'+1)/24$, and a standardized normal deviate, with continuity correction, is given by

$$\frac{|T_+ - \frac{1}{4}n'(n'+1)| - \frac{1}{2}}{\sqrt{[n'(n'+1)(2n'+1)/24]}} \tag{10.1}$$

If some of the observations are numerically equal, they are given tied ranks equal to the mean of the ranks which would otherwise have been used. This feature reduces the variance of T_+ by $(t^3 - t)/48$ for each group of t tied ranks, and the critical values shown in Appendix Table A6 are somewhat conservative (i.e. the result is somewhat more significant than the table suggests).

Example 10.2

The 10 differences in Table 4.2 may be ranked numerically as follows:

	1	2	3	4		6	7		9	10
Rank		$2\frac{1}{2}$			5	$6\frac{1}{2}$		8	$9\frac{1}{2}$	
Numerical value	1	1	1	1	2	3	3	7	8	8
Sign	+	+	+	−	−	−	−	−	+	−

$$T_+ = 2\tfrac{1}{2} + 2\tfrac{1}{2} + 2\tfrac{1}{2} + 9\tfrac{1}{2} = 17,$$
$$T_- = 2\tfrac{1}{2} + 5 + 6\tfrac{1}{2} + 6\tfrac{1}{2} + 8 + 9\tfrac{1}{2} = 38.$$

From Table A6, for $n' = 10$, the 5% point for the minimum of T_+ and T_- is 8. Both T_+ and T_- exceed this critical value, and the effect is clearly non-significant.

For the large-sample test, we calculate

$$E(T_+) = \tfrac{1}{4}(10)(11) = 27.5,$$
$$\text{var}(T_+) = \frac{10(11)(21)}{24} - \frac{1}{48}\left[(4^3 - 4) + (2^3 - 2) + (2^3 - 2)\right]$$
$$= 96 \cdot 25 - 1 \cdot 50$$
$$= 94 \cdot 75,$$
$$\text{SE}(T_+) = \sqrt{94 \cdot 75} = 9 \cdot 73,$$

and the standardized normal deviate is $(10 \cdot 5 - 0 \cdot 5)/9 \cdot 73 = 1 \cdot 03$, clearly non-significant (from Table A1, $P = 0 \cdot 303$). From Lehmann's (1975) table, ignoring the ties, the probability of the observed result or one more extreme is $0 \cdot 322$. Both the P values quoted here are approximate (one because of the normal approximation, the other because of the ties), but they agree reasonably well.

Estimation

Suppose the observations (or differences, in the case of a paired comparison as in Example 10.2) are distributed symmetrically not about zero, as specified by the null hypothesis, but about some other value, μ. How can we best estimate μ? One obvious suggestion is the sample mean. Another is the sample median, which, if subtracted from each observation, would give the null expectation in the sign test, since there would be equal numbers of positive and negative differences. A somewhat better suggestion is related to the signed rank test. We could choose that value $\hat{\mu}$ which, if subtracted from each observation, would give the null expectation in the signed rank test. It is not difficult to see that the test statistic T_+ is the number of positive values amongst the 'pair means', which are formed by taking the mean of each pair of observations (including each observation with itself). The estimate $\hat{\mu}$ is then the median of these pair means.

Confidence limits for μ are the values which, if subtracted from each observation, just give a significantly high or low test result. For this purpose all n readings may be used. The limits may be obtained by ranking the $\frac{1}{2}n(n+1)$ pair means, and taking the values whose ranks are one greater than the appropriate entry in Table A6, and the symmetric rank obtained by subtracting this from $\frac{1}{2}n(n+1)+1$. That is, one excludes the tabulated number of observations from each end of the ranked series. For values of n beyond the range of Table A6 the number of values to be excluded is the integer part of

$$\tfrac{1}{4}n(n+1) - z\sqrt{\left[\frac{n(n+1)(2n+1)}{24}\right]},$$

where $z = 1{\cdot}96$ for 95% confidence limits and $2{\cdot}58$ for 99% limits.

The procedure is illustrated below. Because of the discreteness of the ranking, the confidence coefficient is somewhat greater than the nominal value (e.g. greater than 95% for the limits obtained from the entries for $0{\cdot}05$ in Table A6). If there are substantial ties in the data, as in the example below, a further widening of the confidence coefficient takes place.

Example 10.2, continued

The 10 differences from Table 4.2, used earlier in this example for the signed rank sum test, are shown in the following table, arranged in ascending order in both rows and columns. They give the following $55(=\frac{1}{2}\times 10\times 11)$ pair means:

	−8	−7	−3	−3	−2	−1	+1	+1	+1	+8
−8	−8	−7·5	−5·5	−5·5	−5	−4·5	−3·5	−3·5	−3·5	0
−7		−7	−5	−5	−4·5	−4	−3	−3	−3	+0·5
−3			−3	−3	−2·5	−2	−1	−1	−1	+2·5
−3				−3	−2·5	−2	−1	−1	−1	+2·5
−2					−2	−1·5	−0.5	−0·5	−0·5	+3
−1						−1	0	0	0	+3·5
+1							+1	+1	+1	+4·5
+1								+1	+1	+4·5
+1									+1	+4·5
+8										+8

Note that the numbers of positive and negative pair means (counting zero values as contributing $\frac{1}{2}$ to each sum) are 17 and 38, respectively, agreeing with the values of T_+ and T_- obtained earlier. The estimate $\hat{\mu}$ is the median value of the pair means, namely −1. For 95% confidence limits, note that the entry in Table A6 for $n = 10$ and $P = 0·05$ is 8. The confidence limits are therefore the pair of means whose ranks are 9 and 47 ($= 56 - 9$). From the display above, these values are −4·5 and +1·0. For comparison, the t distribution used for these data in Example 4.3 gave limits of −4·55 and +1·95, not too dissimilar from the present values.

10.3 **Comparison of two independent groups**

Suppose we have two groups of observations: a random sample of n_1 observations, x_i, from population X and a random sample of n_2 observations, y_j, from population Y. The null hypothesis to be tested is that the distribution of x in population X is exactly the same as that of y in population Y. We should like the test to be sensitive to situations in which the two distributions differ primarily in location, so that x tends to be greater (or less) than y.

The normal-theory test is the two-sample (unpaired) t test described in §4.3. Three distribution-free tests in common usage are all essentially equivalent to each other. They are described briefly here.

The Mann–Whitney U test

The observations are ranked together in order of increasing magnitude. There are $n_1 n_2$ pairs (x_i, y_j); of these

U_{XY} is the number of pairs for which $x_i < y_j$,

and U_{YX} is the number of pairs for which $x_i > y_j$.

Any pairs for which $x_i = y_j$, count $\frac{1}{2}$ a unit towards both U_{XY} and U_{YX}.

Either of these statistics may be used for a test, with exactly equivalent results. Using U_{YX}, for instance, the statistic must lie between 0 and $n_1 n_2$. On the null hypothesis its expectation is $\frac{1}{2} n_1 n_2$. High values will suggest a difference between the distributions, with x tending to take higher values than y. Conversely, low values of U_{YX} suggest that x tends to be less than y.

Wilcoxon's rank sum test

Again there are two equivalent statistics:

$$T_1 \text{ is the sum of the ranks of the } x_i\text{s};$$
$$T_2 \text{ is the sum of the ranks of the } y_j\text{s}.$$

Low values assume low ranks (i.e. rank 1 is allotted to the smallest value). Any group of tied ranks is allotted the midrank of the group.

The smallest value which T_1 can take arises when all the xs are less than all the ys; then $T_1 = \frac{1}{2}n_1(n_1 + 1)$. The maximum value possible for T_1 arises when all xs are greater than all ys; then $T_1 = n_1 n_2 + \frac{1}{2}n_1(n_1 + 1)$. The null expectation of T_1 is $\frac{1}{2}n_1(n_1 + n_2 + 1)$.

Kendall's S

This is defined in terms of the two Mann–Whitney statistics:

$$S = U_{XY} - U_{YX}. \tag{10.2}$$

Its minimum value (when all ys are less than all xs) is $-n_1 n_2$; its maximum value (when all xs are less than all ys) is $n_1 n_2$. The null expectation is 0.

Interrelationships between tests

There are, first, two relationships between the two Mann–Whitney statistics and between the two Wilcoxon statistics:

$$U_{XY} + U_{YX} = n_1 n_2, \tag{10.3}$$

$$T_1 + T_2 = \frac{1}{2}(n_1 + n_2)(n_1 + n_2 + 1). \tag{10.4}$$

These show that tests based on either of two statistics in each pair are equivalent; given T_1 and the two sample sizes, for example, T_2 can immediately be calculated from (10.4).

Secondly, the three tests are interrelated by the following formulae:

$$U_{YX} = T_1 - \frac{1}{2}n_1(n_1 + 1), \tag{10.5}$$

$$U_{XY} = T_2 - \frac{1}{2}n_2(n_2 + 1) \tag{10.6}$$

and

$$S = U_{XY} - U_{YX},$$

as already given in (10.2).

The three tests are exactly equivalent. From (10.5) for instance, the probability of observing a value of T_1 greater than or equal to that observed is exactly equal to the probability of a value of U_{YX} greater than or equal to that observed. Significance tests based on T_1 and U_{YX} will therefore yield exactly the same significance level. The choice between these tests depends purely on familiarity with a particular form of computation and accessibility of tables.

The probability distributions of the various statistics are independent of the distributions of x and y. They have been tabulated for small and moderate sample sizes, for situations in which there are no ties. Table A7 gives critical values for T_1 (the samples being labelled so that $n_1 \leq n_2$). The table provides for two-sided tests, at the 5% and 1% levels, for n_1 and n_2 up to 15. More extensive tables are given in the Geigy Scientific Tables (1982, pp. 156–62), and the exact distribution (in terms of U_{XY}) is given by Lehmann (1975, Table B) for some smaller values of n_1 and n_2. Beyond the range of Table A7, the normal approximation based on the variance formulae of Table 10.1 is adequate unless the smaller of n_1 and n_2 is less than 4.

When there are ties the variance formulae are modified as shown in Table 10.1. The summations in the formulae are taken over all groups of tied observations, t being the number of observations in a particular group. As with the signed rank sum test, the tables of critical values are somewhat conservative in the presence of ties.

Example 10.3

We illustrate the use of Kendall's S, and the equivalent Mann–Whitney U test, in a set of data shown in Table 10.2. The observations are measurements of the percentage change in area of gastric ulcers after 3 months' treatment, the comparison being between 32 in-patients and 32 out-patients. A percentage change is an awkward measurement; its minimum value is -100 (when the ulcer has disappeared); each group contains several readings bunched at or near this lower limit. In the other direction very large values may be recorded (when the ulcer was initially very small and increased greatly during the period of observation).

A point which may be noted in the calculation of S when there are ties is that there is no need to count $\frac{1}{2}$ for each (x, y) tie, for these contributions form part of both U_{XY} and U_{YX} and therefore cancel out in S because of (10.2). We can therefore calculate S as $P - Q$, where P and Q are calculated like U_{XY} and U_{YX} except that nothing is added for (x, y) ties.

In this example, denote the in-patients by x and the out-patients by y. To calculate P, take each member of the x sample in turn and count the number of members of the y sample greater than this value. For the first few values of x, we find:

Table 10.1 Some properties of three equivalent two-sample distribution-free tests.

	Bounds		Sampling distribution		
				Variance	
	All $x_i <$ all y_j	All $y_j <$ all x_i	Mean	No ties	Ties
Mann–Whitney U test					
U_{XY} = No. of pairs with $x_i < y_j$	$n_1 n_2$	$\left.\begin{array}{c} 0 \\[2ex] n_1 n_2 \end{array}\right\}$	$\frac{1}{2}n_1 n_2$	$\dfrac{n_1 n_2 (n+1)}{12}$	$\dfrac{n_1 n_2}{12n(n-1)}\left[n^3 - n - \sum_t (t^3 - t)\right]$
U_{YX} = No. of pairs with $y_j < x_i$	0				
Wilcoxon rank sum test					
T_1 = Sum of ranks for x_is	$\frac{1}{2}n_1(n_1 + 1)$	$n_1 n_2 + \frac{1}{2}n_1(n_1 + 1)$	$\frac{1}{2}n_1(n + 1)$	As above	
T_2 = Sum of ranks for y_js	$n_1 n_2 + \frac{1}{2}n_2(n_2 + 1)$	$\frac{1}{2}n_2(n_2 + 1)$	$\frac{1}{2}n_2(n + 1)$		
Kendall's S test					
$S = U_{XY} - U_{YX}$	$n_1 n_2$	$-n_1 n_2$	0	$\dfrac{n_1 n_2 (n+1)}{3}$	$\dfrac{n_1 n_2}{3n(n-1)}\left[n^3 - n - \sum_t (t^3 - t)\right]$

Notation: n_1 = Sample size of x_is.
$\quad\quad\quad\quad n_2$ = Sample size of y_js.
$\quad\quad\quad\quad n = n_1 + n_2$.

Table 10.2 Percentage change in area of gastric ulcer after 3 months' treatment (Doll & Pygott, 1952).

	Number	
X: In-patients	32	$-100^{(12)}$, -93, -92 $-91^{(2)}$, -90, -85, -83, -81, -80, -78, -46, -40, -34, 0, 29, 62, 75, 106, 147, 1321
Y: Out-patients	32	$-100^{(5)}$, -93, -89, -80, -78, -75, -74, -72, -71, -66, -59, -41, -30, -29, -26, -20, -15, 20, 25, 37, 55, 68, 73, 75, 145, 146, 220, 1044

Notation: $-100^{(5)}$ indicates 5 observations at -100, etc.

x_i	$-100^{(12)}$	-93	-92	$-91^{(2)}$	-90	-85	$\ldots$
Number of $y_j > x_i$	27	26	26	26	26	25	$\ldots$

Thus,

$$P = 12(27) + 5(26) + 3(25) + 24 + 23 + 17 + 2(16) + 11 + 9 + 7 + 2(4) + 2 + 0$$
$$= 662,$$
$$Q = 5(20) + 19 + 15 + 11 + 7(10) + 9 + 5(7) + 2(6) + 2(5) + 2(4) + 3 + 2(2) + 2(1)$$
$$= 298,$$

and

$$S = 662 - 298 = 364.$$

From Table 10.1,

$$\text{var}(S) = \frac{(32)(32)}{3(64)(63)} \left[64^3 - 64 - (17^3 - 17) - \ldots \right],$$

where the terms arising from the small groups of ties (like two observations at -93) have been omitted as they can easily be seen to be very much smaller than the other terms.

$$\text{var}(S) = (0 \cdot 084656)(257\,184)$$
$$= 21\,772$$
$$\text{SE}(S) = \sqrt{21\,772} = 147 \cdot 5.$$

Using the normal approximation, the standardized normal deviate is $364/147 \cdot 5 = 2 \cdot 47(P = 0 \cdot 014)$.

For the Mann–Whitney version, each tie contributes $\frac{1}{2}$ to U_{XY} and U_{YX}. Thus, for example,

$$U_{YX} = 5(26) + 19\tfrac{1}{2} + 15 + 11\tfrac{1}{2} + \ldots$$
$$= 330,$$
$$\text{E}(U_{YX}) = \tfrac{1}{2}(32)(32) = 512,$$
$$U_{YX} - \text{E}(U_{YX}) = -182(= \tfrac{1}{2}S),$$
$$\text{var}(U_{YX}) = 5443(= \tfrac{1}{4}\text{var}(S)),$$

and the standardized normal deviate is $-2 \cdot 47$, as before apart from the sign.

This is an example in which the difference between the x and y samples would not have been detected by a t test. The distributions are exceedingly non-normal, and the two-sample t test gives $t = 0 \cdot 51$—clearly non-significant.

The ability of these two-sample tests to handle ties provides an interesting link with some tests for contingency tables described elsewhere in this book. In Example 15.1, for instance, illustrating the test for a trend in proportions, we could ask whether the distribution of time since the last visit is the same for the attenders and non-attenders. Taking the four time periods as the values of a heavily grouped variate, the distribution-free tests just described could be applied. It can be shown (Armitage, 1955) that the resulting normal deviate is exactly the same as X_{1a}, the square root of the statistic given by (15.6), provided that in the latter test the x scores are chosen in a particular way. The scores must be equal to the midranks of the different groups; in Example 15.1, for instance, they would be 78·5, 177·0, 221·5 and 262·0. When these scores, which are referred to as *modified ridits*, are used, the Wilcoxon/Mann–Whitney test and the test for trend in proportions given by (15.6) are entirely equivalent. In this example the $\chi^2_{(1)}$ statistic, X^2_{1a}, is 8·48 ($P = 0 \cdot 003$).

A 2×2 contingency table is an extreme case of this situation, and here the normal deviate from the distribution-free test (making due allowance for the ties) is the same as that for the usual normal approximation of §4.5, apart from a factor of $\sqrt{[(n-1)/n]}$.

Estimation

Suppose the two distributions have the same shape, but differ in their location by a displacement δ along the scale of measurement, this being positive when the xs tend to exceed the ys. The parameter δ, with confidence limits, may be estimated as follows. First note that U_{YX} is the number of pairs for which $x_i > y_j$. Therefore, if all the $n_1 n_2$ differences $x_i - y_j$ are formed, then U_{YX} is the number of positive values (assuming no ties); so U_{YX} is a test statistic for the hypothesis that the median difference is zero. If a constant quantity δ were subtracted from all the xs, and therefore from all the differences, the two samples would be effectively drawn from the same distribution and the null hypothesis would be true. If U_{YX} were recalculated after the subtraction, it would provide a test of the hypothesis that the displacement, or median difference, is in fact δ. Confidence limits for the displacement are thus obtained by finding those values which, if subtracted from all the differences, give a result on the borderline of significance. If the differences are ranked, then the confidence interval is the middle part of the distribution, with a number of differences excluded from both ends according to the critical value of the test of

U_{YX}. The number of values to be excluded can be evaluated by using Table A7 and (10.5), as illustrated in the following example. A point estimate of the parameter δ is given by the median of the differences, since this is the value which, if subtracted from all the differences, would make the test statistic equal to its expectation.

Example 10.4

The data of Table 4.3 may be ranked as follows, denoting the low and high protein as groups 1 and 2, respectively, so that $n_1 = 7$ and $n_2 = 12$.

Values		Ranks	
High protein	Low protein	High protein	Low protein
	70		1
83		2	
	85		3
	94		4
97		5	
	101		6
104		7	
107		8·5	
	107		8·5
113		10	
	118		11
119		12	
123		13	
124		14	
129		15	
	132		16
134		17	
146		18	
161		19	
Sum of ranks		$T_2 = 140 \cdot 5$	$T_1 = 49 \cdot 5$
		$n_2 = 12$	$n_1 = 7$

From Table A7 there would be a significant difference at the 5% level if $T_1 \leq 46$; using (10.5), that is if $U_{YX} \leq 18$. Therefore 18 of the differences are eliminated from each end of the set of ordered differences to give the 95% confidence interval. The 84 differences, high protein minus low protein, are tabulated on p. 284.

The median of these 84 differences is 18·5 and excluding the 18 highest and 18 lowest differences gives a 95% confidence interval from −3 to 40. These values are in close agreement with those found using the t distribution in Example 4.4, as would be expected since the data satisfy the condition for this analysis.

Low protein	High protein											
	83	97	104	107	113	119	123	124	129	134	146	161
70	13	27	34	37	43	49	53	54	59	64	76	91
85	−2	12	19	22	28	34	38	39	44	49	61	76
94	−11	3	10	13	19	25	29	30	35	40	52	67
101	−18	−4	3	6	12	18	22	23	28	33	45	60
107	−24	−10	−3	0	6	12	16	17	22	27	39	54
118	−35	−21	−14	−11	−5	1	5	6	11	16	28	43
132	−49	−35	−28	−25	−19	−13	−9	−8	−3	2	14	29

For values outside the range of Table A7 an approximation to the number of differences to be excluded from each end of the ordered set is given by the integer part of

$$\tfrac{1}{2}n_1 n_2 - z \sqrt{\left[\frac{n_1 n_2 (n_1 + n_2 + 1)}{12} \right]}$$

The method of estimation described above could be applied to the data of Example 10.3. The 95% confidence limits are calculated as −66 and −2, in the units of percentage change used in Table 10.2. However, the method is inappropriate here, since the hypothesis of a constant displacement in the distributions is quite unrealistic in view of the bunching of observations at the lower bound of −100%. Other parameters need to be used to describe the difference between the groups. For instance, one might report the difference in the proportions of observations at the lower bound, or less than −90%. An alternative approach, which is available for any application of the Wilcoxon/Mann–Whitney test, is to note that the statistic $U_{XY}/n_1 n_2$ is clearly an estimate of the probability that a randomly chosen value of x is less than a randomly chosen value of y. However, the variance of this statistic is difficult to evaluate since it depends on the precise way in which the two distributions differ; it is important to realize that the usual binomial variance for a proportion with $n_1 n_2$ observations is wholly inappropriate here since the $n_1 n_2$ differences are not independent.

Normal scores

An alternative approach to the two-sample distribution-free problem is provided by the Fisher–Yates *normal scores*. Instead of using ranks, the observations are transformed to a different set of scores, which depend purely on the ranks in the combined sample of size n. The score for the observation of rank number r is, in fact, numerically equal to the mean value of the rth smallest observation in a sample of n from a standardized normal distribution, N(0, 1). The scores are tabulated for various sample sizes by Fisher and Yates (1963, Table XX).

Now, these scores can be regarded as a method of transforming to normality as a preliminary step to the use of standard normal methods, and this is usually a perfectly adequate use of the method. However, normal methods inevitably introduce an approximation, since the transformed data cannot be regarded as randomly drawn from a normal distribution. If one wished to have an exact distribution-free test, one could calculate the difference between the means of the two sets of scores and use the fact that its sampling distribution does not depend on the distribution of the original observations. Tables are given by Klotz (1964).

An incidental use of normal scores is to provide a graphical test of normality (see §11.9).

Some further general comments about the value of two-sample distribution-free tests are made at the end of §10.4.

10.4 **Comparison of several groups**

Related groups: Friedman's test

Suppose we have more than two groups of observations and the data are also classified by a block structure so that the data form a two-way classification of the type considered in §9.2, where the two-way analysis of variance of a random-ized block design was described. Suppose that there are t treatments and b blocks. A distribution-free test for such a situation was given by Friedman (1937) and this test is a generalization of the sign test to more than two groups. The test is based on ranking the values within each block.

The test procedure can best be explained by considering a two-way analysis of variance of the ranks, using the formulae of §9.2. In such an analysis the sums of squares and their degrees of freedom may be written as follows:

	SSq	DF
Blocks	0	0
Treatments	S_{tr}	$t - 1$
Residual	S_{res}	$(b - 1)(t - 1)$
Total	S_{tot}	$b(t - 1)$

Both the sum of squares and the degrees of freedom for blocks are zero because the sum of the ranks is the same for every block, namely $\frac{1}{2}t(t + 1)$. In the calculation of the sums of squares the correction term (T^2/N in Table 9.2) is $\frac{1}{4}bt(t + 1)^2$. The usual form of the Friedman test statistic is

$$T_1 = \frac{b(t - 1)S_{tr}}{S_{tot}}, \tag{10.7}$$

which is distributed approximately as $\chi^2_{(t-1)}$. This statistic is the ratio of the Treatment sum of squares (SSq) to the Total mean square (MSq) in the analysis of variance. A somewhat preferable test statistic is analogous to the usual variance ratio in the analysis of variance, i.e. the ratio of the Treatment MSq to the Residual MSq:

$$T_2 = \frac{(b-1)S_{tr}}{S_{tot} - S_{tr}}, \tag{10.8}$$

which is distributed as F, with $t-1$ and $(t-1)(b-1)$ DF.

When there are no ties, the Total SSq, S_{tot}, can be calculated directly as $bt(t+1)(2t+1)/6$, and the formulae for the test statistics are often written in forms that make use of this expression. When $t = 2$ the test statistic T_1 is identical to the sign test statistic without a continuity correction.

Example 10.5

Table 10.3 shows the data given in Table 9.3 with the values within each block ranked. The effect of treatments is highly significant by either test, in agreement with the analysis of Example 9.1. Note that T_2 is more significant than T_1; this will generally be true when the effect is in any case highly significant, because the Residual MSq used as the basis for T_2 will then be substantially smaller than the Total MSq used in T_1. This is the reason for the general preference for the second of the two tests.

Table 10.3 Clotting times of plasma from eight subjects, treated by four methods, after ranking the four values within each subject.

Subject	Treatment 1	2	3	4	Total
1	1	2	3	4	10
2	1	4	2	3	10
3	2	1	4	3	10
4	2	1	3	4	10
5	2	1	3·5	3·5	10
6	1	3	2	4	10
7	1	2	3	4	10
8	1	2	3	4	10
Total	11·0	16·0	23·5	29·5	80

Correction term $= 80^2/32 = 200$,
Between-Treatments SSq, $S_{tr} = (11\cdot0^2 + 16\cdot0^2 + 23\cdot5^2 + 29\cdot5^2)/8 - 200$
$\qquad\qquad = 24\cdot9375$,
Total SSq, $S_{tot} = 1^2 + 2^2 + \ldots + 4^2 - 200 = 39\cdot5$,
$\qquad\quad T_1 = 8 \times 3 \times 24\cdot9375/39\cdot5 = 15\cdot15$ (as $\chi^2_{(3)}$; $P = 0\cdot002$),
$\qquad\quad T_2 = 7 \times 24\cdot9375/14\cdot5625 = 11\cdot99$ (as $F_{3,21}$; $P < 0\cdot001$).

In some studies treatments may be compared within strata or blocks, but with more than one observation per treatment in each stratum, and the numbers of replicates may be unbalanced. This situation is referred to later in this section.

Independent groups: the Kruskal–Wallis test

Suppose we have more than two groups of observations and the data form a one-way classification of the type considered in §8.1, where the one-way analysis of variance was described. Suppose that there are t groups. A distribution-free test for such a situation would be a generalization of the Mann–Whitney or Wilcoxon rank sum test to more than two groups. A generalization was given by Kruskal and Wallis (1952). This test is based on ranking all the values and then the test proceeds by a method which has similarities with a one-way analysis of variance on the ranks.

Suppose that there are n_i observations for group i, and let $N = \sum n_i$. The observations are ranked from 1 to N, and the ranks are subjected to a one-way analysis of variance. Let T_i be the sum of the ranks in group i. Denote the corrected sum of squares for groups by S_{tr}, and the corrected total sum of squares by S_{tot}. In these calculations the correction term is given by $\frac{1}{4}N(N+1)^2$. The test statistic is then calculated as

$$T = \frac{(N-1)S_{tr}}{S_{tot}}, \tag{10.9}$$

distributed approximately as $\chi^2_{(t-1)}$. If there are no ties, S_{tot} can be evaluated directly and the formula for the test statistic simplifies to

$$T = \frac{12}{N(N+1)} \sum T_i^2/n_i - 3(N+1). \tag{10.10}$$

Example 10.6

Table 10.4 shows the data from Table 8.1, ranked from 1 to 20. From (10.9), $T = 19 \times 217/664 \cdot 5 = 6 \cdot 20$ (as $\chi^2_{(3)}$; $P = 0 \cdot 10$). If (10.10) is used in spite of the single pair of tied ranks, $T = 12 \times 2422/(20 \times 21) - 3 \times 21 = 6 \cdot 20$ again; the effect of this small degree of tying in the ranks is negligible. The conclusions from the analysis are very similar to those from the analysis of variance in Example 8.1: the differences are non-significant.

When the data are stratified by one or more factors (e.g. if data like those in Table 10.4 are obtained on each of several days), the Kruskal–Wallis test needs to be adapted to take account of the stratification. We shall not attempt a full discussion here, partly because the methods become more arduous and partly because, for complex sets of data, it may be advisable to consider a

Table 10.4 Counts of adult worms in four groups each of five rats, after ranking.

	Experiment			
	1	2	3	4
	6	17	1	18
	14	5	12.5	16
	11	19	12.5	15
	2	4	7	20
	9	8	3	10
Total	42	53	36	79

Correction term $= \frac{1}{4} \times 20 \times 441 = 2205$,

Between-Treatments SSq, $S_{tr} = (42^2 + 53^2 + 36^2 + 79^2)/5 - 2205$
$\qquad\qquad = 217$,

Total SSq, $S_{tot} = 6^2 + 17^2 + \ldots + 10^2 - 2205 = 664 \cdot 5$.

multiple regression approach to the original data or a transformed data set; see §10.8.

Two points may be noted, however. First, if there are two treatments, so that the solution required is a stratified version of the Wilcoxon/Mann–Whitney test, van Elteren (1960) has described a test based on a weighted sum of the Wilcoxon rank sum statistics T_{1h} (where the subscript h refers to a particular stratum). Secondly, data of this sort often arise in situations where the observations are heavily grouped, so that the groups may be regarded as categories in an ordinal categorical variable. The analysis of this type of data will be discussed briefly in §15.7.

General remarks on distribution-free tests of location

Distribution-free tests of location are supported by remarkably strong theoretical arguments. Suppose that one wished to test the null hypothesis that the two samples were drawn from the same distribution, and that one wished the test to have high power against alternative hypotheses specifying that the distributions differed only in their location, i.e. one distribution could be changed into the other by a simple shift along the scale of the measurement. If the distributions are normal with the same variance, the t test is the most efficient test, but the rank test (Wilcoxon, Mann–Whitney or Kendall) has a relative efficiency* of 0·96. If the distributions are not normal, the relative efficiency of the rank test is never less

---

*This measure of efficiency can be interpreted as the ratio of sample sizes needed to provide a certain power of detecting a given small shift in location.

than 0·86 and may be infinitely high. For detecting a shift in location, therefore, the rank test is never much worse than the *t* test, and can be very much better. Furthermore, the distribution-free test based on normal scores has a relative efficiency against the *t* test which is never less than unity and may be infinite.

Why, then, should one not always use either the rank test or the normal score test in preference to the *t* test? The first point to make is that significance tests form only a part of the apparatus of statistical analysis. The main purpose of an analysis is usually to provide as much information as possible about the nature of the random variation affecting a set of observations. This can usually be done only by specifying a model for that variation, estimating the parameters of the model in a reasonably efficient way and informing oneself about the precision of these estimates.

Distribution-free methods were devised initially as significance tests, and they are not always easily adapted for purposes of estimation. We have described a number of estimation methods. None of these is particularly difficult, and the computational effort, which may be substantial in all but quite small samples, is alleviated by computer programs, which are readily available. However, as noted earlier, the methods tend to assume a particular model for the contrasts between samples; for example, the model used in conjunction with the Wilcoxon/Mann–Whitney test assumes a constant displacement in location between the two distributions. If the model is judged to be inappropriate, it may be difficult to find a satisfactory alternative, and hence to decide what should be estimated. A related point is that the theoretical results on power also refer to a particular form of difference between two distributions. In other situations the relative merits of different tests are less clear.

10.5 **Rank correlation**

Suppose that, in a group of *n* individuals, each individual provides observations on two variables, *x* and *y*. The closeness of the association between *x* and *y* is usually measured by the product–moment correlation coefficient *r* (§7.3). The use of this statistic might be thought objectionable on one of the following grounds: (i) it is based on the concept of closeness to linear regression, and its value may be affected drastically by a non-linear transformation; (ii) the measurements to be analysed may be qualitative, although ordered, and the investigator may not wish to assume any particular numerical scale; and (iii) the sampling variation of *r* depends on the distribution of the variables, normality being usually assumed—a distribution-free approach may be desired.

These objections would be overcome by a correlation coefficient dependent only on the ranks of the observations. To preserve comparability with the product–moment correlation coefficient, *r*, a rank correlation coefficient should have at least the following properties:

1   It should lie between -1 and $+1$, taking the value $+1$ when the individuals are ranked in exactly the same order by x as by y, and -1 when the order is reversed.

2   For large samples in which the distribution of x is independent of y (and conversely), the value should be zero.

A satisfactory rank correlation coefficient can be obtained from Kendall's S statistic, described in §10.3, with a generalization of the definition used there. The total number of pairs of individuals is $\frac{1}{2}n(n-1)$. Let P be the number of pairs which are ranked in the same order by x and by y, and Q the number of pairs in which the rankings are in the opposite order. Then

$$S = P - Q.$$

(The previous definition is a particular case of this in which one variable represents a dichotomy into the two groups, with group X being ranked before group Y, and the other variable represents the measurement under test, both x_i and y_j as previously defined being values of this second variable.)

The rank correlation coefficient, τ, is now defined by

$$\tau = \frac{S}{\frac{1}{2}n(n-1)}. \tag{10.11}$$

It is fairly easy to see that for complete agreement of rankings $\tau = 1$, and for complete reversal $\tau = -1$. A significance test of the null hypothesis that the x ranking is independent of the y ranking can conveniently be done on S. The null expectation of S (as of τ) is zero, and, in the absence of ties,

$$\mathrm{var}(S) = n(n-1)(2n+5)/18. \tag{10.12}$$

If there are ties, (10.12) is modified to give

$$\mathrm{var}(S) = \tfrac{1}{18}[n(n-1)(2n+5) - \sum_t t(t-1)(2t+5) - \sum_u u(u-1)(2u+5)]$$

$$+ \frac{1}{9n(n-1)(n-2)}[\sum_t t(t-1)(t-2)][\sum_u u(u-1)(u-2)]$$

$$+ \frac{1}{2n(n-1)}[\sum_t t(t-1)][\sum_u u(u-1)],$$

where the summations are over groups of ties, t being the number of tied individuals in a group of x values and u the number of a group of tied y values.

For further discussion of rank correlation, including tables for the significance of S, see Kendall and Gibbons (1990).

An alternative, and earlier method of rank correlation, due to Spearman, uses the product–moment correlation of the ranks. In the absence of ties the formula for the Spearman coefficient may be simplified by the fact that the ranked observations in each group are the integers from 1 to n, to give

$$r_s = 1 - \frac{6 \sum d^2}{n^3 - n},$$ (10.13)

where the ds are the differences in the paired ranks. Significance may be tested approximately by the usual formula (7.19) for testing product–moment correlation coefficients.

Example 10.7

A sample of 10 students training as clinical psychologists are ranked by a tutor at the end of the course according to (a) suitability for their career, and (b) knowledge of psychology.

Student	A	B	C	D	E	F	G	H	I	J
Rank on (a)	4	10	3	1	9	2	6	7	8	5
Rank on (b)	5	8	6	2	10	3	9	4	7	1

Rearranging according to the (a) ranking, we have:

(a)	1	2	3	4	5	6	7	8	9	10
(b)	2	3	6	5	1	9	4	7	10	8

To calculate P take each of the (b) rankings in turn and count how many individuals to the right of this position have a higher ranking. These counts are then added. Thus, starting with the first individual, with rank 2, there are eight ranks greater than 2 to the right of this; for the next individual with rank 3 there are seven ranks greater than 3 to the right of this; and so on. Similarly, Q is defined by counting lower rather than higher ranks.

$$P = 8 + 7 + 4 + 4 + 5 + 1 + 3 + 2 + 0 + 0 = 34,$$
$$Q = 1 + 1 + 3 + 2 + 0 + 3 + 0 + 0 + 1 + 0 = 11.$$

As a check, $P + Q = \frac{1}{2}n(n-1)$ in the absence of ties; $P + Q = 45 = \frac{1}{2}(10)(9)$.

$$S = P - Q = 23.$$

From Appendix Table 1 of Kendall and Gibbons (1990), the null probability of a value of S equal to 23 or more is 0·023. A one-sided test is perhaps appropriate here. For a two-sided test, the significance probability would be $2 \times 0·023 = 0·046$, still rather low. There is, therefore, a definite suggestion of an association between the two rankings.

The rank correlation coefficient is, by (10.11),

$$\tau = \frac{23}{\frac{1}{2}(10)(9)} = \frac{23}{45} = 0·51.$$

For the normal approximation to the significance test, from (10.12),

$$\text{var}(S) = 10(9)(25)/18 = 125,$$
$$\text{SE}(S) = 11·18.$$

It is useful to apply a continuity correction of 1 unit, since the possible values of S turn out to be separated by an interval of 2 units. The standardized normal deviate is $22/11 \cdot 18 = 1 \cdot 97$, for which $P = 0 \cdot 049$, rather close to the exact value.

For this set of data Spearman's rank correlation coefficient is $0 \cdot 68$. The approximate t test from (7.19) gives $t = 2 \cdot 66$ on 8 DF ($P = 0 \cdot 029$). A more exact significance level, allowing for the discreteness of the distribution, is $0 \cdot 031$. Both these values are smaller, indicating a more significant result, than for Kendall's test. However, different measures of association which are not logically equivalent will necessarily achieve different levels of significance, and the reader will hardly need to be reminded that the method chosen for final presentation should not be selected merely as the one showing the most significance.

10.6 **Permutation and Monte Carlo tests**

In the preceding sections the significance levels of various distribution-free tests have been given by reference to tables specially constructed for the purpose. In most cases these tables only apply to small sample sizes—for larger samples approximations to the appropriate null distribution are generally used (as given in Table 10.1). However, it is instructive to consider in more detail how the special tables have been constructed. This is because an explanation of the tables will illustrate that many of the distribution-free tests can be justified as instances of a more general class of tests known as *permutation tests*.

As an example consider the comparison of two independent samples of sizes 4 (sample 1) and 5 (sample 2) using the Wilcoxon rank sum test. As above, the sum of the ranks from sample 1 is denoted by T_1. Reference to Table A7 shows that the difference between the groups is significant at the 5% level if $T' \leq 11$. As explained in the legend to Table A7, $T' = T_1$ if $T_1 \leq E(T_1)$ and $T' = 2E(T_1) - T_1 (= 40 - T_1$ in this example) if $T_1 > E(T_1)$: T' is considered because the test is two-sided. If, for simplicity, it is assumed that there are no ties, then the ranks of the four values from sample 1 will be four values chosen from $\{1, 2, 3, 4, 5, 6, 7, 8, 9\}$. Under the null hypothesis that both samples were drawn from the same population, any set of four of these values is equally likely. There are, therefore, $\binom{9}{4} = 126$ different sets of four ranks that could have come from sample 1 (see §3.6 for a definition of the binomial coefficient $\binom{n}{r}$). From Table 10.1 it can be seen that the only possible values for T' are from 10 to $E(T_1) = 20$, that is, 11 distinct values. Consequently some values of T' will arise from several sets of ranks. Indeed, because each set of ranks is equally likely, the value of $P(T' = t)$ under the null distribution is simply the number of sets of ranks giving $T' = t$, divided by 126.

The smallest value of T' is 10, which occurs only when sample 1 has the four smallest ranks, or the four largest ranks. The second smallest value of T', 11, also can be obtained in only two ways, namely when the ranks for sample 1 are either $\{1, 2, 3, 5\}$ or $\{5, 7, 8, 9\}$. The next smallest value, 12, can occur in four ways, namely when sample 1 comprises ranks $\{1, 2, 3, 6\}$ or $\{1, 2, 4, 5\}$ or $\{4, 7, 8, 9\}$ or $\{5, 6, 8, 9\}$. It follows that, under the null distribution, $P(T' \le 10) = 2/126 = 0.0159, P(T' \le 11) = (2 + 2)/126 = 0.0317$ and $P(T' \le 12) = (2 + 2 + 4)/ 126 = 0.0635$. Since the probability associated with the smallest value of T' exceeds 0.01, it is not possible to obtain a significance level of 0.01 for the difference between samples of sizes 4 and 5 using a Wilcoxon rank sum test. The entry 11 in Table A7 follows because, under the null distribution, the probability that the observed value of T' is less than or equal to 11 is less than 0.05: in fact, an observed value of T' of 11 actually corresponds to a two-sided significance level of approximately 0.0317. However, as $P(T' \le 12) > 0.05$, a significance level less than 0.05 could not be ascribed to any value of T' greater than 11.

This procedure for evaluating the null distribution of T' can be viewed more generally as follows. Under the null hypothesis, all observations are drawn from the same population and the division into two samples, of sizes n_1 and n_2, say, is arbitrary and the two samples so formed will differ only by sampling variation. No one of the $\binom{n_1 + n_2}{n_1}$ ways of arranging the combined sample into groups of sizes n_1 and n_2 is of special significance. Consequently, if the null hypothesis is true, the observed value of T' is on the same footing as the $\binom{n_1 + n_2}{n_1}$ values that can be computed from the different ways of partitioning the combined sample. If the $\binom{n_1 + n_2}{n_1}$ values of T' are computed and the observed value is found to be in the extremes of the distribution of these values, then this provides evidence against the null hypothesis. Indeed, the significance level of the test is simply the proportion of the $\binom{n_1 + n_2}{n_1}$ values of T' that are as extreme as or more extreme than the observed value. How 'extreme' is interpreted depends whether a one-sided or two-sided test is required. The generality of this approach comes from the observation that the procedure is valid not just for the statistic T' defined above but for any statistic G, say.

If the data from the combined sample are written as a vector, then a second vector of equal length with elements 1 or 2 could be used to contain information about which observation came from which sample. The null distribution for this kind of test can be thought of as being generated by all the possible permutations of the label vector, so they are referred to as *permutation tests*. It is important that the allowed permutations are appropriate to the structure of the data. The above discussion has considered two independent samples, although its extension to more than two such samples is straightforward.

For other structures, such as two paired samples, perhaps comprising measurements taken before and after an intervention, different sets of permutations need to be considered. Under the null hypothesis that the intervention has no effect, there could still be substantial variation between the pairs. Consequently, the only valid permutations are ones which respect the integrity of each pair. Under the null hypothesis, the label 'before' could be applied with equal probability to either element of a pair, with the other element being given the other label. Moreover, this can be repeated independently for each pair. In practice, this means that all possible changes of sign can be applied to each within-pair difference, giving 2^n possible permutations when there are n pairs.

The idea behind permutation tests underlies the justification of several well-known tests. This has just been demonstrated for the Wilcoxon rank sum test and it is also the case for the exact test for 2×2 tables (see §4.5). In the latter case, if there are two binary samples of sizes r_1 and r_2 then, in general, several permutations of the sample labels will give rise to the same table. The number of such permutations, divided by $\binom{r_1+r_2}{r_1}$, will be the probability of obtaining that table under the null hypothesis; this approach gives a combinatorial argument for the justification of (4.35). Fisher (1966, para. 21) also used permutation arguments to justify the use of t tests under certain circumstances, even when the usual assumption of normality might be inappropriate. The same ideas underlie *randomization tests*, which are tests justified by the actual randomization of treatments to experimental units.

In addition to providing theoretical grounds to justify certain types of tests, the ideas behind permutation tests can be used directly in applications. They may be particularly helpful if there is doubt about the validity of other types of tests or when the calculation of quantities, such as standard errors, needed for other approaches, is intractable.

Example 10.8

Suppose it was decided to assess whether the standard deviation of weight gain was the same in the high- and low-protein groups of Example 4·4. The sample standard deviations are 21·39 g in the high-protein group and 20·62 g in the low-protein group, giving a ratio of 1·037. A straightforward approach would be to apply the variance ratio test from §5·1 to $1\cdot037^2 = 1\cdot076$, with degrees of freedom 11 and 6. This gives a two-sided significance level of 0·979. However, as mentioned in §5·1, the variance ratio test is sensitive to the assumption that the gains in weight follow a normal distribution and an alternative which makes no such assumption is a permutation test.

Table 10.5 shows the weight changes and the second column of the table indicates the type of diet fed to each rat. If the null hypothesis that the standard deviations are equal is true then the observed ratio, namely 1·037, will be typical of the ratio of the standard deviations for the groups labelled L and H for any permutation of the column of Ls and Hs. With 12 observations, in one group and seven in the other there are $\binom{19}{12} = 50\,388$ permutations and the ratio of the standard deviations can be computed for each of these; the results are shown in the histogram in Fig. 10.1. As deviations from the null hypothesis in either direction are of equal interest, a value should be considered 'more extreme' than the observed ratio of 1·037 if it exceeds 1·037 or if it is less than $1\cdot037^{-1} = 0\cdot964$. There are 46\,669 such values, so the permutation P value is $46\,669/50\,388 = 0\cdot926$, which is very similar to that obtained from the variance ratio test.

Table 10.5 Some of the permutations in the test of equality of standard deviation: H and L denote the high- and low-protein groups, respectively.

Change in weight (g)	Actual group	Permutation				
		2	3	4	...	50 388
134	H	L	H	H		L
146	H	H	L	H		L
104	H	H	H	L		L
119	H	H	H	H		L
124	H	H	H	H		L
161	H	H	H	H		L
107	H	H	H	H		L
83	H	H	H	H		H
113	H	H	H	H		H
129	H	H	H	H		H
97	H	H	H	H		H
123	H	H	H	H		H
70	L	H	H	H		H
118	L	L	L	L		H
101	L	L	L	L		H
85	L	L	L	L		H
107	L	L	L	L		H
132	L	L	L	L		H
94	L	L	L	L		H
Ratio of SDs	1·037	1·349	1·116	1·653	...	0·942

Monte Carlo tests

The significance level of a permutation test based on a statistic G is found by computing G for each of the N permutations allowed under the null hypothesis and counting the number, M, of these values that are as extreme as, or more extreme than, the value of G computed from the observed data, G_{obs}. The permutation significance level, P_{perm}, is then M/N. While conceptually very attractive, there are often severe practical problems with this approach.

The calculation of the significance level for the permutation test in Example 10.8 required the evaluation of the ratio of standard deviations for 50 388 different permutations. For modern computing machinery this size of task is relatively straightforward, but if G were more difficult and time-consuming to evaluate the task could be more daunting. Similarly, if N were larger, the number of permutations could be substantially greater; even with groups only twice the

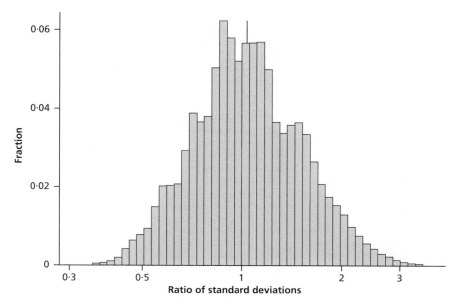

Fig. 10.1 Histogram of ratios of standard deviations for all 50 388 permutations of the group labels: note the log scale and the vertical line at the observed ratio of 1·037.

size of those in Example 10.8 there would be 9 669 554 100 permutations. Also, if the problem were more complicated, as in some spatial or image-processing applications, the approach might not be feasible. Even in the very simple case in Example 10.8, the evaluation of all the possible permutations is not entirely straightforward and requires special software, for example, Chase (1970) or using StatXact (Cytel, 1995).

An alternative approach is to choose a random sample of N_R of the permutations, compute the statistic for the sampled subset and count the number, M_R, of these statistics that are as extreme as, or more extreme than, the observed value. The significance level, $P_R = M_R/N_R$ is an estimate of the permutation significance level P_{perm} and its value will, of course, depend on the particular random sample. Despite the element of chance in the value of the significance level, this approach, widely referred to as a *Monte Carlo test*, can be very useful. Values of N_R much smaller than N are sufficient for virtually all practical purposes and it is also usually easier to generate random permutations of, for example, treatment labels, than it is to produce the full set of all permutations.

As it is based on a sample of permutations, the value P_R will be affected by sampling error. It is clearly important that the size of this error should be sufficiently small for it not to materially affect the inferences that are to be drawn. Perhaps the simplest way to ensure this is to select a sufficiently large sample of permutations. If the null hypothesis is true, then the number of permutations that will result in a statistic that is more extreme than the observed value will have a binomial distribution with parameters N_R and P_{perm}. Consequently there is, approximately, a 95% probability that P_R lies within $2\sqrt{[\{P_{perm}(1 - P_{perm})\}/N_R]}$ of P_{perm}. As there is usually greater interest in smaller significance levels, it is sensible to try to ensure that smaller values of P_{perm} are estimated with greater absolute precision. Sensible values of N_R might be found by requiring the coefficient of variation of P_R, which is

$$\sqrt{[(1 - P_{perm})/(N_R P_{perm})]}, \tag{10.14}$$

to be less than some prescribed value, such as 0·05 or 0·1. To obtain a coefficient of variation of 0·1 when $P_{perm} = 0·5$ requires $N_R = 100$, but this rises to $N_R = 1900$ when $P_{perm} = 0·05$. This is intuitively reasonable: many more simulations will be required to determine, with given relative precision, the probability of a rare event than the probability of a more common event.

Determining N_R from (10·14) requires an estimate of P_{perm}: a conservative approach would be to assume a small value and accept that if this is untrue some unnecessary samples will be drawn. In many applications several thousand permutations can be sampled very rapidly, so this is often acceptable. An alternative, which can be very useful when evaluation of each statistic is time-consuming, is to adopt a sequential approach. The essential idea is that if the observed statistic is not extreme then it is likely that a high proportion of the first few random permutations will result in values of the statistic that are more extreme than G_{obs}. For example, if 40 of the first 100 random permutations gave more extreme statistics than the observed value, then it would be clear that the test will not reject the null hypothesis. There would be no point in continuing to sample permutations in order to obtain a more precise estimate of a value which holds little further interest. On the other hand, if the observed statistic is extreme, then it will be worthwhile continuing sampling until a sufficiently precise estimate of P_{perm} is obtained. These informal ideas are put on a firm foundation by Besag and Clifford (1991), who suggest that sampling continues until h values of the statistic more extreme than the observed value are obtained. If the number of samples needed to achieve this is l then the estimate of P_{perm} is h/l. These authors suggest values for h of 10 or 20, although smaller values could be used if the sampling and evaluations were particularly onerous.

Monte Carlo significance levels are necessarily discrete: non-sequential values being restricted to the set $0/N_R, 1/N_R, \ldots, (N_R - 1)/N_R, 1$. However, for practical purposes N_R will generally be sufficiently large to ensure that this is of no practical importance. An advantage of the sequential approach is that significance levels obtained in this way are restricted to the set 1,

$h/(h+1), h/(h+2), \ldots, h/(h+l), \ldots$ and this set is more finely graded around the smaller, and hence more interesting, significance levels.

Example 10.8, continued

Rather than generate all possible permutations of the group labels, a Monte Carlo approach might be used. If a coefficient of variation in the estimated significance level of 0.1 is prescribed and P_{perm} is taken as 0.05, then 1900 random permutations are needed, whereas, if P_{perm} is taken as 0.1, only 900 have to be generated. An alternative would be to generate random permutations until 20 values of the ratio of the standard deviations that are more extreme than the observed value (1.037) are obtained.

From 1900 permutations, 1760 give more extreme ratios, whereas 844 of the 900 samples are more extreme, giving values for P_R of 0.926 and 0.938, respectively. However, 20 values more extreme than the observed statistic were obtained in the first 22 permutations, giving $P_R = 20/22 = 0.909$. Thus, significance levels of 0.979, 0.962, 0.926, 0.938 and 0.909 have been obtained for testing the equality of the standard deviations in these two groups. The first is based on an assumption, deviations from which are known to be troublesome for this test. The remainder require no assumptions and are based on, respectively, 50 388, 1900, 900 and 22 permutations. It is clear that there are no material differences between these values and there is no evidence at all against the null hypothesis. What does differ between the estimates is the amount of effort needed to obtain them.

Permutation tests are applicable in many circumstances and are based on a procedure that is easily understood. Sampling all possible permutations is seldom practicable but the Monte Carlo approximation can be used widely, especially now that substantial computing power is readily available. Although these tests will be valid for any statistic, the choice of which statistic to use may have an important effect on the power of the test when the null hypothesis is false. Consideration of this aspect is beyond the scope of this discussion and the interested reader is referred to the book by Edgington (1987) and to the relevant parts of Efron and Tibshirani (1993, Chapter 15) and Davison and Hinkley (1997, Chapter 4).

10.7 **The bootstrap and the jackknife**

Permutation tests and Monte Carlo tests make extensive use of random samples and the lack of adequate computational power may have led to their relative neglect in the past. Now that good computational facilities are widely available, permutation and Monte Carlo tests are taking their place in an increasingly important group of techniques collectively known as *computationally intensive methods*. The bootstrap, which will be the main subject of this section, is another member of this class of techniques and plays an important role in estimation. The jackknife is a rather older technique which still has uses and is related to the bootstrap.

The bootstrap—basic ideas and standard errors

Most statistical analyses attempt to make inferences about a population on the basis of a sample drawn from that population. The distribution function F of a variable x in the population is almost always unknown. Analyses usually proceed by focusing attention on specific summaries of F, such as the mean μ_F, which are, of course, also unknown (the subscript F is used to emphasize the dependence of the mean on the underlying distribution). Most analyses estimate parameters such as μ_F from random samples drawn from the population, using estimators that have usually been constructed in a sensible way and which have been found to have good properties (e.g. minimum variance, unbiased, etc.). Naturally the values of the estimates will vary from sample to sample, i.e. the estimates are affected by sampling variation (see §4.1). This source of variability is usually quantified through the relevant standard error, which for the mean is simply $\sigma_F/\sqrt{n}$, or more precisely through the estimate of the standard error, $s/\sqrt{n}$.

The bootstrap approaches this problem from a rather different perspective. For the problem of estimating a mean and its associated standard error, it essentially reproduces the usual estimators. However, the new perspective permits estimation in a very wide variety of situations, including many that have proved intractable for conventional methods. Rather than trying to make inferences about F by estimating summaries such as the mean and variance, the bootstrap approach estimates F directly and then estimates any relevant summaries through the estimated F. Various estimates, $\hat{F}$, of F are possible and some of these will be discussed briefly below. However, the most general form and the only one that we consider in detail is the *empirical distribution function* (EDF), which is a discrete distribution that gives probability $1/n$ to each sample point $x_i (i = 1, \ldots, n)$. Using the formula for the expectation of a probability distribution (3.6) the mean of the EDF is $\mu_{\hat{F}}$, which is

$$\mu_{\hat{F}} = \frac{1}{n} \times x_1 + \frac{1}{n} \times x_2 + \ldots + \frac{1}{n} \times x_n$$

i.e. $\mu_{\hat{F}} = \bar{x}$, the sample mean, which is the usual estimator of μ_F. The same type of argument gives the variance of $\hat{F}$ as $\sigma_{\hat{F}}^2 = n^{-1} \sum (x_i - \bar{x})^2$, which again is the usual estimator, apart from the denominator being n rather than $n - 1$. This discrepancy arises because $\bar{x}$ *is* the mean of $\hat{F}$, rather than merely an estimator of it. The bootstrap estimate of the standard error of the mean is then $\sigma_{\hat{F}}/\sqrt{n}$, which is $s/\sqrt{n}$ but for the factor $\sqrt{[n/(n-1)]}$.

The bootstrap has provided estimators of the mean and its standard error that are virtually the same as the conventional ones but has done so by first estimating the distribution function. Because $\hat{F}$ is a known function, properties such as its mean and variance can be computed and these used as estimators.

This is what has been done above and the estimators obtained are often referred to as *ideal bootstrap estimators* (Efron & Tibshirani, 1993, p. 46). In many applications it is not possible to find the relevant properties of $\hat{F}$ by algebraic methods, but because $\hat{F}$ is a known function, powerful alternatives are now available.

For example, in the conventional quantification of sample-to-sample variation in the value of some estimator, an approach based on the theoretical properties of the estimator was inevitable because only one sample, and hence one value of the estimator, was available. The bootstrap starts by estimating F and then working with $\hat{F}$: since this is known, as many samples as necessary, often referred to as *bootstrap samples*, can be drawn from it and the sample-to-sample variation observed directly.

As an illustration, we now explain how the standard error of a mean could be found in this way. The standard error of the sample mean is simply the standard deviation of the hypothetical population of sample means obtained by repeatedly drawing a sample of a given size. As samples can be repeatedly drawn from $\hat{F}$, the means of each of B samples can be found and the standard deviation of these B means can be computed. This is a bootstrap estimate of the standard error of the mean. The beauty of this approach is its generality. The formula $s/\sqrt{n}$ has not been used, so the technique can be applied in circumstances where no such formula can be found by theoretical means or where there may be doubt about the validity of assumptions that have been used in the calculation of a theoretical expression. Also, because the EDF has been used to estimate F, no assumptions have been made about the form of the distribution.

When F is estimated by the EDF, drawing a sample from $\hat{F}$ is simply a matter of choosing a random sample of size n, *with replacement*, from the values $x_1, x_2, \ldots, x_n$. It follows that some observations may appear several times in a bootstrap sample while others will not be chosen at all.

The ideal bootstrap estimator computed the mean and standard error by working directly with $\hat{F}$. These estimators will be inaccurate because $\hat{F}$ is only an estimator of F. When the means and standard error are calculated from B bootstrap samples, there will be the further inaccuracy that arises from basing inference on a sample from $\hat{F}$. However, this latter source of error can be reduced by ensuring that B is sufficiently large. Efron and Tibshirani (1993, p. 52) and Davison and Hinkley (1997, §2·5·2) suggest that the estimation of standard errors will seldom require values of B in excess of 200.

The bootstrap can be applied to data with more structure than the simple sample considered above, although the appropriate implementation of the bootstrap needs careful consideration. For comparing two groups, one with distribution F and the other with an independent distribution G, then a bootstrap approach would proceed from separate estimates $\hat{F}$ and $\hat{G}$, with bootstrap samples chosen independently from each estimated distribution.

Standard errors for regression coefficients can be obtained using bootstrap methods. However, here several approaches are possible. If the data are $(x_1, y_1), (x_2, y_2), \ldots, (x_n, y_n)$, then a bootstrap sample of size n could be drawn with replacement from these n pairs. This amounts to using the usual bootstrap but with F now taken as the bivariate distribution function of the pairs. This may be entirely natural for cases where it is plausible that the pairs have been drawn from such a distribution, but it is less appealing if the x values were controlled in some way, perhaps by the design of the study. In this case the alternative procedures could be used, in which conventional fitted values and residuals are first obtained. A bootstrap sample of the residuals is drawn: the bootstrap for the regression comprises the x values from the original data and y values computed by adding the fitted values to the bootstrap residuals. For linear regression this method gives the same standard errors as conventional theory, as when using the bootstrap to find the standard error of the sample mean. However, the approach could be used for non-linear regressions and for types of regression other than the classical least squares method, for which closed expressions for standard errors are not available. Further details on applying the bootstrap to more complicated data structures can be found in Efron and Tibshirani (1993, Chapter 9) and Davison and Hinkley (1997, Chapters 6–8).

Example 10.9

In §10.3 it was noted that describing the difference between the distributions of changes in ulcer size for in-patients (X) and out-patients (Y), given in Table 10.2, in a meaningful way was not straightforward. One possibility is to estimate the probability that a randomly chosen value for an in-patient X is less than the corresponding quantity Y for an out-patient, $\mathrm{P}(X < Y)$. This can be estimated by $D = U_{XY}/(n_1 n_2)$ where n_1 denotes the size of the sample of X values, with n_2 similarly defined: in this example both are 32. For the data in Table 10.2 $U_{XY} = 694$, so $D = 0.678$. It was noted in §10.3 that methods for computing the standard error of this quantity were not readily available: expressions based on the binomial distribution are not valid because the pairs that are counted in the numerator of this statistic are not independent. However, a bootstrap estimate of the standard error of D can be found.

A sample of 32 percentage changes in ulcer size is drawn with replacement from the sample of values for in-patients given in Table 10.2. A further sample of 32 is drawn in the same way for the out-patient values. For these bootstrap samples, the Mann–Whitney U statistic can be computed and hence a further estimator of $\mathrm{P}(X < Y)$ is obtained: call this D_1. In total B pairs of bootstrap samples are drawn, yielding B values $D_1, D_2, \ldots, D_B$. The standard deviation of these values is the required estimate of the standard error of D.

Choosing $B = 300$ gave an estimate of the standard error of D of 0.0667. Choosing $B = 2000$ gave 0.0674—virtually the same as for the smaller sample.

Note that the naïve estimate of the standard error based on the binomial distribution, $\sqrt{[D(1 - D)]/32} = 0.0146$ would have been a serious underestimate.

Bootstrap confidence intervals

As explained above, the bootstrap can be a very effective method for estimating a standard error. However, these estimates are frequently not of direct interest themselves, but are useful in constructing confidence intervals. For example, if g is a statistic that estimates a parameter γ, then a confidence interval γ is $g \pm z\,\mathrm{SE}(g)$, where z is a standard normal deviate chosen to give the correct confidence coefficient—for example, $z = 1\cdot96$ gives a 95% confidence interval. This interval would be used if it was believed that

$$\frac{g - \gamma}{\mathrm{SE}(g)}$$

had, at least approximately, a normal distribution with mean 0 and standard deviation 1.

In many circumstances there may be doubt about the validity of this approximation and a bootstrap approach can be used to construct an interval that has wider validity. This proceeds by drawing a bootstrap sample for which the value of the statistic is g^*. The quantity

$$z^* = \frac{g^* - g}{\mathrm{SE}(g^*)}$$

is then computed. This is repeated until B values of z^* are to hand. The appropriate sample quantiles of these values are found: for example, for a symmetric 95% confidence interval, the $0\cdot025B$th largest value z_L and the $0\cdot975B$th largest value z_U would be obtained. The required interval, known as a *bootstrap–t interval*, is $(g - z_U\,\mathrm{SE}(g), g - z_L\,\mathrm{SE}(g))$ (note the minus sign and the use of z_L and z_U in the apparently 'wrong' order).

The method is an improvement on the interval $g \pm z\,\mathrm{SE}(g)$ as it replaces the assumption that $(g - \gamma)/\mathrm{SE}(g)$ is normal with a bootstrap approximation to the true distribution. As interest is usually focused on extreme quantiles of this distribution, the number of bootstrap samples, B, needs to be substantially larger than was necessary for the estimation of a standard error: values of 1000 or 2000 are often needed. A weakness of the approach is that it requires an estimate of the standard error of g and this may be difficult or impossible to compute. The bootstrap could be applied to estimate the standard error—that is, a bootstrap could be nested within a bootstrap. However, even if the standard error were based on a very small value of B, say 25, the total number of bootstrap samples would become very large, typically 20 000–30 000.

An alternative method, which is perhaps more intuitive than that just outlined, can be used. The method, known as the *percentile method*, simply generates B bootstrap samples and computes g for each, giving bootstrap values $g_1^*, g_2^*, \ldots, g_B^*$. These are arranged in ascending order and, for a 95% interval, the $0\cdot025B$th and $0.975B$th largest values are taken as the lower and upper limits, respectively. For a $100(1 - 2\alpha)\%$ interval the limits would be the αBth and $(1 - \alpha)B$th largest values. This is known as the *percentile* method.

It turns out that this kind of interval does not perform all that well: for example, the coverage probability can stray from the nominal value. A refinement of the method, known as the bias-corrected and accelerated method, BC_a for short, has better properties. The method still uses the ordered set of the $g_1^*, g_2^*, \dots, g_B^*$ but chooses the $\alpha_1 B$th and $\alpha_2 B$th largest values for the limits of the interval. The values α_1 and α_2 are defined as

$$\alpha_1 = \Phi\left(w + \frac{w + z^{(\alpha)}}{1 - a(w + z^{(\alpha)})}\right) \tag{10.15}$$

$$\alpha_2 = \Phi\left(w + \frac{w + z^{(1-\alpha)}}{1 - a(w + z^{(1-\alpha)})}\right) \tag{10.16}$$

and here $z^{(\xi)}$ is determined by $\xi = \Phi(z^{(\xi)})$, where Φ is the standard normal distribution function. Note that this differs from the definition of a quantile of the standard normal variable, z_ξ, given in §4.2: the two are related by $z_{2\xi} = -z^{(\xi)}, \xi < \frac{1}{2}$. The quantity w corrects for bias in the distribution of the statistic. The quantity a, known as the acceleration, is related to the behaviour of the variance of the statistic: further details can be found in Efron and Tibshirani (1993, Chapters 14 and 22) and Davison and Hinkley (1997, Chapter 5). If these are both zero, then $\alpha_1 = \alpha$ and $\alpha_2 = 1 - \alpha$ and the BC_a method reduces to the percentile method.

The estimate of w is easily obtained: $\Phi(w)$ is the proportion of the bootstrap values of g that are less than the observed value. The estimation of a is potentially more complicated: for a single sample of size n, suppose that g_{-i} is the value of g obtained from the sample with the ith point omitted. If $\bar{g}$ is the mean of $g_{-1}, g_{-2}, \dots, g_{-n}$ and

$$M_k = \sum_{i=1}^{n} (\bar{g} - g_{-i})^k$$

then $a = M_3/(6M_2^{3/2})$. For more complicated data structures, Davison and Hinkley (1997, Chapter 5) should be consulted.

Example 10.9, continued

A 95% confidence interval for $P(X < Y)$ can be found by generating 2000 bootstrap samples and for each one computing the value of D. The 50th and 1950th largest values are 0·546 and 0·808 and this defines the 95% percentile bootstrap confidence interval for $P(X < Y)$.

The BC_a interval can also be computed. The proportion of the 2000 values of D that are less than the observed value, 0·678, is 0·48, giving $w = -0·0502$. Computation of a is more involved and only a brief outline is given here. The formula depends on the quantities $l_{xi}(i = 1, \ldots, n_1)$ and $l_{yj}(j = 1, \ldots, n_2)$: $l_{xi} = (D_{xi}/n_2) - D$ where

$$D_{xi} = \text{number of } y_j > x_i + \tfrac{1}{2} \times \text{ number of } y_j = x_i.$$

Similarly for l_{yj} with

$$D_{yj} = \text{number of } x_i < y_j + \tfrac{1}{2} \times \text{ number of } x_i = y_j.$$

The value of a is estimated by

$$\frac{\sum\limits_{i=1}^{32} l_{xi}^3 + \sum\limits_{j=1}^{32} l_{yj}^3}{6 \left(\sum\limits_{i=1}^{32} l_{xi}^2 + \sum\limits_{j=1}^{32} l_{yj}^2 \right)^{3/2}}.$$

This follows from equation (5.28) of Davison and Hinkley (1997): it has been possible to simplify the formula because in this application $n_1 = n_2$. This gives $a = -0.0258$. Applying (10.15) and (10·16) gives $\alpha_1 = 0.0150$ and $\alpha_2 = 0.9616$. This implies that the $BC_a 95\%$ confidence interval comprises the 30th and 1923rd largest values of the ordered bootstrap statistics, giving an interval of 0.532 to 0.795. The values 30 and 1923 are rounded values: more sophisticated methods for interpolation are available but are usually not needed in practice.

The jackknife

An estimate for the standard error of a general statistic can be obtained using a technique which predates the bootstrap but is related to it. Suppose the statistic g, based on a sample of size n, is an estimator of a scalar parameter γ. The method, known as the *jackknife*, is based on the values of g that are obtained if g is recalculated n times, each time omitting in turn one of the observations from the original sample: the value of g obtained when the ith observation of the sample is omitted is denoted by g_{-i}. The jackknife is most easily given in terms of the n so-called *pseudo-values* $\tilde{g}_i, i = 1, \ldots, n$,

$$\tilde{g}_i = ng - (n-1)g_{-i}.$$

The standard error of g is then estimated by the usual formula for the standard error of a mean, using the pseudo-values as if they were the data. Indeed, if g is the sample mean, the ith pseudo-value is the ith observation. This method will provide a reasonably good estimator of the standard error without the need for any formula or for hundreds of bootstrap simulations.

One application of both the bootstrap and the jackknife that has not been mentioned hitherto is the estimation of, and correction for, *bias*. If the expectation of g over repeated samples is γ, then g is known as an *unbiased* estimator (see §4.1). If this is not the case, then $E(g) - \gamma$ is known as the bias of the estimator. The jackknife was first introduced, by Quenouille (1949), to correct for bias: its use for the estimation of standard errors described above is based on a remark by Tukey (1958) made almost a decade later. A useful review of early contributions can be found in Miller (1974).

The jackknife estimator of bias is $g - \bar{\bar{g}}$, where the second term is the mean of the pseudo-values. Alternatively, $\bar{\bar{g}}$ can be thought of as a *bias-corrected* estimator of γ, i.e. an estimator of γ based on g but which has reduced bias relative to using g itself. Details of using the bootstrap for this purpose can be found in Chapter 10 of Efron and Tibshirani (1993). Although the jackknife is usually an effective method for reducing bias, the general issue of bias correction is one which is not widely addressed and, when it is, should be approached cautiously. Bias-corrected estimators may have smaller bias but, because the correction is estimated from data, this improvement may be offset by an increase in the standard error of the estimator.

Another use proposed for the jackknife is the formation of confidence intervals. If the ratio

$$\frac{(\bar{\bar{g}} - \gamma)}{\sqrt{\left[n - 1^{-1} \sum_{i=1}^{n} (\tilde{g}_i - \bar{\bar{g}})^2 \right]}} \tag{10.17}$$

is assumed to follow, approximately, a t distribution on $n - 1$ degrees of freedom, then a confidence interval for γ can be constructed.

The jackknife can break down in some circumstances, such as when g is not a smoothly varying function of the data. Thus, the jackknife does not give adequate standard errors or bias correction when g is the sample median. Also the confidence intervals, such as those suggested by the use of (10.17), do not, in practice, perform well. To an extent the jackknife has been superseded in practice by the bootstrap. Part of the reason for this is that the jackknife can, in a certain sense, be viewed as a linear approximation to the bootstrap: when the approximation is good the two techniques give similar answers, but when they are different it is probably the bootstrap version that is to be preferred.

Nevertheless, the jackknife can be useful, often in conjunction with the bootstrap. For example, the jackknife might be a useful way to obtain a standard error in the computation of a bootstrap–t interval. The jackknife can be used to obtain information about details of a bootstrap analysis using a class of methods jointly referred to as *jackknife-after-bootstrap* (see §19.4 of Efron and Tibshirani (1993) and Chapter 3 of Davison and Hinkley (1997)). Quantities related to the jackknife, known as *empirical influence values*, are useful in more sophisticated applications of the bootstrap.

General remarks on the bootstrap

Perhaps because it entails no assumptions about the form of F, the EDF is probably the version of $\hat{F}$ most widely used in applications of the bootstrap.

Sampling from such a distribution might seem rather unnatural, especially if F were a smooth continuous distribution. Modifications of the bootstrap are possible where the EDF is replaced by a smoother alternative. An obvious possibility, but one which falls outside the scope of this chapter, is to assume that F is known up to the values of unknown parameters θ. In this approach, known as the *parametric bootstrap*, θ is estimated using some conventional method and the bootstrap samples are drawn from $\hat{F}(x) = F(x; \hat{\theta})$. This can be very efficient, but if the model $F(x; \theta)$ is inappropriate then the results from the bootstrap can be misleading. There are *non-parametric bootstrap* methods that estimate F other than by simply using the EDF: these involve applying smoothing techniques, such as kernel density estimation (see §12.2): the reader is referred to §3.4 of Davison and Hinkley (1997) for further discussion of this point.

Indeed, the reader is encouraged to consult specialist texts on the bootstrap, such as Efron and Tibshirani (1993) and Davison and Hinkley (1997), for many aspects of the technique. The bootstrap has the potential for such wide application in statistics that the present discussion cannot do it justice. The power of the technique makes it one of the most important advances in statistical methodology made in recent years.

The bootstrap is already widely applied, often as a useful means of checking the validity of estimates obtained by conventional methods. A recent area of application discussed by Thompson and Barber (2000) is to the analysis of cost data from randomized trials. Interest usually centres on the total cost of using a treatment and this can be estimated by multiplying the number of patients using it by the arithmetic mean cost per patient. Consequently interpretation would be hampered if the data were summarized by a geometric mean or median. However, this often happens, because such data are often highly skewed and conventional statistical advice to use logarithmic transformations or distribution-free methods has been followed. Analysing the data using arithmetic means and applying the bootstrap to obtain valid inferences despite the skewed distribution are a promising approach to this kind of data.

10.8 Transformations

This chapter has dealt with various methods that are useful when the data do not have a normal distribution. However, it should be remembered that if X is a random variable with distribution function $F(X)$, the distribution of $Y = g(X)$, a transformation of X, will not, in general, have the same form as F. This leaves open the possibility of an alternative approach to the analysis of data which do not have a normal distribution. It may be possible to find a transformation, g, such that $g(X)$ is normal, or at least sufficiently close to normal for all practical purposes. Analyses using normal-theory methods can be applied to $g(X)$. The results will usually be more meaningful if they can be expressed on the original scale, although the extent to which this will be possible depends on the type of analysis and also on the transformation that has been used. It can occasionally be useful to use transformations which yield data having specific distributions other than the normal distribution, but such applications are much less common.

Transformations in general

The three main reasons why it may be appropriate to transform data are: (i) to change their distributional form (usually to make it closer to that of a normal distribution); (ii) to stabilize variance; and (iii) to linearize relationships.

1   *Transformation to normality.* Deviation from normality can, in principle, arise in many ways and there is seldom much prior guidance that can be gleaned about the appropriate transformation, and in most cases an empirical approach is necessary. A common reason for wanting to normalize the distribution of the data is so that standard normal-theory methods can be applied. However, many of these methods also require that the residual variation does not change as the mean changes (so, for example, in a regression the variance of the residuals does not change with the fitted value). Moreover, many of these techniques are less robust to departures from constant variance than from normality. Consequently a transformation that normalized the data but did not stabilize the variance might be of questionable value.

2   *Variance-stabilizing transformation.* If the variance, σ^2, of a response X depends on the mean, μ, then methods which assume σ^2 is constant may not perform adequately in data sets where the mean varies (as, for example, in a simple linear regression). In these circumstances it is desirable to attempt to find a transformation that will result in a response with a variance that is unrelated to the mean. The form of the transformation will depend on the nature of the mean. The form of the transformation will depend on the nature of the dependence of $\sigma^2 = \sigma^2(\mu)$ on μ. Application of the delta method (5.19) shows that the variance of $g(X)$ is approximately

$$\sigma^2(\mu)[g'(\mu)]^2, \tag{10.18}$$

where $g'(\mu)$ denotes the value of $dg(x)/dx$ evaluated at $x = \mu$. A variance-stabilizing transformation can be found by setting (10.18) to be a constant, k, substituting the specific form for $\sigma^2(\mu)$ and solving the differential equation.

   If the outcome is a proportion, then $\sigma^2(\mu) = \mu(1 - \mu)/n$ and solving (10.18) gives $g(X) = \arcsin(\sqrt{X})$ (in radians), which is sometimes known as the *angular transformation*, and has approximate variance $1/(4n)$. If the variance is equal to the mean, e.g. X has a Poisson distribution, then $g(X) = \sqrt{X}$. If the standard deviation of the response is proportional to the square of the mean, i.e. $\sigma^2(\mu) = \mu^4$—a very severe form of dependence of spread on the mean—then g is the reciprocal transformation. If the standard deviation is proportional to the mean, i.e. the coefficient of variation is constant, then (10.18) leads to the log transformation.

Many transformations have the form $g(X) = X^\lambda$. If this is written in the essentially equivalent form $g_\lambda(X) = (X^\lambda - 1)/\lambda$ (which differs from the first form only by a linear transformation), then $g(X) = \ln(X)$ is included in this family of transformations as the limiting case when $\lambda \to 0$. The general form $g_\lambda(X)$ is known as the Box–Cox transformation (Box & Cox, 1964) and the value of λ can be estimated from the data. This can be useful in exploratory analyses, although final analysis is often best performed using a value of λ which bears a straightforward interpretation, such as $-1, 0, \frac{1}{2}, \frac{1}{3}, 1, 2$. An exception to this can be found in the method for estimating age-related reference ranges (Cole, 1988; see also §12.3).

3 *Linearizing transformations.* Statistical techniques such as multiple regression assume that the effects on a response y of various covariates, e.g. x_1 and x_2, can be expressed using a linear equation, such as $E(y) = \alpha + \beta_1 x_1 + \beta_2 x_2$, i.e. the effects of the covariates are additive. However, in many biological applications a multiplicative form may be more appealing. In the study of the size and shape of individual organisms, the simple bivariate allometric equation $y = \alpha x^\beta$ is commonly used to relate some feature, y, to a measure of size, x. This equation can be expressed in the linear form $\log y = \log \alpha + \beta \log x$: in this case the logarithmic transformation has been used to linearize the form of the equation (see Griffiths & Sandland, 1984, for further details on allometry). Another example is provided by the Michaelis–Menten equation, which describes the rate of many reactions in enzymology (see §20.5 for a fuller discussion). The velocity of a reaction, v, is related to substrate concentrations, s, via the equation

$$v = \frac{V_{max}s}{K + s},$$

which depends on two parameters, K and V_{max}. These parameters can be estimated using linear regression if it is noted that the reciprocal transformation applied to both v and s linearizes the equation, viz.

$$\frac{1}{v} = \frac{1}{V_{max}} + \frac{K}{V_{max}} \frac{1}{s} :$$

a manoeuvre often referred to as the *Lineweaver–Burk* transformation.

In both these illustrations of linearizing transformations, little account has been taken of how the residual terms in the regressions are affected by these transformations. While a transformation may have a desirable effect in one respect, such as bringing an equation into a form that can be handled by standard methods, it may have a far from desirable effect on other aspects, such as the distributional form of the errors. This is the case with the Line-weaver–Burk transformation, which can be a poor method for analysing this model. Generalized linear models (McCullagh & Nelder, 1989) can be useful if this kind of problem arises, as they allow linearizing transformations to be applied to the mean, without it directly affecting the distribution of the errors.

Logarithmic transformation

It was noted above that if a variable X has a constant coefficient of variation, CV, then the logarithmic transformation will stabilize the variance. Very often, if the coefficient of variation is large, then X will exhibit substantial skewness and the log transform will reduce this, usually resulting in a variable that is sufficiently close to being normally distributed to allow standard methods to be applied (see §2.5).

On a heuristic level it is easy to see why, in practice, a large coefficient of variation results in a skewed variable. Many variables encountered in medicine are necessarily positive and, crudely speaking, if the coefficient of variation is large then the mean is too close to the lower bound of 0 to permit a symmetric distribution. It might be argued that a positive variable cannot have a normal distribution, as a normal distribution is defined for all values, whether positive or negative. However, this view is unnecessarily restrictive and, provided the normal distribution involved ascribes negligible probability to the event $X < 0$, then a normal distribution can be an entirely satisfactory way to describe a positive variable. If X is normal, then it can be written as $\mu + \sigma Z$, where Z has a standard normal distribution, so the probability ascribed to $X < 0$ is $P(Z < -\mu/\sigma = -(CV)^{-1})$. If the CV is 1 then this probability is about 0·16, which is too large to be tenable. Not until the coefficient of variation was noticeably smaller, say, less than $\frac{1}{2}$, would it be likely that a normal distribution could prove acceptable. It is therefore inevitable that the distributions of positive variables with large coefficients of variation are skewed.

The distribution of log X will often be close to normal and analyses using normal-theory methods can be applied not to original sample values $x_1, x_2, \ldots, x_n$ but to log x_1, log x_2, $\ldots$, log x_n. The sample arithmetic mean of the logged values is then

$$\frac{\log x_1 + \log x_2 + \ldots + \log x_n}{n} = \log(x_1 \times x_2 \times \ldots \times x_n)^{1/n} = \log G,$$

i.e. it is the log of the sample geometric mean G (see §2.5). This is an alternative measure of location to the arithmetic mean which is less sensitive to the presence of individual large values and therefore better suited to the description of skewed data. The corresponding population geometric mean can be defined as

$\mu_G = $ antilog(E(log X)). If ln X is exactly normal (i.e. X has a *log-normal* distribution), with mean and standard deviation on the log scale of μ_L and σ_L, the geometric mean of X is $\exp(\mu_L)$ whereas the arithmetic mean is $\exp(\mu_L) \times \exp(\frac{1}{2}\sigma_L^2)$, which exceeds the geometric mean, as is always the case. As μ_L is the median of ln X, $\exp(\mu_L)$ is also the median of X.

Differences between arithmetic means on the log scale, for example differences between treatment groups, will estimate differences between logged geometric means; so, for example, when comparing groups 1 and 2, the difference in arithmetic means on the log scale will estimate

$$\log \mu_G(\text{Group 1}) - \log \mu_G(\text{Group 2}) = \log \frac{\mu_G(\text{Group 1})}{\mu_G(\text{Group 2})}.$$

Thus, the antilog of the differences of the arithmetic means on the log scale estimates a *ratio* of geometric means.

While the antilogs of arithmetic means computed on the log scale are readily interpreted, there is no straightforward interpretation available for the antilog of the standard deviation of the log X_i. If confidence intervals for geometric means or ratios of geometric means are required, then the usual confidence intervals should be computed on the log scale. Taking antilogs of the ends of these intervals will yield confidence intervals on the original scale or for the ratio.

Example 10.10

The treatment of some skin diseases involves exposing patients to doses of ultraviolet radiation. Too high a dose of radiation will burn the patient, so before treatment commences it is important to expose small areas of skin to increasing doses to establish at what dose a patient will burn. The minimum dose which just causes reddening of the skin is known as the minimum phototoxic dose, MPD (in J/cm^2). Data on MPD were collected from 51 patients with fair skins and from 44 patients with darker skin (categorized using standard dermatological criteria): the data have kindly been made available by Dr P.M. Farr. The mean and standard deviations are:

	Arithmetic mean (J/cm^2)	Standard deviation (J/cm^2)
Fairer skin	2·60	2·52
Darker skin	3·34	3·56

While patients with fairer skin appear to burn at lower doses, it is also clear that the data are far from normally distributed. Negative MPDs are impossible and the standard deviations are approximately equal to the means. This hampers formal assessment of the difference between the groups. Taking logarithms, to base 10, and computing means and standard deviations of the logged values gives the second and third columns of the following table. MPD has been extensively studied and there is good external evidence that the logarithm of the MPD does closely follow a normal distribution (MacKenzie, 1983).

	Arithmetic mean, logged values	Standard deviation, logged values	Geometric mean, original scale (J/cm^2)
Fairer skin	0·225	0·414	1·68
Darker skin	0·268	0·478	1·85

The antilogs of the arithmetic means of the logged values, i.e. the geometric means, are shown above and can be seen to be noticeably smaller than the arithmetic means in the previous table. The standard deviations on the log scale are similar and the null hypothesis that the population geometric means are equal can be tested using the usual two-sample t test (see §4.3). Applying the t test to the logged values gives $t = -0.47, P = 0.64$. The difference in the arithmetic means of the logged values is -0.043, and a 95% confidence interval for the difference is $(-0.224, 0.139)$. Taking antilogs of the difference, and of the limits of the confidence interval, gives 0·91 for the ratio of geometric means (confirmed by direct calculation because $1.68/1.85 = 0.91$) and the 95% confidence interval for the ratio is $(0.60, 1.38)$.

Of course, a logarithmic transformation can only be applied to a positive number, and associated quantities, such as geometric means are only defined for positive variables. Even if the sample values are generally positive the application of a log transformation can be ruled out because of occasional zero values. Even if a value of zero is physiologically impossible recorded zeros can arise because actual levels are below limits of detection. There are no simple solutions to this difficulty. *Ad hoc* solutions, such as replacing zero values by the limit of detection (or perhaps half the limit of detection) if the limit is known, may prove satisfactory. Adding a constant k to each x_i before taking logs is an alternative, although it can be difficult to decide on the value for k and the results of the analysis can be disconcertingly sensitive to the choice of k. Treating k as a parameter to be estimated by the data is beset by theoretical problems.

11 Modelling continuous data

11.1 **Analysis of variance applied to regression**

In Chapters 8 and 9 the analysis of variance has been used to study the effect, on the mean value of a random variable, of various types of classification of the data into qualitative categories. We now return to the linear regression model of Chapter 7, in which the mean value of y is linearly related to a second variable x, and consider the analysis of variance for this situation.

Suppose, as in §7.2, that there are n pairs of values, $(x_1, y_1), \ldots, (x_i, y_i), \ldots, (x_n, y_n)$, and that the fitted regression line of y on x has the equation

$$Y = a + bx, \tag{11.1}$$

with a and b given by (7.2) and (7.3).

The deviation of y_i from the mean $\bar{y}$ can be divided into two parts:

$$y_i - \bar{y} = (y_i - Y_i) + (Y_i - \bar{y}), \tag{11.2}$$

where Y_i is the value of y calculated from the regression line (11.1) with $x = x_i$ (see Fig. 11.1).

It can be shown that when both sides of (11.2) are squared, and the terms summed from $i = 1$ to n, the sum of the products of the terms on the right is zero, and the following relation holds:

$$\sum(y_i - \bar{y})^2 = \sum(y_i - Y_i)^2 + \sum(Y_i - \bar{y})^2. \tag{11.3}$$

The term on the left is the Total sum of squares (SSq); the first term on the right is the SSq of deviations of observed ys about the regression line, and the second is the SSq about the mean of the values Y_i predicted by the regression line. In short,

Total SSq = SSq about regression + SSq due to regression.

In Fig. 11.1(a), most of the Total SSq is explained by the SSq about regression; in Fig. 11.1(b), in contrast, most of the Total SSq is due to regression.

An expression for $\sum(y_i - Y_i)^2$ has already been given in (7.5). From (2.3) and (7.7) the computing formulae shown in Table 11.1 immediately follow (the subscripts i now being dropped).

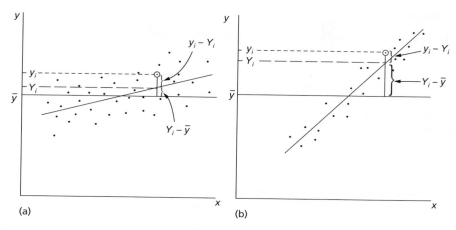

Fig. 11.1 Subdivision of a deviation about the mean into two parts: about regression and due to regression. In (a) the regression of y on x explains a much smaller fraction of the total variation of y than in (b).

Table 11.1 Analysis of variance for linear regression.

	SSq	DF	MSq	VR
Due to regression	$\dfrac{[\sum xy - (\sum x)(\sum y)/n]^2}{\sum x^2 - (\sum x)^2/n}$	1	s_1^2	s_1^2/s_0^2
About regression	By subtraction	$n-2$	s_0^2	
Total	$\sum y^2 - (\sum y)^2/n$	$n-1$		

Suppose, as in §7.2, that the ys are distributed independently and normally, with variance σ^2, about expected values given by

$$E(y) = \alpha + \beta x. \tag{11.4}$$

The null hypothesis that $\beta = 0$ (that is, that the expectation of y is constant, irrespective of the value of x) may be tested by the analysis of variance in Table 11.1. If $\beta = 0$, s_1^2 and s_0^2 are independent unbiased estimates of σ^2. If $\beta \neq 0$, s_0^2 is an unbiased estimate of σ^2 (see (7.6)) but s_1^2 estimates a quantity greater than σ^2. The variance ratio $F = s_1^2/s_0^2$, on 1 and $n-2$ degrees of freedom (DF), may therefore be used to test whether $\beta = 0$.

The significance of the regression slope has previously been tested by

$$t = \frac{b}{\text{SE}(b)} = \frac{b}{s_0 \sqrt{\sum (x - \bar{x})^2}}$$

on $n-2$ DF (as in (7.16) and (7.18)). Using the formula (7.3) for b, it is easy to see that $F = t^2$, and (as noted, for example, in §§5.1 and 8.1) the tests are equivalent.

Example 11.1

The analysis of variance of y, from the data of Example 7.1 (pp. 192 and 199), is as follows:

	SSq	DF	MSq	VR
Due to regression	7 666·39	1	7666·39	24·2 $(P < 0.001)$
About regression	9 502·08	30	316·74	1·00
Total	17 168·47	31		

The SSq have already been obtained on pp. 192 and 199. The value of t obtained previously was -4.92; note that $(4.92)^2 = 24.2$, the value of F.

Test of linearity

It is often important to know not only whether the slope of an assumed linear regression is significant, but also whether there is any reason to doubt the basic assumption of the linearity of the regression.

   If the data provide a number of replicate readings of y for certain values of x, a test of linearity is easily obtained. Suppose that, at the value x_i of x, there are n_i observations on y, with a mean $\bar{y}_i$. Each such group of replicates is called an array. Figure 11.2 illustrates three different situations. In (a), a linear regression seems to be consistent with the observed data in that the array means $\bar{y}_i$ are reasonably close to the regression line. In (b) and (c), however, the array means deviate from the line by more than can easily be explained by the within-arrays variation. In (b) the deviations seem to be systematic, suggesting that a curved regression line is required. In (c) the deviations seem to lack any pattern, suggesting perhaps an extra source of variation associated with each array; for example, if each array referred to observations on animals in a single cage, the positioning of the cage in the laboratory might affect the whole array.

   In discussing Fig. 11.2 we have made a rough comparison between the magnitude of deviations of array means from the regression line and the within-arrays variation. The comparison is made formally as follows. For any value y in the array corresponding to x_i, the residual $y - Y_i$ may be divided into two parts:

$$y - Y_i = (y - \bar{y}_i) + (\bar{y}_i - Y_i). \tag{11.5}$$

When both sides are squared and summed over all observations, the sum of products of the two terms on the right vanishes, and we have a partition of the Residual SSq:

$$\sum (y - Y_i)^2 = \sum (y - \bar{y}_i)^2 + \sum (\bar{y}_i - Y_i)^2, \tag{11.6}$$

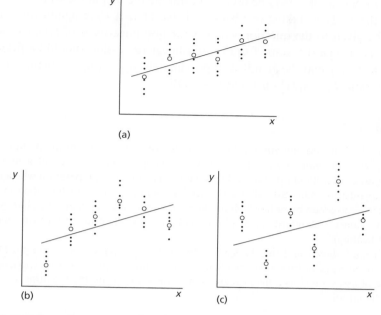

Fig. 11.2 Deviations of array means from linear regression. Those in (a) are explicable by within-arrays variation; those in (b) suggest a systematic departure from linearity; while those in (c) suggest a further source of variation.

the summations being taken over all n observations. The first term on the right is the SSq about array means; the second term is the SSq of deviations of array means from the regression line. The first of these is precisely what would be obtained as the Within-Arrays SSq in a one-way analysis of variance of the ys without reference to the xs.

The computing formulae are given in Table 11.2. Here k is the number of arrays, and T_i is the sum of values of y for the ith array. The variance ratio F_2 tests the deviation of the array means about linear regression, and F_1 tests the departure of β from zero assuming linear regression. If F_2 is not significant and

Table 11.2 Analysis of variance with test of linearity.

	SSq	DF	MSq	VR
Due to regression	(As in Table 11.1)	1	s_1^2	$F_1 = s_1^2/s_3^2$
Deviation of array means from regression	(By subtraction)	$k-2$	s_2^2	$F_2 = s_2^2/s_3^2$
Within-arrays residual	$\sum y^2 - \sum_i (T_i^2/n_i)$	$n-k$	s_3^2	
Total	$\sum y^2 - (\sum y)^2/n$	$n-1$		

$n - k$ is rather small, it may be useful to combine the SSq in the second and third lines of the analysis, taking one back to Table 11.1. If F_2 is significant, thought should be given to the question whether the non-linearity is of type (b) or type (c). If it is of type (b), some form of non-linear regression should be fitted (see §12.1). Type (c) may be handled approximately by testing s_1^2 against s_2^2 by a variance ratio $F_1' = s_1^2/s_2^2$ on 1 and $k - 2$ DF.

Example 11.2

In one method of assaying vitamin D, rats are fed on a diet deficient in vitamin D for 2 weeks so as to develop rickets. The diet is then supplemented by one of a number of different doses of a standard vitamin D preparation or of a test preparation which is to be assayed against the standard. After a further 2 weeks the degree to which the rickets has been healed is assessed by radiographing the right knee of each animal. The photograph is matched against a standard set of photographs numbered from 0 to 12 (in increasing order of healing).

The results shown in Table 11.3 were obtained with three doses of vitamin D. Each score is the average of four assessments of a single photograph. General experience with this type of assay suggests a linear regression of the score, y, on the log dose, x.

The Total SSq is

$$314 \cdot 2500 - (89 \cdot 00)^2/31 = 58 \cdot 7339,$$

and the Within-Doses Residual SSq is

$$314 \cdot 2500 - (32 \cdot 4000 + 87 \cdot 7813 + 152 \cdot 3269) = 41 \cdot 7418.$$

The calculation of the SSq due to regression makes use of the fact that only three values of x occur. Thus,

$$\sum x = 10(0 \cdot 544) + 8(0 \cdot 845) + 13(1 \cdot 146) = 27 \cdot 098,$$
$$\sum (x - \bar{x})^2 = 10(0 \cdot 544)^2 + 8(0 \cdot 845)^2 + 13(1 \cdot 146)^2 - (27 \cdot 098)^2/31 = 2 \cdot 0576$$

and

$$\sum (x - \bar{x})(y - \bar{y}) = (0 \cdot 544)(18 \cdot 00) + (0 \cdot 845)(26 \cdot 50) + (1 \cdot 146)(44 \cdot 50)$$
$$- (27 \cdot 098)(89 \cdot 00)/31 = 5 \cdot 3840,$$

from which

$$\text{SSq due to regression} = (5 \cdot 3840)^2/2 \cdot 0576 = 14 \cdot 0880.$$

The variance ratio for deviations of dose means is not significant, and the conclusion that the regression is effectively linear is reinforced by general experience with this assay method. The regression slope is, of course, highly significant.

If the observations do not fall into arrays at fixed values of x, the testing of linearity is less simple. It is often adequate to form groups along the x-scale, and

Table 11.3 Radiographic assessments of bone healing for three doses of vitamin D.

Dose (i.u.)	3·5	7	14	
Log dose, x_i	0·544	0·845	1·146	Total
	0	1·50	2·00	
	0	2·50	2·50	
	1·00	5·00	5·00	
	2·75	6·00	4·00	
	2·75	4·25	5·00	
	1·75	2·75	4·00	
	2·75	1·50	2·50	
	2·25	3·00	3·50	
	2·25		3·00	
	2·50		2·00	
			3·00	
			4·00	
			4·00	
T_i	18·00	26·50	44·50	89·00
n_i	10	8	13	31
$\bar{y}_i$	1·8000	3·3125	3·4231	
$\sum y^2$	43·1250	106·3750	164·7500	314·2500
T_i^2/n_i	32·4000	87·7813	152·3269	

Analysis of variance

	SSq	DF	MSq	VR	
Due to regression	14·0880	1	14·0880	9·45	($P = 0{\cdot}005$)
Deviations of dose means	27·9041	1	2·9041	1·95	($P = 0{\cdot}17$)
Within-doses residual	41·7418	28	1·4908	1.00	
Total	58·7339	30			

treat the data as though the arrays corresponded to the mid-points of the groups of x. Alternatively one can use the methods of §12.1 and fit a non-linear regression curve by including an extra term, such as $\log x$, $\sqrt{x}$, $x \log x$, or x^2. A test of the significance of the extra term is a test of the linearity.

11.2 **Errors in both variables**

In studying the regression of y on x it has not been necessary to consider any form of random variation in the values of x. Clearly, in many sets of data, the values of x do vary randomly—either because the individual units on which the measurements are made are selected by an effectively random process, or because any observation on x is affected by measurement error or some other form of random perturbation. In the standard regression formulation these

considerations are irrelevant. There are, however, some questions rather different from those answered by regression analysis, in which random errors in x are
relevant. These are, basically, questions involving the values of x which would
have been observed had there been no random error.

Suppose that any pair of observed values (x, y) can be regarded as differing by
random errors from a pair of 'true values' (X, Y) which are linearly related. Thus,

$$Y = \alpha + \beta X, \tag{11.7}$$

where we observe

$$\left.\begin{array}{l} x = X + \delta \\[2ex] y = Y + \varepsilon, \end{array}\right\} \tag{11.8}$$

and

and δ and ε are distributed independently of each other and also independently
of X and Y. Suppose that δ is distributed as $N(0, \sigma_\delta^2)$ and ε as $N(0, \sigma_\varepsilon^2)$ (see
Fig. 11.3).

The first point to emphasize is that, if the problem is to predict the behaviour
of y or Y in terms of x (the observed value), ordinary regression analysis is
appropriate. In many situations this is the case. If y is a measure of clinical
change and x is a biochemical measurement, the purpose of an analysis may be
to study the extent to which y can be predicted from x. Any value of x used in the
analysis will be subject to random variation due to physiological fluctuations and
measurement error, but this fact can be disregarded because predictions will be
made from values of x which are equally subject to such variation.

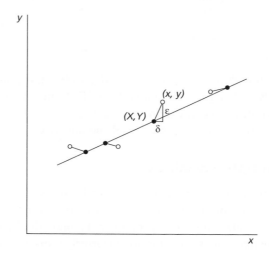

Fig. 11.3 Deviations of observed values from a linear functional relationship with errors in both
variables.

Suppose, however, that the purpose is to estimate the value of β, the slope of the line relating Y to X (not to x). This problem is likely to arise in two different circumstances.

1 The 'true' value X may be of much more interest than the 'observed' value, x, because future discussions will be in terms of X rather than x. For instance, in a geographical survey, x may be the mean household size of a certain town as estimated from the survey and y some measure of health in that town. The size of the random error component in x may be peculiar to this particular survey and of no relevance in future work. Any arguments should be based on the effect, on y, of changes in the true mean household size, X.

2 The equation (11.7) may express a *functional relationship* between the true values X and Y which is of particular scientific importance. For instance, if X and Y are, respectively, the volume and mass of different specimens of a metal, equation (11.7) with $\alpha = 0$ would clearly represent the relationship between X and Y with β measuring the density. The estimation of β would be a reasonable objective, but the complication arises that both X and Y are affected by random measurement errors, so the investigator observes pairs of values (x, y).

The estimation of α and β from pairs of observed values (x, y) is a difficult problem (Kendall, 1951, 1952; Sprent, 1969). One general result is that b, the regression coefficient of y on x, underestimates β on the average. The expected value of b is approximately

$$\beta' = \beta \left[1 - \frac{\sigma_\delta^2}{\text{var}(x)} \right]. \tag{11.9}$$

If it were known that σ_δ^2 is small in comparison with var(x), that is, that the measurement error in x is small relative to the total variation in x, then the correction term in square brackets would be close to unity and the underestimation small. If σ_δ^2 can be estimated (for example, by a special experimental study involving replicate observations of the same X), the correction term can be estimated, and a correction applied to the estimated slope b. If the ratio $\lambda = \sigma_\varepsilon^2 / \sigma_\delta^2$ is known then the relationship may be fitted by maximum likelihood (see (3.4.12) of Draper & Smith, 1998).

In many situations no direct estimate of σ_δ^2 will be possible because there is no way of selecting observations with different values of x but the same value of X. Usually the situation here is that a set of pairs (x, y) shows some general linear trend which the investigator wishes to represent by a single straight line without making the distinction between x and y required in a regression analysis. The investigator should make quite sure that any subsequent use of the line will not put either variable in the role of a predictor variable, and that a single line will perform a useful function in representing the general trend. A fuller discussion of this situation is given by Draper and Smith (1998, §3.4). If there is insufficient basis for any reasonable assumptions about σ_δ^2 and σ_ε^2, a simple visual approach is probably best: draw a freehand line through the cluster and refrain from any assertions of sampling error. This process may be made more objective by dividing the sample into three groups by quantiles (§2.6) of the x values, and drawing a line through the mean of the middle group with slope equal to that of the line joining the means of the upper and lower groups (Bartlett, 1949).

Other possibilities are to use the geometric mean functional relationship. In this approach the slope is equal to the ratio of the standard deviations of y and x, that is $b = \pm s_y/s_x$ with the sign determined by the sign of the correlation coefficient. This slope is the geometric mean of the slopes of the regression lines of y on x and of x on y (see Fig. 7.4 and (7.11)). It corresponds to the solution when $\lambda = \mathrm{var}(y)/\mathrm{var}(x)$. Another possibility is when $\lambda = 1$ and this gives a line for which the sum of squares of the perpendicular distances of the points from the line is minimized. The geometric mean functional relationship has been criticized as being based on an unrealistic assumption. An important point is that since λ is unknown no particular solution can be justified and, therefore, basing the solution on any particular value of λ is arbitrary.

An interesting special situation is that in which x is a *controlled variable*. Suppose that x is known to differ from X by a random error, as in (11.8), but that the value of x is selected by the experimenter. For example, in drawing liquid into a pipette the experimenter may aim at a specified volume x, and would assume that the experimental value was x, although the true value X would differ from x by a random error. If there is no systematic bias, (11.8) will represent the situation, but the important difference between this problem and that considered earlier is that the random error δ is independent of x, whereas previously δ was independent of X. It follows, as Berkson (1950) pointed out, that the regression coefficient of y on x does in this case provide an unbiased estimate of β, and standard methods of regression analysis are appropriate.

11.3 **Straight lines through the origin**

Sometimes there may be good reason to suppose that a regression line must pass through the origin, in the sense that when $x = 0$ the mean value of y must also be 0. For instance, in a psychological experiment the subject may be asked to guess how far a certain light falls to the left or to the right of a marker. If the guessed distance to the right is y (distances to the left corresponding to $y < 0$) and the true distance is x, a subject whose responses showed no bias to left or right would have $\mathrm{E}(y) = 0$ when $x = 0$.

The regression of y on x will then take the form

$$Y = \beta x, \tag{11.10}$$

and the least squares solution is similar to that of the ordinary regression formulae, except that sums of squares and products are not corrected for deviations about mean values. Thus, β is estimated by

$$b = \sum xy / \sum x^2,$$ (11.11)

and the SSq about regression is

$$\sum y^2 - \left(\sum xy\right)^2 / \sum x^2$$

on $n - 1$ (not $n - 2$) DF.

This result assumes, as usual, that the residual variance of y is independent of x. In many problems in which a line through the origin seems appropriate, particularly for variables which take positive values only, this is clearly not so. There is often a tendency for the variability of y to increase as x increases. Two other least squares solutions are useful here.

1 If the residual var(y) increases in proportion to x, the best estimate of β is $b_1 = \sum y / \sum x = \bar{y}/\bar{x}$, the ratio of the two means. An example of this situation would occur in a radioactivity counting experiment where the same material is observed for replicate periods of different lengths. If x_i is a time interval and y_i the corresponding count, Poisson theory shows that var(y_i) = E(y_i/x_i) ∝ x_i. The estimate of the mean count per unit time is, as would be expected, $\sum y_i / \sum x_i$, the total count divided by the total time period.

2 If the residual *standard deviation* of y increases in proportion to x, the best estimate of β is $b_2 = \sum(y/x)/n$, the mean of the individual ratios.

Care should be taken to enquire whether a regression line, rather than a functional relationship (§11.2), is really needed in such problems. Suppose that x and y are estimates of a biochemical substance obtained by two different methods. If y is the estimate by the more reliable method, and x is obtained by a rapid but rather less reliable method, it may be reasonable to estimate y from x, and one of the above methods may be appropriate. If the question is rather 'How big are the discrepancies between x and y?' there is no reason to treat the problem as one of the regression of y on x rather than x on y. A useful device here is to rewrite (11.10) as

$$\log Y = \log \beta + \log x,$$

and to take the individual values of $z = \log y - \log x$ as estimates of $\log \beta$ (see also p. 707). If random variation in z is approximately independent of x or y (and this can be checked by simple scatter diagrams), the mean value of z will be the best estimate of $\log \beta$, confidence limits being obtained by the t distribution, as is usual for a mean value. This situation is roughly equivalent to **2** above. If random variation in z depends heavily on x or y, the observations could be grouped and some form of weighted average taken (see §8.2).

11.4 **Regression in groups**

Frequently data are classified into groups, and within each group a linear regression of y on x may be postulated. For example, the regression of forced expiratory volume on age may be considered separately for men in different occupational groups. Possible differences between the regression lines are then often of interest.

In this section we consider comparisons of the slopes of the regression lines. If the slopes clearly differ from one group to another, then so, of course, must the mean values of y—at least for some values of x. In Fig. 11.4(a), the slopes of the regression lines differ from group to group. The lines for groups (i) and (ii) cross. Those for (i) and (iii), and for (ii) and (iii) would also cross if extended sufficiently far, but here there is some doubt as to whether the linear regressions would remain valid outside the range of observed values of x.

If the slopes do not differ, the lines are parallel, as in Fig. 11.4(b) and (c), and here it becomes interesting to ask whether, as in (b), the lines differ in their height above the x axis (which depends on the coefficient α in the equation

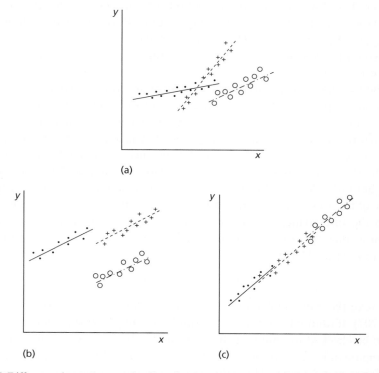

(a)

(b)   (c)

Fig. 11.4 Differences between regression lines fitted to three groups of observations. The lines differ in slope and position in (a), differ only in position in (b), and coincide in (c). (——) (i); (- - -) (ii); (- · -) (iii).

$E(y) = \alpha + \beta x)$, or whether, as in (c), the lines coincide. In practice, the fitted regression lines would rarely have *precisely* the same slope or position, and the question is to what extent differences between the lines can be attributed to random variation. Differences in position between parallel lines are discussed in §11.5. In this section we concentrate on the question of differences between slopes.

Suppose that there are k groups, with n_i pairs of observations in the ith group. Denote the mean values of x and y in the ith group by $\bar{x}_i$ and $\bar{y}_i$, and the regression line, calculated as in §7.2, by

$$Y_i = \bar{y} + b_i(x - \bar{x}_i). \tag{11.12}$$

If all the n_i are reasonably large, a satisfactory approach is to estimate the variance of each b_i by (7.16) and to ignore the imprecision in these estimates of variance. Changing the notation of (7.16) somewhat, we shall denote the residual mean square for the ith group by s_i^2 and the sum of squares of x about $\bar{x}_i$ by $\sum_{(i)}(x - \bar{x}_i)^2$. Note that the parenthesized suffix i attached to the summation sign indicates summation only over the specified group i; that is,

$$\sum_{(i)}(x - \bar{x}_i)^2 = \sum_{j=1}^{n_i}(x_{ij} - \bar{x}_i)^2.$$

To simplify the notation, denote this sum of squares about the mean of x in the ith group by

$$S_{xxi}, \tag{11.13}$$

the sum of products of deviations by S_{xyi}, and so on. Then following the method of §8.2, we write

$$w_i = \frac{1}{\text{var}(b_i)} = \frac{S_{xxi}}{s_i^2}, \tag{11.14}$$

and calculate

$$G = \sum w_i b_i^2 - \left(\sum w_i b_i\right)^2 / \sum w_i. \tag{11.15}$$

On the null hypothesis that the true slopes β_i are all equal, G follows approximately a $\chi^2_{(k-1)}$ distribution. High values of G indicate departures from the null hypothesis, i.e. real differences between the β_i. If G is non-significant, and the null hypothesis is tentatively accepted, the common value β of the β_i is best estimated by the weighted mean

$$\bar{b} = \sum w_i b_i / \sum w_i, \tag{11.16}$$

with an estimated variance

$$\text{var}(\bar{b}) = 1/\sum w_i. \tag{11.17}$$

The sampling variation of $\bar{b}$ is approximately normal.

It is difficult to say how large the n_i must be for this 'large-sample' approach to be used with safety. There would probably be little risk in adopting it if none of the n_i fell below 20.

A more exact treatment is available provided that an extra assumption is made—that the residual variances σ_i^2 are all equal. Suppose the common value is σ^2. We consider first the situation where $k = 2$, as a comparison of two slopes can be effected by use of the t distribution. For $k > 2$ an analysis of variance is required.

Two groups

The residual variance σ^2 can be estimated, using (7.5) and (7.6), either as

$$\begin{aligned} s_1^2 &= \frac{\sum_{(1)}(y - Y_1)^2}{n_1 - 2} \\ &= \frac{S_{yy1} - S_{xy1}^2/S_{xx1}}{n_1 - 2} \end{aligned}$$

or by the corresponding mean square for the second group, s_2^2. A pooled estimate may be obtained (very much as in the two-sample t test (p. 107)), as

$$s^2 = \frac{\sum_{(1)}(y - Y_1)^2 + \sum_{(2)}(y - Y_2)^2}{n_1 + n_2 - 4}. \tag{11.18}$$

To compare b_1 and b_2 we estimate

$$\text{var}(b_1 - b_2) = s^2\left[\frac{1}{S_{xx1}} + \frac{1}{S_{xx2}}\right]. \tag{11.19}$$

The difference is tested by

$$t = \frac{b_1 - b_2}{\text{SE}(b_1 - b_2)} \quad \text{on } n_1 + n_2 - 4 \text{ DF}, \tag{11.20}$$

the DF being the divisor in (11.18).

If a common value is assumed for the regression slope in the two groups, its value β may be estimated by

$$b = \frac{S_{xy1} + S_{xy2}}{S_{xx1} + S_{xx2}}, \tag{11.21}$$

with a variance estimated as

$$\text{var}(b) = \frac{s^2}{S_{xx1} + S_{xx2}}. \tag{11.22}$$

Equations (11.21) and (11.22) can easily be seen to be equivalent to (11.16) and (11.17) if, in the calculation of w_i in (11.14), the separate estimates of residual variance s_i^2 are replaced by the common estimate s^2. For tests or the calculation of confidence limits for β using (11.22), the t distribution on $n_1 + n_2 - 4$ DF should be used. Where a common slope is accepted it would be more usual to estimate s^2 as the residual mean square about the parallel lines (11.34), which would have $n_1 + n_2 - 3$ DF.

Example 11.3

Table 11.4 gives age and vital capacity (litres) for each of 84 men working in the cadmium industry. They are divided into three groups: A_1, exposed to cadmium fumes for at least 10 years; A_2, exposed to fumes for less than 10 years; B, not exposed to fumes. The main purpose of the study was to see whether exposure to fumes was associated with a change in respiratory function. However, those in group A_1 must be expected to be older on the average than those in groups A_2 or B, and it is well known that respiratory test performance declines with age. A comparison is therefore needed which corrects for discrepancies between the mean ages of the different groups.

We shall first illustrate the calculations for two groups by amalgamating groups A_1 and A_2 (denoting the pooled group by A) and comparing groups A and B.

The sums of squares and products of deviations about the mean, and the separate slopes b_i are as follows:

Group	i	n_i	S_{xxi}	S_{xyi}	S_{yyi}	b_i
A	1	40	4397·38	−236·385	26·5812	−0·0538
B	2	44	6197·16	−189·712	20·6067	−0·0306
Total			10594·54	−426·097	47·1879	(−0·0402)

The SSq about the regressions are

$$\sum_{(1)}(y - Y_1)^2 = 26 \cdot 5812 - (-236 \cdot 385)^2 / 4397 \cdot 38 = 13 \cdot 8741$$

and

$$\sum_{(2)}(y - Y_2)^2 = 20 \cdot 6067 - (-189 \cdot 712)^2 / 6197 \cdot 16 = 14 \cdot 7991.$$

Thus,

$$s^2 = (13 \cdot 8741 + 14 \cdot 7991)/(40 + 44 - 4) = 0 \cdot 3584,$$

and, for the difference between b_1 and b_2 using (11.19) and (11.20),

$$t = \frac{-0 \cdot 0538 - (-0 \cdot 0306)}{\sqrt{\left[(0 \cdot 3584)\left(\dfrac{1}{4397 \cdot 38} + \dfrac{1}{6197 \cdot 16}\right)\right]}}$$
$$= -0 \cdot 0232/0 \cdot 0118$$
$$= -1 \cdot 97 \text{ on } 80 \text{ DF.}$$

Table 11.4 Ages and vital capacities for three groups of workers in the cadmium industry. x, age last birthday (years); y, vital capacity (litres).

Group A₁, exposed > 10 years		Group A₂, exposed < 10 years		Group B, not exposed			
x	y	x	y	x	y	x	y
39	4·62	29	5·21	27	5·29	43	4·02
40	5·29	29	5·17	25	3·67	41	4·99
41	5·52	33	4·88	24	5·82	48	3·86
41	3·71	32	4·50	32	4·77	47	4·68
45	4·02	31	4·47	23	5·71	53	4·74
49	5·09	29	5·12	25	4·47	49	3·76
52	2·70	29	4·51	32	4·55	54	3·98
47	4·31	30	4·85	18	4·61	48	5·00
61	2·70	21	5·22	19	5·86	49	3·31
65	3·03	28	4·62	26	5·20	47	3·11
58	2·73	23	5·07	33	4·44	52	4·76
59	3·67	35	3·64	27	5·52	58	3·95
		38	3·64	33	4·97	62	4·60
		38	5·09	25	4·99	65	4·83
		43	4·61	42	4·89	62	3·18
		39	4·73	35	4·09	59	3·03
		38	4·58	35	4·24		
		42	5·12	41	3·88		
		43	3·89	38	4·85		
		43	4·62	41	4·79		
		37	4·30	36	4·36		
		50	2·70	36	4·02		
		50	3·50	41	3·77		
		45	5·06	41	4·22		
		48	4·06	37	4·94		
		51	4·51	42	4·04		
		46	4·66	39	4·51		
		58	2·88	41	4·06		
Sums 597	47·39	1058	125·21			1751	196·33
n	12		28				44
$\sum x^2$	30 613		42 260				75 879
$\sum xy$	2 280·01		4 624·93				7 623·33
$\sum y^2$	198·8903		572·4599				896·6401

The difference is very nearly significant at the 5% level. This example is continued on p. 329.

The scatter diagram in Fig. 11.5 shows the regression lines with slopes b_A and b_B fitted separately to the two groups, and also the two parallel lines with slope b. The steepness of

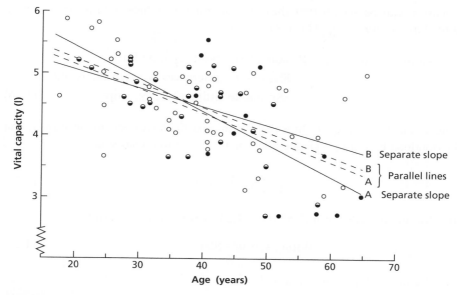

Fig. 11.5 Scatter diagram showing age and vital capacity of 84 men working in the cadmium industry, divided into three groups (Table 11.4). (●) Group A_1; (◖) Group A_2; (○) Group B.

the slope for group A may be partly or wholly due to a curvature in the regression: there is a suggestion that the mean value of y at high values of x is lower than is predicted by the linear regressions (see p. 330). Alternatively it may be that a linear regression is appropriate for each group, but that for group A the vital capacity declines more rapidly with age than for group B.

More than two groups

With any number of groups the pooled slope b is given by a generalization of (11.21):

$$b = \frac{\sum_i S_{xyi}}{\sum_i S_{xxi}}. \tag{11.23}$$

Parallel lines may now be drawn through the mean points $(\bar{x}_i, \bar{y}_i)$, each with the same slope b. That for the ith group will have this equation:

$$Y_{ci} = \bar{y}_i + b(x - \bar{x}_i). \tag{11.24}$$

The subscript c is used to indicate that the predicted value Y_{ci} is obtained using the common slope, b.

The deviation of any observed value y from its group mean $\bar{y}_i$ may be divided as follows:

$$y - \bar{y}_i = (y - Y_i) + (Y_i - Y_{ci}) + (Y_{ci} - \bar{y}_i). \tag{11.25}$$

Again, it can be shown that the sums of squares of these components can be added in the same way. This means that

Within-Groups SSq = Residual SSq about separate lines
+ SSq due to differences between the b_i and b
+ SSq due to fitting common slope b. (11.26)

The middle term on the right is the one that particularly concerns us now. It can be obtained by noting that the SSq due to the common slope is

$$\left(\sum_i S_{xyi}\right)^2 / \sum_i S_{xxi}; \qquad (11.27)$$

this follows directly from (7.5) and (11.23). From previous results,

$$\text{Within-Groups SSq} = \sum_i S_{yyi} \qquad (11.28)$$

and Residual SSq about separate lines

$$= \sum_i [S_{yyi} - (S_{xyi})^2 / S_{xxi}]. \qquad (11.29)$$

From (11.26) to (11.29),

$$\text{SSq due to differences in slope} = \sum_i \frac{(S_{xyi})^2}{S_{xxi}} - \frac{\left(\sum_i S_{xyi}\right)^2}{\sum_i S_{xxi}}. \qquad (11.30)$$

It should be noted that (11.30) is equivalent to

$$\sum_i W_i b_i^2 - \frac{\left(\sum_i W_i b_i\right)^2}{\sum_i W_i}, \qquad (11.31)$$

where $W_i = S_{xxi} = \sigma^2/\text{var}(b_i)$, and that the pooled slope b equals $\sum W_i b_i / \sum W_i$, the weighted mean of the b_i. The SSq due to differences in slope is thus essentially a weighted sum of squares of the b_i about their weighted mean b, the weights being (as usual) inversely proportional to the sampling variances (see §8.2).

The analysis is summarized in Table 11.5. There is only one DF for the common slope, since the SSq is proportional to the square of one linear contrast, b. The $k - 1$ DF for the second line follow because the SSq measures differences between k independent slopes, b_i. The residual DF follow because there are $n_i - 2$ DF for the ith group and $\sum_i (n_i - 2) = n - 2k$. The total DF within groups are, correctly, $n - k$. The F test for differences between slopes follows immediately.

Table 11.5 Analysis of variance for differences between regression slopes.

	SSq	DF	MSq	VR
Due to common slope	$\dfrac{\left(\sum_i S_{xyi}\right)^2}{\sum_i S_{xxi}}$	1		
Differences between slopes	$\sum_i \dfrac{(S_{xyi})^2}{S_{xxi}} - \dfrac{\left(\sum_i S_{xyi}\right)^2}{\sum_i S_{xxi}}$	$k-1$	s_A^2	$F_A = s_A^2/s^2$
Residual about separate lines	$\sum_i S_{yyi} - \sum_i \dfrac{(S_{xyi})^2}{S_{xxi}}$	$n-2k$	s^2	
Within groups	$\sum_i S_{yyi}$	$n-k$		

Example 11.3, continued

We now test the significance between the three slopes. The sums of squares and products of deviations about the mean, and the separate slopes, are as follows:

Group	i	n_i	S_{xxi}	S_{xyi}	S_{yyi}	b_i
A_1	1	12	912·25	−77·643	11·7393	−0·0851
A_2	2	28	2282·71	−106·219	12·5476	−0·0465
B	3	44	6197·16	−189·712	20·6067	−0·0306
Total		84	9392·12	−373·574	44·8936	(− 0·0398)

The SSq due to the common slope is

$$(-373\cdot574)^2/9392\cdot12 = 14\cdot8590.$$

The Residual SSq about the separate lines using (11.29) are:

$$\sum\nolimits_{(1)}(y - Y_1)^2 = 5\cdot1310; \sum\nolimits_{(2)}(y - Y_2)^2 = 7\cdot6050; \sum\nolimits_{(3)}(y - Y_3)^2 = 14\cdot7991.$$

The total Residual SSq about separate lines is therefore

$$5\cdot1310 + 7\cdot6050 + 14\cdot7991 = 27\cdot5351.$$

The Within-Groups SSq is 44·8936. The SSq for differences between slopes may now be obtained by subtraction, as

$$44\cdot8936 - 14\cdot8590 - 27\cdot5351 = 2\cdot4995.$$

Alternatively, it may be calculated directly as

$$\frac{(-77\cdot643)^2}{912\cdot25} + \frac{(-106\cdot219)^2}{2282\cdot71} + \frac{(-189\cdot712)^2}{6197\cdot16} - \frac{(-373\cdot574)^2}{9392\cdot12} = 2\cdot4995.$$

The analysis of variance may now be completed.

	SSq	DF	MSq	VR
Common slope	14·8590	1	14·8590	42·09 ($P < 0.001$)
Between slopes	2·4995	2	1·2498	3·54 ($P = 0.034$)
Separate residuals	27·5351	78	0·3530	
Within groups	44·8936	81		

The differences between slopes are more significant than in the two-group analysis. The estimates of the separate slopes, with their standard errors calculated in terms of the Residual MSq on 78 DF, are

$$b_{A1} = -0.0851 \pm 0.0197, \quad b_{A2} = -0.0465 \pm 0.0124, \quad b_B = -0.0306 \pm 0.0075.$$

The most highly exposed group, A_1, provides the steepest slope. Figure 11.6 shows the separate regressions as well as the three parallel lines.

The doubt about linearity suggests further that a curvilinear regression might be more suitable; however, analysis with a quadratic regression line (see §11.1) shows the non-linearity to be quite non-significant.

The analysis of variance test can, of course, be applied even for $k = 2$. The results will be entirely equivalent to the t test described at the beginning of this section, the value of F being, as usual, the square of the corresponding value of t.

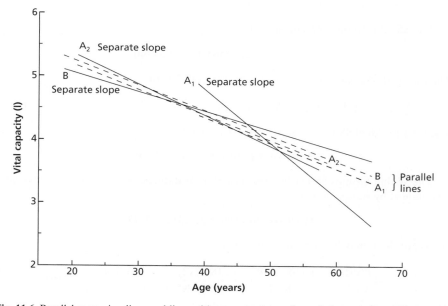

Fig. 11.6 Parallel regression lines and lines with separate slopes, for cadmium workers (Fig. 11.5).

11.5 **Analysis of covariance**

If, after an analysis of the type described in the last section, there is no strong reason for postulating differences between the slopes of the regression lines in the various groups, the following questions arise. What can be said about the relative position of parallel regression lines? Is there good reason to believe that the true lines differ in position, as in Fig. 11.4(b), or could they coincide, as in Fig. 11.4(c)? What sampling error is to be attached to an estimate of the difference in positions of lines for two particular groups? The set of techniques associated with these questions is called the *analysis of covariance*.

Before describing technical details, it may be useful to note some important differences in the purposes of the analysis of covariance and in the circumstances in which it may be used.

1 *Main purpose.*

(a) *To correct for bias.* If it is known that changes in x affect the mean value of y, and that the groups under comparison differ in their values of $\bar{x}$, it will follow that some of the differences between the values of $\bar{y}$ can be ascribed partly to differences between the $\bar{x}$s. We may want to remove this effect as far as possible. For example, if y is forced expiratory volume (FEV) and x is age, a comparison of mean FEVs for men in different occupational groups may be affected by differences in their mean ages. A comparison would be desirable of the mean FEVs at the same age. If the regressions are linear and parallel, this means a comparison of the relative position of the regression lines.

(b) *To increase precision.* Even if the groups have very similar values of $\bar{x}$, precision in the comparison of values of $\bar{y}$ can be increased by using the residual variation of y about regression on x rather than by analysing the ys alone.

2 *Type of investigation.*

(a) *Uncontrolled study.* In many situations the observations will be made on units which fall naturally into the groups in question—with no element of controlled allocation. Indeed, it will often be this lack of control which leads to the bias discussed in **1**(a).

(b) *Controlled study.* In a planned experiment, in which experimental units are allocated randomly to the different groups, the differences between values of $\bar{x}$ in the various groups will be no greater in the long run than would be expected by sampling theory. Of course, there will occasionally be large fortuitous differences in the $\bar{x}$s; it may then be just as important to correct for their effect as it would be in an uncontrolled study. In any case, even with very similar values of $\bar{x}$, the extra precision referred to in **1**(b) may well be worth acquiring.

Two groups

If the t test based on (11.20) reveals no significant difference in slopes, two parallel lines may be fitted with a common slope b given by (11.23). The equations of the two parallel lines are (as in (11.24)),

$$Y_{c1} = \bar{y}_1 + b(x - \bar{x}_1)$$

and

$$Y_{c2} = \bar{y}_2 + b(x - \bar{x}_2).$$

The difference between the values of Y at a given x is therefore

$$
\begin{aligned}
d &= Y_{c1} - Y_{c2} \\
&= \bar{y}_1 - \bar{y}_2 - b(\bar{x}_1 - \bar{x}_2)
\end{aligned}
\tag{11.32}
$$

(see Fig. 11.7).

The sampling error of d is due partly to that of $\bar{y}_1 - \bar{y}_2$ and partly to that of b (the term $\bar{x}_1 - \bar{x}_2$ has no sampling error as we are considering x to be a non-random variable). The three variables, $\bar{y}_1, \bar{y}_2$ and b, are independent; consequently

$$
\begin{aligned}
\text{var}(d) &= \text{var}(\bar{y}_1) + \text{var}(\bar{y}_2) + (\bar{x}_1 - \bar{x}_2)^2 \text{var}(b) \\
&= \sigma^2 \left[\frac{1}{n_1} + \frac{1}{n_2} + \frac{(\bar{x}_1 - \bar{x}_2)^2}{S_{xx1} + S_{xx2}} \right],
\end{aligned}
$$

which is estimated as

$$
s_c^2 \left[\frac{1}{n_1} + \frac{1}{n_2} + \frac{(\bar{x}_1 - \bar{x}_2)^2}{S_{xx1} + S_{xx2}} \right],
\tag{11.33}
$$

where s_c^2 is the residual mean square about the parallel lines:

$$
s_c^2 = \frac{S_{yy1} + S_{yy2} - \dfrac{(S_{xy1} + S_{xy2})^2}{S_{xx1} + S_{xx2}}}{n_1 + n_2 - 3}.
\tag{11.34}
$$

Note that s_c^2 differs from the s^2 of (11.18). The latter is the Residual mean square (MSq) about separate lines, and is equivalent to the s^2 of Table 11.5. The Residual MSq s_c^2 in (11.34) is taken about parallel lines (since parallelism is an initial assumption in the analysis of covariance), and would be obtained from Table 11.5 by pooling the second and third lines of the analysis. The resultant DF would be $(k-1) + (n-2k) = n - k - 1$, which gives the $n_1 + n_2 - 3 \, (= n - 3)$ of (11.34) when $k = 2$.

The standard error (SE) of d, the square root of (11.33), may be used in a t test. On the null hypothesis that the regression lines coincide, $\text{E}(d) = 0$, and

$$t = d/\text{SE}(d) \tag{11.35}$$

has $n_1 + n_2 - 3$ DF. Confidence limits for the true difference, $\text{E}(d)$, are obtained in the usual way.

The relative positions of the lines are conveniently expressed by the calculation of a *corrected* or *adjusted* mean value of y for each group. Suppose that group 1 had had a mean value of x equal to some arbitrary value x_0 rather than $\bar{x}_1$. Often x_0 is given the value of the mean of x over all the groups. From (11.24) we should estimate that the mean y would have been

$$\bar{y}'_1 = \bar{y}_1 + b(x_0 - \bar{x}_1), \tag{11.36}$$

with a similar expression for $\bar{y}'_2$. The difference between $\bar{y}'_1$ and $\bar{y}'_2$ can easily be seen to be equal to d given by (11.32). If the regression lines coincide, $\bar{y}'_1$ and $\bar{y}'_2$ will be equal. If the line for group 1 lies above that for group 2, at a fixed value of x, $\bar{y}'_1$ will be larger than $\bar{y}'_2$ (see Fig. 11.7).

The sampling variance of $\bar{y}'_i$ is estimated by

$$\text{var}(\bar{y}'_i) = \text{var}(\bar{y}_i) + (x_0 - \bar{x}_i)^2 \text{var}(b)$$
$$= s_c^2 \left[\frac{1}{n_i} + \frac{(x_0 - \bar{x}_i)^2}{S_{xx1} + S_{xx2}} \right], \tag{11.37}$$

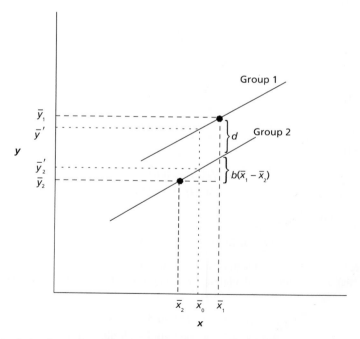

Fig. 11.7 Analysis of covariance for two groups, illustrating the formula for vertical difference, d, between parallel lines, and showing the corrected (adjusted) means $\bar{y}'$ for each group.

which varies with group not only through n_i but also because of the term $(x_0 - \bar{x}_i)^2$, which increases as $\bar{x}_i$ gets further from x_0 in either direction. The arbitrary choice of x_0 is avoided by concentrating on the difference between the corrected means, which is equal to d for all values of x_0.

Example 11.4

The data of Example 11.3 will now be used in an analysis of covariance. We shall first illustrate the calculations for two groups, the pooled exposed group A and the unexposed group B.

Using the sums of squares and products given earlier we have:

$$S_{xxA} + S_{xxB} = 10\,594 \cdot 54$$
$$S_{xyA} + S_{xyB} = -426 \cdot 097$$
$$S_{yyA} + S_{yyB} = 47 \cdot 1879.$$

Also

$$n_A = 40 \qquad n_B = 44$$
$$\bar{x}_A = 41 \cdot 38 \quad \bar{x}_B = 39 \cdot 80$$
$$\bar{y}_A = 4 \cdot 315 \quad \bar{y}_B = 4 \cdot 462.$$

From (11.23),

$$b = -0 \cdot 0402;$$

from (11.32),

$$d = -0 \cdot 0835;$$

from (11.34),

$$s_c^2 = 0 \cdot 3710;$$

from (11.33),

$$\text{var}(d) = 0 \cdot 01779,$$
$$\text{SE}(d) = 0 \cdot 1334,$$

and from (11.35),

$$t = -0 \cdot 0835/0 \cdot 1334 = -0 \cdot 63 \text{ on 81 DF.}$$

The difference d is clearly not significant ($P = 0 \cdot 53$).

Corrected values can be calculated, using (11.36), with $x_0 = 40 \cdot 5$, the overall mean. Thus,

$$\bar{y}'_A = 4 \cdot 315 - 0 \cdot 0402(40 \cdot 5 - 41 \cdot 38) = 4 \cdot 35;$$
$$\bar{y}'_B = 4 \cdot 462 - 0 \cdot 0402(40 \cdot 5 - 39 \cdot 80) = 4 \cdot 43.$$

The difference is $d = -0 \cdot 08$, as above.

This analysis is based on the assumption that the regression lines are parallel for groups A and B but, as noted in Example 11.3, there is at least suggestive evidence that the slopes differ. Suppose we abandon the assumption of parallelism and fit lines with separate slopes, b_A and b_B. The most pronounced difference between predicted values occurs at high ages. The difference at, say, age 60 is

$$d' = \bar{y}_A - \bar{y}_B + b_A(60 - \bar{x}_A) - b_B(60 - \bar{x}_B)$$
$$= -0.5306,$$

and

$$\mathrm{var}(d') = \mathrm{var}(\bar{y}_A) + \mathrm{var}(\bar{y}_B) + (60 - \bar{x}_A)^2 \mathrm{var}(b_A) + (60 - \bar{x}_B)^2 \mathrm{var}(b_B)$$
$$= (0.3584) \left\{ \frac{1}{40} + \frac{1}{44} + \frac{(18.62)^2}{4397.38} + \frac{(20.20)^2}{6197.16} \right\}$$
$$= 0.06896.$$

Thus $t = d'/\mathrm{SE}(d') = -2.02$ on 80 DF ($P = 0.05$).

This test suggests, therefore, that in spite of the non-significant result in the main analysis of covariance test, there may nevertheless be a difference in mean vital capacity, at least at the higher ages. The statistical significance of this finding is, of course, a reflection of the difference between the slopes, which had a similar level of statistical significance.

More than two groups

Parallel lines may be fitted to several groups, as indicated in §11.4. The pooled slope, b, is given by (11.23) and the line for the ith group is given by (11.24).

The relative positions of the lines are again conveniently expressed in terms of corrected mean values (11.36). On the null hypothesis that the true regression lines for the different groups coincide, the corrected means will differ purely by sampling error. For two groups the test of this null hypothesis is the t test (11.35). With $k(>2)$ groups this test becomes an F test with $k - 1$ DF in the numerator. The construction of this test is complicated by the fact that the sampling errors of the corrected means $\bar{y}'_i$ are not independent, since the random variable b enters into each expression (11.36). The test is produced most conveniently using multiple regression, which is discussed in the next section, and we return to this topic in §11.7. Other aspects of the analysis are similar to the analysis with two groups. The data of Example 11.4 are analysed in three groups as Example 11.7 (p. 353) using multiple regression.

In considering the possible use of the analysis of covariance with a particular set of data, special care should be given to the identification of the dependent and independent variables. If, in the analysis of covariance of y on x, there are significant differences between groups, it does not follow that the same will be true of the regression of x on y. In many cases this is an academic point because the investigator is clearly interested in differences between groups in the mean value of y, after correction for x, and not in the reverse problem. Occasionally, when x and y have a symmetric type of relation to each other, as in §11.2, both of the analyses of covariance (of y on x, and of x on y) will be misleading. Lines representing the general trend of a functional relationship may well be coincident (as in Fig. 11.8), and yet both sets of regression lines are non-coincident. Here the difficulties of §11.2 apply, and lines drawn by eye, or the other methods discussed on p. 319, may provide the most satisfactory description of the data. For a fuller discussion, see Ehrenberg (1968).

The analysis of covariance described in this section is appropriate for data forming a one-way classification into groups. The method is essentially a combination of linear regression (§7.2) and a one-way analysis of variance (§8.1). Similar problems arise in the analysis of more complex data. For example, in the analysis of a variable y in a Latin square one may wish to adjust the apparent treatment effects to correct for variation in another variable x. In particular, x may be some pretreatment characteristic known to be associated with y; the covariance adjustment would then be expected to increase the precision with which the treatments can be compared. The general procedure is an extension of that considered above and the details will not be given.

The methods presented in this and the previous section were developed before the use of computers became widespread, and were designed to simplify

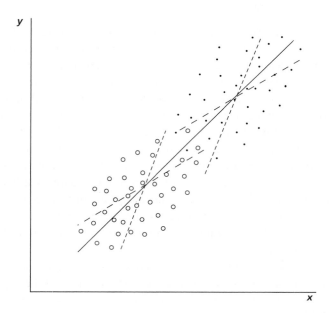

Fig. 11.8 Scatter diagram showing a common trend for two groups of observations but with non-coincident regression lines. (— —) Regression of y on x; (– – –) regression of x on y.

the calculations. Nowadays this is not a problem and the fitting of regressions in groups, using either separate non-parallel lines or parallel lines, as in the analysis of covariance, may be accomplished using multiple regression, as discussed in the next two sections.

11.6 **Multiple regression**

In the earlier discussions of regression in Chapter 7 and the earlier sections of this chapter, we have been concerned with the relationship between the mean value of one variable and the value of another variable, concentrating particularly on the situation in which this relationship can be represented by a straight line.

It is often useful to express the mean value of one variable in terms not of one other variable but of several others. Some examples will illustrate some slightly different purposes of this approach.

1   The primary purpose may be to study the effect on variable y of changes in a particular single variable x_1, but it may be recognized that y may be affected by several other variables x_2, x_3, etc. The effect on y of simultaneous changes in x_1, x_2, x_3, etc., must therefore be studied. In the analysis of data on respiratory function of workers in a particular industry, such as those considered in Examples 11.3 and 11.4, the effect of duration of exposure to a hazard may be of primary interest. However, respiratory function is affected by age, and age is related to duration of exposure. The simultaneous effect on respiratory function of age and exposure must therefore be studied so that the effect of exposure on workers of a fixed age may be estimated.

2   One may wish to derive insight into some causative mechanism by discovering which of a set of variables $x_1, x_2, \ldots$, has apparently most influence on a dependent variable y. For example, the stillbirth rate varies considerably in different towns in Britain. By relating the stillbirth rate simultaneously to a large number of variables describing the towns—economic, social, meterological or demographic variables, for instance—it may be possible to find which factors exert particular influence on the stillbirth rate (see Sutherland, 1946). Another example is in the study of variations in the cost per patient in different hospitals. This presumably depends markedly on the 'patient mix'— the proportions of different types of patient admitted—as well as on other factors. A study of the simultaneous effects of many such variables may explain much of the variation in hospital costs and, by drawing attention to particular hospitals whose high or low costs are out of line with the prediction, may suggest new factors of importance.

3   To predict the value of the dependent variable in future individuals. After treatment of patients with advanced breast cancer by ablative procedures, prognosis is very uncertain. If future progress can be shown to depend on several variables available at the time of the operation, it may be possible to

predict which patients have a poor prognosis and to consider alternative methods of treatment for them (Armitage *et al.*, 1969).

The appropriate technique is called *multiple regression*. In general, the approach is to express the mean value of the *dependent* variable in terms of the values of a set of other variables, usually called *independent* variables. The nomenclature is confusing, since some of the latter variables may be either closely related to each other logically (e.g. one might be age and another the square of the age) or highly correlated (e.g. height and arm length). It is preferable to use the terms *predictor* or *explanatory* variables, or *covariates*, and we shall usually follow this practice.

The data to be analysed consist of observations on a set of n individuals, each individual providing a value of the dependent variable, y, and a value of each of the predictor variables, $x_1, x_2, \ldots, x_p$. The number of predictor variables, p, should preferably be considerably less than the number of observations, n, and the same p predictor variables must be available for each individual in any one analysis.

Suppose that, for particular values of $x_1, x_2, \ldots, x_p$, an observed value of y is specified by the linear model:

$$y = \beta_0 + \beta_1 x_1 + \beta_2 x_2 + \ldots + \beta_p x_p + \varepsilon, \qquad (11.38)$$

where ε is an error term. The various values of ε for different individuals are supposed to be independently normally distributed with zero mean and variance σ^2. The constants $\beta_1, \beta_2, \ldots, \beta_p$ are called *partial regression coefficients*; β_0 is sometimes called the *intercept*. The coefficient β_1 is the amount by which y changes on the average when x_1 changes by one unit and all the other x_is remain constant. In general, β_1 will be different from the ordinary regression coefficient of y on x_1 because the latter represents the effect of changes in x_1 on the average values of y with no attempt to keep the other variables constant.

The coefficients $\beta_0, \beta_1, \beta_2, \ldots, \beta_p$ are idealized quantities, measurable only from an infinite number of observations. In practice, from n observations, we have to obtain estimates of the coefficients and thus an estimated regression equation:

$$Y = b_0 + b_1 x_1 + b_2 x_2 + \ldots + b_p x_p. \qquad (11.39)$$

Statistical theory tells us that a satisfactory method of obtaining the estimated regression equation is to choose the coefficients such that the sum of squares of residuals, $\sum(y - Y)^2$, is minimized, that is, by the method of least squares, which was introduced in §7.2. Note that here y is an observed value and Y is the value predicted by (11.39) in terms of the predictor variables. A consequence of this approach is that the regression equation (11.39) is satisfied if all the variables are given their mean values. Thus,

$$\bar{y} = b_0 + b_1\bar{x}_1 + b_2\bar{x}_2 + \ldots + b_p\bar{x}_p,$$

and consequently b_0 can be replaced in (11.39) by

$$\bar{y} - b_1\bar{x}_1 - b_2\bar{x}_2 - \ldots - b_p\bar{x}_p$$

to give the following form to the regression equation:

$$Y = \bar{y} + b_1(x_1 - \bar{x}_1) + b_2(x_2 - \bar{x}_2) + \ldots + b_p(x_p - \bar{x}_p). \tag{11.40}$$

The equivalent result for simple regression was given at (7.4).

We are now left with the problem of finding the partial regression coefficients, b_i. An extension of the notation introduced in §11.4 will be used; for instance,

$$S_{x_jx_j} = \sum(x_j - \bar{x}_j)^2$$
$$= \sum x_j^2 - \left(\sum x_j\right)^2/n,$$

$$S_{x_jy} = \sum(x_j - \bar{x}_j)(y - \bar{y})$$
$$= \sum x_jy - \left(\sum x_j\right)\left(\sum y\right)/n,$$

and so on.

The method of least squares gives a set of p simultaneous linear equations in the p unknowns, $b_1, b_2, \ldots, b_p$ as follows:

$$(S_{x_1x_1})b_1 + (S_{x_1x_2})b_2 + \ldots + (S_{x_1x_p})b_p = S_{x_1y}$$
$$(S_{x_2x_1})b_1 + (S_{x_2x_2})b_2 + \ldots + (S_{x_2x_p})b_p = S_{x_2y}$$
$$\vdots$$
$$(S_{x_px_1})b_1 + (S_{x_px_2})b_2 + \ldots + (S_{x_px_p})b_p = S_{x_py}. \tag{11.41}$$

These are the so-called *normal equations*; they are the multivariate extension of the equation for b in §7.2. In general, there is a unique solution. The numerical coefficients of the left side of (11.41) form a *matrix* which is symmetric about the diagonal running from top left to bottom right, since, for example, $S_{x_1x_2} = S_{x_2x_1}$. These coefficients involve only the xs. The terms on the right also involve the ys.

The complexity of the calculations necessary to solve the normal equations increases rapidly with the value of p but, since standard computer programs are available for multiple regression analysis, this need not trouble the investigator. Those familiar with matrix algebra will recognize this problem as being soluble in terms of the *inverse matrix*. We shall return to the matrix representation of multiple regression later in this section but, for now, shall simply note that the equations have a solution which may be obtained by using a computer with statistical software.

Sampling variation

As in simple regression, the Total SSq of y may be divided into the SSq due to regression and the SSq about regression with (11.2) and (11.3) applying and illustrated by Fig. 11.1, although in multiple regression the corresponding figure could not be drawn, since it would be in $(p + 1)$-dimensional space. Thus, again we have

$$\text{Total SSq} = \text{SSq about regression} + \text{SSq due to regression},$$

which provides the opportunity for an analysis of variance. The subdivision of DF is as follows:

$$\text{Total} = \text{About regression} + \text{Due to regression}$$
$$n - 1 = (n - p - 1) \quad\quad + p$$

The variance ratio

$$F = \frac{\text{MSq due to regression}}{\text{MSq about regression}} \tag{11.42}$$

provides a composite test of the null hypothesis that $\beta_1 = \beta_2 = \ldots = \beta_p = 0$, i.e. that all the predictor variables are irrelevant.

We have so far discussed the significance of the joint relationship of y with the predictor variables. It is usually interesting to study the sampling variation of each b_j separately. This not only provides information about the precision of the partial regression coefficients, but also enables each of them to be tested for a significant departure from zero.

The variance and standard error of b_j are obtained by the multivariate extension of (7.16) as

$$\left.\begin{array}{l} \text{var}(b_j) = s^2 c_{jj}, \\ \text{SE}(b_j) = \sqrt{(s^2 c_{jj})} \end{array}\right\}, \tag{11.43}$$

where s^2 is the Residual MSq about regression and c_{ij} is the general term of the inverse of the matrix on the left side of (11.41) (see also (11.51)), which is calculated during the solution of the normal equations. Tests and confidence limits are obtained in the usual way, with the t distribution on $n - p - 1$ DF. We note also, for future reference, that the *covariance* of b_j and b_h is

$$\text{cov}(b_j, b_h) = s^2 c_{jh}. \tag{11.44}$$

If a particular b_j is not significantly different from zero, it may be thought sensible to call it zero (i.e. to drop it from the regression equation) to make the equation as simple as possible. It is important to realize, though, that if this is done the remaining b_js would be changed; in general, new values would be obtained by doing a new analysis on the remaining x_js.

The ratio

$$\frac{\text{SSq due to regression}}{\text{Total SSq}} \qquad (11.45)$$

is often denoted by R^2 (by analogy with the similar result (7.10) for r^2 in simple regression). The quantity R is called the *multiple correlation coefficient*. R^2 must be between 0 and 1, and so must its positive square root. In general, no meaning can be attached to the direction of a multiple correlation with more than one predictor variable, and so R is always given a positive value. The appropriate test for the significance of the multiple correlation coefficient is the F test described above.

R^2 must increase as further variables are introduced into a regression and therefore cannot be used to compare regressions with different numbers of variables. The value of R^2 may be adjusted to take account of the chance contribution of each variable included by subtracting the value that would be expected if none of the variables was associated with y. The adjusted value, R_a^2, is calculated from

$$
\begin{aligned}
R_a^2 &= R^2 - \frac{p}{n-p-1}(1-R^2) \\
&= \frac{(n-1)R^2 - p}{n-p-1}.
\end{aligned} \qquad (11.46)
$$

R^2 is not a satisfactory measure of goodness of fit of the fitted regression. Where there are replicate values of y for certain values of the explanatory variables, then the goodness of fit may be assessed by subdividing the SSq about the regression into two components, one representing deviations of the mean of the replicates about the regression, and the other variability within replicates (Healy, 1984; see also §11.1). Without replication, goodness of fit cannot be strictly tested but methods of assessing the adequacy of the model are discussed later in this section.

Example 11.5

The data shown in Table 11.6 are taken from a clinical trial to compare two hypotensive drugs used to lower the blood pressure during operations (Robertson & Armitage, 1959). The dependent variable, y, is the 'recovery time' (in minutes) elapsing between the time at which the drug was discontinued and the time at which the systolic blood pressure had

Table 11.6 Data on the use of a hypotensive drug: x_1, log (quantity of drug used, mg); x_2, mean level of systolic blood pressure during hypotension (mmHg); y, recovery time (min).

x_1	x_2	y	Y	$y - Y$	x_1	x_2	y	Y	$y - Y$
Group A: 'Minor' non-thoracic ($n_A = 20$)					*Group B: (continued)*				
2·26	66	7	29·3	−22·3	2·70	73	39	34·7	4·3
1·81	52	10	28·6	−18·6	1·90	56	28	27·9	0·1
1·78	72	18	13·6	4·4	2·78	83	12	29·4	−17·4
1·54	67	4	11·5	−7·5	2·27	67	60	28·8	31·2
2·06	69	10	22·4	−12·4	1·74	84	10	4·1	5·9
1·74	71	13	13·4	−0·4	2·62	68	60	36·3	23·7
2·56	88	21	20·6	0·4	1·80	64	22	19·8	2·2
2·29	68	12	28·5	−16·5	1·81	60	21	22·9	−1·9
1·80	59	9	23·4	−14·4	1·58	62	14	16·0	−2·0
2·32	73	65	25·7	39·3	2·41	76	4	25·7	−21·7
2·04	68	20	22·6	−2·6	1·65	60	27	19·1	7·9
1·88	58	31	26·0	5·0	2·24	60	26	33·1	−7·1
1·18	61	23	7·3	15·7	1·70	59	28	21·0	7·0
2·08	68	22	23·6	−1·6					
1·70	69	13	13·9	−0·9	*Group C: Thoracic* ($n_C = 13$)				
1·74	55	9	24·8	−15·8	2·45	84	15	20·9	−5·9
1·90	67	50	20·0	30·0	1·72	66	8	16·5	−8·5
1·79	67	12	17·4	−5·4	2·37	68	46	30·4	15·6
2·11	68	11	24·3	−13·3	2·23	65	24	29·3	−5·3
1·72	59	8	21·5	−13·5	1·92	69	12	19·1	−7·1
					1·99	72	25	18·6	6·4
Group B: 'Major' non-thoracic ($n_B = 20$)					1·99	63	45	25·0	20·0
1·74	68	26	15·5	10·5	2·35	56	72	38·5	33·5
1·60	63	16	15·8	0·2	1·80	70	25	15·5	9·5
2·15	65	23	27·4	−4·4	2·36	69	28	29·5	−1·5
2·26	72	7	25·0	−18·0	1·59	60	10	17·7	−7·7
1·65	58	11	20·6	−9·6	2·10	51	25	36·2	−11·2
1·63	69	8	12·2	−4·2	1·80	61	44	22·0	22·0
2·40	70	14	29·7	−15·7					

Summary statistics for all subjects

$n = 53$

$\bar{x}_1 = 1 \cdot 9925$ $\qquad \bar{x}_2 = 66 \cdot 34$ $\qquad \bar{y} = 22 \cdot 70$

$\text{SD}(x_1) = 0 \cdot 3402$ $\qquad \text{SD}(x_2) = 7 \cdot 73$ $\qquad \text{SD}(y) = 16 \cdot 29$

returned to 100 mmHg. The data shown here relate to one of the two drugs used in the trial. The recovery time is very variable, and a question of interest is the extent to which it depends on the quantity of drug used and the level to which blood pressure was lowered during hypotension. The two predictor variables are:

x_1: log (quantity of drug used, mg);

x_2: mean level of systolic blood pressure during hypotension (mmHg).

The 53 patients are divided into three groups according to the type of operation. Initially we shall ignore this classification, the data being analysed as a single group. Possible differences between groups are considered in §11.7.

Table 11.6 shows the values of x_1, x_2 and y for the 53 patients. The columns headed Y and $y - Y$ will be referred to later. Below the data are shown the means and standard deviations of the three variables.

Using standard statistical software for multiple regression, the regression equation is

$$Y = 23 \cdot 011 + 23 \cdot 639 x_1 - 0 \cdot 71467 x_2.$$

The recovery time increases on the average by about 24 min for each increase of 1 in the log dose (i.e. each 10-fold increase in dose), and decreases by 0·71 min for every increase of 1 mmHg in the mean blood pressure during hypotension.

The analysis of variance of y is

	SSq	DF	MSq	VR
Due to regression	2 783·2	2	1391·6	6·32 ($P = 0·004$)
About regression	11 007·9	50	220·2	
Total	13 791·2	52		

The variance ratio is highly significant and there is thus little doubt that either x_1 or x_2 is, or both are, associated with y. The squared multiple correlation coefficient, R^2, is $2783·2/13791·2 = 0·2018$; $R = \sqrt{0·2018} = 0·45$. Of the total sum of squares of y, about 80% ($0·80 = 1 - R^2$) is still present after prediction of y from x_1 and x_2. The predictive value of x_1 and x_2 is thus rather low, even though it is highly significant.

From the analysis of variance, $s^2 = 220·2$ so that the SD about the regression, s, is 14·8. The standard errors of the partial regression coefficients are

$$SE(b_1) = 6·85$$
$$SE(b_2) = 0·301.$$

To test the significance of b_1 and b_2 we have the following values of t on 50 DF:

$$\text{For } b_1: t = 23·64/6·85 = 3·45 \quad (P = 0·001)$$
$$\text{For } b_2: t = -0·7147/0·301 = -2·37 \quad (P = 0·022).$$

Both partial regression coefficients are thus significant. Each predictor variable contributes separately to the effectiveness of the overall regression.

Analysis of variance test for deletion of variables

The t test for a particular regression coefficient, say, b_j, tests whether the corresponding predictor variable, x_j, can be dropped from the regression equation without any significant effect on the variation of y.

Sometimes we may wish to test whether variability is significantly affected by the deletion of a group of predictor variables. For example, in a clinical study there may be three variables concerned with body size: height (x_1), weight (x_2) and chest measurement (x_3). If all other variables represent quite different characteristics, it may be useful to know whether all three of the size variables can be dispensed with. Suppose that q variables are to be deleted, out of a total of p. If two multiple regressions are done, (a) with all p variables, and (b) with the reduced set of $p - q$ variables, the following analysis of variance is obtained:

(i) *Due to regression* (*a*)	p
(ii) Due to regression (b)	$p - q$
(iii) Due to deletion of q variables	q
(iv) *Residual about regression* (*a*)	$n - p - 1$
Total	$n - 1$

The SSq for (i) and (iv) are obtained from regression (a), that for (ii) from regression (b) and that for (iii) by subtraction: (iii) = (i) − (ii). The variance ratio from (iii) and (iv) provides the required F test.

It is usually very simple to arrange for regressions to be done on several different subsets of predictor variables, using a multiple regression package on a computer. The 'TEST' option within the SAS program PROC REG gives the F test for the deletion of the variables.

When only one variable, say, the jth, is to be deleted, the same procedure could, in principle, be followed instead of the t test. The analysis of variance would be as above with $q = 1$. If this were done, it would be found that the variance ratio test, F, would be equal to t^2, thus giving the familiar equivalence between an F test on 1 and $n - p - 1$ DF, and a t test on $n - p - 1$ DF.

It will sometimes happen that two or more predictor variables all give non-significant partial regression coefficients, and yet the deletion of the whole group has a significant effect by the F test. This often happens when the variables within the group are highly correlated; any one of them can be dispensed with, without appreciably affecting the prediction of y; the remaining variables in the group act as effective substitutes. If the whole group is omitted, though, there may be no other variables left to do the job. With a large number of interrelated predictor variables it often becomes quite difficult to sort out the meaning of the various partial regression coefficients (see p. 358).

Weighted analysis

Sometimes the various values of y are known to have different residual variances. Suppose the variance of y_i is known, or can be assumed to be σ^2/w_i, where the σ^2 is, in general, unknown, but the weights w_i are known. In other words, we know the *relative* precisions of the different observations. The correct procedure is to follow the general multiple regression method, replacing all sums like $\sum x_j$ and $\sum y$ by $\sum wx_j$ and $\sum wy$ (the subscript i, identifying the individual observation, has been dropped here to avoid confusion with j, which identifies a particular explanatory variable). Similarly, all sums of squares and products are weighted: $\sum y^2$ is replaced by $\sum wy^2$, $\sum x_j x_k$ by $\sum wx_j x_k$, and in calculating corrected sums of squares and products n is replaced by $\sum w$ (see (8.15) and (8.16)).

The standard t tests, F tests and confidence intervals are then valid. The Residual MSq is an estimate of σ^2, and may, in certain situations, be checked against an independent estimate of σ^2. For example, in the situation discussed on p. 360, where the observations fall into groups with particular combinations of values of predictor variables, y_i may be taken to be the mean of n_i observations at a specified combination of xs. The variance of y_i is then σ^2/n_i, and the analysis may be carried out by weighted regression, with $w_i = n_i$. The Residual MSq will be the same as that derived from line (iii) of the analysis on p. 360, and may be compared (as indicated in the previous discussion) against the Within-Groups MSq in line (iv).

Matrix representation

As noted, the normal equations (11.41) may be concisely written as a matrix equation, and the solution may be expressed in terms of an inverse matrix. In fact, the whole theory of multiple regression may be expressed in matrix notation and this approach will be indicated briefly. A fuller description is given in Chapters 4 and 5 of Draper and Smith (1998); see also Healy (2000) for a general description of matrices as applied in statistics. Readers unfamiliar with matrix notation could omit study of the details in this subsection, noting only that the matrix notation is a shorthand method used to represent a multivariate set of equations. With the more complex models that are considered in Chapter 12, the use of matrix notation is essential.

A *matrix* is a rectangular array of elements. The size of the array is expressed as the number of rows and the number of columns so that an $r \times c$ matrix consists of r rows and c columns. A matrix with one column is termed a *vector*. We shall write matrices and vectors in bold type, with vectors in lower case and other matrices in upper case.

A theory of matrix algebra has been developed which defines operations that may be carried out. Two matrices, A and B may be multiplied together provided that the number of columns of A is the same as the number of rows of B. If A is an $r \times s$ matrix and B is an $s \times t$ matrix, then their product C is an $r \times t$ matrix. A matrix with the same number of rows and columns is termed a *square* matrix. If A is a square $r \times r$ matrix then it has an inverse A^{-1} such that the products AA^{-1} and $A^{-1}A$ both equal the $r \times r$ *identity matrix*, I, which has ones on the diagonal and zeros elsewhere. The identity matrix has the property that when it is multiplied by any other matrix the product is the same as the original matrix, that is, $IB = B$.

It is convenient to combine the intercept b_0 and the regression coefficients into a single set so that the $(p+1) \times 1$ vector b represents the coefficients, $b_0, b_1, b_2, \ldots, b_p$. Correspondingly a dummy variable x_0 is defined which takes the value of 1 for every individual. The data for each individual are the x variables, $x_0, x_1, x_2, \ldots, x_p$, and the whole of the data may be written as the $n \times (p+1)$ matrix, X, with element $(i, j+1)$ being the variable x_j for individual i.

If y represents the vector of n observations on y then the multiple regression equation (11.38) may be written as

$$y = X\beta + \varepsilon. \qquad (11.47)$$

The normal equations are then

$$(X^T X)b = X^T y \qquad (11.48)$$

where X^T is the transpose of X, that is the $(p+1) \times n$ matrix formed by interchanging rows and columns of X. Equation (11.48) corresponds to (11.41), except that it also incorporates the intercept term. The elements of the $p+1$ square matrix $X^T X$ on the left side are the uncorrected sums of squares and products of the x variables. These form a symmetric matrix and, since $x_0 = 1$, the first row and column consist of the sums of the x variables and the element in the first column of the first row is n. Similarly on the right side, $X^T y$ is the $p+1$ vector of uncorrected sums of products of y with the x variables, the first element being simply $\sum y$.

The solution of (11.48) is then given by

$$b = (X^T X)^{-1} X^T y. \qquad (11.49)$$

In matrix notation the SSq about the regression may be written as

$$(y - Xb)^T (y - Xb) = y^T y - b^T X^T y \qquad (11.50)$$

and dividing this by $n - p - 1$ gives the residual mean square, s^2, as an estimate of the variance about the regression. The estimated variance–covariance matrix of b is

$$s^2 (X^T X)^{-1}. \qquad (11.51)$$

It can be shown that (11.51) gives the same variances and covariances for $b_1, b_2, \ldots, b_p$ as (11.43) and (11.44), even though (11.51) involves the inverse of a $p+1$ square matrix of uncorrected sums of squares and products, whilst (11.43) and (11.44) involve the inverse of a p square matrix of corrected sums of squares and products.

Using (11.49), the right side of (11.50) may be rewritten as

$$y^T y - y^T H y = y^T (I - H) y \qquad (11.52)$$

where the $(n \times n)$ matrix $H = X(X^T X)^{-1} X^T$, and I is the $(n \times n)$ identity matrix.

Weighted regression may be expressed in matrix notations as follows. First define a square $n \times n$ matrix, V, with diagonal elements equal to $1/w_i$, where w_i is the weight for the ith subject, and all off-diagonal terms zero. Then the normal equations (11.48) become

$$(X^T V^{-1} X) b = X^T V^{-1} y \qquad (11.53)$$

and their solution (11.49) becomes

$$b = (X^T V^{-1} X)^{-1} X^T V^{-1} y. \qquad (11.54)$$

Since V^{-1} has diagonal elements equal to w_i and off-diagonal terms zero, it is clear that this formulation brings in the weights in all the sums and sums of squares and products.

Further generalizations are possible. Suppose that the usual assumption that the error terms, ε, of different subjects are independent does not apply, and that there are correlations between them. Then the matrix V could represent this situation by non-zero off-diagonal terms corresponding to the covariances between subjects. The matrix V is termed the *dispersion matrix*. Then (11.53) and (11.54) still apply and the method is termed *generalized least squares*. This will not be pursued here but will be taken up again in the context of multilevel models (§12.5) and in the analysis of longitudinal data (§12.6).

11.7 **Multiple regression in groups**

When the observations fall into k groups by a one-way classification, questions of the types discussed in §§11.4 and 11.5 may arise. Can equations with the same partial regression coefficients (b_is), although perhaps different intercepts (b_0s), be fitted to different groups, or must each group have its own set of b_is? (This is a generalization of the comparison of slopes in §11.4.) If the same b_is are appropriate for all groups, can the same b_0 be used (thus leading to one equation for the whole data), or must each group have its own b_0? (This is a generalization of the analysis of covariance, §11.5.)

The methods of approach are rather straightforward developments of those used previously and will be indicated only briefly. Suppose there are, in all, n observations falling into k groups, with p predictor variables observed throughout. To test whether the same b_is are appropriate for all groups, an analysis of variance analogous to Table 11.5 may be derived, with the following subdivision of DF:

	DF
(i) Due to regression with common slopes (b_is)	p
(ii) Differences between slopes (b_is)	$p(k-1)$
(iii) Residual about separate regressions	$n-(p+1)k$
Within groups	$n-k$

The DF agree with those of Table 11.5 when $p=1$. The SSq within groups is exactly the same as in Table 11.5. The SSq for (iii) is obtained by fitting a separate regression equation to each of the k groups and adding the resulting Residual SSq. The residual for the ith group has $n_i-(p+1)$ DF, and these add to $n-(p+1)k$. The SSq for (i) is obtained by a simple multiple regression calculation using the pooled sums of squares and products *within groups* throughout; this is the appropriate generalization of the first line of Table 11.5. The SSq for (ii) is obtained by subtraction. The DF, obtained also by subtraction, are plausible as this SSq represents differences between k values of b_1, between k values of b_2, and so on; there are p predictor variables, each corresponding to $k-1$ DF.

It may be more useful to have a rather more specific comparison of some regression coefficients than is provided by the composite test described above. For a particular coefficient, b_j, for instance, the k separate multiple regressions will provide k values, each with its standard error. Straightforward comparisons of these, e.g. using (11.15) with weights equal to the reciprocals of the variances of the separate values, will often suffice.

The analysis of covariance assumes common values for the b_is and tests for differences between the b_0s. The analysis of covariance has the following DF:

	DF
(iv) Differences between b_0s	$k-1$
(v) Residual about within-groups regression	$n-k-p$
(vi) Residual about total regression	$n-p-1$

The corrected Total SSq (vi) is obtained from a single multiple regression calculation for the whole data; the DF are $n-p-1$ as usual. That for (v) is obtained as the residual for the regression calculation using within-groups sums of squares and products; it is in fact the residual corresponding to the regression term (i) in the previous table, and is the sum of the SSq for (ii) and (iii) in that table. That for (iv) is obtained by subtraction.

As indicated in §11.5, multiple regression techniques offer a convenient approach to the analysis of covariance, enabling the whole analysis to be done by one application of multiple regression. Consider first the case of two groups. Let us introduce a new variable, z, which is given the value 1 for all observations in group 1 and 0 for all observations in group 2. As a model for the data as a whole, suppose that

$$E(y) = \beta_0 + \delta z + \beta_1 x_1 + \beta_2 x_2 + \ldots + \beta_p x_p. \tag{11.55}$$

Because of the definition of z, (11.55) is equivalent to assuming that

$$E(y) = \begin{cases} \beta_0 + \delta + \beta_1 x_1 + \beta_2 x_2 + \ldots + \beta_p x_p & \text{for group 1} \\ \beta_0 + \beta_1 x_1 + \beta_2 x_2 + \ldots + \beta_p x_p & \text{for group 2,} \end{cases} \tag{11.56}$$

which is precisely the model required for the analysis of covariance. According to (11.56) the regression coefficients on the xs are the same for both groups, but there is a difference, δ, between the intercepts. The usual significance test in the analysis of covariance tests the hypothesis that $\delta = 0$. Since (11.55) and (11.56) are equivalent, it follows from (11.55) that the whole analysis can be performed by a single multiple regression of y on $z, x_1, x_2, \ldots, x_p$. The new variable z is called a *dummy*, or *indicator*, variable. The coefficient δ is the partial regression coefficient of y on z, and is estimated in the usual way by the multiple regression analysis, giving an estimate d, say. The variance of d is estimated as usual from (11.43) or (11.51), and the appropriate tests and confidence limits follow by use of the t distribution. Note that the Residual MSq has $n - p - 2$ DF (since the introduction of z increases the number of predictor variables from p to $p + 1$), and that this agrees with (v) on p. 348 (putting $k = 2$).

When $k > 2$, the procedure described above is generalized by the introduction of $k - 1$ dummy variables. These can be defined in many equivalent ways. One convenient method is as follows. The table shows the values taken by each of the dummy variables for all observations in each group.

| Group | Dummy variables | | | |
	z_1	z_2	...	z_{k-1}
1	1	0	...	0
2	0	1	...	0
⋮	⋮	⋮	⋮	⋮
$k-1$	0	0	...	1
k	0	0	...	0

The model specifies that

$$E(y) = \beta_0 + \delta_1 z_1 + \ldots + \delta_{k-1} z_{k-1} + \beta_1 x_1 + \ldots + \beta_p x_p \tag{11.57}$$

and the fitted multiple regression equation is

$$Y = b_0 + d_1 z_1 + \ldots + d_{k-1} z_{k-1} + b_1 x_1 + \ldots + b_p x_p. \tag{11.58}$$

The regression coefficients $d_1, d_2, \ldots, d_{k-1}$ represent contrasts between the mean values of y for groups $1, 2, \ldots, k-1$ and that for group k, after correction for differences in the xs. The overall significance test for the null hypothesis that $\delta_1 = \delta_2 = \ldots = \delta_{k-1} = 0$ corresponds to the F test on $k-1$ and $n-k-p$ DF ((iv) and (v) on p. 348). The equivalent procedure here is to test the composite significance of $d_1, d_2, \ldots, d_{k-1}$ by deleting the dummy variables from the analysis (p. 344). This leads to exactly the same F test.

Corrected means analogous to (11.36) are obtained as

$$\bar{y}'_i = \bar{y}_i + b_1(x_{01} - \bar{x}_{i1}) + b_2(x_{02} - \bar{x}_{i2}) + \ldots + b_p(x_{0p} - \bar{x}_{ip}) \qquad (11.59)$$

or equivalently

$$\bar{y}'_i = b_0 + d_i + b_1 x_{01} + b_2 x_{02} + \ldots + b_p x_{0p} \qquad (11.60)$$

where $\bar{x}_{ij}$ is the mean of x_j in the ith group, and for the kth group d_k is taken as zero. The corrected difference between two groups—say, groups 1 and 2—is

$$\bar{y}'_1 - \bar{y}'_2 = (\bar{y}_1 - \bar{y}_2) - \sum_j b_j(\bar{x}_{1j} - \bar{x}_{2j}). \qquad (11.61)$$

Its estimated variance is obtained from the variances and covariances of the ds. For a contrast between group k and one of the other groups, i, say, the appropriate d_i and its standard error are given directly by the regression analysis; d_i is in fact the same as the difference between corrected means $\bar{y}'_i - \bar{y}'_k$. For a contrast between two groups other than group k, say, groups 1 and 2, we use the fact that

$$\bar{y}'_1 - \bar{y}'_2 = d_1 - d_2, \qquad (11.62)$$

and

$$\mathrm{var}(d_1 - d_2) = \mathrm{var}(d_1) + \mathrm{var}(d_2) - 2\mathrm{cov}(d_1, d_2), \qquad (11.63)$$

the variances and covariances being given as usual by (11.43) and (11.44), or (11.51).

Example 11.6

The data of Table 11.6 have so far been analysed as a single group. However, Table 11.6 shows a grouping of the patients according to the type of operation, and we should clearly enquire whether a single multiple regression equation is appropriate for all three groups. Indeed, this question should be raised at an early stage of the analysis, before too much effort is expended on examining the overall regression.

An exploratory analysis can be carried out by examining the residuals, $y - Y$, in Table 11.6. The mean values of the residuals in the three groups are:

A: $-2{\cdot}52$ B: $-0{\cdot}46$ C: $4{\cdot}60$.

These values suggest the possibility that the mean recovery time, at given values of x_1 and x_2, increases from group A, through group B, to group C. However, the residuals are very variable, and it is not immediately clear whether these differences are significant. A further question is whether the regression coefficients are constant from group to group.

As a first step in a more formal analysis, we calculate separate multiple regressions in the three groups. The results are summarized as follows:

	Group A	Group B	Group C
n	20	20	13
$b_1 \pm \mathrm{SE}(b_1)$	$7\cdot83 \pm 13\cdot78$	$22\cdot76 \pm 9\cdot19$	$36\cdot16 \pm 15\cdot86$
$b_2 \pm \mathrm{SE}(b_2)$	$0\cdot300 \pm 0\cdot553$	$-1\cdot043 \pm 0\cdot469$	$-1\cdot197 \pm 0\cdot550$
Res. SSq	3995·8	3190·3	2228·8
Res. MSq (DF)	235·0 (17)	187·7 (17)	222·9 (10)
$\bar{x}_1$	1·9150	2·0315	2·0515
$\bar{x}_2$	66·250	66·850	65·692
$\bar{y}$	18·400	22·800	29·154

The values of $\bar{y}$ show differences in the same direction as was noted from the overall residuals. However, the differences are explained in part by differences in the values of $\bar{x}_1$ and $\bar{x}_2$. Predicted values from the three multiple regressions, for values of x_1 and x_2 equal to the overall means, 1·9925 and 66·340, respectively, are:

$$\text{A: } 19\cdot03 \qquad \text{B: } 22\cdot44 \qquad \text{C: } 26\cdot24,$$

closer together than the unadjusted means shown in the table above.

There are substantial differences between the estimated regression coefficients across the three groups, but the standard errors are large. Using the methods of §11.4, we can test for homogeneity of each coefficient separately, the reciprocals of the variances being used as weights. This gives, as approximate χ^2 statistics on 2 DF, 1·86 for b_1 and 4·62 for b_2, neither of which is significant at the usual levels. We cannot add these $\chi^2_{(2)}$ statistics, since b_1 and b_2 are not independent. For a more complete analysis of the whole data set we need a further analysis, using a model like (11.57). We shall need two dummy variables, z_1 (taking the value 1 in group A and 0 elsewhere) and z_2 (1 in group B and 0 elsewhere). Combining the Residual SSqs from the initial overall regression, the new regression with two dummy variables, and the regressions within separate groups (pooling the three residuals), we have:

	DF	SSq	MSq	VR
Residual from overall regression	50	11 007·9		
Between intercepts	2	421·3	210·7	0·96
Residual from (11.57)	48	10 586·6	220·6	
Between slopes	4	1 171·7	292·9	1·37
Residual from separate regressions	44	9 414·9	214·0	

In the table on p.351, the SSq between intercepts and between slopes are obtained by subtraction. Neither term is at all significant. Note that the test for differences between slopes is approximately equivalent to $\chi^2_{(4)} = 4 \times 1\cdot37 = 5\cdot48$, rather less than the sum of the two $\chi^2_{(2)}$ statistics given earlier, confirming the non-independence of the two previous tests. Note also that even if the entire SSq between intercepts were ascribed to a trend across the groups, with 1 DF, the variance ratio (VR) would be only $421\cdot33/220\cdot6 = 1\cdot91$, far from significant. The point can be made in another way, by comparing the intercepts, in the model of (11.57), for the two extreme groups, A and C. These groups differ in the values taken by z_1 (1 and 0, respectively). In the analysis of the model (11.57), the estimate d_1, of the regression coefficient on z_1 is $-7\cdot39 \pm 5\cdot39$, again not significant. Of course, the selection of the two groups with the most extreme contrast biases the analysis in favour of finding a significant difference, but, as we see, even this contrast is not significantly large.

In summary, it appears that the overall multiple regression fitted initially to the data of Table 11.6 can be taken to apply to all three groups of patients.

The between-slopes SSq was obtained as the difference between the residual fitting (11.57) and the sum of the three separate residuals fitting regressions for each group separately. It is often more convenient to do the computations as analyses of the total data set, as follows.

Consider first two groups with a dummy variable for group 1, z, defined as earlier. Now define new variables w_j, for $j = 1$ to p, by $w_j = zx_j$. Since z is zero in group 2, then all the w_j are also zero in group 2; $z = 1$ in group 1 and therefore $w_j = x_j$ in group 2. Consider the following model

$$E(y) = \beta_0 + \delta z + \beta_1 x_1 + \ldots + \beta_p x_p + \gamma_1 w_1 + \ldots + \gamma_p w_p. \tag{11.64}$$

Because of the definitions of z and the w_j, (11.64) is equivalent to

$$E(y) = \begin{cases} \beta_0 + \delta + (\beta_1 + \gamma_1)x_1 + \ldots + (\beta_p + \gamma_p)x_p & \text{for group 1} \\ \beta_0 + \beta_1 x_1 + \ldots + \beta_p x_p & \text{for group 2,} \end{cases}$$

$$\tag{11.65}$$

which gives lines of different slopes and intercepts for the two groups. The coefficient γ_j is the difference between the slopes on x_j in the two groups. The overall significance test for the null hypothesis that $\gamma_1 = \gamma_2 = \ldots = \gamma_p = 0$ is tested by deleting the w_j variables from the regression to give the F test on p and $n - 2p - 2$ DF.

When $k > 2$, the above procedure is generalized by deriving $p(k-1)$ variables, $w_{ij} = z_i x_j$, and an overall test of parallel regressions in all the groups is given by the composite test of the regression coefficients for all the w_{ij}. This is an F test with $p(k-1)$ and $n - (p+1)k$ DF.

In the above procedure the order of introducing (or deleting) the variables is crucial. The w_{ij} should only be included in regressions in which the corresponding z_i and x_j variables are also included. Three regressions are fitted in sequence on the following variables:

(i) $x_1, \ldots, x_p,$

(ii) $x_1, \ldots, x_p, z_1, \ldots, z_k,$

(iii) $x_1, \ldots, x_p, z_1, \ldots, z_k, w_{11}, \ldots, w_{kp}.$

These three regressions in turn correspond to Fig. 11.4(c), 11.4(b) and 11.4(a), respectively.

Example 11.7

The three-group analysis of Examples 11.3 and 11.4 may be done by introducing two dummy variables: z_1, taking the value 1 in Group A_1 and 0 otherwise; and z_2, taking the value 1 in group A_2 and 0 otherwise. As before, y represents vital capacity and x age. Two new variables are derived: $w_1 = xz_1$ and $w_2 = xz_2$. The multiple regressions of y on x, of y on x, z_1 and of z_2, and of y on x, z_1, z_2, w_1 and w_2 give the following analysis of variance table.

		DF	SSq	MSq	VR
(1)	Due to regression on x	1	17·4446		
(2)	Due to introduction of z_1 and z_2 $(= (4) - (1))$	2	0·1617	0·0808	0·22
(3)	Residual about regression on x, z_1 and z_2	80	30·0347	0·3754	
(4)	Due to regression on x, z_1 and z_2	3	17·6063		
(5)	Due to introduction of w_1 and w_2 $(= (6) - (4))$	2	2·4994	1·2497	3·54
(6)	Due to regression on $x, z_1, z_2 w_1$ and w_2	5	20·1057		
(7)	Residual about regression on x, z_1, z_2, w_1 and w_2	78	27·5352	0·3530	
	Total	83	47·6410		

Apart from rounding errors, lines (5) and (7) agree with the analysis of variance in Example 11.3 on p. 330.

For the analysis of covariance model, the partial regression coefficients and their standard errors are

$$b_0 = 6\cdot0449$$
$$d_1 = -0\cdot1169 \pm 0\cdot2092$$
$$d_2 = -0\cdot0702 \pm 0\cdot1487$$
$$b_1 = -0\cdot0398 \pm 0\cdot0063 (t = -6\cdot29).$$

The coefficients d_1 and d_2 are estimates of the corrected differences between Groups A_1 and A_2, respectively, and Group B; neither is significant. The coefficient b_1, representing the age effect, is highly significant.

For the model with separate slopes the coefficients are (using c to represent estimates of γ)

$$b_0 = 5\cdot6803$$
$$d_1 = 2\cdot5031 \pm 1\cdot0418$$
$$d_2 = 0\cdot5497 \pm 0\cdot5759$$
$$b_1 = -0\cdot0306 \pm 0\cdot0075$$
$$c_1 = -0\cdot0545 \pm 0\cdot0211$$
$$c_2 = -0\cdot0159 \pm 0\cdot0145.$$

The coefficients c_1 and c_2 represent estimates of the differences in the slope on age between Groups A_1 and A_2, respectively, and Group B. As noted earlier there are significant differences between the slopes ($F = 3\cdot54$ with 2 and 78 DF, $P = 0\cdot034$). The estimates of the slopes for Groups A_1, A_2 and B are $-0\cdot0306 - 0\cdot0545 = -0\cdot0851$, $-0\cdot0306 - 0\cdot0159 = -0\cdot0465$, and $-0\cdot0306$, respectively, agreeing with the values found earlier from fitting the regressions for each group separately.

11.8 Multiple regression in the analysis of non-orthogonal data

The analysis of variance was used in Chapter 9 to study the separate effects of various factors, for data classified in designs exhibiting some degree of balance. These so-called *orthogonal designs* enable sums of squares representing different sources of variation to be presented simultaneously in the same analysis.

Many sets of data follow too unbalanced a design for any of the standard forms of analysis to be appropriate. The trouble here is that the various linear contrasts which together represent the sources of variation in which we are interested may not be orthogonal in the sense of §8.4, and the corresponding sums of squares do not add up to the Total SSq. We referred briefly to the analysis of unbalanced block designs in §9.2, and also to some devices that can be used if a design is balanced except for a small number of missing readings. Non-orthogonality in a design often causes considerable complication in the analysis.

Multiple regression, introduced in §11.6, is a powerful method of studying the simultaneous effect on a random variable of various predictor variables, and no special conditions of balance are imposed on their values. The effect of any variable, or any group of variables, can, as we have seen, be exhibited by an analysis of variance. We might, therefore, expect that the methods of multiple regression would be useful for the analysis of data classified in an unbalanced design. In §11.7 the analysis of covariance was considered as a particular instance of multiple regression, the one-way classification into groups being represented by a system of dummy variables. This approach can be adopted for any factor with two or more levels. A significance test for any factor is obtained by performing two multiple regressions: first, including the dummy variables representing the factor and, secondly, without those variables. For a full analysis of any set of data, many multiple regressions may be needed.

Many statistical packages have programs for performing this sort of analysis. The name *general linear model* is often used, and should be distinguished from the more complex *generalized linear model* to be described in Chapters 12 and 14. In interpreting the output of such an analysis, care must be taken to ensure that the test for the effect of a particular factor is not distorted by the presence or absence of correlated factors. In particular, for data with a factorial structure, the warning given on p. 255, against the testing of main effects in the presence of interactions involving the relevant factors, should be heeded.

Freund *et al.* (1986) describe four different ways in which sums of squares can be calculated in general linear models, and the four different types are particularly relevant to output from **PROC GLM** of SAS. Briefly, Type I is appropriate when factors are introduced in a predetermined order; Type II shows the contribution of each factor in the presence of all others except interactions involving that factor; in Types III and IV, any interactions defined in the model are retained even for the testing of main effects.

In the procedure recommended on p. 353 to distinguish between different forms of multiple regression within groups, we noted that the order of introducing the variables is critical. This procedure corresponds to Type I SSq since the variables are introduced in a predetermined order. The Type I SSq for differences between groups, in the analysis of covariance model with no interactions between the effects of the covariates and the groups, is also a Type II SSq, since the group differences are then tested in a model that excludes interactions. Type I SSq are also useful in split-unit designs, where it is necessary to introduce terms for the treatments allocated to main unit, before terms for the subunit treatments and interactions (§9.6).

The rationale of Type III and IV SSq is to try and reproduce the same type of analysis for main effects and interactions that would have occurred if the design had been balanced. In a balanced design, as we saw in §9.3, the SSq for main effects and interactions are orthogonal and this means that the value of the SSq for a main effect is the same whether an interaction involving that main effect is included or not. Type III SSq arise when contrasts are created corresponding to main effects and interactions, and these contrasts are defined to be orthogonal. Another feature of an orthogonal design is that if there is an interaction involving a main effect, then the estimate of that main effect is effectively the average value of the effect of that factor over the levels of the other factors with which it interacts. Type IV SSq are defined to reproduce this property. Type III and IV SSq will be identical unless there are some combinations of factors with no observations.

If there are interactions then the Type III and IV SSq for main effects correspond to averages of heterogeneous effects. The use of Type II SSq corresponds to a more commendable strategy of testing interactions in the presence of main effects, and either testing main effects without interactions (if the latter can safely be ignored) or not testing main effects at all (if interactions are regarded as being present), since it would rarely be useful to correct a main effect for an interaction. Type I SSq are also useful since they allow an effect to be corrected for any other effects as required in the context of the nature of the variables and the purpose of the analysis; in some cases the extraction of all the required Type I SSq may require several analyses, with the variables introduced in different orders. To summarize, in our view, appropriately chosen Type I SSq and Type II SSq are useful, but Types III and IV are unnecessary.

11.9 Checking the model

In this section we consider methods that can be used to check that a fitted regression model is valid in a statistical sense, that is, that the values of the regression coefficients, their standard errors, and inferences made from test statistics may be accepted.

Selecting the best regression

First we consider how the 'best' regression model may be identified. For a fuller discussion of this topic see Berry and Simpson (1998), Draper and Smith (1998, Chapter 15) or Kleinbaum *et al.* (1998, Chapter 16).

The general form of the multiple regression model (11.38), where the variables are labelled $x_1, x_2, \ldots, x_p$, includes all the explanatory variables on an apparently equal basis. In practice it would rarely, if ever, be the case that all variables had equal status. One or more of the explanatory variables may be of particular importance because they relate to the main objective of the analysis. Such a variable or variables should always be retained in the regression model, since estimation of their regression coefficients is of interest irrespective of whether or not they are statistically significant. Other variables may be included only because they may influence the response variable and, if so, it is important to correct for their effects but otherwise they may be excluded. Other variables might be created to represent an interactive effect between two other explanatory variables—for example, the w_i variables in (11.64)—and these variables must be assessed before the main effects of the variables contributing to the interaction may be considered. All of these considerations imply that the best regression is not an unambiguous concept that could be obtained by a competent analyst without consideration of what the variables represent. Rather, determination of the best regression requires considerable input based on the purpose of the analysis, the nature of the possible explanatory variables and existing knowledge of their effects.

As an example, suppose an analysis is being carried out to determine if lung function, measured by the FEV, is associated with years of exposure to fumes in an occupational environment. Then estimation of the regression coefficient of FEV on years of exposure is the purpose of the analysis but, since FEV is dependent on age, height and smoking and possibly on other variables, then these variables would also be included in the regression model. Estimation of their effects is not important *per se*, but it is required to allow for their effects when assessing the association between FEV and exposure. Moreover, the effect of smoking may increase with years of smoking, and hence with age, so that there is an interactive effect of age and smoking on FEV. This would be included by creating an interaction variable defined as the product of the age and smoking variables.

Automatic selection procedures

A number of procedures have been developed whereby the computer selects the 'best' subset of predictor variables, the criterion of optimality being somewhat arbitrary. There are four main approaches.

1   *Step-up (forward-entry) procedure.* The computer first tries all the p simple regressions with just one predictor variable, choosing that which provides the highest Regression SSq. Retaining this variable as the first choice, it now tries all the $p - 1$ two-variable regressions obtained by the various possibilities for the second variable, choosing that which adds the largest increment to the Regression SSq. The process continues, all variables chosen at any stage being retained at subsequent stages. The process stops when the increments to the Regression SSq cease to be (in some sense) large in comparison with the Residual SSq.

2   *Step-down (backward-elimination) procedure.* The computer first does the regression on all predictor variables. It then eliminates the least significant and does a regression on the remaining $p - 1$ variables. The process stops when all the retained regression coefficients are (in some sense) significant.

3   *Stepwise procedure.* This is an elaboration of the step-up procedure (**1**), but allowing elimination, as in the step-down procedure (**2**). After each change in the set of variables included in the regression, the contribution of each variable is assessed and, if the least significant makes insufficient contribution, by some criterion, it is eliminated. It is thus possible for a variable included at some stage to be eliminated at a later stage because other variables, introduced since it was included, have made it unnecessary. The criterion for inclusion and elimination of variables could be, for example, that a variable will be included if its partial regression coefficient is significant

at the 0·05 level and eliminated if its partial regression coefficient fails to be significant at the 0·1 level.

4   *Best-subset selection procedure*. Methods **1, 2** and **3** do not necessarily reach the same final choice, even if they end with the same number of retained variables. None will necessarily choose the best possible regression (i.e. that with the largest Regression SSq) for any given number of predictor variables. Computer algorithms are available for selecting the best subset of variables, where 'best' may be defined as the regression with the largest adjusted R^2 (11.46) or the related Mallows C_p statistic (see Draper & Smith, 1998, §15.1).

All these methods of model selection are available in the SAS program PROC REG under the SELECTION option; method **4** requires much more computer time than the others and may not be feasible for more than a few explanatory variables.

None of these methods provides infallible tactics in the difficult problem of selecting predictor variables. As discussed earlier in this section, sometimes certain variables should be retained even though they have non-significant effects, because of their logical importance in the particular problem. Sometimes logical relationships between some of the variables suggest that a particular one should be retained in preference to another. In some cases a set of variables has to be included or eliminated as a group, rather than individually—for example, a set of dummy variables representing a single characteristic (§11.7). In other cases some variables can only logically be included if one or more other variables are also included; for example, an interaction term should only be included in the presence of the corresponding main effects (§11.8). Many statistical computing packages do not allow the specification of all of these constraints and a sequence of applications may be necessary to produce a legitimate model. Nevertheless, automatic selection is often a useful exploratory device, even when the selected set of variables has to be modified on common-sense grounds.

Collinearity

We mentioned on p. 344 that difficulties may arise if some of the explanatory variables are highly correlated. This situation is known as *collinearity* or *multi-collinearity*. More generally, collinearity arises if there is an almost linear relationship between some of the explanatory variables in the regression. In this case, large changes in one explanatory variable can be effectively compensated for by large changes in other variables, so that very different sets of regression coefficients provide very nearly the same residual sum of squares. This leads to the consequences that the regression coefficients will have large standard errors and, in extreme cases, the computations, even with the precision achieved by computers, may make nonsense of the analysis. The regression coefficients may be numerically quite implausible and perhaps largely useless.

Collinearity is a feature of the explanatory variables independent of the values of the dependent variable. Often collinearity can be recognized from the correlation matrix of the explanatory variables. If two variables are highly correlated then this implies collinearity between those two variables. On the other hand, it is possible for collinearity to occur between a set of three or more variables without any of the correlations between these variables being particularly large, so it is useful to have a more formal check in the regression calculations. A measure of the collinearity between x_i and the other explanatory variables is provided by the proportion of the variability in x_i that is explained by the other variables, R_i^2, when x_i is the dependent variable in a regression on all the other xs. The variance of b_i, in the regression of y on x_1 to x_p, is proportional to the reciprocal of $1 - R_i^2$ (see Wetherill *et al.*, 1986, §4.3), so values of R_i^2 close to 1 will lead to an increased variance for the estimate of b_i. The *variance inflation factor* (VIF) for variable i is defined as

$$\text{VIF} = \frac{1}{1 - R_i^2} \tag{11.66}$$

and the *tolerance* is the reciprocal of the VIF, that is,

$$\text{Tolerance} = 1 - R_i^2.$$

A high value of the VIF, or equivalently a low value of the tolerance, indicates a collinearity problem. Wetherill *et al.* (1986) suggest that, as a rule of thumb, a VIF higher than 10 is of concern.

The problems of collinearity may be overcome in several ways. In some situations the collinearity has arisen purely as a computational problem and may be solved by alternative definitions of some of the variables. For example, if both x and x^2 are included as explanatory variables and all the values of x are positive, then x and x^2 are likely to be highly correlated. This can be overcome by redefining the quadratic term as $(x - \bar{x})^2$, which will reduce the correlation whilst leading to an equivalent regression. This device is called *centring*. When the collinearity is purely computational, values of the VIF much greater than 10 can be accepted before there are any problems of computational accuracy, using a modern regression package, such as the SAS program. This is demonstrated in the following example.

Example 11.8

In Example 11.6 when the analysis is carried out using the model defined by (11.64), extended to three groups, then there are high correlations between w_{ij}, z_i and x_j. For the full model with eight variables fitted, the values of the VIF for the z_i were both greater than 140, and two of the w_{ij} had similar VIFs, whilst the other two had VIFs of 86 and 92. Thus, six of the eight VIFs were particularly large and this might cause some concern about collinearity. These high VIFs can be avoided by centring x_1 and x_2, when the maximum VIF was 6.8. However, the original analysis lost no important precision, using SAS regression PROC REG, so that the collinearity was of no practical concern.

In other situations the correlation is an intrinsic feature of the variables; for example, if both diastolic and systolic blood pressure were included, then a high correlation between these two measures may lead to a collinearity problem. The appropriate action is to use only one of the measures or possibly replace them by the mean of the pair. This leads to no real loss because the high correlation effectively means that only one measure is needed to use almost all the information.

In most situations the reasons for collinearity will be readily identified from the variance inflation factors and the nature of the variables, but where this is not the case more complex methods based on the principal components (§13.2) of the explanatory variables may be used (see Draper & Smith, 1998, §§16.4–16.5, or Kleinbaum et al., 1998, §12.5.2).

Another approach, which we shall not pursue, is to use *ridge regression*, a technique which tends to give more stable estimates of regression coefficients, usually closer to zero, than the least squares estimates. For a fuller discussion, see Draper and Smith (1998, Chapter 17). As they point out, this is an entirely reasonable approach from a Bayesian standpoint if one takes the view that numerically large coefficients are intrinsically implausible, and prior knowledge, or belief, on the distribution of the regression coefficients may be formally incorporated into the method. In other circumstances the method might be inappropriate and we agree with Draper and Smith's advice against its indiscriminate use.

Adequacy of model

Sometimes, particularly in experimental work, data will be available in groups of replicates, each group corresponding to a particular combination of values of $x_1, x_2, \ldots, x_p$, but providing various values of y. The adequacy of the model can then be tested, as in §11.1, by comparing the variation of the group mean values of y about the predicted values Y, with the variation within groups (obtained from a one-way analysis of variance). The method is a straightforward generalization of that of §11.1. In general, with a total of n observations falling into k groups, the DF are partitioned as follows:

	DF	
(i) *Between groups*	$k-1$	
(ii) Due to regression		p
(iii) Deviations from regression		$k-p-1$
(iv) *Within groups*	$n-k$	
Total	$n-1$	

The SSq for (iii) is obtained by subtraction, (i) − (ii), and the adequacy of the model is tested by the variance ratio from lines (iii) and (iv).

In general, the above approach will not be feasible since the observations will not fall into groups of replicates.

Residual plots

Much information may be gained by graphical study of the residuals, $y − Y$. These values, and the predicted values Y, are often printed in computer output. The values for the data in Example 11.5 are shown in Table 11.6. We now describe some potentially useful scatter diagrams involving the residuals, illustrating these by Fig. 11.9, which relates to Example 11.5.

1 Plot of $y − Y$ against Y (Fig. 11.9a). The residuals are always uncorrelated with the predicted value. Nevertheless, the scatter diagram may provide some useful pointers. The distribution of the residuals may be markedly non-normal; in Fig. 11.9(a) there is some suggestion of positive skewness. This positive skewness and other departures from normality can also be detected by constructing a histogram of the residuals or a normal plot (see p. 371; Example 11.10 is for the data of Example 11.5). The variability of the residuals may not be constant; in Fig. 11.9(a) it seems to increase as Y increases. Both these deficiencies may sometimes be remedied by transformation of the y variable and reanalysis (see §10.8). There is some indication in this example that it would be appropriate to repeat the analysis after a logarithmic transformation (§2.5) of y and this is explored in §11.10, In some cases the trend in variability may call for a weighted analysis (§11.6). Even though the correlation is zero there may be a marked non-linear trend; if so, it is likely to appear also in the plots of type **2** below.

2 Plot of $y − Y$ against x_j (Fig. 11.9b,c). The residuals may be plotted against the values of any or all of the predictor variables. Again, the correlation will always be zero. There may, however, be a non-linear trend—for example, with the residuals tending to rise to a maximum somewhere near the mean, $\bar{x}_j$, and falling away on either side, as is perhaps suggested in Fig. 11.9(c); or showing a trend with a minimum value near $\bar{x}_j$. Such trends suggest that the effect of x_j is not adequately expressed by the linear term in the model. The simplest suggestion would be to add a term involving the square of x_j as an extra predictor variable. This so-called *quadratic* regression is described in §12.1.

3 Plot of $y − Y$ against product $x_j x_h$ (Fig. 11.9d). The model (11.38) postulates no interaction between the xs, in the sense of §9.3. That is, the effect of changing one predictor variable is independent of the values taken by any other. This would not be so if a term $x_j x_h$ were introduced into the model. If such a term is needed, but has been omitted, the residuals will tend to be

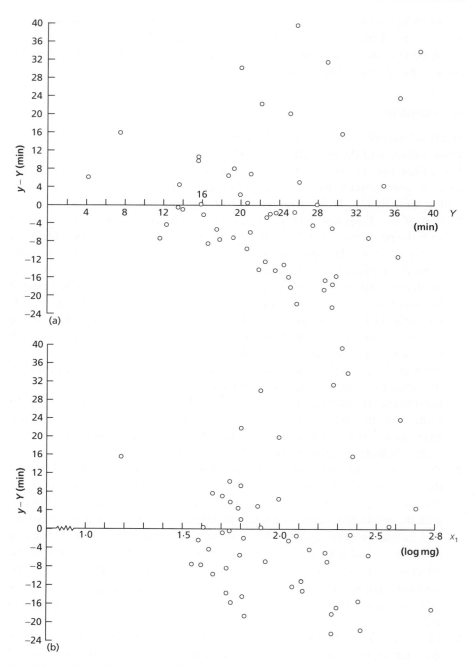

Fig. 11.9 Residuals of recovery time from multiple regression data of Table 11.6 plotted against (a) predicted value; (b) x_1, log quantity of drug;

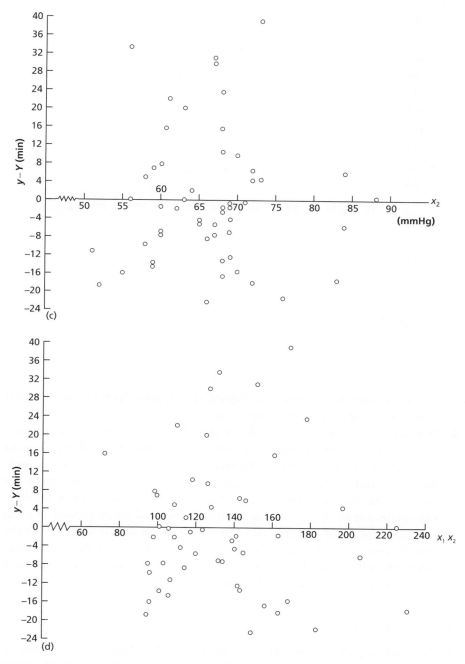

Fig. 11.9 (*continued*) (c) x_2, mean systolic level during hypotension; (d) the product $x_1 x_2$ (*continued, p. 364*);

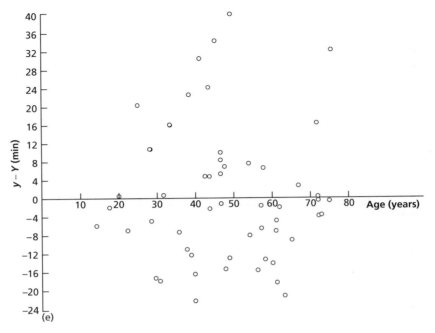

Fig. 11.9 (*continued*) (e) Age.

correlated with the product $x_j x_h$. Figure 11.9(d) provides no suggestion that interaction is important in our example.

4 Plot of $y - Y$ against a new variable x' (Fig. 11.9e). If x' is a variable not used in the regression, the presence of correlation in this plot will give a good visual indication that it should be included. In Fig. 11.9(e) we have introduced a variable not previously used in the calculations, i.e. the age of the patient. The diagram gives no suggestion of a correlation. A more sensitive examination is to plot $y - Y$ against the residuals of the regression of x' on the same explanatory variables used in the regression of y; this plot shows the partial association of y and x' for given values of the explanatory variables.

Atkinson (1985) describes methods of checking the adequacy of regression models, particularly by graphical diagnostics.

Statistical checking of residuals

Whilst residual plots can be very informative in identifying possible outliers, more formal methods are also useful. Some *regression diagnostic methods* are directed towards the identification of individual points that are either discrepant from the regression through the remaining points, or have a disproportionate influence on the fitted regression equation, or both. The concepts are illustrated in Fig. 11.10 in terms of a univariate regression, although it is in multivariate regression, where graphical representations are not easy to construct, that these diagnostic methods are most useful. In Fig. 11.10(a), a regression through nine points is shown. Figure 11.10(b) shows an additional point which is distant from the other nine points but nevertheless is near to the regression through these nine points; this point does not influence the slope of the fitted regression. In Fig. 11.10(c), there is an additional point that is distant from the other nine points and lies below the regression line through these nine points; it is not clearly an

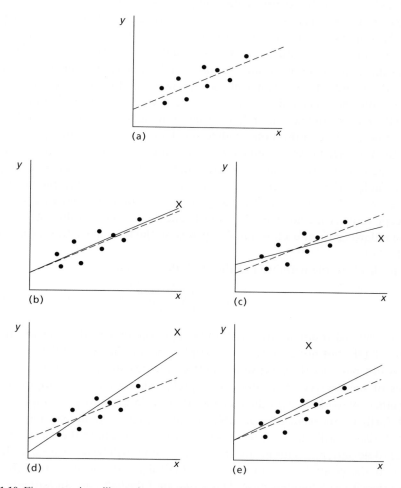

Fig. 11.10 Five regressions illustrating the effect of an extra point which may be an outlier, an influential point, or both. In (a), the regression through nine points is shown. In each of (b) to (e) a 10th point has been added, indicated by ×, and the regression through the set of 10 points (——) is shown together with the regression through the original nine points (– – –).

outlier but inclusion of this point reduces the slope of the fitted line to two-thirds of its value; the additional point is influential in determining the regression. In Fig. 11.10(d), the additional point is again influential in changing the regression but also appears to be an outlier with respect to the regression through the other nine points. Finally, in Fig. 11.10(e), the extra point is within the range of the x values of the other nine points; it is clearly an outlier but does not have a marked effect on the slope of the fitted line. We consider first the identification of outlying points.

For each point the residual is given by $e_i = y_i - Y_i$. The *standardized residual* is defined as $z_i = e_i/s$. At first sight it might seem that e_i is an estimate of ε_i in (11.38). However, this is not strictly the case since the residuals are not independent—this follows because the observed points have been used to fit the regression and the sum of the residuals is zero. Although, if n is much larger than p, the standardized residuals have an average standard deviation of approximately unity, the standard deviation will vary from point to point. A point that is distant from the other points in terms of the x values is especially important in fixing the regression line since relatively large changes in the position of the fitted line can be achieved at this point with lesser changes at all the other points; this is illustrated in Fig. 11.9(b, c and d). Such a point is said to have a high *leverage*, where the leverage is a measure of the standardized distance between the point in the multivariate x space and the mean in this space over all the points. The leverage, h_i, lies within the range $1/n$ to 1 for the usual case where an intercept term is included in the model, and has a mean value of $(p+1)/n$. The standard error of each residual depends on the leverage, and is estimated as $s_i\sqrt{(1 - h_i)}$.

This leads to the definition of the *studentized residual*,

$$r_i = \frac{e_i}{s\sqrt{(1 - h_i)}}. \tag{11.67}$$

The studentized residuals are distributed approximately as the t distribution on $n - p - 1$ DF, but not exactly since e_i and s are correlated, and the approximation is not particularly good in the tails of the distribution even for moderate values of the degrees of freedom. It is preferable to avoid the approximation altogether by working with the residuals defined in the next paragraph.

A further improvement is possible by noting that if a point, say the ith point, is an outlier it will have a large residual, which will inflate the estimate of the standard deviation, s. This means that both z_i and r_i will be decreased, so that the fact that the point is an outlier is, paradoxically, making it more difficult to detect that it has a high residual. The way round this is to use an estimate of the standard deviation that is independent of the ith point. Such an estimate can be obtained by fitting the regression to the data excluding the ith point. Denoting this estimate of the standard deviation by $s_{(-i)}$ and defining the residual as

$$t_i = \frac{e_i}{s_{(-i)}\sqrt{(1 - h_i)}} \tag{11.68}$$

gives the *externally studentized residual* or *jackknife residual*. From (11.67),

$$t_i = r_i\left(\frac{s}{s_{(-i)}}\right) \tag{11.69}$$

and it can be shown mathematically that

$$t_i = r_i\sqrt{\left[\frac{n - p - 2}{n - p - 1 - r_i^2}\right]}. \tag{11.70}$$

so that the jackknife residuals are easily computed for every point without having to fit the n separate regressions, each excluding one point. The numerator and denominator of (11.68) are uncorrelated and the jackknife residuals are distributed exactly as the t distribution on $n - p - 2$ DF.

The definition of t_i might seem to be no more than an adjustment using a more appropriate estimate of standard deviation, but it is in fact much more than this. Suppose the residual were redefined as the difference between the observed y_i and the value, $Y_{(-i)}$, that would be predicted for the ith point using the regression based on all the points except that point. The standard error of this residual could be calculated, using the multivariate extension of (7.22). Then define as a standardized residual

$$t_i = \frac{y_i - Y_{(-i)}}{SE(y_i - Y_{(-i)})}. \tag{11.71}$$

The residual defined in this way, as an externally studentized residual, is mathematically equivalent to the jackknife residual as defined in (11.70). Therefore each jackknife residual is a standardized residual about the regression fitted using all the data except the point under consideration. This rather remarkable mathematical property hinges on the leverage. From (11.70) the studentized residual, r_i, cannot exceed $\sqrt{(n - p - 1)}$, and this limit is only reached when deletion of the ith point results in a regression that is a perfect fit to all the other points (Gray & Woodall, 1994). In this extreme case the jackknife residual has an infinitely high value. Mathematically inclined readers are referred to the books by Cook and Weisberg (1982) and Belsley (1991) for a full mathematical treatment.

These residuals are given in Table 11.7 for the data shown in Fig. 11.10. The column headed D_{10} will be referred to later. Since all the residuals are standardized and independent of the scale on which y and x are measured, these scales have been chosen so that the slope of the line and the standard deviation in Fig. 11.10(a) are both unity. For Fig. 11.10(b to e) the residual diagnostic statistics are given for the extra 10th point. When judged against the t distribution with 8

Table 11.7 Residual diagnostic statistics for Fig. 11.10.

Fig. 11.10	Fitted slope	s	r_{10}	t_{10}	Leverage h_{10}	Cook's D_{10}
(a)	1·00	1·00				
(b)	1·03	0·94	0·14	0·13	0·54	0·01
(c)	0·64	1·11	−1·51	−1·68	0·54	1·37
(d)	1·61	1·37	2·07	2·84	0·54	2·55
(e)	1·21	2·15	2·55	5·49	0·11	0·41

and 7 DF, respectively, the studentized and jackknife residuals are clearly not remarkable for either Fig. 11.10(b) or (c). The greater sensitivity of the jackknife residual is shown for Fig. 11.10(d and e); the lower values of the studentized residual, r_{10}, in these two cases is a consequence of the increase in standard deviation due to the outlier under test. For Fig. 11.10(d and e), the extra point is suggested as a possible outlier by the values of the jackknife residual. We now consider the formulation of a significance test of the residuals.

For Fig. 11.10(d), $t_{10} = 2 \cdot 84$ and if this is assessed as a t statistic with 7 DF then $P = 0 \cdot 025$. However, this takes no account of the fact that this residual has been chosen as the largest, in absolute magnitude, and the effect of this is quite considerable and increases with increasing n. The required significance level is then the probability that the largest residual in a set of n residuals will be as large as or larger than the observed value. This probability is the probability that not all 10 residuals are in the central part of the distribution and is given approximately by $P = 1 - (1 - 0 \cdot 025)^{10} = 0 \cdot 22$, since the jackknife residuals are almost independent. This is the Bonferroni correction (see §13.3). An equivalent means of assessment is to work with a lower critical significance probability, and the largest residual would be significant at level α only if the t statistic gave $P < \alpha/n$. For Fig. 11.10(d), and a significance test at the 0·05 level, we would require $P < 0 \cdot 005$ so that the largest residual with a nominal P of 0·025 is not significant. In Fig. 11.10(e) the largest residual has a nominal P of just less than 0·001 and so there is significant evidence $(P < 0 \cdot 01 (= 10 \times 0 \cdot 001))$ that the 10th point is an outlier. Kleinbaum *et al.* (1998) give a table (Table A–8A) to facilitate the assessment of the significance of jackknife residuals and from this table the significance level is slightly less than 0·01 (critical value 5·41).

Checking for influential points

A point may be regarded as *influential* if it exerts more than its fair share in determining the values of the regression coefficients. Conceptually the influence of the ith point may be envisaged in terms of the changes in the estimates of the regression coefficients when the ith point is excluded from the analysis—that is, in terms of the change in the position and slope of the regression in multivariate space. A standardized measure was proposed by Cook (1977) and is known as *Cook's distance*. This measure, D_i, consists of the squares of the changes in each regression coefficient, standardized by the variances and covariances of these regression coefficients. Cook's distance is always positive but has no upper limit. Cook and Weisberg (1982) suggested that values of D_i greater than 1 should be examined. This corresponds to a point whose removal changes the regression coefficients to outside the 50% confidence region of the estimates, using the full data set. Draper and Smith (1998, §8.3) suggest examining points with the largest values of D_i when these largest values are extreme with respect to the bulk of the values. The values of the leverage, h_i, are important in determining D_i. It can be shown mathematically that

$$D_i = \frac{r_i^2 h_i}{(p+1)(1-h_i)}. \tag{11.72}$$

From Table 11.7 the extra points in both Fig. 11.10(c) and (d) have Cook's distances greater than 1, and this confirms the impression from the plots that these points are influential in determining the regression coefficients.

The mean value of the leverage is $(p+1)/n$ and it is sometimes suggested that points with high leverage, say, greater than $2(p+1)/n$, should be scrutinized. Such points are especially distant from the mean position of the points in terms of the x variables. Whilst it is good practice to check data carefully, a point with a high leverage, but for which there is no evidence that it is either an outlier or an influential point, is not a cause for alarm. Such points are beneficial in reducing the standard errors of the regression coefficients and, if it were possible to supplement a set of data by collecting more data, then a good choice of x values would be those with high leverages.

Multiple regression does not involve any assumptions on the distribution of the x values. Since the leverages depend only on the x values, there is no significance test for the largest leverage which is pertinent to checking the validity of the multiple regression model. The same applies to the Cook's distances, since they depend on the leverages. If the x values are assumed to follow a multivariate normal distribution then tests are available for the maximum leverage and the largest Cook's distance (Kleinbaum *et al.*, 1998, §12-4-2), but these tests identify outliers in the space of the x variables rather than necessarily discrepant points in the multiple regression.

Example 11.9

Residuals, leverages and Cook's distances are given below for some of the points in Example 11.5. The points with studentized residuals greater than 2 in absolute magnitude

Patient	x_1	x_2	y	r	t	h	D
A_1	2·26	66	7	−1·53	−1·55	0·035	0·028
A_7	2·56	88	21	0·03	0·03	0·173	0·000
A_{10}	2·32	73	65	2·71	2·90	0·041	0·104
A_{13}	1·18	61	23	1·14	1·14	0·133	0·066
A_{17}	1·90	67	50	2·04	2·11	0·021	0·030
B_{10}	2·78	83	12	−1·27	−1·28	0·150	0·095
B_{11}	2·27	67	60	2·14	2·22	0·034	0·053
B_{12}	1·74	84	10	0·44	0·44	0·200	0·016
C_1	2·45	84	15	−0·42	−0·42	0·121	0·008
C_8	2·35	56	72	2·41	2·53	0·123	0·270
C_{12}	2·10	51	25	−0·81	−0·81	0·133	0·033
C_{13}	1·80	61	44	1·51	1·53	0·029	0·023

have all been included, as well as the points with leverages greater than 0·11, and the two points with the highest Cook's distances.

The largest studentized residual is 2·71, for the 10th patient in Group A. The jackknife residual is 2·90. Is this point an outlier? The jackknife residual is assessed as a t value on 49 DF. This gives $P = 0.0056$ and an adjusted P value of $1 − 0.9944^{53} = 0.26$. Alternatively, referring to Table A–8A in Kleinbaum *et al.* (1998), the critical value for a significance level of 0·1 is 3·28. Since the jackknife residual is less than this, we have $P > 0.1$. The largest residual is not at all exceptional after adjusting for the fact that it is the largest of the 53 residuals.

Examination of Cook's distance for the 53 points shows that the largest value of D_i is 0·27 for the eighth subject in Group C. This point is that to the top and left in Fig. 11.9(c). The next largest D_i is 0·10 so that the point C is clearly the most influential.

The mean leverage is $3/53 = 0.057$. There are seven points with a leverage greater than twice this value but only one of these has an exceptional residual. This is the point with the highest Cook's distance identified above, but even for this point the residual is not particularly high, given that there are 53 points. Thus, although this point is the most influential, it is not so discrepant from the regression line fitted to the other points as to cause particular concern.

All the calculations and plots discussed above for the detection of outliers and influential points are conveniently carried out on a computer. For example, values of the residuals, leverage and Cook's distance are all available in SAS program PROC REG and may be plotted or analysed.

A discussion of the circumstances in which it may be legitimate to exclude outliers is given in §2.7. The same considerations apply to influential points. Certainly data should not be excluded simply because they appear discrepant from the remainder of the data in some way, but such data should be checked especially carefully in case there has been an error at some stage between the data collection stage and the transfer of data to the computer. When this is not the case, it is important to recognize such discrepant data and assess how they influence the interpretations that might be made.

Testing normality

Although one should not expect real data to follow exactly a normal distribution, it is usually convenient if continuous variables do not depart too drastically from normality. Transformations to improve the approximation to normality have been discussed in §10.8. It is useful to have a quick visual device for checking the approximate normality of an observed distribution, either in an initial study of the raw data or after transformation. This may be done by plotting the standardized normal deviate (§3.8), also known as the *normal equivalent deviate* (NED), corresponding to the cumulative distribution against the variable values. If the observations are grouped, the boundary points between the groups may be plotted horizontally and the cumulative frequencies below each boundary point are plotted on the transformed probability scale. Any systematic departure from a normal distribution will produce a systematic deviation from a straight line in this graph. If the observations are not grouped, one can either: (i) introduce a convenient system of group intervals; (ii) arrange the individual observations in order of magnitude and plot on probability paper, the ordinate for the ith observation out of n being the proportion $p' = (2i - 1)/2n$; or (iii) plot the individual observations *on ordinary graph paper* against the so-called *normal scores* (see §10.3).

Normal plots are particularly useful for checking the adequacy of fit of a model, such as a multiple regression, in which the error terms are normally distributed. If the model is fitted by standard methods, the residuals should behave rather like a sample from a normal distribution, and this can be checked from a normal plot. Most computer packages will provide listings of residuals and many will provide normal plots.

Example 11.10

Residuals, after fitting a multiple regression, are given in Table 11.6 (p. 342). Are these normally distributed? It is preferable to work with the studentized residuals, r, which have mean very near to zero and standard deviation very near to 1. The normal probability plot is shown in Fig. 11.11, plotted following method (ii). This figure shows some deviations from normality with a deficit of low values and an excess of high values, that is, an indication of positive skewness.

A further application of normal plots arises in 2^p factorial experiments, where it is often useful to test the joint significance of a large number of main effects and interactions (see p. 255). On the null hypothesis that none of the relevant effects are present, the observed contrasts should follow approximately a normal

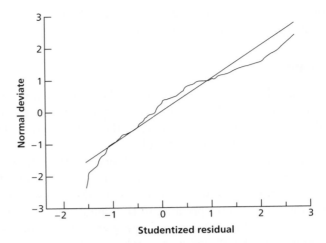

Fig. 11.11 Normal plot of studentized residuals. The cumulative probability is plotted on the ordinate in terms of the normal deviate against the residual on the abscissa.

distribution. The signs of the contrasts are, however, arbitrary, and it is useful to have a visual test which ignores these signs. In the *half-normal plot* (Daniel, 1959), the observed contrasts are put into order of absolute magnitude (ignoring sign) and plotted on the upper half of a sheet of probability paper. The value $\frac{1}{2}(1 + p')$, which lies between $\frac{1}{2}$ and 1, is used for the ordinate. The half-normal plot should indicate which, if any, of the contrasts suggest the presence of real effects.

In general, a theoretical probability distribution can be fitted using simple statistics calculated from the data. For a normal distribution the fitted distribution is obtained using the estimated mean and standard deviation, which for standardized residuals would be approximately zero and 1. If the range of values is divided into k grouping intervals then the observed frequency, O_i, and expected frequency, E_i, may be compared for an interval. From general theory (§5.1) we should expect the familiar statistic

$$X^2 = \sum \frac{(O_i - E_i)^2}{E_i} \tag{11.73}$$

to follow a χ^2 distribution. With efficient methods of estimating the parameters used to fit the distribution, the degrees of freedom for (11.73) are $(k - 1 -$ number of independent parameters estimated from the data). The term 1 accounts for the equality of observed and expected totals. For residuals from a multiple regression with p explanatory variables, the degrees of freedom are $k - 1 - (p + 1) = k - p - 2$. Using the χ^2 distribution is an approximation and it is wise not to use more than a small proportion of values of E_i less than 5, and to avoid values smaller than 2, by choice of grouping intervals. There is no unique way of doing this.

An alternative test which avoids this difficulty is the Kolmogorov–Smirnov test, which is a significance test of the goodness of fit of observations to a hypothesized distribution. The basis of this test is a comparison of the observed and hypothesized distribution functions. The observations, x, are first put into ascending order and then the observed distribution function, $S(x)$, is calculated at each point. The hypothesized distribution function, $F(x)$, is calculated. Then the Kolmogorov–Smirnov test statistic is

$$T = \max {}_{(x)} |F(x) - S(x)| \tag{11.74}$$

where $\max_{(x)}$ indicates the maximum value over the whole range of x, and the vertical lines indicate that the sign of the difference is ignored. This test statistic is referred to tables—for example, Table A13 in Conover (1999).

The Kolmogorov–Smirnov test in its original form applies when $F(x)$ is completely specified independently of the data. Usually this is not the case. When testing if a series of observations fits a normal distribution, the particular normal distribution would be the one with mean and standard deviation estimated from the data, and a modified version of the Kolmogorov–Smirnov test, due to H.W. Lilliefors, is used. The test statistic is calculated exactly as in (11.74) but the critical values are different. Table A14 of Conover (1999) gives critical values for n up to 30, and for larger values of n the critical values for a test at levels of 0·10, 0·05 and 0·01 are approximately $0·805/\sqrt{n}$, $0·886/\sqrt{n}$ and $1·031/\sqrt{n}$, respectively.

Example 11.11

Consider the studentized residuals used in Example 11.10. The concept of the test can be expressed in graphical form (Fig. 11.12) by plotting $F(r)$ and $S(r)$ against r, where $S(r)$ is plotted as a series of steps. Again, the positive skewness is revealed by the plot.

The value of the test statistic is the maximum vertical difference between the two distribution functions and this equals 0·131. This exceeds the critical value for a significance level of 5%, $0·886/\sqrt{53} = 0·122$, but not that for a level of 1%, 0·142. Therefore there is evidence ($P < 0·05$) that the assumption that the observed values are normally distributed with constant variance about the predicted values does not hold.

Another test for normality that is commonly used is the Shapiro–Wilk test. The basis for this test is to compare two measures of the variability of the data, which would be equal for a normal distribution but not otherwise. The first such measure is the sum of squares about the mean, whilst the second is the square of a weighted sum of differences between pairs of values, where each pair consists of corresponding values from each side of the median. The data values are denoted

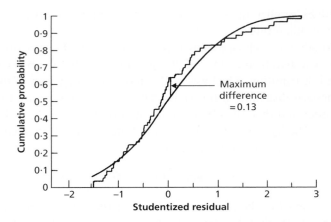

Fig. 11.12 Plot of observed and expected distribution functions plotted against studentized residual.

by $x_1, x_2, \ldots, x_n$, and after sorting into ascending order by $x_{(1)}, x_{(2)}, \ldots, x_{(n)}$. Then the test statistic is

$$W = \frac{\left[\sum_{i=1}^{k} a_i(x_{(n-i+1)} - x_{(i)})\right]^2}{\sum_{i=1}^{n}(x_i - \bar{x})^2}, \tag{11.75}$$

where k is the integral part of $\frac{1}{2}n$. The coefficients a_i depend on n and are tabulated by Conover (1999, Table A16). The test statistic has to be in the range $0 < W \leq 1$, and would be 1 for a normal distribution. Low values of W indicate non-normality and critical values are given by Conover (1999, Table A17).

Example 11.12

The gains in weight of seven rats on a low-protein diet are 70, 85, 94, 101, 107, 118 and 132 g (Table 4.3). The sum of squares about the mean, 101·0, is 2552·0. The difference between the two extreme values, $132 - 70 = 62$ is a measure of variability, as are the differences between the next two extreme values, $118 - 85 = 33$, and the next $107 - 94 = 13$. These differences are combined, using coefficients from Table A16 of Conover (1999), to give

$$(0·6233)(62) + (0·3031)(33) + (0·1401)(13) = 50·47,$$

and

$$W = 2552·0/(50·47)^2 = 0·9981.$$

Referring to Table A17 in Conover (1999) we find that these seven values are exceptionally close to a normal distribution, $P > 0·99$.

Both the Shapiro–Wilk and Lilliefors modification of the Kolmogorov–Smirnov test are extremely tedious to calculate by hand and would normally be obtained using statistical software; for example, SAS allows the calculation of one or other of these test statistics in its UNIVARIATE procedure.

Example 11.11, continued

The value of W is 0.9320, $P = 0.006$. This test also shows significant evidence of non-normality.

Although tests of normality have a place in checking the assumptions of an analysis, their importance should not be overestimated, since many of the methods are valid because the sample size is sufficient to take care of non-normality through operation of the central limit theorem. For example, a two-sample t test (§4.3) is exactly correct if the two samples are from normal distributions with equal variances, and otherwise is approximately valid, where the approximation improves with increasing n_1 and n_2 and the closer the distributions are to normality. The larger n_1 and n_2 then the more non-normality can be tolerated, but it is precisely in this situation that non-normality is easiest to detect. It is likely that the value of the Shapiro–Wilk statistic, W, is more relevant than its statistical significance.

11.10 **More on data transformation**

One of the assumptions of multiple regression is that the distribution of the residuals about the regression is normal with constant variance. In Example 11.5 the analysis of the residuals has revealed that this assumption does not hold; that is, there is evidence that the recovery time is not normally distributed with constant variance about the regression line, from the Shapiro–Wilk test ($P = 0.006$). The distribution of residuals is positively skewed and it was suggested, when discussing Fig. 11.9(a), that it would be appropriate to reanalyse the data after a logarithmic transformation of the y variable.

A discussion of transformations is given in §10.8 and there it was noted that the logarithmic transformation is often appropriate to convert a positive skew distribution to a symmetrical distribution.

Example 11.13

The analyses of the data of Table 11.6 (Examples 11.5 and 11.6) have been repeated using $\log(y)$ instead of y as the response variable. Some features of the analyses are compared in Table 11.8.

First, it may be noted that the basic conclusions are unaltered. That is, there is no evidence that the regression slopes differ between groups; there is no evidence in the

Table 11.8 Comparison of regression models for data of Table 11.6 with untransformed response variable (recovery time, y), and with the logarithmic transformation of the response variable (log y).

	Untransformed	Log transformation
Test of parallelism ($F_{4,44}$)	$1\cdot37$ ($P = 0\cdot26$)	$1\cdot91$ ($P = 0\cdot13$)
Test of group differences ($F_{2,48}$)	$0\cdot96$ ($P = 0\cdot39$)	$1\cdot40$ ($P = 0\cdot26$)
Test of b_1 (t_{50})	$3\cdot45$ ($P = 0\cdot001$)	$2\cdot87$ ($P = 0\cdot006$)
Test of b_2 (t_{50})	$-2\cdot37$ ($P = 0\cdot022$)	$-2\cdot19$ ($P = 0\cdot033$)
Largest jackknife residuals	$2\cdot90$ (A_{10}) ($P = 0\cdot26$)	$-2\cdot67$ (B_{17}) ($P = 0\cdot41$)
	$2\cdot53$ (C_8)	$1\cdot98$ (A_{10})
Largest Cook's distances	$0\cdot27$ (C_8)	$0\cdot13$ (B_{17})
	$0\cdot10$ (A_{10})	$0\cdot09$ (A_{13})
Shapiro–Wilk test of normality, W	$0\cdot932$ ($P = 0\cdot006$)	$0\cdot977$ ($P = 0\cdot61$)

analysis of covariance model that the groups differ in mean level after allowing for x_1 and x_2, and there is strong evidence that both x_1 and x_2, especially x_1, influence the recovery time.

Secondly, the largest jackknife residuals are lower with the log transformation, although in neither case is the largest significant. Thirdly, the largest Cook's distance after the log transformation is only half that with the untransformed recovery time, and the slightly troublesome point in the untransformed analysis, C_8, is no longer so; its jackknife residual is now $1\cdot30$ and the Cook's distance $0\cdot08$. The point with the largest Cook's distance after the log transformation, B_{17}, also has the largest jackknife residual. The Cook's distance is, however, small and not particularly extreme when judged against the bulk of the values, and the residual is clearly not significant. Finally, the Shapiro–Wilk test of normality is not at all significant for the transformed analysis ($P = 0\cdot6$). The transformation has proved effective.

In view of the highly significant rejection of the hypothesis of normality of residuals from the untransformed data ($P = 0\cdot006$), it may seem surprising that the untransformed analysis gives such similar conclusions to the transformed analysis. This illustrates the robustness of the analysis to some non-normality. However, it clearly cannot be expected that failure of the assumptions will necessarily leave the conclusions inviolate, and the conclusions from an analysis which satisfies the assumptions must clearly be preferred.

As noted in §10.8, three main reasons for a transformation are to give a distribution closer to normal, to stabilize variance and to linearize relationships. In Example 11.13 the logarithmic transformation has been successful in the first of these aims with respect to the residuals about the regression. The regression fitted is of log(y) on x_1 and x_2 and, therefore, the relationship between y and x_1 and x_2 is curvilinear. Over the range of x_1 and x_2 the curvature is not great but nevertheless the transformation has changed the form of the relationship, as well as leading to normality of the residuals. McCullagh and Nelder (1989) observe that there is no a priori reason why a single transformation should achieve all three aims, and in §10.8 an example is given of a transformation that leads to a linear relationship but not to normality. In such cases classical multiple regression, as described in this chapter, cannot be applied, but generalized linear models which allow a general form for the distribution of errors about the regression are appropriate.

12 Further regression models for a continuous response

12.1 **Polynomial regression**

Reference was made in §11.6 to the possibility of creating new predictor variables defined as the squares of existing variables, to cope with non-linear or *curvilinear* relationships. This is an important idea, and is most easily studied in situations in which there is originally only one predictor variable x. Instead of the linear regression equation

$$E(y) = \alpha + \beta x \tag{12.1}$$

introduced in §7.2, we consider the *polynomial* model

$$E(y) = \alpha + \beta_1 x + \beta_2 x^2 + \ldots + \beta_p x^p. \tag{12.2}$$

The highest power of x, denoted here by p, is called the *degree* of the polynomial. Some typical shapes of low-degree polynomial curves are shown in Fig. 12.1. The curve for $p = 2$, when the term in x^2 is added, is called *quadratic*; that for $p = 3$ *cubic*, and that for $p = 4$ *quartic*. Clearly, a wide variety of curves can be represented by polynomials. The quadratic curve has one peak or trough; the cubic has at most two peaks or troughs; and so on. A particular set of data may be fitted well by a portion of a low-degree polynomial even though no peaks or troughs are present. In particular, data showing a moderate amount of curvature can often be fitted adequately by a quadratic curve.

The general principle of polynomial regression analysis is to regard the successive powers of x as separate predictor variables. Thus, to fit the p-degree polynomial (12.2), we could define $x_1 = x, x_2 = x^2, \ldots x_p = x^p$ and apply the standard methods of §11.6. It will often be uncertain which degree of polynomial is required. Considerations of simplicity suggest that as low an order as possible should be used; for example, we should normally use linear regression unless there is any particular reason to use a higher-degree polynomial. The usual approach is to use a slightly higher degree than one supposes to be necessary. The highest-degree terms can then be dropped successively so long as they contribute, separately or together, increments to the sum of squares (SSq) which are non-significant when compared with the Residual SSq. Some problems arising from this approach are illustrated in Example 12.1, p. 379.

378

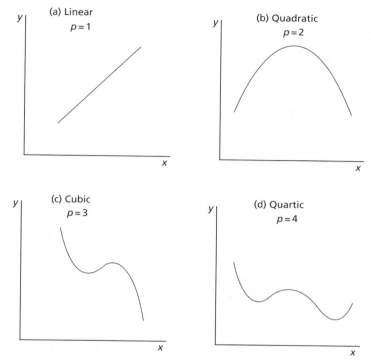

Fig. 12.1 Illustrations of polynomials of up to the fourth degree.

Note that, with n observations, all with different values of x, a polynomial of degree $p = n - 1$ would have $n - p - 1 = n - (n - 1) - 1 = 0$ DF. It is always possible to fit a polynomial of degree $n - 1$, so as to pass through n points with different values of x, just as a straight line ($p = 1$) can be drawn through any two points. The Residual SSq is, therefore, also zero, and no significance tests are possible. To provide a test of the adequacy of the model, the degree of the polynomial should be considerably lower than the number of observations.

Example 12.1

Table 12.1 gives the population size of England and Wales (in millions) as recorded at decennial censuses between 1801 and 1971; there is a gap in the series at 1941, as no census was taken in that year. It is of some interest to fit a smooth curve to the trend in population size, first, to provide estimates for intermediate years and, secondly, for projection beyond the end of the series, although demographers would in practice use more sophisticated methods of projection. The figure for 1981 is given at the foot of the main series to provide a comparison with estimates obtained by extrapolation from the main series.

Table 12.1 Trend in population of England and Wales between 1801 and 1971 fitted by polynomials up to the sixth degree.

Year	Population, England and Wales (millions)	Values predicted by polynomial of degree:					
		1	2	3	4	5	6
1801	8·89	6·88	7·42	9·11	9·20	8·61	8·78
11	10·16	9·36	9·71	10·19	10·18	10·63	10·38
21	12·00	11·84	12·02	11·68	11·62	12·20	12·05
31	13·90	14·32	14·36	13·52	13·45	13·73	13·80
41	15·91	16·80	16·72	15·66	15·61	15·50	15·69
51	17·93	19·28	19·10	18·05	18·04	17·64	17·82
61	20·07	21·76	21·51	20·64	20·66	20·18	20·24
71	22·71	24·24	23·94	23·39	23·43	23·06	22·97
81	25·97	26·71	26·40	26·23	26·29	26·16	25·98
91	29·00	29·19	28·88	29·13	29·18	29·34	29·17
1901	32·53	31·67	31·38	32·03	32·06	32·45	32·37
11	36·07	34·15	33·91	34·87	34·88	35·34	35·40
21	37·89	36·63	36·46	37·61	37·58	37·92	38·10
31	39·95	39·11	39·04	40·20	40·14	40·16	40·36
41	—						
51	43·76	44·07	44·26	44·72	44·64	43·95	43·83
61	46·10	46·55	46·91	46·55	46·52	46·00	45·76
71	48·75	49·03	49·58	48·02	48·10	48·73	48·89
(81	49·15)	(51·51	52·28	49·09	49·36	52·82	54·64)
Multiple correlation coefficient		0·9964	0·9966	0·9991	0·9991	0·9997	0·9998
Residual MSq		1·354	1·346	0·365	0·392	0·139	0·109
DF		15	14	13	12	11	10
t for highest-degree term		45·23	1·05	−6·21	0·34	4·78	2·02
P		<0·001	0·31	<0·001	0·74	<0·001	0·071

The data are plotted in Fig. 12.2. The trend is not too far from linear, but there are obvious systematic deviations which suggest that a polynomial curve might fit quite well.

Table 12.1 shows the predicted values from polynomials up to the sixth degree, and Fig. 12.2 illustrates the fits obtained by linear ($p = 1$), cubic ($p = 3$) and fifth-degree ($p = 5$) curves. The entries at the foot of Table 12.2 show that the Residual mean square (MSq) is reduced substantially by the introduction of the cubic term, and this curve seems from Fig. 12.2 to provide an excellent fit. However, there are slight systematic fluctuations of groups of adjacent points about the cubic, and Table 12.1 shows that the introduction of the fifth-degree term produces a significant decrease in the Residual MSq (since the t value for this coefficient is significant).

The process could be continued beyond this stage, but it is doubtful whether any useful purpose would be achieved. We are left in a slight dilemma. There is no theoretical reason for expecting precisely a polynomial curve plus random error. The cubic is a close approximation to the best-fitting smooth curve, but slight (yet significant) improvement

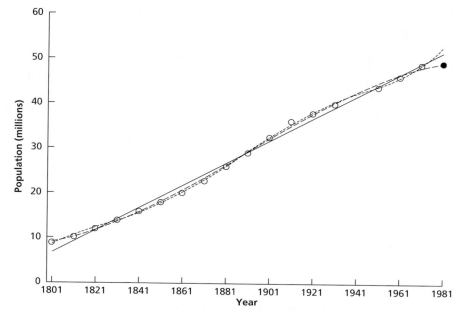

Fig. 12.2 Polynomial regressions fitted to population trend data (Table 12.1). (——) $p = 1$; (– –) $p = 3$; (- - -) $p = 5$.

can be made by introducing a higher-degree term. Note that the improvement is evident in the agreement between observed and predicted values within the range 1801–1971. Extrapolation, or prediction outside this range, is a different matter. The cubic curve gives adequate agreement between the predicted and observed value for 1981. The fifth-degree curve is much less satisfactory. This is a rather common finding, and argues strongly for the use of a polynomial with as low a degree as possible for an acceptable fit, even though higher-degree terms provide noticeable reductions in residual variation within the fitted range.

The various powers of x, which form the predictor variables in (12.2), are correlated with each other, often quite highly so. This occasionally causes some computational difficulties due to collinearity (§11.8). Such difficulties can usually be overcome by redefining the powers of x as deviations from their own means or by centring (Healy, 1963).

These intercorrelations of the powers of x mean that the coefficient of a particular power in the fitted regression equation will depend on which other powers are present in the equation, as indeed is usually the case in multiple regression. If the powers were transformed to an equivalent set of predictor variables which were uncorrelated, we should be able to fit successively higher-order polynomials by relatively simple methods, without recalculating the coefficients previously obtained. This is particularly convenient when the xs are equally spaced, as often happens in controlled experiments (where the xs may represent quantities of some substance) or in time series (where the xs may be equally spaced points of time). The method uses what are called *orthogonal polynomials*. Full details and the necessary reference tables are given in Fisher and Yates (1963).

Orthogonal polynomials provide a useful way of incorporating curvilinear regression in the analysis of variance of balanced data. Suppose that a certain factor is represented by a variable, x, which is observed at k equally spaced values,

$$x_1, \, x_2 = x_1 + h, \, \ldots, \, x_k = x_1 + (k-1)h.$$

Suppose that there are n observations in each group, and that the observed totals of y are

$$T_1, T_2, \ldots, T_k.$$

If $k = 2$, the regression coefficient, b, of y on x, is clearly estimated by

$$\frac{T_2 - T_1}{nh}$$

and the SSq due to regression on 1 DF coincides with the SSq between groups, namely,

$$\frac{(T_2 - T_1)^2}{2n}$$

(as in (8.10)).

If $k = 3$, we could consider a quadratic regression on x which would exactly fit the data, since a quadratic curve can always be found to go through three points. To obtain the regression equation, define two new variables (the orthogonal polynomials),

$$\begin{aligned} X_1 &= (x - \bar{x})/h \\ X_2 &= 3X_1^2 - 2 \end{aligned} \tag{12.3}$$

so that X_1 takes the values -1, 0 and 1, and X_2 takes the values 1, -2 and 1. The regression equation can be written

$$Y = \bar{y} + b_1 X_1 + b_2 X_2, \tag{12.4}$$

where

$$b_1 = (T_3 - T_1)/2n$$

and

$$b_2 = (T_3 - 2T_2 + T_1)/6n.$$

The equation may be written in terms of x and x^2 by substituting (12.3) in (12.4).

The SSq due to the linear and quadratic terms (which are independent, each on 1 DF, and add to the SSq between groups) are

$$S_1 = \frac{(T_3 - T_1)^2}{2n}$$

and

$$S_2 = \frac{(T_3 - 2T_2 + T_1)^2}{6n}.$$

The method can clearly be generalized for higher values of k (see Table A18 of Snedecor & Cochran, 1989). The most useful features of the generalization are the SSq for the linear and quadratic terms. These take the form $(\sum \lambda_i T_i)^2 / \sum \lambda_i^2$, where for the linear term the λ_is are integers centred about zero (e.g. $-1, 0, 1$ for $k = 3$; $-3, -1, 1, 3$ for $k = 4$). For the quadratic term each λ_i is obtained by squaring the corresponding λ_i for the linear term, subtracting the mean of the values thus obtained and multiplying by a convenient constant if this is necessary to give integer values. These SSq account for 2 DF out of the total $k - 1$ DF between groups. The remaining $k - 3$ DF represent deviations about the quadratic curve and can be tested against the appropriate residual in the analysis. If necessary, the cubic and higher terms can be successively isolated until the MSq for deviations reaches a sufficiently low level.

Fractional polynomials

While polynomials offer a family of curves that can be fitted easily using the methods of §11.7, the range of shapes of these curves is rather limited and consequently less useful to the data analyst than might at first be thought. Quadratic terms are widely used, but frequently this is as a simple assessment of the adequacy of a linear fit, rather than as a model in its own right. Cubic and higher terms rarely offer useful alternative models: higher-order polynomials can lead to curves with too many turning-points and which yield inappropriately large or small fitted values at the extremes of the data.

Curves similar to polynomials such as:

$$y = \alpha + \frac{\beta_2}{\sqrt{x}} + \beta_3 \log x + \beta_1 x$$

might usefully enrich the family of curves available to fit data. This is an example of a family of curves known as *fractional polynomials*, introduced by Royston and Altman (1994). The link with the form in (12.1) can be seen by writing this in the form

$$y = \alpha + \sum_{j=1}^{m} \beta_j x^{(p_j)}, \tag{12.5}$$

where $m = 3$ and $(p_1, p_2, p_3) = (1, -\frac{1}{2}, 0)$. The parentheses around the powers of x are because $x^{(0)}$ is interpreted as $\log x$, as in the Box–Cox transformation (see §10.8).

The form (12.5), with powers $p_1 < p_2 < \ldots p_m$ taking real, rather than just non-negative, integer values, provides a wider selection of curves than conventional polynomials. However, the family can be widened further by allowing equality between some of the powers. If $p_j = p_{j+1}$ then at first sight the term

$$\beta_j x^{(p_j)} + \beta_{j+1} x^{(p_j)}$$

reduces to

$$(\beta_j + \beta_{j+1}) x^{(p_j)};$$

in other words, the expression really has degree $m - 1$. However, if $p_{j+1} = p_j + \delta$, then

$$\beta_j x^{(p_j)} + \beta_{j+1} x^{(p_j + \delta)}$$
$$= \beta_j^* x^{(p_j)} + \beta_{j+1}^* x^{(p_j)} (x^\delta - 1)/\delta \rightarrow \beta_j^* x^{(p_j)} + \beta_{j+1}^* x^{(p_j)} \log x$$

as $\delta \rightarrow 0$ for suitable β_{j+1}^*, β_j^*. This rather heuristic argument suggests that the family can be extended to include products of the form

$$x^{(p)} \log x$$

and also (see Royston & Altman, 1994) to include

$$x^{(p)} (\log x)^j, \quad j = 2, \ldots, m - 1.$$

The full definition of a fractional polynomial of degree m, $\phi_m(x; \boldsymbol{\beta}, \mathbf{p})$, depends on a real-valued m-dimensional vector $\boldsymbol{p}$ with elements $p_1 \leq p_2 \leq \ldots \leq p_m$:

$$\phi_m(x; \boldsymbol{\beta}, \mathbf{p}) = \alpha + \sum_{j=1}^{m} \beta_j H_j(x)$$

where

$$H_j(x) = x^{(p_j)} \text{ if } p_j \neq p_{j-1} \text{ and } H_j(x) = H_{j-1}(x) \log x, \text{ if } p_j = p_{j-1}.$$

Since the coefficients β_j enter fractional polynomials linearly they can be fitted in exactly the same manner as conventional polynomials—namely, using the methods of §11.7. The appearance of terms in $\log x$ and the possibility of terms such as $\sqrt{x}$ mean that some fractional polynomials cannot be used directly if some x are negative or zero. A simple way out of this difficulty is to work with $x + \zeta$ rather than x, where ζ is such that $x + \zeta$ is positive for all cases. However, the choice of ζ can be a delicate matter.

There is only one conventional polynomial of a given degree but the presence of the vector p means that there is an infinite number of fractional polynomials of degree m. On the one hand, this enriches the family of curves available to the analyst but, on the other, it complicates the fitting of a fractional polynomial. As pointed out above, the coefficients β_j can be found using linear regression techniques, but this is not the case unless the elements of p are effectively taken to be fixed. Treating p as another collection of parameters to be estimated from the data removes the simplicity from the fitting procedure that is one of the most attractive features of fractional polynomials. Royston and Altman (1994) propose the following simple, heuristic approach to fitting fractional polynomials. The elements of p are assumed to belong to a small discrete set of possible powers, which is usually taken to be $\mathcal{P} = \{-2, -1, -\frac{1}{2}, 0, \frac{1}{2}, 1, 2, \ldots, M\}$ where M could be 3 or possibly max $\{3, m\}$. Each m-tuple taken from $\mathcal{P}$ with replacement defines a fractional polynomial and the m-tuple which gives rise to the smallest residual mean square defines the best-fitting fractional polynomial of degree m. It is also suggested that fractional polynomials of degree m and $m + 1$ can be compared using the usual F-ratio statistic for the ratio of residual mean squares, but it must be remembered that the fractional polynomial of higher degree has *two* extra parameters, a power and a coefficient, so the numerator DF for the F statistic must be 2.

Figure 12.3 shows the population trend data with the cubic polynomial previously fitted and the best-fitting fractional polynomial of degree 3. The fractional polynomial has $p = (0, 0, \frac{1}{2})$—that is, a quadratic in log(year) together with a term $\sqrt{\text{year}}$. The residual mean square for the fractional polynomial is 0·300 compared with 0·365 for the cubic. The improvement in fit for a model which at least nominally has the same number of terms may be very worthwhile for some purposes. Interpolation and smoothing within the range of the data may be two such purposes. However, some caution is also advisable.

The fractional polynomial shown in Fig. 12.3 has been found as a result of considering 120 fractional polynomials of degree 3 and a further 44 of degree 2 or 1. The number of fractional polynomials considered obviously depends on the size of the set $\mathcal{P}$. If $\mathcal{P}$ has P elements then there are P fractional polynomials of degree 1, $P(P + 1)/2$ of degree 2 and $P(P + 1)(P + 2)/6$ of degree 3. Some of the statistical features of a fractional polynomial fitted using the method outlined, such as the standard errors of the coefficients β_j that are reported by the regression program, will be unreliable because they will not take account of the number of models that have been considered. This is, of course, true of conventional polynomials, but the number of alternatives that are available from consideration here is so much smaller that its effect is likely to be much less important. For some purposes, the standard errors are unimportant; in other cases it may be sensible to check the reliability of standard errors using techniques such as the bootstrap (see §10.7). When so many models are considered, it

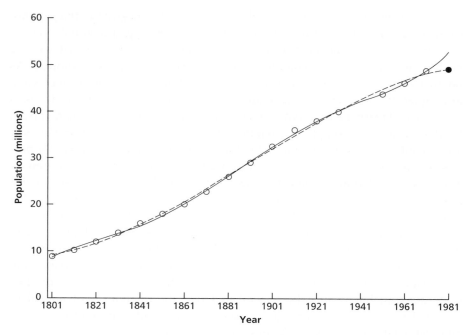

Fig. 12.3 Cubic (– – –) and degree 3 fractional polynomial with $\boldsymbol{p} = (0, 0, \frac{1}{2})$ fitted to population trend data.

may be sensible to inspect all models with residual mean squares that are close to the minimum, with the choice between such models being made on grounds related to the nature of the application.

It was noted that successive terms in a conventional polynomial are likely to be highly correlated and that this can have implications for the numerical stability of the estimated coefficients and the size of the associated standard errors. This problem also applies to fractional polynomials. The estimated coefficients in the $(0, 0, \frac{1}{2})$ polynomial shown in Fig. 12.3 are all large and all the correlations between them exceed 0·99. When using fractional polynomials, the data analyst must keep such numerical features in mind and ensure that they do not have an untoward effect on the purpose of the analysis.

Fractional polynomials offer a useful extension to conventional polynomials as a means of smoothing and interpolating data and for exploring the nature of possible non-linear effects of continuous variables. An important asset is that they can be fitted, at least heuristically, using exactly the same straightforward methods that are used for conventional polynomials. They can be used alone or in combination with other covariates, which can be categorical or continuous, and the latter can be simple linear terms or further fractional polynomials. If deviance rather than residual mean square is used in the fitting, then fractional polynomials can be used for generalized linear models (§4.1) and, indeed, wherever a linear predictor is used to summarize the information from covariates, such as a Cox regression (§17.8).

Polynomials, even when they are extended to include fractional polynomials, have limitations as a source of smooth curves for the description and interpretation of data. Their fitting is global rather than local, so changes in coefficient values to accommodate the response in one part of the data can have consequences (often unwanted) in other parts. Moreover, their explanatory power is low: applications where there is background theory to guide the choice of curve will rarely point to the use of polynomials. Methods for smoothing that avoid many of the problems associated with polynomials are discussed in the next section and more general aspects are considered in §12.4.

12.2 **Smoothing and non-parametric regression**

It is often useful to think of data as having been generated by a process that could be represented by the equation:

$$\text{Data} = \text{Signal} + \text{Noise}.$$

The statistician's task is often to prise apart these two components of the data: quantification of the 'Signal' may be of primary interest but measurement of the amount of noise is usually a necessary adjunct in an analysis. Indeed, the usual multiple regression model (11.1) can be thought of in these terms, with 'Signal' associated with $x_1\beta_1 + x_2\beta_2 + \ldots + x_p\beta_p$ and 'Noise' with the random term ε. However, simple linear regression techniques, even with the extensions described in §12.1, are not always the most suitable method. Even if an approach based on §12.1 is ultimately adopted, it is useful to be able to employ a number of approaches to an analysis, to find the most appropriate method and to assess the robustness of any inferences being made.

There has been considerable progress in recent years in the theoretical and practical development of smoothing techniques and much fuller treatments can be found in, for example, Hastie and Tibshirani (1990), Green and Silverman (1994) and Bowman and Azzalini (1997).

Moving averages, lines and kernel smoothing

Suppose that data of the form $(x_i, y_i), i = 1, \ldots, n$ have been observed and it is desired to produce some estimate of the signal, which might be thought of in this case to be the relationship between y and x. Suppose the signal at the ith data point is S_i and the noise is ε_i, so

$$y_i = S_i + \varepsilon_i,$$

and S could be thought of as y_i without the noise. There is no way of removing the noise from an observation but we know that its effect can be reduced by taking averages. An obvious way to estimate S_i is by averaging the ys, but if the signal changes with x then it is clearly wrong to include ys whose corresponding x values are far from x_i. On these grounds, a simple and useful estimate of the signal might be found by averaging those ys with x values close to x_i. This will give rise to an estimate of the signal that is *local*, as it is based only on points in the vicinity of where the signal is being estimated and contrasts with the global nature of the regression methods in §12.1.

The idea of the last paragraph and relatively simple extensions of it give rise to many ways of estimating S. Since an underlying notion is that the observed data are more variable, or jagged, than the underlying signal, because of the presence of the noise, it is natural to refer to these general methods of estimating S as 'smoothing'. Perhaps the oldest and simplest smoother is the *moving average* or *running average*. It is, of course, necessary to decide what is meant by x_j being close to x_i. If the x_is are in ascending order, then a five-point moving average would estimate S_i by

$$\frac{y_{i-2} + y_{i-1} + y_i + y_{i+1} + y_{i+2}}{5}.$$

Although this definition is intuitively appealing, it lacks the detail to be useful and relies on the unhelpful assumption that the xs are in ascending order. Moreover, the above definition only allows the signal to be estimated at values of x in the data. For many purposes, including interpolation and prediction it is essential to be able to provide an estimate $s(x)$ of the signal at any x within the range of the data. The decision to use five data points is also arbitrary and is related to the degree of smoothing required, which in turn will depend on the purpose of the analysis and expectations about the nature of the signal. It will become clear that most smoothing methods include an arbitrary component that controls the degree of smoothing achieved.

An important step in devising a more useful definition is to define the neighbourhood $N(x)$ of x to be the k points closest to x. Sometimes symmetric neighbourhoods, $N^s(x)$, are chosen, which comprises the $\frac{1}{2}k$ points nearest to and below x together with the same number of points closest to and above x. The definition of symmetric neighbourhoods is complicated by end effects when x is close to the extremes of the data and $N(x)$ is generally preferred over $N^s(x)$. Another way of determining the neighbourhood of a point x is the function $d_k(x)$, which is the distance from x to its kth nearest neighbour: so the elements of $N(x)$ are the x_i with $|x - x_i| \le d_k(x)$. The *k-running average* estimate $s(x)$ is then simply the mean of the y_is with $x_i \le d_k(x)$. In determining k, it is sometimes useful to think in terms of $b = k/n$, which is the proportion of the data which contributes to the estimate and is often called the *span* of the estimator.

Although appealingly simple, the running average has serious drawbacks. The resulting estimate $s(x)$ is usually not very smooth, and the estimate at the extremes of the data can be badly biased, as trends there tend to be flattened out. A modification that overcomes the problem of bias is to use a *running line* smoother. This sets

$$s(x) = a(x) + b(x)x,$$

where $a(x)$, $b(x)$ are the least squares estimates of intercept and slope for the linear regression of y on x using points in $N(x)$.

A way of writing the running average smoother is in the form of a weighted mean, namely:

$$s(x) = \frac{\sum_{i=1}^{n} w(x - x_i, d_k(x))y_i}{\sum_{i=1}^{n} w(x - x_i, d_k(x))}, \tag{12.6}$$

where $w(u, h) = 1$ if $|u| \le h$ and 0 otherwise. The running line smoother is defined in terms of $a(x)$ and $b(x)$, which are the solutions of the minimization problem

$$\min_{a, b} \sum_{i=1}^{n} (y_i - a - bx_i)^2 \, w(x - x_i, d_k(x)). \tag{12.7}$$

Not only is this a more compact notation but it suggests a way in which the definition can be extended. The running average provides a local estimate $s(x)$ by giving points close to x weight 1 and points away from x weight 0. A similar effect could be had by choosing a weight function that was large close to x and small far from x but did not change so abruptly from large to small values. It is plausible that such estimators constructed in this way may be smoother than the running average. Such estimators are known as *kernel smoothing estimators*, with the function $w(u, h)$ being the kernel.

In general $d_k(x)$ is not used as the second argument of the kernel, which is usually an adjustable smoothing parameter h, sometimes referred to as a bandwidth. A common kernel smoother, known as a Gaussian kernel smoother, uses

$$w(u, h) = h^{-1} \exp(-\tfrac{1}{2} u^2 / h^2). \tag{12.8}$$

With this kernel, points which are close to x will figure largely in the weighted mean (12.6), with the weight decreasing steadily and symmetrically according to the familiar bell-shaped curve. Unlike the running average, all points do, in theory, contribute to the estimate $s(x)$, but those more than $3h$ distant from x will receive negligible weight. If h is large compared with the range of the x values in the data, then a substantial proportion of the points will receive noticeable weight in the estimate given by (12.6). The result is an

$s(x)$ that varies smoothly but slowly and does not follow the data closely. In the limit, as h becomes very large, $(x - x_i)^2/h^2$ will be close to zero for all data points, the weights will be nearly equal and $s(x) = \bar{y}$, the sample mean of the ys, for all x. For small h, only points close to x will be given noticeable weight, which will result in an $s(x)$ that follows the data much more closely but for many purposes may be an unconvincing representation of a plausible signal in the data. It is the analyst's task to choose a value for h that constitutes a sensible compromise between the extremes. The task is similar to (and, in fact, closely related to) the task of choosing the interval width in a histogram.

Other kernels are available and each has its advantages. Some, like the Gaussian kernel, give decreasing but positive weight to all points in the data, whereas others explicitly give a zero weight to points that are more than a given distance from x. One such is the *tri-cube* weight function, $w(u, h) = \max[0, (1 - (|u|/h)^3)^3]$.

A widely used method for smoothing data, introduced by Cleveland (1979), goes by the name of the *lowess* smoother (from locally weighted smoother). The method uses a weighted running line smoother, as in (12.7), with the tri-cube weight function. The parameter h in this weight function is taken to be $d_k(x)$, so only the k points closest to x are used in estimating the smoothed value at x. The analyst adjusts the degree of smoothing by specifying k, or possibly more usefully by specifying the bandwidth k/n.

Example 12.2

Figure 12.4(a) shows data on the conduction velocity (in m/s) of nerve signals in the human arm. The data were collected to investigate how the conduction velocity changes with age, particularly over developmentally important ages: 406 determinations were made—70 on preterm babies (whose gestational ages were estimated), 92 between term and 3 months, 49 between 3 months and 1 year, 75 between 1 and 5 years, 42 between 5 and 10, 29 between 10 and 18 and 49 over 18, with the oldest subject being 53. With ages of the subjects being clustered at the lower end of the scale, the data are more clearly displayed by plotting conduction velocity against log(age + 0·75): age is in years and preterm babies have a negative age, so the constant 0·75 is included to convert the postbirth ages to approximate postconceptional ages. The conduction velocity rises throughout childhood, possibly levelling off in adulthood. The data are from O'Sullivan *et al.* (1991), where further details can be found.

The plot in Fig. 12.4(b) shows the results of fitting a running average, running line and lowess smoother, each with bandwidth 0·2, so that each point on the smoothed curve is derived from the 81 (approx. 0·2 × 406) subjects whose ages are closest to the point (except near the extremes of the range). The running average is clearly the least smooth and does not follow the data well near the extremes. As might be expected for data in which there is a clear trend the running line smoother does rather better. As x changes, the data points used in the computation of $s(x)$ change abruptly as a new data point comes into $N(x)$. However, with the lowess smoother, the new and old points receive little

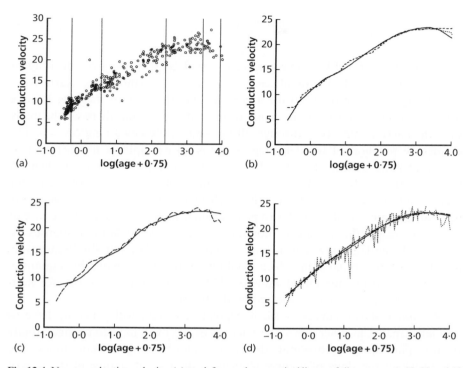

Fig. 12.4 Nerve conduction velocity: (a) top left, raw data, vertical lines at full term, age 1, 10, 30 and 50 years; (b) top right, running mean (- - -), running line (· · · · ·), lowess (——); (c) bottom left, Gaussian kernel smoothing with smoothing parameter 0·06 (– – –) and 0·37 (——); (d) bottom right, penalized least squares $\alpha = 1 \cdot 0$ (continuous), GCV (· · · · ·) and fractional polynomial degree 2, $p = (1, 3)$ (–––).

weight, so the effect on $s(x)$ is far less abrupt. This explains why the lowess smoother is the smoothest of the three estimates of $s(x)$ in this figure.

Figure 12.4(c) shows the effect of fitting two Gaussian kernel smoothers to the data. The parameter h in (12·8) is set at 0·06 and 0·37. It seems implausible that mean conduction velocities should go up and down with age in the rather 'wiggly' way predicted by the estimate of $s(x)$ for the smaller h, suggesting that a larger value of h, such as in the other estimate shown in Fig. 12.4(c), is to be preferred.

Penalized least squares and smoothing splines

The local nature of the smoothing methods just described is achieved quite directly—the methods deliberately construct estimates of $s(x)$ that rely only, or largely, on those observations that are within a certain distance of x. Regression lines, on the other hand, are obtained by optimizing a suitable criterion that expresses a desirable property for the estimator. So, for example, in the case of normal errors, regression lines are obtained by minimizing

$$SS = \sum_{i=1}^{n} [y_i - s(x_i)]^2 \qquad (12.9)$$

over functions defined by a few parameters, such as $s(x) = a + bx$, or a higher polynomial as in §12.1. An alternative approach to smoothing starts from attempting to minimize (12.9) for a general smooth function $s(x)$ (i.e. a curve with a continuous slope). If the x_is are distinct, it is clear that there will be many smooth functions that pass through all the points, thereby giving $SS = 0$. The nth-degree polynomial fitted by regression is an example of a function that *interpolates* the data in this way. If the data points are not distinct, then SS will be minimized by any of the curves that interpolate the means of the y_is for each distinct x_i. However, it is clear that such curves, while smooth, will generally have to oscillate rapidly in order to pass through each point. Such curves are of limited interest to the statistician, not only because such oscillatory responses are intrinsically implausible as a measure of a signal in the data but also because any measure of error in the data, which would naturally be estimated by a quantity proportional to the minimized value of (12.9), is necessarily zero (or, for non-distinct abscissae, a value unaffected by the fitted curve).

As noted above, curves which interpolate the data will generally have to oscillate rapidly, in other words, as x increases, $s(x)$ will have to change rapidly from sloping upwards to sloping downwards and back again many times. The rate at which the slope of a curve changes is the rate of change of the rate of change of the curve. The rate of change of the curve is the derivative of $s(x)$, so the rate of change of the rate of change is the derivative of this, or the second derivative of $s(x)$, which is denoted by $s''(x)$. Consequently, curves that oscillate rapidly will have large numerical values for $s''(x)$, whether positive or negative. If this is true for a large portion of the curve, $\int [s''(u)]^2 \, du$ will also be large; functions for which this is true are often described as *rough*. It may help to note that in this area 'smoothness' is often used in two subtly different ways and care is sometimes needed. Smoothness can refer to the slope of $s(x)$ changing smoothly, that is, without any abrupt changes or *discontinuities*: this is a common mathematical use of the term. On the other hand, it can refer to functions that change smoothly in the sense of not oscillating rapidly: here smooth is being used in its colloquial sense of the opposite of rough, i.e. to describe a function with low $\int [s''(u)]^2 \, du$. Functions that are smooth in the mathematical sense can be very rough, and the sense in which smooth is being used often needs to be judged from the context.

An approach to smoothing that is intermediate between methods based on minimizing (12.9), subject to $s(x)$ being determined by a few adjustable parameters and the locally based methods described above, is to combine the measures of fit to the data, SS, and of roughness. Suppose a function $s(x)$ is chosen which minimizes

$$SSp = \sum_{i=1}^{n} [y_i - s(x_i)]^2 + \alpha \int [s''(x)]^2 \, dx, \qquad (12.10)$$

where SSp is used to denote a sum of squares *penalized* by the addition of the *roughness penalty* $\int [s''(u)]^2 \, du$. The constant $\alpha > 0$ is a smoothing parameter analogous to the parameter h in kernel smoothing. A curve which follows the data closely will make the first term on the right of (12.10) small but will generally oscillate sufficiently rapidly for the second term to be large. A curve which does not oscillate rapidly will have a lower roughness penalty but may fit the data poorly, giving a large value for the sum of squares in (12.10). The curve that minimizes (12.10) will represent a compromise between these extremes. The nature of the compromise is determined by the value of α. A large value of α would mean that the roughness component would dominate SSp. In the limit as α becomes very large, SSp would be minimized by a function for which $s''(x) = 0$, that is $s(x) = a + bx$, so the usual simple linear regression is the limit for large α. A small value of α would put little emphasis on roughness, so the resulting curve would follow the data closely. In the limit as α tends to 0, $s(x)$ would interpolate the data exactly (for distinct abscissae).

At first sight, the optimization posed by minimizing (12.10) is daunting, as the optimal $s(x)$ does not appear to have to belong to any class of functions that can be described by a finite number of parameters. However, it turns out (Reinsch, 1967) that the $s(x)$ which minimizes (12.10) must be a natural *cubic spline*, with knots at the distinct values of the x_i. This means that $s(x)$ is a cubic polynomial between successive knots. A *natural* cubic spline is a cubic spline which is linear below the smallest and above the largest knot. Different cubics can be used between different successive pairs of knots, but the successive cubics must join smoothly and continuously at the knots, so where two cubics join their values must be the same, as must the values of their first and second derivatives. So, while at first sight it looks as though the method uses four parameters between successive data points, these are subject to three constraints, reducing the effective number of parameters. The largest effective number of parameters is n, for the interpolating spline obtained when $\alpha = 0$, and the smallest is two, when α is infinite.

Their genesis through the optimization of a penalized sum of squares, and the ability to tune the degree of smoothing in the estimate, means that splines share features with both conventional regression and locally based smoothing techniques. Indeed, the optimization (12.10) is often referred to as *non-parametric regression*. This intermediate position persists at a more technical level. It can be shown (Silverman, 1984) that, at least approximately, there exists a kernel such that the spline smoothing method obtained from minimizing (12.10) can be written as a kernel smoothing method. On the other hand, it can be shown that the estimates $s(x_i) = s_i$, say, can be written in matrix form as $s = A(\alpha)y$, where s and y are vectors of the s_is and y_is, respectively, and

$$A(\alpha) = (I + \alpha Q R^{-1} Q^{\mathrm{T}})^{-1}.$$

Q, an $n \times (n-2)$ matrix, and R, an invertible matrix of order $n-2$, have elements that are simple functions of the intervals between the x_i: see Green and Silverman (1994, pp. 12–13) for details. This is analogous to the equation determining fitted values from observations in linear regression, where $H = X(X^{\mathrm{T}}X)^{-1}X^{\mathrm{T}}$ would have the role of $A(\alpha)$. If the model is thought of as $y_i = s(x_i) + \varepsilon_i$, then a particular use of this analogy is in the estimation of the variance of the errors ε_i. The usual method is to use:

$$\frac{RSS}{n-p} = \frac{RSS}{\mathrm{tr}(I - H)}$$

where, as usual, RSS is the residual sum of squares. Here, $\mathrm{tr}(A)$ is used to denote the *trace* of a square matrix A, which is the sum of the elements on the leading diagonal of A. By analogy, non-parametric regression uses:

$$\frac{\sum_{i=1}^{n}[y_i - s(x_i)]^2}{\mathrm{tr}[I - A(\alpha)]}$$

as the estimate of $\mathrm{var}(\varepsilon_i)$.

The analogy between H and $A(\alpha)$ can usefully be pursued further. The trace of $I - H$ is the degrees of freedom for error, and $\mathrm{tr}[I - A(\alpha)]$ is often referred to as the *effective degrees of freedom*, EDF, of the spline. Once the abscissae are known, $A(\alpha)$ is determined by α, so specifying EDF is equivalent to specifying α. When α is zero, the fitted curve interpolates the data, so there are no degrees of freedom for error and, indeed, EDF is zero in this case. When α is infinite, the fitted curve is a straight line and EDF $= n-2$, as would be expected. In a sense, EDF, or more accurately $n-$ EDF, measures the number of parameters that the spline is effectively using, and some analysts find it more intuitive to specify EDF, rather than α, to determine the amount of smoothing to be applied to the data. For certain purposes, some authors prefer to use $\mathrm{tr}([I - A(\alpha)][I - A(\alpha)^{\mathrm{T}}])$ as the effective degrees of freedom, but the two definitions are closely related: see Appendix B of Hastie and Tibshirani (1990) for details.

Thus far, for both non-parametric regression and locally weighted methods, it has been assumed that the statistician will determine the smoothing parameter subjectively, perhaps by repeatedly plotting the fitted line. There may be some circumstances in which it is useful for the smoothing parameter to be chosen automatically, essentially to allow the data to determine how much they should be smoothed. Such circumstances might, for example, arise when there are many data sets to be analysed, or when smoothing data sets occurs as part of a larger, automatic procedure.

In this context it is useful to extend the notation for the fitted value to $s(x_i; \alpha)$ to emphasize the dependence of the estimate on α. The most common approach to the automatic choice of α is to view $s(x; \alpha)$ as a prediction of y at a new point, x, that has been uninvolved in the fitting procedure, and choose α to minimize $[y - s(x; \alpha)]^2$. As new points are generally unavailable, they are synthesized by attempting to minimize $[y_i - s_{-i}(x_i; \alpha)^2]$, where $s_{-i}(x; \alpha)$ is the estimate of s obtained from the data set with point i omitted. As i is arbitrary, the method actually chooses α to minimize:

$$CV(\alpha) = n^{-1} \sum_{i=1}^{n} [y_i - s_{-i}(x_i; \alpha)]^2. \tag{12.11}$$

This method of artificially generating 'new' observations is known as *cross-validation* and has wider application in statistics.

On the surface, it appears that n regressions would have to be fitted in order to evaluate (12.11), but, as with jackknife residuals (§11.6), this is not, in fact, necessary. It can be shown that

$$CV(\alpha) = n^{-1} \sum_{i=1}^{n} \frac{[y_i - s(x_i; \alpha)]^2}{[1 - A_{ii}(\alpha)]^2},$$

where $A_{ii}(\alpha)$ is the ith diagonal element of $A(\alpha)$. A similar and widely used alternative that avoids the need to calculate the individual diagonal elements of $A(\alpha)$ is known as *generalized cross-validation*, and seeks to minimize

$$GCV(\alpha) = n^{-1} \frac{\sum_{i=1}^{n} [y_i - s(x_i; \alpha)]^2}{[1 - n^{-1}\mathrm{tr}A(\alpha)]^2}.$$

Similar thinking can be applied to choosing the value of h in kernel smoothing methods—see Bowman and Azzalini (1997, pp. 32–6) for details.

Example 12.2, continued

The continuous line in Fig. 12.4(d) shows a non-parametric regression fitted to the nerve conduction velocity data with a smoothing parameter of 1·0, which is equivalent to an EDF of 5·5. The dotted line is the result of applying cross-validation, using the GCV criterion, which has arrived at a value of 167 for EDF and a smoothing parameter of $5·6 \times 10^{-9}$. This very small value has produced a curve that oscillates rapidly and is unattractive as a summary of the change with age in mean response. Silverman (1986, §3.4.3) explains that cross-validation, at least in the context of kernel smoothing, is particularly sensitive to clustering in the data. Although there are 406 observations of velocity, these occur at only 171 different ages, so there is considerable clustering in the ages in at least parts of the data set. This may be the explanation of the apparently poor performance of cross-validation in this application. Also in Fig. 12.4(d) is a dashed line which is a fractional polynomial with $m = 2$ and $p = (1, 3)$. The spline with an EDF of 5·5 and the fractional polynomial are virtually indistinguishable. The fractional polynomial has been fitted by the method outlined in §12.1. The close agreement with the entirely independent fitting of a smoothing spline may give the statistician considerable encouragement. It also illustrates how a non-parametric approach can often be reproduced with a parametric alternative and the former may act as a useful guide to the selection of the latter.

General remarks

While it will often be adequate to describe the relationship between two or more variables using the methods based on a straight line that were described in Chapters 7 and 11, there are many circumstances when more elaborate models are needed. When the aim is to produce a smooth representation of a relationship, perhaps for interpolation or prediction, or to summarize a relationship succinctly, the methods outlined in this and the previous section are of value. If a parametric model based on polynomials fits the data adequately, then it has the advantages that it can be described by a simple equation and predictions at new x values can calculated simply. Moreover, the statistical properties will essentially be those of linear models, which are well understood to be generally good, although the effect of the way the model was selected may be less than transparent. However, the family of polynomials gives a limited repertory of curves and, although this is usefully extended by fractional polynomials, it is valuable to have access to further methods. More general parametric models, discussed in §12.4, can be useful, as can the smoothing methods discussed above.

Techniques for smoothing data are a large and expanding part of modern statistical methodology and the foregoing description has mentioned only a few of the more widespread methods. One of the disadvantages of the methodology is that the fitted curve is not easily described in a way that others could use. Most of the software that will fit a non-parametric or locally weighted regression will compute $s(x)$ for values of x specified by the user that are not in the data set. However, publishing $s(x)$ in an accessible form is currently less straightforward. In this respect, parametric methods retain an advantage. Careful combination of parametric and non-parametric approaches may prove the most effective way forward.

Many of the more sophisticated methods for smoothing, such as those using basis functions, have not been mentioned. Nor have extensions to the methods that were discussed. Examples of these include the addition of variability bands to give some indication of the uncertainty that attends a given curve, allowing the smoothing parameter to vary with the data and weighted non-parametric regression. For more information on these and other topics, the reader is referred to the texts by Silverman (1986), Hastie and Tibshirani (1990), Green and Silverman (1994) and Bowman and Azzalini (1997).

The present discussion has been entirely in terms of the relationship between a continuous response and a single continuous covariate. When more than one continuous covariate is to be modelled, there are various ways to proceed. An obvious approach is to extend equation (11.38) to

$$y_i = \alpha + s_1(x_{1i}) + s_2(x_{2i}) + s_3(x_{3i}) + \ldots + s_p(x_{pi}) + \varepsilon_i,$$

where $s_1, s_2, \ldots, s_p$ are smooth functions. This equation is the starting point for the subject of additive models, which is considered in great detail in Chapters 4 and 5 of Hastie and Tibshirani (1990). A surprisingly useful class of models are *semi-parametric* models, which are quite explicit combinations of regression and smoothing techniques. In these the effect of a single continuous covariate x_1 is modelled by a general smooth function, while the remaining covariates $x_2, x_3, \ldots, x_p$ (which need not all be continuous) are fitted linearly. This is accomplished by choosing $s, \beta_2, \beta_3, \ldots, \beta_p$ to minimize

$$\sum_{i=1}^{n} [y_i - \beta_2 x_{2i} - \beta_3 x_{3i} \ldots - \beta_p x_{pi} - s(x_{1i})]^2 + \alpha \int s''(x_1)^2 \, dx_1.$$

Both the basic methods and these extensions to more than one covariate can be extended to allow discrete responses and continuous responses with variances that depend on the mean. This is done by extending the way the class of generalized linear models incorporate information from covariates; details can be found in Hastie and Tibshirani (1990) and Green and Silverman (1994).

12.3 **Reference ranges**

In medical practice, it is common for a doctor to guide or confirm a diagnosis by measuring some characteristics of the patient. Examples include weight or height, a haematological variable, such as haemoglobin concentration, blood chemistry, such as serum sodium, or a physiological quantity, such as blood pressure. This is usually done so that the doctor can assess whether the measurement provides evidence of a departure from a healthy state. Because a healthy state is usually compatible with a range of values for a variable, this assessment has an inescapable statistical component. The basis of the interpretation of different variables is different. Anaemia occurs when haemoglobin concentration falls too low for the blood to deliver sufficient oxygen to the body. High blood pressure is thought of in terms of the morbidity that goes with certain levels of hypertension, as determined by epidemiological studies. However, for many variables, such as height and several important clinical chemistry measurements, the assessment is made in terms of the position of the observation relative to that of the patient's peers. The value in a healthy population is estimated by taking a sample of presumably healthy individuals and describing the resulting distribution. The usual approach is to estimate some extreme percentiles so that the range between them covers a substantial and central proportion of the population. The interval between these percentiles is often called a reference range or a normal range, although the latter terminology has disadvantages.

Reference ranges determined by estimating high and low percentiles of the distribution will, by definition, exclude a small proportion of the healthy population. Observations must always be interpreted in the light of this aspect of the definition. Equally, there is a tacit assumption that those within the central part of the distribution, who are undoubtedly normal in the sense of 'commonly occurring', are healthy. This issue often arises when assessing heights of children: in deprived communities all the children may be smaller than would be ideal and, conforming with this distribution, will merely ensure that the individual shares the problems of his or her peers. A fuller discussion of this important issue is beyond our present scope, but it serves to warn that reference ranges should be used thoughtfully. To describe them as normal ranges, with the implication that those within the range are normal and those outside are abnormal in a colloquial sense, is clearly too simplistic.

Once a sample of n observations on a variable X has been obtained from a healthy population, there remains the problem of how to estimate the extreme percentiles. It will be helpful to discuss some of the issues in terms of the estimate, x_α, of the percentile which cuts off the bottom $100\alpha\%$ of the population. In practice, two such percentiles are needed and it is usual to use symmetrical values $100\alpha\%$ and $100(1 - \alpha)\%$, typically with $\alpha = 0\cdot025$, so that the resulting reference range covers the central 95% of the population.

A simple method for estimating x_α is to sort the sample into ascending order and then take the observation $n\alpha$ from the smallest (interpolating between adjacent observations if $n\alpha$ is not an integer). This method does not make any assumptions about the distributional form of the data but depends on the smallest few observations taken. If X has a normal distribution then this fact can be exploited to provide the estimate $x_\alpha = m + z_\alpha s$ (here and throughout this subsection z_α is the $100\alpha\%$ percentile of the standard normal distribution) which, through the sample mean m and standard deviation s, is based on the whole sample and might therefore be thought to be more efficient. This is confirmed by calculating standard deviations of the two estimates.

The standard deviation of x_α using the former method is

$$\frac{1}{f} \sqrt{\left[\frac{\alpha(1 - \alpha)}{n}\right]} \tag{12.12}$$

where $f = f(x_\alpha)$ is the density of X evaluated at x_α. The standard deviation of $x_\alpha = m + z_\alpha s$ can be found using methods outlined in Chapter 5. An approximation to the standard error of s is found by noting that:

$$\text{var}(s) = \text{var}(\sqrt{s^2}) \approx \text{var}(s^2)/(2\sqrt{\sigma^2})^2 = [2\sigma^4/(n - 1)]/(4\sigma^2) \simeq \sigma^2/(2n),$$

using the method in §5.3, the variance of s^2 from §5.1 and approximating $n - 1$ by n. (Note that the variance of s can be found exactly from the χ^2 distribution but the expression is cumbersome and the above approximation is adequate for practical purposes.) Consequently, the standard error of $x_\alpha = m + z_\alpha s$ is given by

$$\sqrt{\left(\frac{\sigma^2}{n} + z_\alpha^2 \frac{\sigma^2}{2n} \right)} = \frac{\sigma}{\sqrt{n}} \sqrt{\left(1 + \frac{1}{2} z_\alpha^2 \right)}. \tag{12.13}$$

When $\alpha = 0\cdot025$ and X has a normal distribution then $f(x_\alpha)^{-1} = \sigma\sqrt{(2\pi)}$ $\exp(\frac{1}{2}z_\alpha^2)$ and (12.12) becomes $\sigma\sqrt{(7\cdot14/n)}$ whereas (12.13) is $\sigma\sqrt{(2\cdot92/n)}$. While (12.12) is valid for any distribution, using it when a normal distribution obtains amounts to throwing away $100(7\cdot14 - 2\cdot92)/7\cdot14 \simeq 60\%$ of your sample. Using the distributionally based method does place considerable stress on the assumption of normality, but its potential benefits are so large that many statistical methods in this area take this approach.

The interpretation of a variable is often impossible until further information about the patient becomes available. For example, knowing that a child has a height of 105 cm is of no value until the age and sex of the child are known. Separate reference ranges, often known as *growth standards* when applied to anthropometric data, for boys and girls overcome one of these problems. Allowing for age requires the relationship between X and age, T, to be incorporated into the reference range. While T could be any covariate such that clinical interest centres on the conditional distribution of X given T, it is so common for this problem to arise in paediatric practice with T being age that the methodology has often been developed under the heading of age-dependent or age-specific reference ranges, and we shall adopt this terminology. Of course, other types of reference ranges, such as standards of height for weight, share the same statistical methodology.

In the remainder of this section, methods for the construction of age-specific reference ranges will be discussed, largely from the viewpoint of the various regression methods discussed earlier in this chapter. It will generally be assumed that the data used for determining the ranges will be cross-sectional, i.e. the sample has been chosen by selecting individuals from some population at more or less a single time and each individual is only measured once. Strictly speaking, such ranges can only be used for the first presentation of a patient. There are many other statistical aspects to this subject, such as the construction of growth standards on which individual patients can be followed up, conditional standards and velocity standards; useful references in this area include Healy (1974, 1989) and Cole (1995, 1998). The issue of the simultaneous interpretation of two measurements is a further extension of this thinking which requires particular care but will not be considered here; Healy (1979, 1981) gives enlightening discussions of some of the main issues.

Regression and the LMS method

Suppose that data are available on some variable X, and the corresponding age T from a sample of size n, and it is required to describe the distribution of X given T (written shortly as $X \mid T$) for a range of ages. At first sight this appears a familiar task to which the methods of regression described in Chapter 7 and §§12.1–12.2 are well suited. If the mean of the distribution of $X \mid T$ is a linear function of T then the $100\alpha\%$ percentile is simply $a + bT + z_\alpha s$, where a and b are estimated regression coefficients and s^2 is the estimated residual mean square. If the dependence of X on T is not linear, the methods of §§12.1–12.2 could be deployed.

A problem of using this familiar regression framework is that it assumes that the distribution $X \mid T$ is normal and that it has a constant standard deviation. This is seldom likely to be true. However, in standard applications of regression methods, such as inference about the regression coefficients or its use to adjust related means, quite substantial deviations from normality and constant variance will not be troublesome. This is not the case when constructing reference ranges, and much more attention needs to be paid to the dependence of the variance and distributional form on age.

If the statistician is confident that $X \mid T$ is normal with mean μ_T and standard deviation σ_T, then joint modelling of the mean and variance, as described by Aitkin (1987) and McCullagh and Nelder (1989, Chapter 10), may be all that is needed. However, it is more often the case that normality cannot be taken for granted and then one approach to the problem is that taken by Cole (1988) in a method that applies a Box–Cox transformation (§10.8), $X^{(\lambda)} = (X^\lambda - 1)/\lambda$, with age-dependent transformation parameter $\lambda = \lambda(T)$ in the hope that the transformed variable follows a normal distribution. The method involves computing three curves, $L(T)$, $M(T)$ and $S(T)$, which record the changing values of λ, of the median of X and of a form of coefficient of variation of X: these curves are fundamental to the technique and give rise to its name, the LMS method.

The original description of the application of the method given by Cole (1988) can be summarized as follows. The method starts by dividing the data into k contiguous groups. Within the ith group it is necessary to compute l_i, an estimates of λ, m_i, the median of X, and s_i, a form of coefficient of variation of X. Given that the method assumes that X^λ is normally distributed, the most efficient way to compute the median of X is as the l_i^{-1} power of the mean of the values of X^{l_i} over the ith group. The value of s_i is actually the standard deviation, over the ith group, of $\xi(l_i)$ where

$$\xi(\lambda) = \frac{X^{(\lambda)}}{\lambda G^\lambda}, \tag{12.14}$$

where G is the geometric mean of the X values in the group. If $\lambda = 0$, then the above is replaced by $\log(X)$ and the median of X is simply G. Once values for l_i,

m_i and s_i have been found, they are plotted against the mean age in the ith group and smoothed, using whatever technique the statistician chooses, to provide the $L(T)$, $M(T)$ and $S(T)$ curves.

In order to start the method, estimates of l_i are needed. The maximum likelihood estimate of λ for the ith group is found when the residual variation of the transformed values is minimized. This is not found simply when the standard deviation of the transformed Xs is minimized, because standard deviations cannot be combined across different scales of measurement. However, working with the transformed variables, (12.14), effectively overcomes this point (technically it is a device which essentially incorporates the Jacobian of the transformation) and the standard deviations of the $\xi(\lambda)$ can be compared for different λ. Cole proposed that the standard deviation of the $\xi(\lambda)$ be computed for a range of values of λ and that a quadratic be fitted to the resulting set of points. The estimate l_i is then the point at which the quadratic is a minimum. If the values of -1, 0 and 1 are chosen for λ then this approach gives the simple formula

$$l_i = \frac{\log[s(-1)/s(1)]}{2\log[s(1)s(-1)/s(0)^2]},$$

where $s(\lambda)$ is the standard deviation of $\xi(\lambda)$ in the ith group.

Once the L, M and S curves have been found, their values at any age, T, can be read off. The 100αth percentile for X at this age can then be found because $X^{L(T)}$ has a normal distribution with mean $M(T)^{L(T)}$ and standard deviation approximately $S(T)L(T)M(T)^{L(T)}$ and consequently the required percentile is

$$M(T)[1 + z_\alpha S(T)L(T)]^{1/L(T)}.$$

Equally, this equation can be inverted to give z_α for an observed value of X, a quantity sometimes called the SD-score or Z-score, and hence α, a percentile value. It is quite common in some areas of medicine, such as when studying a child's growth, to place a patient relative to his or her peers by quoting an SD-score or percentile value.

Example 12.3

Cole (1988) reports the Cambridge infant growth study, in which 132 babies born in 1983–84 were seen every 4 weeks from 4 weeks to 52 weeks of age and then again at 78 weeks. Several variables were measured including weight; full details can be found in Whitehead *et al.* (1989).

The data on weight were analysed using the LMS method. The sample was divided into 15 groups and smoothed using the following curves:

$$L(T) = 1\cdot44 - 0\cdot187T + 0\cdot00383T^2 - 0\cdot000023T^3$$
$$\log S(T) = -2\cdot015 - 0\cdot015T + 0\cdot000315T^2 - 0\cdot00000225T^3$$

$$M(T) = 7 \cdot 59 + 0 \cdot 046T - 4 \cdot 5(0 \cdot 943)^T \text{(Boys)}$$
$$M(T) = 7 \cdot 50 + 0 \cdot 037T - 4 \cdot 3(0 \cdot 953)^T \text{(Girls)}$$

The curves for L and S and the M curve for girls are shown in Fig. 12.5. Note that the M curve was fitted separately to males and females, whereas the L and S curves were based on the combined data because there was no evidence of a difference between the sexes in these curves. This is one of the potential advantages of the LMS method: if it is thought that the distribution and dispersion of some characteristic is constant across levels of a variable, then better estimates of them can be obtained by pooling data. This can be done even when the M curve does differ between levels of the variable. Regional growth standards might be developed on the basis of common L and S curves but using regional M curves. However, while the LMS method offers efficient technical means for implementing this approach, its desirability is a much deeper question.

The LMS method is now widely used, but its original implementation had the disadvantage of requiring *ad hoc* smoothing of points obtained from an arbitrary division of the data. A modification of the method was proposed by Cole and Green (1992) which did not require the data to be divided into groups and which applied spline techniques to obtain smooth L, M and S curves. The

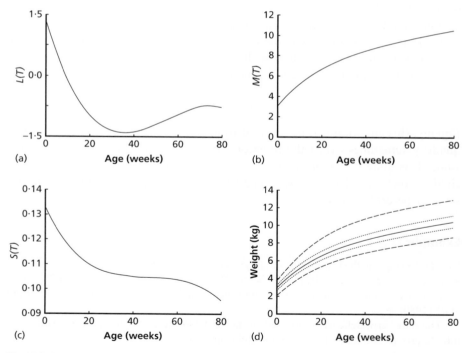

Fig. 12.5 (a) L curve, (b) M curve, (c) S curve and (d) percentiles for weight from the Cambridge growth study as reported by Cole (1988). In (d) – – – are 98th and 2nd percentiles, · · · · · are 25th and 75th percentiles and ——— is the median. The M curve and the percentiles are for girls.

method achieves this by using maximum likelihood, penalized by roughness penalties for each of the curves, as described in §12.2.

Although the approach of Cole and Green is attractive inasmuch as some arbitrary features of the original LMS method have been removed or made more systematic, the resulting curves are more complicated to describe in a succinct mathematical form and this may be a limitation in some applications. Alternative methods using a similar approach, namely transforming data to normality and smoothing the dependence on age, are emerging. Royston and Wright (1998) describe a method which makes use of fractional polynomials.

Distribution-free methods

The LMS method and other methods mentioned hitherto determine percentiles on the basis that the data, perhaps after transformation, have a given distributional form, usually the normal distribution. The percentiles are then computed by substituting estimates of parameters into the expression for the percentiles derived from the form of the distribution. If the data do not have this distribution and if the transformation fails to make them have this distribution, then the derived percentiles may be wrong. In view of this, some statisticians may prefer an approach which does not make such assumptions.

One class of methods is based around the observation that the value of θ which minimizes the mean deviation

$$\frac{1}{n}\sum_{i=1}^{n}|x_i - \theta|$$

over a sample $x_1, \ldots, x_n$ is the sample median. This result can be extended; the $100p$th percentile can be found by minimizing

$$\frac{1}{n}\sum_{i=1}^{n}[(1-p)|x_i - \theta| + (2p-1)(x_i - \theta)^+],$$

where $z^+ = \max\{z, 0\}$. The method can be used to determine age-related percentiles by allowing θ to be a function of age. Details are in Koenker and Bassett (1978), with further work in Newey and Powell (1987). This method seems to have been little used in medical applications.

Another approach altogether is described by Healy *et al.* (1988) and it will be convenient to refer to this method as the HRY (Healy, Rasbash and Yang) method. In this model the median is described by a pth-order polynomial in age, where p is chosen by the statistician on the basis of the data. For illustrative purposes, suppose $p = 1$ and the median at age t is $a_0 + a_1 t$. If the data actually follow a normal distribution, then this will also be the mean. Furthermore, if the standard deviation, σ, does not change with age, then the ith percentile can be written as:

$$a_0 + a_1 t + \sigma z_i = (a_0 + \sigma z_i) + a_1 t, \tag{12.15}$$

where z_i is the standard normal deviate corresponding to the ith percentile. If the standard deviation increases with age—that is, $\sigma = \sigma_0 + \sigma_1 t$ at age t—then (12.15) can be written as:

$$(a_0 + \sigma_0 z_i) + (a_1 + \sigma_1 z_i) t; \tag{12.16}$$

in other words, the expression for the mean is extended to arbitrary percentiles by allowing the coefficients of the polynomial for the mean themselves to be linear polynomials in the standard normal deviate. If the dependence of either the mean or standard deviation on age were not linear, then this could be accommodated by allowing higher-order terms in t.

Whatever the degree of terms in t, provided the dependence on z_i remains linear then the distribution represented by (12.15), (12.16) and their extensions remains the normal distribution. However, if the ith percentile can be expressed as:

$$(a_0 + \sigma_{01} z_i + \sigma_{02} z_i^2) + a_1 t, \quad \sigma_{02} \neq 0,$$

then the distribution is clearly not normal: percentiles represented by $\pm z_i$ are not equally spaced above and below the mean.

The HRY method takes advantage of this implicit method for describing non-normal distributions. In general, the ith percentile is taken to be

$$a_{0i} + a_{1i} t + a_{2i} t^2 + \ldots + a_{pi} t^p, \tag{12.17}$$

where

$$a_{ji} = b_{j0} + b_{j1} z_i + \ldots + b_{jq_j} z_i^{q_j}. \tag{12.18}$$

The user needs to choose values for p and $q_0, q_1, \ldots, q_p$: non-normality is recognized and accommodated if any $q_j > 1$. By substituting (12.18) into (12.17), a set of equations results for the ith percentile at age t. If an estimate of the ith percentile at age t is available for a set of percentiles and a range of ages, then the unknown b_{ij} can be estimated by least squares. Of course, estimates of percentiles are not generally available and the HRY method is a two-stage process. In the first stage, irregular and unusable estimates of percentiles are determined for a specified set of m percentiles; a common choice is to use $m = 7$ and estimate the 3rd, 10th, 25th, 50th, 75th, 90th and 97th percentiles. This produces estimates of these seven percentiles at each age within a range that is slightly less than that in the original data set. The equations arising from substituting (12.18) into (12.17) can then be fitted to these points to yield much smoother and usable percentile curves.

The rough percentiles are computed by using locally weighted methods, similar to those described in §12.2 but adapted to produce a range of percentiles rather than a single measure of central tendency. The data set, which is of size n, is arranged in ascending order of age and points 1 to kn are selected (where k is a fraction, usually between 0·05 and 0·2). For these points the simple linear regression of the variable on age is determined and the residuals are calculated. The m selected percentiles of these residuals are determined by sorting and counting and the m percentiles for the variable found by adding the m residual percentiles to the fitted value of the regression calculated at the median of the kn ages. These percentiles are plotted against the median age and then the whole process is repeated using points 2 to $kn + 1$. The process continues until the whole range of ages is covered. This approach means that no percentiles are computed for the range of ages covered by the smallest $\frac{1}{2}kn$ points and the largest $\frac{1}{2}kn$ points.

Example 12.4

Ultrasound measurements of the kidneys of 560 newborn infants were obtained in a study reported by Scott *et al.* (1990). Measurements of the depth, length and area of each kidney were made and interest was focused on the range of kidney sizes, as certain pathologies are associated with larger kidneys. However, the assessment of what is a large kidney depends on the size of the baby and, to allow for this, birth-weight- and head-circumference-specific percentiles were derived using the HRY method. For each of depth and length, the percentiles were estimated for the maximum of the measurements on the right and left kidney.

Figure 12.6 shows the data on maximum kidney depth plotted against birth weight. The seven percentiles, namely, 3rd, 10th, 25th, 50th, 75th, 90th and 97th are estimated. The unsmoothed percentiles are computed using $k = 0·2$: the results for the 3rd, 50th and 97th percentiles are illustrated. The unsmoothed percentiles are smoothed using (12.17) and (12.18) with $p = 1$, $q_0 = 2$ and $q_1 = 1$: the fitted percentiles are given by

$$a_{0i} = 1·594 + 0·220z_i + 0·013z_i^2 \quad \text{and} \quad a_{1i} = 0·201 + 0·002z_i.$$

These values are arrived at after extensive fitting of the data and assessment of the shape and goodness of fit of the resulting percentiles. The quadratic term of a_{0i} provides evidence of slight non-normality. The linear term for a_{1i} suggests that dispersion increases with birth weight but the size of this effect is modest.

Once the values of the b coefficients in (12.18) have been found, percentile charts can readily be produced. Moreover, if a new subject presents with value x for the variable at age t, then the Z-score or percentile can be found by solving a polynomial equation for z, namely,

$$x = \left(\sum_{r=0}^{q_0} b_{0r}z^r \right) + \left(\sum_{r=0}^{q_1} b_{1r}z^r \right) t + \ldots + \left(\sum_{r=0}^{q_p} b_{pr}z^r \right) t^p.$$

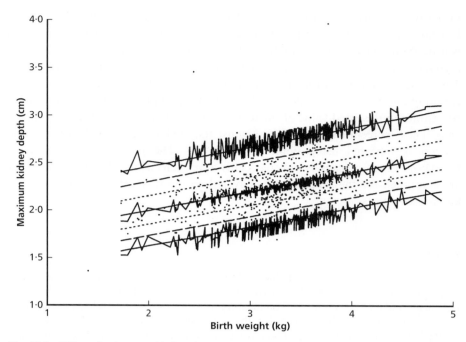

Fig. 12.6 Kidney depth versus birth weight for 560 newborn infants. Points indicate raw data and 3rd, 50th and 97th unsmoothed percentiles are shown. —— shows smoothed versions of these percentiles, – – – shows 10th and 90th percentiles and · · · · · 25th and 75th percentiles.

The HRY method does not rely on any distributional assumptions for its validity. The main weakness of the method is its reliance on polynomials for smoothing. Polynomials are used for two purposes in this method. The polynomial of order p in t (12.17), which describes the median ($z_i = 0$), is affected by the usual difficulties of polynomial smoothing which arise from the global nature of polynomial fits, described in §12.1. This is likely to be especially problematic if the variable changes markedly across the age range being analysed. Some of these difficulties can be overcome by the extension of the method proposed by Pan *et al.* (1990) and Goldstein and Pan (1992), which uses piecewise polynomial fits.

The second use of polynomials—in particular, non-linear polynomials—is to accommodate non-normality in the distribution of the variable. This use of polynomials has some theoretical foundation: approximations to non-normal distribution functions can be made by substituting measures of skewness, kurtosis (degree of 'peakedness') and possibly higher moments in the Cornish–Fisher expansion (Cornish & Fisher, 1937; see also Barndorff-Nielsen & Cox, 1989, §4.4). However, it is probably unwise to expect severe non-normality, or at least non-normality which arises from values of moments higher than kurtosis, to be adequately accommodated by the method. In such cases it may be sensible to try to find a transformation to make the distribution of the data closer to normal before applying the HRY method.

Goodness of fit

At the beginning of this section the benefit of taking advantage of specific distributional forms in deriving percentiles was explained. The LMS method takes advantage of the normal distribution of $X^{L(T)}$ where $L(T)$ has been estimated from the data. However, in practice, variables do not arise with labels on them telling the analyst that they do or do not have a normal distribution. For some variables, such as height, the variable has been measured so often in the past and always found to be normally distributed that a prior assumption of normality may seem quite natural. In other cases, there may be clear evidence from simple plots of the data that the normal distribution does not apply.

If a method for determining percentiles is proposed that assumes the normality of the variable, then it is important that this assumption be examined. If the LMS or some similar method which estimates transformations that are purported to yield data with a normal distribution is to be used, then the normality of the transformed data must be examined. It may be that the wrong $L(T)$ has been chosen or it may be that no Box–Cox transformation will yield a variable that has a normal distribution.

It could be argued that it is important to examine the assumption of a normal distribution that attends many statistical techniques, and this may be so. However, slight departures from the normal distribution in the distribution of, for example, residuals in an analysis of variance are unlikely to have a serious effect on the significance level of hypothesis tests or widths of confidence intervals. However, when the assumption underpins estimated percentiles, matters are rather different. In practice, it is the extreme percentiles, such as the 3rd, 95th or 0·5th percentile, that are of use to the clinician and slight departures of the true distribution from the normal distribution, particularly in the tails of the distribution, can give rise to substantial errors. It is therefore of the utmost importance that any distributional assumptions made by the method are properly checked.

This is a difficult matter which has been the subject of little research. Indeed, it may be almost impossible to detect important deviations of distributional form because they occur precisely in those parts of the distribution where there is least information. Probably the best global test for normality is that due to Shapiro and Wilk (1965). This test computes an estimate of the standard deviation using a linear combination of the data that will be correct only if the data follow a normal distribution. The ratio of this to the usual estimate, which is always valid, is $W, 0 < W < 1$, and is the basis of the test. Significance levels can be found using algorithms due to Royston (1992). However, even this test lacks power. Moreover, if it is the transformed data that are being assessed, and the test is applied to the same data that were used to determine the transformation, then the test will be conservative.

A useful graphical approach to the assessment of the goodness of fit of the percentiles is to use the fitted percentiles to compute the Z-score for each point in the data set. If the percentiles are a good fit, then the Z-scores will all share the standard normal distribution. If these scores and their associated ages are subjected to the first part of the HRY method, then the unsmoothed percentiles should show no trend with age and should be centred around the values of the percentiles, which the HRY method requires. This is a most useful tool for a visual assessment of the adequacy of percentile charts, but its detailed properties do not seem to have been considered. It can be applied to any method which determines percentiles and which allows the computation of Z-scores, not just methods which assume normality. In particular, it can be used to assess percentiles determined by the HRY method itself.

A useful comparison of several methods for deriving age-related reference ranges can be found in Wright and Royston (1997).

12.4 **Non-linear regression**

The regression of a variable y on a set of covariates $x_1, x_2, \ldots, x_p$, $E(y|x_1, x_2, \ldots, x_p)$, can be determined using the multiple regression techniques of §11.6, provided that

$$E(y|x_1, x_2, \ldots, x_p) = \beta_0 + \beta_1 x_1 + \beta_2 x_2 + \ldots + \beta_p x_p. \qquad (12.19)$$

This equation not only encompasses a straight-line relationship with each of several variables, but, as was seen in §12.1, it allows certain types of curves to be fitted to data. If y represents the vector of n observations on y and X is the $n \times (p+1)$ matrix with element (i, j) being the observation of x_{j-1} on unit i (to accommodate the term in β_0, the first element of each row of X is 1), then (12.19) can be written $E(y) = X\beta$ where β is the vector of β_is. The estimate of β can be written as

$$(\mathbf{X}^T\mathbf{X})^{-1}\mathbf{X}^T y, \qquad (12.20)$$

and its dispersion matrix is

$$\sigma^2(\mathbf{X}^T\mathbf{X})^{-1}, \qquad (12.21)$$

where σ^2 is the variance of y about (12.19).

These results depend on the linearity of (12.19) in the parameters, not the covariates, and it is this feature which allows curves to be fitted by this method.

As pointed out in §12.1, polynomial curves in x_1, say, can be fitted by identifying x_2, x_3, etc., with powers of x_1 and the linearity in the βs is undisturbed. The same applies to fractional polynomials and, although this is less easy to see, it also applies to many of the smoothing methods of §12.2.

However, for many curves that a statistician may wish to fit, the parameters do not enter linearly; an example would be an exponential growth curve:

$$E(y|x) = \beta_0(1 - e^{-\beta_1 x}).$$

Suppose n pairs of observations (y_i, x_i) are thought to follow this model, with $y_i = E(y_i|x_i) + \varepsilon_i$, where ε_is are independent, normally distributed residuals with common variance σ^2. Estimates of β_0, β_1 can be found using the same method of least squares used for (12.19)—that is, β_0, β_1 are chosen to minimize

$$\sum_{i=1}^{n}[y_i - \beta_0(1 - e^{-\beta_1 x_i})]^2. \tag{12.22}$$

Unlike the situation with (12.19), the equations which determine the minimizing values of these parameters cannot be solved explicitly as in (12.20), and numerical methods need to be used.

A more general non-linear regression can be written as

$$y_i = f(x_i, \boldsymbol{\beta}) + \varepsilon_i, \tag{12.23}$$

where f is some general function, usually assumed differentiable, $\boldsymbol{\beta}$ is a vector of p parameters and x_i is the covariate for the ith case. In general, x_i can be a vector but in much of the present discussion it will be a scalar, often representing time or dosage. The error terms ε_i will be taken as independently and normally distributed, with zero mean and common variance σ^2, but other forms of error are encountered.

It turns out that some of the properties of the estimates in (12.23) can be written in a form very similar to (12.20) and (12.21), namely,

$$\hat{\boldsymbol{\beta}} = (\boldsymbol{F}^{\mathrm{T}}\boldsymbol{F})^{-1}\boldsymbol{F}^{\mathrm{T}}\boldsymbol{y}, \tag{12.24}$$

$$\mathrm{var}(\hat{\boldsymbol{\beta}}) = \sigma^2(\boldsymbol{F}^{\mathrm{T}}\boldsymbol{F})^{-1}, \tag{12.25}$$

$$E(\hat{\boldsymbol{\beta}}) = \boldsymbol{\beta}, \tag{12.26}$$

where the (i, j)th element of F is $\partial f(x_i, \beta)/\partial\beta_j$ evaluated at $\hat{\boldsymbol{\beta}}$. The similarity stems in part from a first-order Taylor expansion of (12.23) and, as such, the results in (12.24) and (12.25) are approximations, but for large samples the approximations are good and they are often adequate for smaller samples. Indeed, X from (12.20) and (12.21) is F if $f(x_i, \boldsymbol{\beta}) = \beta_0 + \beta_1 x_{i1} + \ldots + \beta_{ip}x_p$, so (12.24) and (12.25) are exact in the linear case and it is not unreasonable to suppose that the closeness of the above approximations depends on the departure of $f(x, \boldsymbol{\beta})$ from linearity.

Much work has been done on the issue of the degree of non-linearity or *curvature* in non-linear regression; important contributions include Beale (1960) and Bates and Watts (1980). Important aspects of non-linearity can be described by a measure of curvature introduced by the latter authors. The measurement of curvature involves considering what happens to $f(x, \boldsymbol{\beta})$ as $\boldsymbol{\beta}$ moves through its allowed values. The measure has two components, namely the *intrinsic* curvature and the *parameter-effects* curvature. These two components are illustrated by the model $f(x, \boldsymbol{\beta}) = 1 - e^{-\beta x}$. The same response curve results from $g(x, \gamma) = 1 - \gamma^x$ if $\gamma = e^{-\beta}$, so in a clear sense these response curves have the same curvature. However, when fitting this curve to data, the statistician searches through the parameter space to find a best-fitting value and it is clear, with one parameter logarithmically related to the other, that the rate at which fitted values change throughout this search will be highly dependent on the parameterization adopted. Thus, while the intrinsic curvatures are similar, their parameter-effects values are quite different.

Indeed, many features of a non-linear regression depend importantly on the parameterization adopted. Difficulties in applying numerical methods to find $\hat{\boldsymbol{\beta}}$ can often be alleviated by altering the parameterization used. Also, the shape of likelihood surfaces and the performance of likelihood ratio tests can be sensitive to the parameterization. More information on these matters can be found in the encyclopaedic work by Seber and Wild (1989).

The foregoing discussion has assumed that a value $\hat{\boldsymbol{\beta}}$ which minimizes (12.22) is available. As pointed out previously, there is no general closed-form solution and numerical methods must be used. Equation (12.24) suggests an iterative approach, with $\boldsymbol{F}$ evaluated at the current estimate being applied as in this equation to give a new estimate of $\boldsymbol{\beta}$. Indeed, this approach is closely related to the Gauss–Newton method for obtaining numerical estimates. However, the numerical analysis of non-linear regression can be surprisingly awkward, with various subtle problems giving rise to unstable solutions. The simple Gauss–Newton is not to be recommended and more sophisticated methods are widely available in the form of suites of programs or, more conveniently, in major statistical packages and these should be the first choice. Much more on this problem can be found in Chapters 3, 13 and 14 of Seber and Wild (1989).

Uses of non-linear regression

The methods described in Chapter 7 and §§12.1–12.2 are used, in a descriptive way, to assess associations between variables and summarize relationships between variables. Non-linear methods can be used in this context, but they

$$f(x, \boldsymbol{\beta}) = -\delta e^{-\kappa x} \qquad \text{Mono-exponential}$$

$$f(x, \boldsymbol{\beta}) = A + \frac{B}{1 + e^{-\lambda - \kappa x}} \qquad \text{Four-parameter logistic}$$

$$f(x, \boldsymbol{\beta}) = \alpha \exp(-e^{-\kappa(x-\gamma)}) \qquad \text{Gompertz}$$

While these, and many other curves, can be thought of as solutions to differential equations they may prove useful as empirical curves, with little or no guidance on the choice of equation available from considerations of the underlying subject-matter.

Sometimes the guidance for choosing a curve is very general and does not wholly specify the form of the curve. Matthews *et al.* (1999) fit the pair of curves:

$$\left. \begin{aligned} f(x, \boldsymbol{\beta}) &= A(1 - e^{-k_a x}) \\ f(x, \boldsymbol{\beta}) &= A(1 - e^{-k_v x}) \end{aligned} \right, \tag{12.29}$$

where the first curve is fitted to the arterial data and the second to the venous data from the Kety–Schmidt technique for the measurement of cerebral blood flow. The Kety–Schmidt technique required a pair of curves starting from 0 and rising to a common asymptote. The method did not indicate the form of curves in any more detail. The above choice was based on nothing more substantial than the appearance of exponential functions in a number of related studies of gaseous diffusion in cerebral tissue and the fact that these curves gave a good fit in a large number of applications of the method.

A further instance of this use of non-linear functions comes from the nerve conduction data analysed in Example 12.2. The data seem to indicate that the conduction velocity increases through childhood, tending to a limit in adulthood. There was some interest in estimating the mean adult conduction velocity. Figure 12.8 shows the data, with variable t on the horizontal axis being the age since conception, together with two plausible models, both of which model the mean conduction velocity as an increasing function of t tending to a limit A, which is the parameter of interest. The first curve is the exponential $A(1 - e^{-\beta t})$ and the second is the hyperbola $A[1 - \beta/(\beta + t)]$. Both of these are zero at $t = 0$ and tend to A as $t \to \infty$.

The fit of both models can be criticized but, nevertheless, one feature of the models deserves careful attention. The estimate A and its standard error are 22·00 (0·16) for the exponential and 24·53 (0·16) for the hyperbola, giving approximate 95% confidence intervals of (21·69, 22·31) and (24·22, 24·84). Both models give plausible but entirely inconsistent estimates for A. The standard errors measure the sampling variation in the parameter estimate, given that the model is correct. Uncertainty in the specification of the model has not been incorporated into the standard error. Situations, such as the use of (12.27) for the Michaelis–Menten equation, where the prior guidance is sufficiently strong to

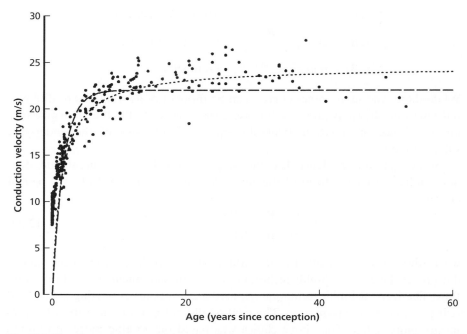

Fig. 12.8 Fits of mono-exponential (– – –) and hyperbola (- - -) to nerve conduction velocity data of Example 12.2.

dictate a specific model are the exception rather than the rule. Once some element of choice enters then the statistician must be aware that, while some parameters may appear to have an interpretation that is independent of the model, such as mean adult velocity, the estimates and standard errors of such parameters are certainly not model-independent. In these circumstances the statistician would be unwise to rely on an estimate from a single model. Methods for accommodating model uncertainty, so that the above standard errors might be appropriately inflated, have been developed, but it remains a matter of debate whether they offer a remedy that is more appropriate and helpful than simply presenting results from a range of plausible models. Details on these methods can be found in Chatfield (1995) and Draper (1995).

Model dependence and model uncertainty are issues which clearly have significance across statistical modelling and are not restricted to non-linear models. However, the rarity of circumstances which, a priori, prescribe a particular model means that the statistician is wise to be especially aware of its effects in non-linear modelling. Models are often fitted when the intention of an analysis is to determine a quantity such as a blood flow rate or a cell birth rate and it is hoped that the value estimated does not rest heavily on an arbitrarily chosen model that has been fitted.

The sensitivity of the estimate of a quantity to the model used can depend on the nature of the quantity. The interest in the model fitted by Matthews *et al.* (1999) given in (12.29) focused on the reciprocal of the area between the fitted curves. Slight changes in the curves are unlikely to lead to major changes in the computed area, so major model dependence would not be anticipated. Quantities such as rates of change, computed as derivatives of fitted curves, are much more likely to be highly model-dependent. Such an example, concerning the rate of growth of tumours, is given by Gratton *et al.* (1978).

Linearizing non-linear equations

Attempts to exploit any resemblance a non-linear equation has to a linear counterpart can often prove profitable but must be made with care.

Many non-linear equations include parameters that appear linearly. An example is equation (12.29) with $f(x, \boldsymbol{\beta}) = \beta_0(1 - e^{-\beta_1 x})$. If β_1 is taken as known, the regression equation is a simple linear regression through the origin (see §11.3). The estimate of β_0 can be found by minimizing the following, with β_1 taken as fixed.

$$RSS(\beta_0, \beta_1) = \sum_{i=1}^{n}(y_i - \beta_0 g_i)^2 = \sum_{i=1}^{n} y_i^2 - 2\beta_0 \sum_{i=1}^{n} y_i g_i + \beta_0^2 \sum_{i=1}^{n} g_i^2 = A - 2\beta_0 B + \beta_0^2 C,$$

say, where $g_i = 1 - e^{-\beta_1 x_i}$. The minimum value of RSS occurs when $\beta_0 = B/C$, a function of β_1 written as $\hat{\beta}_0(\beta_1)$. The minimum value is $A - B^2/C$. Thus, the residual sum of squares for fixed β_1 is

$$RSS(\hat{\beta}_0(\beta_1), \beta_1) = \sum_{i=1}^{n} y_i^2 - \frac{(\sum_{i=1}^{n} y_i g_i)^2}{\sum_{i=1}^{n} g_i^2}. \tag{12.30}$$

The full problem can now be solved by minimizing this expression as a univariate function of β_1. The manoeuvre might be thought pointless, as it has simply produced another intractable non-linear problem. However, reducing the problem to minimizing a function of a reduced number of parameters can make an important contribution to overcoming awkward numerical problems. Perhaps more importantly, in many practical cases, there are only one or two non-linear parameters and being able to plot functions such as that in (12.30) against one or two arguments can give the user valuable information about the behaviour of the problem. It can also be a useful step in the application of *profile likelihood* methods: a full discussion of these is beyond the scope of the present discussion, but an example can be found in the Appendix of Matthews *et al.* (1999).

Perhaps a more common way to attempt to use methods for linear regressions in a non-linear problem is to attempt to apply a transformation that makes the problem accessible to linear methods. A simple example is the non-linear equation $y = \alpha\beta^x$, which becomes the linear equation $\log y = a + bx$ with $a = \log\alpha$ and $b = \log\beta$. However, there is some need for care here with regard to the way residuals are handled.

If the full regression equation is actually $y = E(y|x) + \varepsilon$, with ε being independent residuals with zero mean and constant variance, then taking logs will result in a regression with an error term

$$\log\left(1 + \frac{\varepsilon}{\alpha\beta^x}\right).$$

In general, this does not even have zero mean. If the variance of ε is small compared with the values of $\alpha\beta^x$, then the above is approximately $\varepsilon/(\alpha\beta^x)$, so, in this case, a residual with approximately zero mean is recovered but it no longer has constant variance (except in the trivial case where $\beta = 1$), so estimation by ordinary least squares is inappropriate. The problem has arisen because a transformation which would linearize $E(y|x)$ has instead to be applied to y, because $E(y|x)$ is unknown. Consequently, both the mean and the associated residual term are transformed together. Generalized linear models handle the definition of error and the scale of the mean separately (see McCullagh & Nelder, 1989, and §14.4 for details) and this can alleviate the problem. This issue is discussed in Example 12.5.

Of course, if the errors are not additive with constant variance on the original scale then the problem may not obtain. If the model for y is more realistically written as $y = E(y|x) \times \varepsilon$, where ε is now a positive random variable with mean 1, then an analysis taking logs of the data will be much less likely to be affected than in the case mentioned previously.

Example 12.5

In the course of a study of aspects of the cerebral metabolism of glucose, Forsyth *et al.* (1993) collected data on reaction rates that followed the Michaelis–Menten equation (12.27). This equation can be rewritten as

$$\frac{1}{v} = \frac{1}{V_{\max}} + \frac{K}{V_{\max}}\frac{1}{s}, \tag{12.31}$$

so, if the linear regression of v^{-1} on s^{-1} is computed, the intercept will be an estimate of $1/V_{\max}$ and the slope will estimate $K/V_{\max}$, so K can be found as the ratio of these estimates. For obvious reasons this method of analysing Michaelis–Menten data is known as the double-reciprocal method, or the Lineweaver–Burk method, after those who proposed its use. Equation (12.31) is a rather loose expression of the regression equation as it does not specify the scale on which residuals will most nearly be additive with constant variance. If $v^{-1} = E(v|s)^{-1} + \varepsilon$, where ε has constant variance and $E(v|s)$ is given by (12.27), then this method will have good properties. However, if the equation is thought more likely to be of the form $v = E(v|s) + \varepsilon$, then the double-reciprocal method will not have good properties. Essentially, the reciprocal of velocity will not have constant variance and the equal weighting used in the simple regression of v^{-1} on s^{-1} will give too much weight to observations with low substrate concentrations.

An alternative approach is to use a generalized linear model with normal errors and a reciprocal link. This fits the model $v = E(v|s) + \varepsilon$, with ε having constant variance, and allows a linear model to be fitted to the reciprocal of $E(v|s)$, namely,

$$\frac{1}{E(v|s)} = \alpha + \beta x,$$

so if s^{-1} is used for x, α will correspond to $1/V_{max}$ and β to K/V_{max}. The use of generalized linear models for enzyme-kinetic data appears to have been proposed first by Nelder (1991).

The estimates from the Lineweaver–Burk method are $-6·59 \times 10^{-4}$ for $1/V_{max}$ and $0·0290$ for K/V_{max}. This clearly indicates the shortcomings of the method, as it has provided negative estimates for two necessarily positive parameters. It can be seen from Fig. 12.9(a) that the value of the velocity for the point with the smallest substrate concentration (largest reciprocal) has had a substantial influence on the fitted line. It is often the case that estimates from this method are unduly influenced by points corresponding to small substrate concentrations.

The estimates from the generalized linear model with reciprocal link are $8·98 \times 10^{-4}$ for $1/V_{max}$ and $0·01015$ for K/V_{max} giving $1114·0$ for V_{max} and $11·31$ for K. Figure 12.9(a) shows that this method adopts a system of weights that gives the point with smallest substrate concentration much less influence. Although this model appears to fit poorly in Fig. 12.9(a), the fit appears much better on the original scales shown in Fig. 12.9(b).

Fitting the model $v = E(v|s) + \varepsilon$ with a general non-linear regression method gives identical estimates to those obtained from the generalized linear model. The latter gives standard errors for the parameters K ($2·91$) and V_{max} ($101·2$) directly, as opposed to the standard errors for $1/V_{max}$ ($8·16 \times 10^{-5}$) and K/V_{max} ($1·92 \times 10^{-3}$) that are available from the generalized linear model: the correlation of these estimates is $-0·652$. The methods of §5.3 could be applied to provide estimates of the standard errors of K and V_{max} from these values if required. This will not always be necessary because occasionally primary interest is focused on K/V_{max}.

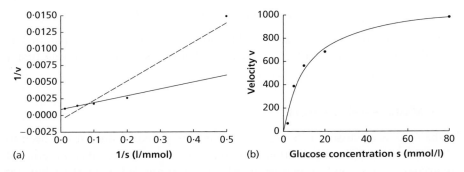

Fig. 12.9 Michaelis–Menten data from the study by Forsyth *et al.* (1993): (a) is a double reciprocal plot with a Lineweaver–Burk regression line (– – –) and a line fitted as a generalized linear model (———); (b) is a plot of the data on their original scale and shows the fitted curve from the generalized linear model.

To be fair to methods which apply transformations directly to data from studies of Michaelis–Menten kinetics, there are several different linearizing transformations, most of which are superior to the Lineweaver–Burk method. One of the best of these is obtained by noting that (12.27) can be written as:

$$\frac{s}{v} = \frac{K}{V_{\max}} + \frac{1}{V_{\max}} s,$$

so a linear regression of the ratios s/v against s has slope $1/V_{\max}$ and intercept $K/V_{\max}$. An extended discussion of several methods for analysing data from Michaelis–Menten studies can be found in Cornish-Bowden (1995a, b).

In some cases linearization techniques effect a valuable simplification without causing any new problems. An example of this is periodic regression, where the response exhibits a cyclic or seasonal nature. A model which comes to mind would be

$$E(y|x) = \alpha_0 + \alpha_1 \sin(\beta x + \gamma). \tag{12.32}$$

While a cyclic trend cannot always be captured by a simple sinusoidal curve, it can be a useful alternative to a null hypothesis that no cyclical trend exists; a fuller discussion is given by Bliss (1958). An example of the use of this model is given by Edwards (1961), who tested a series of counts made at equally spaced intervals for periodicity. Suppose there are k counts, N_i. For example, neurological episodes may be classified by the hour of the day ($k = 24$), or congenital abnormalities by the month of the year ($k = 12$).

In (12.32) α_0 is the mean level about which the N_i fluctuate, α_1 is the amplitude of the variation, β determines the period of the variation and γ is the phase. If the equation (12.32) is to have a complete cycle of k time intervals then $\beta = 360/k$ (degrees). Even though this deals with one non-linear parameter, the resulting equation is still non-linear because γ does not appear linearly. However, expanding the sine function gives the alternative formula

$$E(y|x) = \alpha_0 + \zeta_1 \sin(\beta x) + \zeta_2 \cos(\beta x),$$

where $\zeta_1 = \alpha_1 \cos\gamma$ and $\zeta_2 = \alpha_1 \sin\gamma$. This equation is linear in these parameters and the regression can be fitted by recalling that β is known and noting that x successively takes the values $1, 2, \ldots, k$.

12.5 Multilevel models

In the models discussed so far in this chapter the primary concern has been to allow the mean of the distribution of an outcome, y, to be described in terms of covariates x. A secondary matter, which has been alluded to in §12.3 but not discussed in detail, is the modelling of the variance of y in terms of covariates. In all cases it is assumed that separate observations are quite independent of one another. The distributions of different *y*s may be similar because the correspond-ing *x*s are similar, but knowledge of one of the *y*s will provide no further information about the value of the others.

However, many circumstances encountered in medical research give rise to data in which this level of independence does not obtain and a valid analysis requires richer models than those considered hitherto. For example, it is quite reasonable to assume that observations on the blood pressure of different patients are independent, but it may well be quite unreasonable to make the same assumption about measurements made on the same patient. This could be because the patient may have a familial tendency to hypertension and so usually has a high blood pressure. Consequently the value on one occasion will give information about subsequent observations. To analyse a series of such observa-tions as if they were independent would lead to bias: e.g. the serial dependence would give rise to an inappropriately small estimate of variance. Another ex-ample would be the level of glycaemic control amongst patients with Type II diabetes attending a particular general practice. All patients with this disease in the practice will receive advice on managing their condition from a practice nurse or one of the doctors—that is, the patients share a common source for their advice. If the advisers are particularly good, or particularly bad, then all patients in the practice will tend to benefit or suffer as a consequence.

In these examples the dependence between observations has arisen because the measurements at the most basic level, the individual measurements of blood pressure or the glycaemic control of an individual patient, occur within groups, the individual patient or the general practice, and such data are often referred to as *hierarchical*. It is common for dependence to arise by this means and the class of *multilevel models* provides a family of models that can address the statistical problems posed by this kind of data. In this section only multilevel models for a continuous outcome will be considered, but they can be very usefully employed to analyse other types of outcome. A full discussion of this family of models can be found in Goldstein (1995).

Hierarchical data formed by the serial measurement of a quantity on an individual, also known as *longitudinal data*, occur throughout medicine and can be addressed by a wide variety of methods in addition to those provided by multilevel models. Consequently, discussion of this kind of data is deferred until §§12·6 and 12·7. However, it should be borne in mind that the methods described in this section can often be used fruitfully in the study of longitudinal data.

Random effects and building multilevel models

Rather than attempting to model variances and correlations explicitly, multilevel models make extensive use of random effects in order to generate a wide variety of dependence structures. A simple illustration of this can be found in Example

9.5. The number of swabs positive for *Pneumococcus* is recorded in families. A simple model might assume that the mean number of swabs is μ and the observation on the jth member of the ith family can be modelled by:

$$y_{ij} = \mu + \varepsilon_{ij}, \tag{12.33}$$

where ε_{ij} is a simple error term, with zero mean and variance σ^2, that is independent from observation to observation. However, this model does not reflect the fact that the observations are grouped within families. Moreover, if the variation between families is larger than that within families, then this cannot be modelled because only one variance has been specified. An obvious extension is to add an extra term, ξ_i, to (12.33) to accommodate variation between families. This term will be a random variable that is independent between families and of the ε_{ij}, has zero mean and variance σ_F^2. Thus, the new model for the jth member of the ith family is:

$$\mu + \xi_i + \varepsilon_{ij}.$$

It should be noted that it is the same realization of the random variable that is applied to each observation within a family; a consequence of this is that observations within a family are correlated. Two observations within a family have covariance σ_F^2 and, as each observation has variance $\sigma_F^2 + \sigma^2$, the correlation is

$$\sigma_F^2 / (\sigma_F^2 + \sigma^2). \tag{12.34}$$

This is not surprising; the model is such that families with a propensity to exhibit pneumococcal infection will have a large value for ξ_i and as this is applied to each member of the family, each family member will tend to report a large value—that is, the values are correlated. Clearly, this tendency will be less marked if the within-family variation is substantial relative to that between families; this is reflected in (12.34) because, as σ^2/σ_F^2 becomes larger, (12.34) becomes smaller. It should be noted that correlations generated in this way cannot be negative: they are examples of the *intraclass correlation* discussed in §19.11.

Because they are random variables, the terms ξ and ε are referred to as *random effects* and their effect is measured by a variance or, more accurately, a *component of variance*, such as σ^2 and σ_F^2. More elaborate models can certainly be built. One possibility is to add extra terms that are not random (and so are often referred to as fixed effects) to elaborate on the simple mean μ. In Example 9.5 the families were classified into three categories measuring how crowded their living conditions were. The model could be extended to

$$\mu + \beta_1 x_{1i} + \beta_2 x_{2i} + \xi_i + \varepsilon_{ij}, \tag{12.35}$$

where $x_{1i} = 1$ if the ith family lives in crowded conditions and is 0 otherwise, and $x_{2i} = 1$ if the ith family lives in uncrowded conditions and is 0 otherwise. The parameter μ now measures the mean number of swabs positive for *Pneumococcus* in families living in overcrowded conditions. Note that the variables x_1 and x_2 need only a single subscript i because they measure quantities that only vary at the level of the family.

If the age of the family member was thought to affect the number of positive swabs then this could be incorporated into the model by allowing a suitable term in the model, such as

$$\mu + \beta_1 x_{1i} + \beta_2 x_{2i} + \beta_3 x_{3ij} + \xi_i + \varepsilon_{ij}, \tag{12.36}$$

where x_{3ij} is the age of the jth member of family i. As age varies between members of a family, the variable x_3 requires two subscripts: i, to indicate family, and j, to indicate the individual within the family. Of course, given the typical age differences within a family, the use of a linear term in this example is questionable but this can be overlooked for the purpose of illustration. Not only might the age of an individual affect the outcome but the rate of increase might vary between families. This can be incorporated by allowing the coefficient of age, β_3, to vary randomly between families. This can be built into the model by extending (12.36) to

$$\mu + \beta_1 x_{1i} + \beta_2 x_{2i} + (\beta_3 + \eta_i) x_{3ij} + \xi_i + \varepsilon_{ij}, \tag{12.37}$$

where β_3 is now the mean slope and η_i varies randomly between families with variance σ_b^2. The analyst can decide whether to insist that the random effects η_i and ξ_i are uncorrelated or to allow them to have covariance σ_{bF}. For the latter model the variance of the jth member of family i is

$$\sigma_b^2 x_{3ij}^2 + 2\sigma_{bF} x_{3ij} + \sigma_F^2 + \sigma^2. \tag{12.38}$$

It should be noted that allowing the slope to vary randomly has induced a variance that changes quadratically with age. Also, responses from members of the same family, say j and j', now have a correlation that depends on their ages, namely,

$$\frac{\sigma_b^2 x_{3ij} x_{3ij'} + \sigma_{bF}(x_{3ij} + x_{3ij'}) + \sigma_F^2}{\sqrt{[(\sigma_b^2 x_{3ij}^2 + 2\sigma_{bF} x_{3ij} + \sigma_F^2 + \sigma^2)(\sigma_b^2 x_{3ij'}^2 + 2\sigma_{bF} x_{3ij'} + \sigma_F^2 + \sigma^2)]}}.$$

In this way a family of models can be defined which allow many forms of data to be analysed.

Method of Estimation

For some purposes and sufficiently regular problems, apparently *ad hoc* methods are optimal. For example, suppose the aim is to compare the mean number of swabs positive for *Pneumococcus* between crowded and overcrowded families in Example 9.5. A simple analysis would be to compute the mean number of swabs in each family and compare the two groups, using the six family means in each group as the outcome variable. If model (12.35) obtained, then the difference in group means would estimate β_1 and the pooled within-group variance would estimate $\sigma_F^2 + n^{-1}\sigma^2$, where n is the (constant) size of each family. It is perhaps not surprising that no new methodology is needed for this analysis, as the split-unit analysis of variance described in §9.6 can provide a complete analysis of these data.

The split-unit analysis of variance could still cope if the number of families at each level of crowding were unequal, but the method would fail if the number of people within each family were not constant. The mean for the ith family would have variance $\sigma_F^2 + n_i^{-1}\sigma^2$, where n_i is the size of family i. As this varies between families, an unweighted mean of the families would not necessarily be the optimal way to compare levels of crowding. However, the optimal weighting will depend on the unknown value of the ratio σ_F^2/σ^2; in general, the optimal weighting will depend on several parameters whose values will have to be estimated. A satisfactory approach to the general problem of analysing hierarchical data requires methodology that can handle this kind of problem. A more sophisticated problem is that the analysis should not only be able to estimate the parameters that determine the appropriate weights, but should allow estimates of error to be obtained that acknowledge the uncertainty in the estimates of the weights.

Suppose the 90 observations in Example 9.5 are written as a 90×1 vector y, then the model in (12.35) can be written:

$$y = X\beta + \delta, \tag{12.39}$$

where δ is a 90×1 vector of error terms that subsume the terms ξ and ε from (12.35), X is a 90×2 matrix and β is a 2×1 vector. Consequently δ has zero mean and dispersion matrix V. The form of V is determined by the structure of the random effects in the model and will be specified in terms of the variance parameters. In this example, V has the form:

$$V = \begin{pmatrix} V_1 & & & \\ & V_2 & & \\ & & \ddots & \\ & & & V_{18} \end{pmatrix}, \tag{12.40}$$

i.e. V has a block-diagonal structure where the only non-zero elements are those in the submatrices, V_i, shown. The matrix V_i is the dispersion matrix of the observations from family i. In general, this could be an $n_i \times n_i$ matrix but, as all the families in this example are of size 5, each V_i is a 5×5 matrix. As has been noted, the variance of each response is $\sigma_F^2 + \sigma^2$ and the covariance between any two members of the same family is σ_F^2, so each V_i is

$$\begin{pmatrix} \sigma_F^2 + \sigma^2 & \sigma_F^2 & \sigma_F^2 & \sigma_F^2 & \sigma_F^2 \\ \sigma_F^2 & \sigma_F^2 + \sigma^2 & \sigma_F^2 & \sigma_F^2 & \sigma_F^2 \\ \sigma_F^2 & \sigma_F^2 & \sigma_F^2 + \sigma^2 & \sigma_F^2 & \sigma_F^2 \\ \sigma_F^2 & \sigma_F^2 & \sigma_F^2 & \sigma_F^2 + \sigma^2 & \sigma_F^2 \\ \sigma_F^2 & \sigma_F^2 & \sigma_F^2 & \sigma_F^2 & \sigma_F^2 + \sigma^2 \end{pmatrix}.$$

If the values of σ^2, σ_F^2 were known, then the estimator of the $\boldsymbol{\beta}$ parameters in (12.39) having minimum variance would be the usual generalized least squares estimator (see (11.54)):

$$\hat{\boldsymbol{\beta}} = (X^T V^{-1} X)^{-1} X^T V^{-1} y. \tag{12.41}$$

As σ^2, σ_F^2 are unknown, the estimation proceeds iteratively. The first estimates of $\boldsymbol{\beta}$ are usually obtained using ordinary least squares, that is assuming V is the identity matrix. An estimate of $\boldsymbol{\delta}$ can then be obtained as $\hat{\boldsymbol{\delta}} = y - X\hat{\boldsymbol{\beta}}$. The 90×90 matrix $\hat{\boldsymbol{\delta}}\hat{\boldsymbol{\delta}}^T$ has expectation V and the elements of both these matrices can be written out as vectors, simply by stacking the columns of the matrices on top of one another. Suppose the vectors obtained in this way are W and Z, respectively, then Z can in turn be written $\sum \sigma_k^2 z_k$, where the z_i are vectors of known constants. In the case of Example 9.6, $\sigma_1^2 = \sigma_F^2, \sigma_2^2 = \sigma^2$ and the z vectors comprise 0s and 1s. A second linear model can now be fitted using generalized least squares with W as the response, the *design matrix* comprising the z vectors and the parameter estimates being the estimates of the variance components defining the random effects in the model; further details can be found in Appendix 2.1 of Goldstein (1995). New estimates of the $\boldsymbol{\beta}$s can be obtained from (12.41), with V now determined by the new estimates of the variance components. The whole process can then be repeated until there is little change in successive parameter estimates. This is essentially the process used by the program MLwiN (Goldstein *et al.*, 1998) and is referred to as *iterative generalized least squares* (IGLS).

If the approach outlined above is followed exactly, then the resulting estimates of the variance components will be biased downwards. This is because in the part of the algorithm that estimates the random effects the method uses estimates of fixed effects as if they were the correct values and takes no account of their associated uncertainty. This is essentially the same problem that arises because a standard deviation must be estimated by computing deviations about the sample mean rather than the population mean. In that case, the solution is to use $n-1$ in the denominator rather than n. A similar solution, often referred to as restricted maximum likelihood (see Patterson & Thompson, 1971), can be applied in more general circumstances, such as those encountered in multilevel models, and is then called *restricted iterative generalized least squares* (RIGLS).

A complementary problem arises from neglecting uncertainty in estimates of the random effects. Standard theory allows values for the standard errors of the parameter estimates to be obtained; for example, the dispersion matrix of the estimates of the fixed parameters can be found as $(X^T V^{-1} X)^{-1}$. In practice, V is evaluated using the estimated values of the variance components but the foregoing formula takes no account of the uncertainty in these estimates and is therefore likely to underestimate the required standard errors. For large data sets this is unlikely to be a major problem but it could be troublesome for small data sets. A solution is to put the whole estimation procedure in a Bayesian framework and use diffuse priors. Estimation using Markov chain Monte Carlo (MCMC) methods will then provide estimates of error that take account of the uncertainty in the parameter estimates. For a fuller discussion of the application of MCMC methods to multilevel models, see Appendix 2.4 of Goldstein (1995) and Goldstein *et al.* (1998). The use of MCMC methods in Bayesian methodology is discussed in §16.4.

More generally, this matter does, of course, raise the question of what constitutes a small or large data set, as this is not entirely straightforward when dealing with hierarchical data. There is no longer a single measure of the size of a data set; the implications of having 400 observations arising from a measurement on each of 20 patients in each of 20 general practices will be quite different from those arising from measuring 100 patients in each of four practices. Broadly speaking, it is important to have adequate replication at the highest levels of the hierarchy. If the model in (12.35) were applied to the example of data from general practices, with ξ representing practice effects, only one realization of ξ would be observed from each practice, and a good estimate of σ_F^2 therefore requires that an adequate number of practices be observed. Attempts to try to compensate for using an inadequate number of practices by observing more patients in each practice will, in general, be futile.

Estimation of residuals

In §11.9 simple regression models were checked by computing residuals. Residuals also play an important role in the more elaborate circumstances of multilevel models, and indeed have more diverse uses.

The residuals are clearly useful for checking the assumptions of the model; for example, normal probability plots of the residual effects at each level allow the assumptions underlying the random effects within the model to be assessed. It should, however, be noted that there may be more than one set of residuals at a given level, since there will be a separate set corresponding to each random effect. For example, in (12.37) there will be a set of residuals at the level of the individual, corresponding to ε_{ij}, but there will also be two sets of residuals at the level of the family, corresponding to η_i and ξ_i.

However, in addition to their role in model checking, the residuals can be thought of as estimates of the realized values of random effects. This can be potentially useful, especially for residuals at levels above the lowest; for example, in a study of patients in general practices the practice-level residual might be used to help place the specific practice in the context of other practices, once the influence of other effects in the model had been taken into account. In particular, they might be used in attempts to rank practices. However, attempts to rank units in this way are fraught with difficulty and should be undertaken only with great circumspection; see Goldstein and Spiegelhalter (1996) for a fuller discussion.

The extension of the idea of residuals beyond those for a standard multiple regression (see §11.9) gives rise to complexities in both their estimation and their definition. There is considerable merit in viewing the process as *estimating random effects* rather than as an exercise in extending the definition of a residual in non-hierarchical models. Indeed, there is much relevant background material in the article by Robinson (1991) on estimating random effects.

As a brief and incomplete illustration of the issues, consider model (12.35). The family-level residuals are $\{\hat{\xi}_i\}$ and these are 'estimates' of the random variables $\{\xi_i\}$ that appear in the model. As Robinson (1991) discusses, some statisticians are uneasy about this, seeing it as lying outside the realm of parameter estimation. However, even if such objections are accepted, there is likely to be little objection to the notion of predicting a random effect and the usual definition for residuals in a multilevel model is often put in this way, namely,

$$\hat{\xi}_i = \mathrm{E}(\xi_i | y, \hat{\mu}, \hat{\beta}_1, \hat{\beta}_2, \hat{\sigma}_F^2, \hat{\sigma}^2).$$

If the 'raw' residuals are defined as $r_{ij} = y_{ij} - \hat{\mu} - \hat{\beta}_1 x_{1i} - \hat{\beta}_2 x_{2i}$ and the mean raw residual for family i is $\bar{r}_i = \sum_{j=1}^{n_i} r_{ij}/n_i$ then the above expectation can be expressed as:

$$\hat{\xi}_i = \frac{\hat{\sigma}_F^2}{\hat{\sigma}_F^2 + \hat{\sigma}^2/n_i} \bar{r}_i. \tag{12.42}$$

It might have been expected that the family-level residual would simply be $\bar{r}_i$ but (12.42) is used instead. The difference, namely the factor $\hat{\sigma}_F^2/(\hat{\sigma}_F^2 + \hat{\sigma}^2/n_i)$, is often referred to as a shrinkage factor, as its effect is to 'shrink' $\bar{r}_i$ towards zero because the factor is always between 0 and 1. If the within-family variation is small compared with that between families, or if the size of the family is large, the shrinkage is minor. However, for small families the effect can be noticeable. The reasons for the appearance of this factor can best be appreciated if the procedure is considered in the context of estimation. Information on the term ξ_i is obtained from observation on family i. If substantial information is available from the family, then the estimate $\bar{r}_i$ is essentially sound. However, if few observations are available within a given family the method provides an estimate that is a compromise between the observed values and the population mean of the ξs, namely, 0. It should be noted that this definition naturally leads to individual-level residuals being defined to be $r_{ij} - \hat{\xi}_i$ rather than $r_{ij} - \bar{r}_i$.

If the residuals at levels above the lowest are to be used in their own right, perhaps in a ranking exercise for higher-level units, it may be necessary to compute appropriate standard errors and interval estimates. For discussion of these issues, the reader should consult Appendix 2.2 in Goldstein (1995).

Example 12.6

A trial was conducted to assess the benefit of two methods of giving care to patients who had recently been diagnosed as having Type II diabetes mellitus. The trial was run in general practices in the Wessex region of southern England with 250 patients from 41 practices, 21 randomized to the group in which nurses and/or doctors in the practice received additional training on patient-centred care (the *intervention* group) and patients in the other 20 practices received routine care (the *comparison* group). As the data comprise patients within practices, it is appropriate to use a method of analysis for hierarchical data and a multilevel model is used for the analysis of data on body-mass index (BMI: weight of patient over the square of their height, in kg/m^2). Several outcomes were measured and further details can be found in Kinmonth *et al.* (1998). In that report simpler methods were used because, as will be demonstrated, the variation between practices is not substantial compared with that within a practice.

The modelling approach reported here is based on a subset of 37 practices and 220 patients. The model fitted has four fixed effects and two random effects. The four fixed effects are a general mean and three binary variables: (i) a variable indicating the treatment group to which the practice was allocated in the randomization, $x_1 = 0$ for comparison and $x_1 = 1$ for the intervention group; (ii) a variable indicating whether the number of patients registered with the practice was above 10 000, $x_2 = 0$, or below, $x_2 = 1$; and (iii) a variable indicating whether care was always given to these patients by a nurse, $x_3 = 0$, or otherwise, $x_3 = 1$. There are random effects for the practices, with variance σ_P^2, and for the patients, with variance σ^2, so the full model is

$$y_{ij} = \mu + \beta_1 x_{1i} + \beta_2 x_{2i} + \beta_3 x_{3i} + \xi_i + \varepsilon_{ij}.$$

The term for a treatment effect obviously must be present in the model and the terms for the size of the practice and the care arrangements within a practice are included because these were used to stratify the allocation procedure. In this instance, no fixed effects vary at the patient level. If the model is fitted using RIGLS, the estimates of the parameters are as follows (fixed effects in kg/m^2, variances in kg^2/m^4):

Parameter	μ	β_1	β_2	β_3	σ_P^2	σ^2
Estimate	28.67	1·69	0·11	0·90	0·99	34·85
SE	1·15	0·90	0·95	1·18	1·57	3·58

The mean BMI is estimated to be 1·7 kg/m^2 higher in the intervention group than in the comparison group.

The estimate of σ_P^2 is considerably smaller than its standard error, which is the basis for noting that an analysis which ignores the clustering of patients into practices is unlikely to be misleading. Confidence intervals for the parameters, in particular the treatment effect, can be constructed in the usual way provided that the random effects can be assumed to follow normal distributions. This is checked in Fig. 12.10; note that panel (a) contains 220 points, as it corresponds to the random effects for patients, while panel (b), which corresponds to the practice random effect, has only 37 points. The plots are certainly reasonable confirmation of the assumption of normality, although the pattern for larger residuals at the patient level suggests that some further analysis may be helpful. Note the different scales, which reflect the marked difference in the sizes of the estimates of σ^2 and σ_P^2.

The estimates given above are from a method, RIGLS, that takes account of the uncertainty in the fixed effects when these are used to find estimates of random effects, but the quoted standard errors take no account of the uncertainty in the estimates of random effects. To do this a method based on a Bayesian approach, with diffuse priors and estimation using a Gibbs sampler (see §16.4), would be required. The estimate of treatment effect, its standard error and a 95% confidence interval were computed for each of three methods of estimation. The first is IGLS, the second is RIGLS and the last is a Bayesian formulation with fixed effects having normal prior distributions, with very large variance, and random effects having priors that are uniform between 0 and a very large value.

Method	Treatment effect	Standard error	95% confidence interval estimate
IGLS	$1 \cdot 64$ kg/m^2	$0 \cdot 85$ kg/m^2	$(-0 \cdot 03, 3 \cdot 31)$ kg/m^2
RIGLS	$1 \cdot 69$ kg/m^2	$0 \cdot 90$ kg/m^2	$(-0 \cdot 07, 3 \cdot 45)$ kg/m^2
Gibbs sampler	$1 \cdot 76$ kg/m^2	$1 \cdot 01$ kg/m^2	$(-0 \cdot 19, 3 \cdot 79)$ kg/m^2

The point estimates of treatment effect are very similar and, for all practical purposes, identical. The Gibbs sampler is based on a chain of length 40 000, and technical diagnostic values suggest that this is adequate to ensure convergence of the method. In this case, the 95% confidence interval estimate is derived from the distribution of estimates of treatment effect found from the chain. It is also clear that as the estimation method takes into account sources of variation neglected in other approaches, the estimate of standard error, and hence the width of the interval estimate, increases.

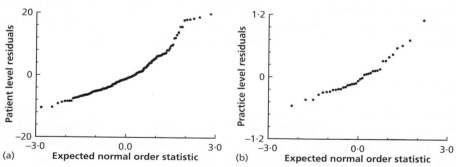

Fig. 12.10 Normal probability plots for the estimated residuals at the patient and practice levels from the trial of patient-centred care in general practice.

All the interval estimates demonstrate that any advantage the intervention group might have over the comparison group is practically negligible, whereas the comparison group could be substantially better than the intervention group.

Other uses of multilevel models

It has already been mentioned that multilevel models can be very useful in the analysis of hierarchical data when the response is not continuous, but even with continuous responses there is still scope for useful extensions. A few of these are outlined below.

Variations in random effects

In model (12.37) the variance increases with the square of age according to (12.38). However, it may be that this is inappropriate and a linear dependence is required. In this case the same model can be fitted, but in the fitting procedure the parameter σ_b^2 is held at 0. This is perhaps best regarded as a device for fitting the appropriate model, as the notion of a variable with a non-zero covariance but zero variance is not easy to interpret.

It should also be pointed out that the variation at the lowest level of the hierarchy, which hitherto has been assumed to be constant, can be made more elaborate. For example, allowing different variances at the lowest level of the hierarchy for different groups is possible.

As will be seen in the next section, observations made longitudinally on, for example, a patient are often serially correlated. A reasonable supposition is that the correlation is larger between measurements made closer together in time than further apart. However, the correlations induced between measurements on the same patient by a model which is of the form (12.34) are the same regardless of their separation in time. A model which overcomes this is known as the *autocorrelation* or *autoregressive model*, and a simple version of this leads to a correlation of $\rho^{|r-s|}$ between observations at times r and s. This kind of feature can be accommodated in multilevel models; see Goldstein *et al.* (1994) for details and §12.7 for a further discussion of autoregressive processes.

Non-linear models

In all the multilevel models discussed hitherto the response has depended linearly on the covariates. Non-hierarchical non-linear models were discussed in §12.4 and these can be extended to hierarchical data. Such models can be particularly useful for growth data; the data are hierarchical because individuals are measured longitudinally, but adequate modelling of the form of the response usually requires non-linear functions.

Non-linear models can be accommodated by repeatedly using Taylor expansions to linearize the model. There are close connections between this way of extending linear multilevel models and the types of model obtained by extending non-linear models to hierarchical data. Models generated in this way have recently been widely used to model pharmacokinetic data and this alternative approach is well described by Davidian and Giltinan (1995).

Multivariate analysis

Multivariate analysis, which is considered at greater length in Chapter 13, is the term used to describe a collection of statistical techniques which can be used when each observation comprises several variables, that is, each observation is a vector of, say, p dimensions. For example, the concentrations of creatinine, sodium and albumin in the blood of a patient may be measured, yielding as an observation a three-dimensional vector, which will have a mean that is also a three-dimensional vector and its 'variance' is a 3×3 dispersion matrix of variances and covariances. Of course, each component of this vector will be on its own scale and it will not, in general, be possible to specify common parameters across components of the vector.

Deployment of a certain amount of ingenuity means that multivariate observations of this kind can be analysed as multilevel models, and it turns out that there are some attractive benefits to viewing such data in this way. Suppose that y_i is a p-dimensional vector observed on patient i. It is assumed that if y were a scalar then this would be the lowest level of a hierarchy but, despite the single subscript, there is no implication that the patient is the top level of a hierarchy; the subscript might, for example, be elaborated to describe a hierarchy in which the patient is from a hospital, which in turn belongs to a given health authority. The multivariate nature of y is accommodated by the device of constructing a new lowest level to the hierarchy, which describes the variables within each vector y_i. This makes extensive use of dummy, i.e. 0–1, variables. To be specific, suppose the scalar y_{ij} is the jth variable observed on patient i (so, for example, in the above instance, y_{i1} might be the creatinine, y_{i2} the sodium and y_{i3} the albumin on patient i); the model used is then

$$y_{ij} = \beta_1 z_{1ij} + \beta_2 z_{2ij} + \beta_3 z_{3ij} + \xi_{1i} z_{1ij} + \xi_{2i} z_{2ij} + \xi_{3i} z_{3ij},$$

where z_{1ij} is 1 if y_{ij} is an observation on creatinine (i.e. the first variable in the vector y_i) and 0 otherwise. Similarly z_{kij} is 1 or 0 and is 1 only if y_{ij} is an observation on the kth variable in the vector. The random effects are at the level one up from the lowest level, i.e. the patient level in this example, and, in general, have arbitrary variances and covariances. Note that there are no random effects at the lowest level as this level is simply a device to distinguish between the different variables within each observed vector.

A notable advantage to this way of specifying multivariate data is that there is no requirement that each variable is present in all the vectors—that is, the vector can be only partially observed for some patients. If, for example, the albumin is not measured on patient i then the model simply has no entry for y_{i3}. This can be very useful because incomplete vectors can cause serious difficulties for standard approaches to multivariate analysis. It can be helpful if an element of a vector is inadvertently missing, although the analyst must then be satisfied that the omission is not for a reason that could bias the analysis (related concerns to this arise in the analysis of longitudinal data and are discussed at more length in the next section and also in clinical trials (see §18.6)). It can also be useful to arrange to collect data in a way that deliberately leads to the partial observation of some or all vectors. If the creatinine, sodium and albumin of the foregoing example are to be observed on premature infants then it may not be permissible to take sufficient blood for all items to be observed on each baby. It may then be helpful to observe just two of the variables on each infant, to arrange the patients into three groups and take just one of the three possible pairs of measurements on each baby. This is a simple example of a *rotation design*, in which predetermined subgroups of the variables of interest are observed on particular individuals. Further details on rotation designs and on the application of multilevel models to multivariate methods can be found in Goldstein (1995, Chapter 4).

12.6 **Longitudinal data**

In many medical studies there is interest not only in observing a variable at a given instant but in seeing how it changes over time. This could be because the investigator wishes to observe how a variable evolves over time, such as the height of a growing child, or to observe the natural variation that occurs in a clinical measurement, such as the blood pressure of a volunteer on successive days. A very common reason is to observe the time course of some intervention, such as a treatment: for example the respiratory function of a patient at a series of times after the administration of a bronchodilator, or the blood glucose of a diabetic patient in the two hours after a glucose challenge.

Data collected successively on the each of several units, whether patients, volunteers, animals or other units, are variously referred to as *longitudinal data, serial data* or *repeated measurements*, although many other terms are encountered from time to time. Typically the data will be collected on several, say, g, groups of individuals, perhaps defined by allocation to different treatments; typically there will be n_i units in the ith group. The jth unit in the ith group will be observed k_{ij} times. There is wide variation between studies in the timing and number of the observations on an individual. The observations on each individual constitute a *time series*, and in the next section methods that are traditionally described as applying to time series are discussed. However, such methods apply to a single long series, perhaps comprising hundreds of observations, whereas the data discussed in this section typically arise from many shorter series, often of two to 20 measurements per individual.

Another feature that varies widely between studies is why observations are made when they are. Most studies attempt to make observations at preplanned times; those which do not—for example, taking observations opportunistically, or perhaps when some clinical event occurs—are likely to present formidable problems of interpretation. For preplanned observations there is no requirement that they be taken at regular intervals, and in fact it may often not be sensible to do so; for example, observations may need to be taken more frequently when the response is changing rapidly, provided, of course, that that aspect of the response is of interest. For example, in the study of the profile of the blood level of a short-acting drug, measurements may be made every 10 or 15 min in the initial stages when the profile is changing rapidly, but then less frequently, perhaps at 1, 2 and 3 h post-administration. In many studies in the medical literature the reasons behind the timing of observations are seldom discussed, and it may be that this aspect of research involving the collection of longitudinal data would benefit from greater reflection.

Often it will be intended to measure individuals at the same set of times, but this is not achieved in every case. Such *missing data* give rise to two separate problems, which are often not distinguished from one another as clearly as they might be. The first, which is largely technical, is that the varying number of observations per individual may influence the type of analysis performed, as some methods are less tractable, or even impossible, when the number of observations varies between individuals. The second problem, which is more subtle and, because it can evade an unwary analyst, potentially more serious, is that the missing data are absent for reasons related to the purpose of the study, so an analysis of only the available data may well be biased and possibly misleading. The second of these problems will be discussed at greater length towards the end of the present section.

As with any statistical analysis, it is important when dealing with longitudinal data that their structure is respected. The two most important aspects for longitudinal data are: (i) that the method should take account of the link between successive measurements on a given individual; and (ii) that it should recognize that successive measurements on an individual will not, in general, be independent. Despite warnings to the contrary (Matthews *et al.*, 1990; Matthews, 1998), both these aspects appear to be frequently overlooked in the medical literature, where it is common to see separate analyses performed at the different times when measurements were made. Such analyses ignore the fact that the same individuals are present in successive analyses and makes no allowance for within-individual correlation.

Appropriate methods for the analysis of longitudinal data have been studied intensively in recent years and there is now a very large statistical literature on the subject. Some topics will be discussed in more detail below, but the reader should be aware that it is a highly selective account. The selection has largely been guided by consideration of the issues outlined in the previous paragraph, and in particular focuses on methods available for studying correlated responses. Important areas, such as growth curves, which are concerned with the shape of the response over time, are not mentioned and the reader should consult one of the excellent specialist texts in the field, such as Crowder and Hand (1990) or Diggle *et al.* (1994). Methods for graphing longitudinal data are also not covered. This is a surprisingly awkward but practically important problem, which has received much less attention than analytical methods; articles which contain some relevant material include Jones and Rice (1992), and Goldstein and Healy (1995), as does Chapter 3 of Diggle *et al.* (1994).

Repeated measures analysis of variance

As was remarked in §12.5, the multiple measurements taken on a patient means that longitudinal data can be viewed as a form of hierarchical data. It was also noted in the previous section that a split-unit analysis of variance (see §9.6) could analyse certain forms of sufficiently regular hierarchical data. It follows that split-unit analysis of variance can be pressed into service to analyse longitudinal data, with the whole units corresponding to the individuals and the subunits corresponding to measurement occasion. When used in this context the technique is usually referred to as *repeated measures analysis of variance*.

This method requires that each individual be measured on the same number of occasions, say, k times, that is, $k_{ij} = k$. There is no requirement that the number of individuals in each group is the same. If the total number of individuals in the study is denoted by $N = \sum_{i=1}^{g} n_i$, the analysis of variance table breaks down as follows into two strata, one between individuals and one within individuals.

Source of variation	DF	
Between-individuals stratum	$N-1$	
Groups		$g-1$
Residual between individuals		$N-g$
Within-individuals stratum	$N(k-1)$	
Occasions		$k-1$
Occasions × groups		$(g-1)(k-1)$
Residual within individuals		$(N-g)(k-1)$
Grand total	$Nk-1$	

Use of this technique therefore allows the analyst to assess not only effects of time (the Occasions row) and differences between groups (the Groups row), but whether or not the difference between groups changes with time (the Occasions × groups interaction). This is often the row of most interest in this technique. However, some care is needed; for example, if the groups arise through random allocation of individuals to treatments and the first occasion is a pretreatment baseline measurement, then any treatment effect, even if it is constant across all times post-randomization, will give rise to an interaction because there will necessarily be no difference between the groups on the first occasion. A minor problem is that, if there is a significant interaction between occasions and groups, then it is natural to ask when differences occur. If there is a prior belief of a particular pattern in the response, then this can be used to guide further hypothesis tests. In the absence of such expectations, techniques that control the Type I error rate need to be considered; the discussion in §8.4 is relevant here. However, in applying these methods, it is important that the user remembers the ordering implicit in the Occasions term and the fact that, in general, the response is likely to change smoothly rather than abruptly with time.

A further problem with the method is that the variance ratios formed in the within-individuals stratum will not, in general, follow an F distribution. This is a consequence of the dependence between successive measurements on the same individual. The use of an F test is valid under certain special circumstances but these are unlikely to hold in practice. Adjustments to the analysis can be made to attempt to accommodate the dependence under other circumstances and this can go some way to salvaging the technique. The adjustments amount to applying the usual method but with the degrees of freedom for the hypothesis tests for occasions and occasions × groups reduced by an appropriate factor. More details of this are given below, but a heuristic explanation of why this is a suitable approach is because within-individual correlation means that a value on an individual will contain some information about the other values, so there are fewer independent pieces of information than a conventional counting of degrees of freedom would lead you to believe. It is therefore sensible to apply tests with a reduced number of degrees of freedom.

In order to be more specific, suppose that y_i is the k-dimensional vector of observations on individual i and the dispersion matrix of this vector is Σ. The between-individuals stratum of the repeated measures analysis of variance can be viewed as a simple one-way analysis of variance between groups on suitably scaled individual totals, namely, the values proportional to $\mathbf{1}^T y_i$, where $\mathbf{1}$ is a k-dimensional vector of ones. The within-individual stratum is a simultaneous analysis of the within-individual contrasts, namely, of the $a_j^T y_i$, where $a_1, \ldots a_{k-1}$ are $k - 1$ independent vectors each of whose entries sum to zero, i.e. $a_j^T \mathbf{1} = 0$. The variance ratios in this analysis will be valid if the dispersion matrix is such that $a_j^T \Sigma a_j$ is proportional to the identity matrix (see §11.6). One form for Σ that satisfies this is the *equi-correlation structure*, where all variances in Σ are equal, as are all the covariances. However, this implies that pairs of observations taken close together in time have the same correlation as pairs taken at widely separated times, and this is unlikely to hold in practice.

By using the work of Box (1954a, b), Greenhouse and Geisser (1959) devised an adjustment factor that allows the technique to be applied for an arbitrary dispersion matrix. The adjustment is to reduce the degrees of freedom in the hypothesis tests for occasions and for occasions $\times$ groups by a factor ε, so, for example, the test for an effect of occasions compares the usual variance ratio statistic with an F distribution on $(k-1)\varepsilon$ and $(N-g)(k-1)\varepsilon$ degrees of freedom. The factor ε, often called the Greenhouse–Geisser ε, is defined as

$$\varepsilon = \frac{\{\mathrm{tr}(\Sigma H)\}^2}{(k-1)\mathrm{tr}(\Sigma H \Sigma H)}, \qquad (12.43)$$

where $H = I_k - \frac{1}{k}J_k$, where I_k is a $k \times k$ identity matrix and J_k is a $k \times k$ matrix of ones. If this correction is applied, then the variance ratios in the within-patient stratum still do not follow an F distribution but the discrepancy is less than would be the case without the correction. Of course, in practice ε must be estimated by substituting an estimate of Σ into (12.43) and the properties of the test based on an estimated ε may not be the same as those using the true value. Huyhn and Feldt (1976) devised an alternative correction of similar type whose sampling properties might be preferable to those of (12.43).

Calculation of (12.43) is awkward, requires an estimate of Σ and may have uncertain properties when ε has to be estimated. A practically useful device is available because it can be shown that (12.43) must lie between $(k-1)^{-1}$ and 1. As the degrees of freedom decrease, any critical point, say the 5% point, of the F distribution will increase. So, if an effect is not significant in an uncorrected test in the within-individual stratum, then it will not become significant when the correction is applied. Similarly, if an effect is significant when a correction using $(k-1)^{-1}$ is used rather than ε, then it would be significant at that level if the correction in (12.43) were used. Using this approach the analyst only has to compute an estimate of ε for effects which are significant under the uncorrected analysis but not under the analysis using the factor $(k-1)^{-1}$.

The between-individuals stratum is also not without problems. The test for equality of group means, which would only sensibly be considered in the absence of an occasion by group interaction, is generally valid (given usual assumptions about normality and equality of variances) because it is essentially the one-way analysis of variance of the means of the responses on an individual. This amounts to summarizing the response of an individual by the mean response, and this is an automatic consequence of using repeated measures analysis of variance. However, the mean response over time may not be an appropriate way to measure a relevant feature of the response. The idea of reducing the k

responses on an individual to a suitable scalar quantity, which can then be analysed simply, is the key idea behind the important approach to the analysis of longitudinal data that is outlined in the next subsection.

Summary measures

Perhaps the principal difficulty in analysing longitudinal data is coping with the dependency that is likely to exist between responses on the same individual. However, there is no more difficulty in assuming that responses from different individuals are independent than in other areas of data analysis (this assumes, for simplicity, that the individuals in the analysis are not embedded in a larger design, such as a complex survey (see §19.2) or a cluster-randomized trial (see §18.9), which may itself induce dependence). Consequently, if the responses on individual i, y_i, together with other information, such as the times of the responses, t_i, say, are used to compute a suitable scalar (i.e. a single value), s_i, say, then the s_i are independent and can be analysed using straightforward statistical methods. The value of this approach, which can be called the *summary measures method*, rests on the ability of the analyst to be able to specify a suitable function of the observations that can capture an important feature of the response of each individual. For this reason the method is sometimes referred to as *response feature analysis* (Crowder & Hand, 1990). The method has a long history, an early use being by Wishart (1938). More recent discussions can be found in Healy (1981), Yates (1982) and Matthews *et al.* (1990).

If, for example, the response of interest is the overall level of a blood chemistry measurement, then the simple average of the responses on an individual may be adequate. If the effect of some treatment on this quantity is being assessed then it may be sensible to omit the first few determinations from the average, so as to allow the treatment time to have its effect. A rate of change might best be summarized by defining s_i to be the regression slope of y_i on t_i. Summaries based on the time-scale may be particularly important from a clinical point of view: the time that a quantity, such as a drug concentration, is above a therapeutic level or the time to a maximum response may be suitable summaries. It may be that more than one feature of the data is of interest and it would then be legitimate to define and analyse a summary for each such feature. Simple bivariate analyses of summaries are also possible, although they seem to be little used in practice. Judgement should be exercised in the number of summaries that are to be analysed; summaries should correspond to distinct features of the response and in practice there are unlikely to be more than two or three of these.

The choice of summary measure should be guided by what is clinically or biologically reasonable and germane to the purpose of the study. Indeed, it is preferable to define the summary before the data are collected, as this may help to focus attention on the purpose of the investigation and the most appropriate times at which to make observations. This is particularly important when time-based summaries, such as time above a therapeutic level, are considered. Any prior information on when concentrations are likely to reach and decline from therapeutic levels can lead the investigators to placing more observations around these times. Occasionally, theoretical background can inform a choice of summary measure; the maximum response and the area under the response versus time curve are summaries that have long been used in pharmacology for such reasons. Choice of summary on the basis of the observed responses can be useful but, unless the summary ultimately chosen has a clear biological or clinical interpretation, the value of this approach is much reduced. Healy (1981) outlines the role of orthogonal polynomials in the method, although this is probably of greater theoretical importance in relating the method to other approaches than of practical interest.

There are, of course, drawbacks to the method. The most obvious is that in some circumstances it may not be possible to define a summary that adequately captures the response over time. Other problems in longitudinal data analysis are not naturally approached by this method; assessing whether changes in the blood concentration of a beta-blocker are related to changes in blood pressure is an example. Also there are technical problems. Many of the simple statistical methods that it is assumed will be used for the analysis of the summaries suppose that they share a common distribution, except perhaps for a few parameters such as those describing differences in the mean between treatment groups. In particular, the variances will often be assumed equal. This can easily be violated and this is illustrated by the following situation. Suppose the summary chosen is the mean and that the model for the elements of y_i is

$$y_{ij} = \mu_i + \xi_i + \varepsilon_{ij}, \tag{12.44}$$

where ξ_i and ε_{ij} are random variables with zero mean and $\text{var}(\xi_i) = \sigma_B^2$ and $\text{var}(\varepsilon_{ij}) = \sigma^2$. The mean of the elements of y_i has variance $\sigma_B^2 + n_i^{-1}\sigma^2$ and this will differ between individuals unless all the n_i are equal. While the intention at the outset of the study may have been to ensure that all the n_i were equal, it is almost inevitable that some individuals will be observed incompletely. However, even if there are marked differences between the n_i, there will be little important difference in the variances if the between-individuals variance, σ_B^2, is substantial relative to the within-individual variance, σ^2. Obviously there may be circumstances when concerns about distributional aspects of summary measures may be less easy to dismiss.

The problem with unequal variance for the mean response arose from unequal replication, which can commonly be attributed to occasional missing data. This leads naturally to the problem of dealing with missing values, which are of concern throughout statistics but seem to arise with especial force and frequency in longitudinal studies. On a naïve level the method of summary measures is sufficiently flexible to deal with missing data; a summary such as a mean or regression slope can often be computed from the observations that are available. However, to do so ignores consideration of *why* the unavailable observations are missing and this can lead to a biased analysis. This is clearly illustrated if the summary is the maximum observed response: if the response is measured at weekly visits to an out-patient clinic and large values are associated with feeling especially unwell, then it is precisely when the values of most interest arise that the patient may not feel fit to attend for observation. The problem of missing data, which is discussed in more detail at the end of this section, is only a special problem for the method of summary measures in so far as the method may make it too easy to overlook the issue altogether, and this should not be a problem for the alert analyst.

Modelling the covariance

A natural method for dealing with longitudinal data is to view the response on an individual as a vector from a suitable multivariate distribution, typically a multivariate normal distribution. In this way the dependence is handled by assuming each vector has a dispersion matrix Σ; if each vector has k elements then the $\frac{1}{2}k(k+1)$ parameters describing the dispersion are estimated from the data in the usual way for multivariate analysis. For example, two groups could be compared using Hotelling's T^2 statistic (see Mardia *et al.*, 1979, pp. 139 ff.). A good discussion of the application of multivariate methods to longitudinal data can be found in Morrison (1976).

There are, however, good reasons why this approach is seldom adopted. As with many medical applications of multivariate methods (see multiple outcomes in clinical trials, §18.3), these general methods are rather inefficient for specialized application. In the case of longitudinal data analysis the dispersion matrix may plausibly take forms in which correlations between occasions closer in time are higher, rather than the general form allowed by this class of methods. Differences in mean vectors might also be expected to change smoothly over time. In addition, the ever-present problem of missing values means that in practice not all vectors will be of the same length and this can cause substantial problems for standard multivariate methods.

An alternative way to view substantially the same analysis, but which readily accommodates unequal replication within each individual, is to put the analysis in terms of a linear model. If the vectors y_i from the N individuals in the study are stacked to form a single M-dimensional vector y (where M is the number of observations in the study), then this can be written with some generality as $y = X\beta + \epsilon$, where X is an $M \times p$-dimensional design matrix and β is a p-dimensional vector describing the mean response. The longitudinal nature of the data is described by the form of the dispersion matrix of ϵ, namely Σ. This is block diagonal, as in (12.40), now with N blocks on the diagonal, and the dispersion matrix for the ith individual in the study, $\mathbf{\Sigma}_i$, is the ith block. Usually the $\mathbf{\Sigma}_i$ are different because of missing data, so each $\mathbf{\Sigma}_i$ comprises the available rows and columns from a common 'complete case' matrix $\mathbf{\Sigma}_c$.

General statistical theory tells us that the best estimator of $\boldsymbol{\beta}$ is

$$\hat{\boldsymbol{\beta}} = \left(\sum_{i=1}^{N} X_i^{\mathrm{T}} \mathbf{\Sigma}_i^{-1} X_i \right)^{-1} \left(\sum_{i=1}^{N} X_i^{\mathrm{T}} \mathbf{\Sigma}_i^{-1} y_i \right), \qquad (12.45)$$

where X_i is the matrix comprising the rows of X that relate to individual i. However, this estimator is only available if the $\mathbf{\Sigma}_i$ are known and this will hardly ever be the case. An obvious step is to use (12.45) with an estimate, $\hat{\mathbf{\Sigma}}_i$, in place of $\mathbf{\Sigma}_i$. If all $\mathbf{\Sigma}_i$ were the same, such an estimator would be:

$$\frac{1}{N-p} \sum_{i=1}^{N} (y_i - X_i \hat{\boldsymbol{\beta}})(y_i - X_i \hat{\boldsymbol{\beta}})^{\mathrm{T}}.$$

In the case of missing data there is no simple solution; a sensible approach is to estimate the (u, v)th element of $\mathbf{\Sigma}_c$ from the terms $(y_i - X_i \hat{\boldsymbol{\beta}})(y_i - X_i \hat{\boldsymbol{\beta}})^{\mathrm{T}}$ in which the (u, v)th element is present.

It should be pointed out that when $\boldsymbol{\beta}$ is estimated using (12.45), but with an estimated dispersion matrix, there is no longer any guarantee that the estimator is optimal. If the data can provide a good estimate of the dispersion matrices, then the loss is unlikely to be serious. However, a general dispersion matrix such as $\mathbf{\Sigma}_c$ comprises $\frac{1}{2}k(k+1)$ parameters that need to be estimated, and it would effect a useful saving if the information in the data could be used to estimate fewer parameters. In addition, a general dispersion matrix may well be inappropriate for data collected over time; for example, it may be plausible to expect correlations to decrease as the time between when they were recorded increases. Therefore it may be useful to attempt to provide a model for the dispersion matrix, preferably one using substantially fewer than $\frac{1}{2}k(k+1)$ parameters.

There are various approaches to this task. One is to introduce random effects which induce a particular form for the dispersion matrix. This is the approach outlined in the previous section in the more general setting of multilevel models. An important reference to the application of this approach in the analysis of longitudinal data is Laird and Ware (1982); further details can be found in Chapter 6 of Crowder and Hand (1990).

In some applications the random effects method will be sufficient. However, if the model, for example, for serial measurements of blood pressure on patient i, is as in (12.44), then it may be inadequate to assume that the terms $\varepsilon_{i1}, \varepsilon_{i2}, \ldots, \varepsilon_{ik}$, are independent and some further modelling may be required. It may be that ε_{ij} could be decomposed as $\varepsilon_{ij} = \zeta_{ij} + \eta_{ij}$. The second of these terms may well be considered to be independent from one measurement occasion to the next, with constant variance σ_M^2, and would represent items such as measurement error. The first term would have a more complicated dispersion matrix, $\Sigma(\theta)$ defined in terms of a vector of parameters θ, preferably of low dimension. The dependence between the different elements $\zeta_{i1}, \zeta_{i2}, \ldots, \zeta_{ik}$ measures the genuine serial correlation between the measurements of blood pressure within patient i.

Many different models have been suggested in the literature as candidates for $\Sigma(\theta)$. Only one type is discussed here, the widely used *first-order autoregression model* (see §12.7), which for observations taken at equally spaced intervals, say, times $1, 2, \ldots, k$, has

$$\Sigma(\theta)_{ij} = \sigma_W^2 \theta^{|i-j|} \text{ for a scalar} - 1 < \theta < 1. \tag{12.46}$$

This form is used because it arises from the following equation for generating the $\zeta_{i1}, \zeta_{i2}, \ldots, \zeta_{ik}$, namely,

$$\zeta_{ij} = \theta \zeta_{i,j-1} + \omega_{ij} \, j = 2, \ldots, k, \tag{12.47}$$

in which each term is related to the previous term through the first part of the equation, but with a random perturbation from the innovation term ω_{ij}. This term comprises independent terms with zero mean and variance $\sigma_W^2(1 - \theta^2)$. It should be noted that the above equation does not specify ζ_{i1} and in order to complete matters it is necessary to supplement the equation with $\zeta_{i1} = \omega_{i1}$ and, if the above equation for $\Sigma(\theta)_{ij}$ is to be obtained, then it is further required to set the variance of ω_{i1} to σ_W^2. This rather clumsy manoeuvre, which appears more natural if the time index in (12.47) is extended indefinitely in the negative direction, is required to obtain a *stationary* autoregression, in which the variance of the ζ term does not change over time, and the correlations depend only on the interval between the occasions concerned. If ω_{i1} had the same variance as the other innovation terms, then a *non-stationary first-order* autoregression would result.

If the matrix in (12.46) is inverted, then the result is a matrix with non-zero entries only on the leading diagonal and the first subdiagonal. This is also true for the dispersion matrix that arises from the non-stationary first-order autoregression. This reflects a feature of the dependence between the observations known as the *conditional independence structure*, which also arises in more advanced techniques, such as graphical modelling (Whittaker, 1990; Cox & Wermuth, 1996). The structure of the inverse dispersion matrix bears the following interpretation. Suppose the blood pressure of a patient had been measured on each day of the week; then, provided the value on Thursday was known, the value on Friday is independent of the days before Thursday. In other words, the information about the history of the process is encapsulated in the one preceding measurement. This reflects the fact that (12.47) is a first-order process, which is also reflected in there being only one non-zero diagonal in the inverse dispersion matrix.

This can be extended to allow second- and higher-order processes. A process in which, given the results of the two previous days, the current observation is then independent of all earlier values is a second-order process, and an rth-order process if the value of the r days preceding the present need to be known to ensure independence. The inverse dispersion matrix would have, respectively, two or r subdiagonals with non-zero entries. Generally, this is referred to as an ante-dependence process, and the two first-order autoregressions described above are special cases. If the total number of observations on an individual is k, then the $(k-1)$th-order process is a general dispersion matrix and the zero-order process corresponds to complete independence. The theory of ante-dependence structures was propounded by Gabriel (1962). An important contribution was made by Kenward (1987), who realized that these complicated models could be fitted by using analysis of covariance, with the analysis at any time using some of the previous observations as covariates.

Although a very useful contribution to the modelling of the covariance of equally spaced data, the ante-dependence models are less useful when the intervals between observations vary. Diggle (1988) proposes a modified form of (12.46) suitable for more general intervals.

The way a covariance model is chosen is also important but is beyond the scope of this chapter. Excellent descriptions of ways to approach empirical modelling of the covariance structure, involving simple random effects and measurement error terms, as well as the serial dependence term, can be found in Diggle *et al.* (1994), especially Chapters 3 and 5.

Generalized estimating equations

Although modelling the covariance structure has considerable logical appeal as a thorough approach to the analysis of longitudinal data, it has some drawbacks. Identifying an appropriate model for the dispersion matrix is often difficult and, especially when there are few observations on each patient or experimental unit, the amount of information in the data on the parameters of the dispersion matrix can be limited. A consequence is that analyses based on (12.44) with estimated dispersion matrices can be much less efficient than might be imagined because of the uncertainty in the estimated dispersion matrices. Another difficulty is that most of the suitable and tractable models are based on the multivariate normal distribution.

An alternative approach is to base estimation on a postulated dispersion matrix, rather than to attempt to identify the correct matrix. The approach, which was proposed by Liang and Zeger (1986) and Zeger and Liang (1986), uses *generalized estimating equations* (GEEs) (see, for example, Godambe, 1991) and has been widely used for longitudinal data when the outcome is categorical. However, it is useful for continuous data and will be described in this context.

This discussion is rather more mathematical than many other parts of the book, although it is hoped that appreciation of the more detailed parts of the argument is not necessary to gain a general understanding of this topic.

It is most convenient for the following discussion to assume that the data have been written in the succinct form of (12.39), the longitudinal aspect of the data being represented by the block diagonal nature of the dispersion matrix of the residual term. The true dispersion matrix which is, of course, unknown, is denoted by V_T. If the data are analysed by ordinary least squares, that is, the longitudinal aspect is ignored, then the estimate of the parameters of interest, $\boldsymbol{\beta}$, is

$$\hat{\boldsymbol{\beta}}_O = (X^T X)^{-1} X^T y, \tag{12.48}$$

where the subscript O indicates that the estimator uses ordinary least squares. Despite the implicit misspecification of the dispersion matrix, this estimator is unbiased and its variance is

$$(X^T X)^{-1} X^T V_T X (X^T X)^{-1}. \tag{12.49}$$

If ordinary least squares were valid and $V_T = \sigma^2 I$, then (12.49) would reduce to the familiar formula (11.51). However, in the general case, application of (11.51) would be incorrect, but (12.49) could be used directly if a suitable estimator of V_T were available. Provided that the mean, $X\boldsymbol{\beta}$, is correctly specified, then a suitable estimator of the ith block within V_T is simply:

$$(y_i - X_i \hat{\boldsymbol{\beta}}_O)(y_i - X_i \hat{\boldsymbol{\beta}}_O)^T, \tag{12.50}$$

and, if these N estimators are collected together in $\hat{V}_T$ and this is used in place of V_T in (12.49), then a valid estimator of the variance of $\hat{\boldsymbol{\beta}}_O$ is obtained. The estimator is valid because, regardless of the true dispersion matrix, the variance of y is correctly estimated by the collection of matrices in (12.50). This estimator of variance is occasionally called a robust estimator because it is valid independently of model assumptions; the estimator of the variance of $\hat{\boldsymbol{\beta}}_O$ is referred to as a 'sandwich estimator' because the estimator of the variance of y is 'sandwiched' between other matrices in (12.49) (see Royall, 1986).

Although using (12.49) in conjunction with (12.50) yields a valid estimate of error, the estimates may be inefficient in the sense that the variances of elements of $\hat{\boldsymbol{\beta}}_O$ are larger than they would have been using an analysis which used the correct variance matrix. The unbiasedness of (12.48) does not depend on using ordinary least squares and an alternative would be to use

$$\hat{\boldsymbol{\beta}}_G = (X^T V_W^{-1} X)^{-1} X^T V_W^{-1} y, \tag{12.51}$$

with the associated estimator of variance being

$$(X^T V_W^{-1} X)^{-1} X^T V_W^{-1} V_T V_W^{-1} X (X^T V_W^{-1} X)^{-1}.$$

Here V_W is a postulated or working dispersion matrix specified by the analyst. It is at least plausible that if V_W is, in some sense, closer to V_T than $\sigma^2 I$ then the estimator (12.51) will be more efficient than (12.48).

The above discussion has outlined the main ideas behind GEEs but has done so using a normal regression model that underestimates the range of applications of the technique, and is rather oversimplified. Rather than equations such as (12.48) and (12.51), and in line with their name, it is more usual for estimators to be written implicitly, as solutions to systems of equations. Reverting to the format of (12.44), an equivalent way to write (12.51) is as the solution of

$$\sum_{i=1}^{N} X_i^{\mathrm{T}} V_{Wi}^{-1} (y_i - X_i \beta) = 0, \qquad (12.52)$$

where V_{Wi} is the ith block of V_W. A further modification is to separate the specification of the variances and correlations in V_W by writing $V_{Wi} = \Delta_i R_i \Delta_i = V_i$, say, where Δ_i is a diagonal matrix with the kth element equal to the standard deviation of the kth element of y_i (y_{ik}, say) and R_i is a 'working' correlation matrix specified by the analyst. This separation is useful when the outcome does not have a normal distribution: the variance will then be readily specified through the mean–variance relationship of the distribution concerned and this defines Δ_i, leaving the analyst only to postulate the correlation structure. For example if the outcome were a 0–1 variable then the variance of y_{ik} would be $E(y_{ik})\{1 - E(y_{ik})\}$ and the square root of this would be the kth element of Δ_i. An example with a continuous outcome would be if the data had a gamma distribution then the kth element of Δ_i would be $E(y_{ik})$. This leads to the form of (12.52),

$$\sum_{i=1}^{N} D_i^{\mathrm{T}} \Delta_i^{-1} R_i^{-1} \Delta_i^{-1} (y_i - \mu_i) = 0, \qquad (12.53)$$

where it should be noted that among other changes D_i has replaced X_i and μ_i has replaced $X_i \beta$. For normal error models where the mean is $X_i \beta$, D_i and X_i are identical. For other models, $D_i = B_i X_i$, where B_i is determined by the dependence of the variance on the mean and the way the mean is related to covariates; see Liang and Zeger (1986) or Diggle *et al.* (1994) for details. It should also be noted that dependence of D_i and Δ_i on β (through the former's dependence on the mean of the outcomes) means that there is no longer a closed form for the solution of (12.53), which explains why the superficially attractive forms (12.48) and (12.51) do not appear in the general theory of GEEs.

Solutions of (12.52) for β, $\hat{\beta}_G$, say, were shown to be useful by Liang and Zeger (1986), in so far as they are approximately unbiased (technically, they are consistent (see Cox & Hinkley, 1974, p. 287)), and the variance of $\hat{\beta}_G$ can be validly estimated by

$$H^{-1}\left(\sum_{i=1}^{N} D_i^T V_i^{-1}(y_i - \hat{\mu}_i)(y_i - \hat{\mu}_i)^T V_i^{-1} D_i\right) H^{-1}, \qquad (12.54)$$

where $H = \sum_{i=1}^{N} D_i^T V_i^{-1} D_i$. As discussed above, the validity of (12.54) arises from its use of the robust estimator of variance, which stems from the appearance of $(y_i - \hat{\mu}_i)(y_i - \hat{\mu}_i)^T$ in (12.54). The drawback is that the standard errors will be greater than if the true covariance structure were known and modelled directly—that is, the estimator may lack efficiency.

A way to improve the efficiency of GEEs is to use a working correlation matrix that is as close as possible to the true matrix. Any fixed correlation matrix can be used, and the case $R = I$—that is, the assumption of independent errors—is often adopted in practice. Indeed, Kenward and Jones (1994), writing in the context of crossover trials, remark that this assumption often performs well. Of course, it will be rare for the analyst to know what would be a good choice for R, and a possibility is to specify R up to a number of unknown parameters. Simple cases include the equi-correlation matrix, $R_{ij} = \alpha$, $i \neq j$ and the case $R_{i,i+1} = \alpha_i$, $R_{ij} = 0$, $|i - j| > 1$. Liang and Zeger (1986) discuss *ad hoc* ways to estimate the parameters in R and more sophisticated approaches are outlined in Liang *et al.* (1992).

It is important to remember, when dealing with GEEs that require estimation of parameters in the correlation matrix, that this does not amount to the same kind of analysis outlined in the previous subsection, where the aim was to model the covariance. This is because in this technique the variances of the parameters of interest are obtained robustly, and remain valid even if the working correlation matrix is not an estimate of the true correlation matrix.

Missing data

It is often the case in the course of a study that the investigator is unable to obtain all the data that it was intended to collect. Such 'missing data' arise, and cause difficulties, in almost all areas of research: individuals who were sampled in a survey but refuse to respond are naturally a concern as they will undermine the representativeness of the sample (see §19.2); patients in clinical trials who fail to comply with the protocol can lead to problems of comparability and/or interpretation (see §18.6).

In the context of longitudinal data, it will often be the case that some of the data that should have been collected from an individual are missing but that the remainder are to hand. Data could, of course, be missing intermittently throughout the planned collection period, or the data might be complete up to some time, with all the subsequent measurements missing; the second case is often referred to as a 'drop-out' because it is the pattern that would arise if the individual concerned dropped out of a study at a given time and was then lost to follow-up. This particular pattern is distinguished from other patterns because it has recently been studied quite extensively, and will be discussed below.

With missing values in longitudinal data, the analyst is confronted with the problem of whether or not the values on an individual that are available can be used in an analysis and, if so, how. A naïve approach would simply be to analyse the data that were available. This could present technical problems for some methods; for example, repeated measures analysis of variance cannot deal with unbalanced data in which different individuals are measured different numbers of times. There are techniques which allow the statistician to impute values for the missing observations, thereby 'completing' the data and allowing the analysis that was originally intended to be performed. These methods were widely used in the days before substantial computing power was as readily available as it is now, because many methods for unbalanced data used to present formidable computational obstacles. However, this approach is clearly undesirable if more than a very small proportion of the data is missing. Other methods, for example, a summary measures analysis using the mean of the responses on an individual, have no difficulty with unbalanced data. However, regardless of the ability of any technique to cope with unbalanced data, analyses which ignore the reasons why values are missing can be seriously misleading. For example, if the outcome is a blood chemistry measurement that tends to be high when some chronic condition is particularly active and debilitating, then it may be on just such occasions that the patient feels too unwell to attend the clinic, so the missing values are generally the high values. A summary measures mean of the available values would be biased downwards, as would be the results from the interindividual stratum in a repeated measures analysis of variance.

It is clear that there are potentially severe difficulties in dealing with missing values. It is important to know if the fact that an observation is missing is related to the value that would have been obtained had it not been missing. It is equally clear that unequivocal statistical evidence is unlikely to be forthcoming on this issue. Nevertheless, a substantial body of statistical research has recently emerged on this topic, stemming from the seminal work of Little (1976) and Rubin (1976), and this will be discussed briefly below. It should also be noted that, although the problem of missing data can be severe, it does not have to be, and it is important to keep matters in perspective. If the number of missing values is small as a proportion of the whole data set, and if the purpose of the analysis is not focused on extreme aspects of the distribution of the response, such as determining the top few percentiles, then it is unlikely that naïve approaches will be seriously misleading.

Almost all of the formal methods discussed for this problem stem from the classification of missing data mechanisms into three groups, described by Little and Rubin (1987). These are: (i) *missing completely at random* (MCAR); (ii) *missing at random* (MAR); and (iii) processes not in (i) or (ii). The final group has been given various names, including *informative missing, non-ignorable, missing not at random* (MNAR). The differences between these groups are quite subtle in some areas, and precise definition requires some careful notation to be established and, for a full understanding, a certain level of mathematics is probably inescapable. Nevertheless, it is hoped that the general importance of this topic and the advantage and limitations of recent developments can be appreciated without fully absorbing all of the following detail.

Suppose that the k measurements on an individual are denoted by the vector y; this comprises *all* measurements, whether or not they were observed—that is, this framework assumes, at least conceptually, that there are values for all elements of y, it is just that some of them are not observed. There is another k-dimensional vector, r, comprising 0s and 1s, with a 1 indicating that the corresponding element of y was observed and a 0 indicating that it was missing; this vector will occasionally be referred to as the 'missing value process'. The implied partition of y into components of observed and missing observations is $y = (y_o, y_m)$ with subscripts standing for 'observed' and 'missing', respectively.

The joint density of y and r is written as $f(y, r)$, but analyses can only start from the observed data, (y_o, r), which has density

$$f(y_o, r) = \int f(y, r)\ \mathrm{d}y_m = \int f(y_o, y_m, r)\mathrm{d}y_m. \tag{12.55}$$

The classification of Little and Rubin (1987) largely revolves around the nature of the dependence between y and r and the subsequent simplifications in (12.55) that follow. It is also convenient to suppose that the marginal density of y is more fully described by $f(y|\theta)$, where θ is a vector of parameters, and the marginal density of r by $f(r|\beta)$, where β is another vector of parameters. It is supposed that there is no functional connection between the elements of the two parameter vectors, i.e. it is assumed that a connection such as $\beta_1 = \phi = \theta_2$ is not specified. In practice, such connections are very unlikely to be needed, so this assumption is not very restrictive. It is important to realize that, when covariates are introduced to explain the observations and the missing value process, this restriction does not stop the same covariate, e.g. 'age', from being used in both parts of the model. The vector θ governs the distribution of the outcomes, whether observed or not. In the development of this area of methodology it is supposed that the aim of the analysis is inference about θ, although this will not always be the case, as will be discussed below.

The first group, MCAR, is when the probability that an observation is missing is independent of the outcomes—that is, it is independent both of the particular missing observation and of all the other data, whether missing or observed. An example might be the random failure of some recording apparatus, entirely unconnected with the data. In this case, $f(y, r) = f(y)f(r)$, from which it follows that $f(y_o, r) = f(y_o|\theta)f(r|\beta)$, and, as the observed outcomes and the missing value process are independent, inferences about θ can be made from the observed data.

The second group, MAR, assumes that the missing value process can depend on observed values of the outcome, so the conditional density $f(r|y)$ does not depend on unobserved values, i.e. $f(r|y) = f(r|y_o)$. In this case, the 'missingness' may be related to observed data, but given that dependence, it does not depend further on the missing observations. An example might be a tendency for old people to miss occasional hospital visits, age being related to other observed data, but where the specific missing observation does not otherwise influence the 'missingness'. It follows that $f(y,r) = f(r|y_o)f(y_o, y_m)$ and, after substituting in (12.55), the first factor can be removed from the integration, giving $f(y_o, r) = f(y_o|\theta)f(r|y_o, \beta)$. If inferences are to be made using the method of maximum likelihood, the contribution to the log-likelihood from this individual is

$$\log f(y_o|\theta) + \log f(r|y_o, \beta). \qquad (12.56)$$

So, from (12.56), it is seen that the log-likelihood comprises two terms, one containing information on θ and depending only on observed outcomes, and another term which does not depend on θ. Therefore, if MAR holds, inference about θ can be based on the likelihood of the observed outcomes and, to an extent, the missing value process can be ignored. However, while certain aspects of a likelihood analysis can proceed simply—for example, a maximum likelihood estimate of θ can certainly be obtained by maximizing a sum of terms of the form $\log f(y_o|\theta)$—other aspects need more care; see Kenward and Molenberghs (1998) for an excellent discussion.

The final group, MNAR, is where neither MCAR nor MAR holds, so in particular the probability that an item is missing depends on at least some of the unobserved values, $f(y,r) = f(y)f(r|y_o, y_m)$ and no further simplification is possible. This is perhaps the most realistic scenario, and would occur, for instance, if a patient's failure to report for a follow-up visit was caused by a deterioration in health, which would have been reflected in an extreme value of a clinical test measurement on the occasion in question.

While this classification provides a useful framework within which the issues of missing data can be discussed, it does not in itself take matters forward in a practical way. In recent times, there have been numerous papers addressing the practical implications; these include, among many others, Diggle and Kenward (1994), Fitzmaurice *et al.* (1995), Diggle (1998), Kenward (1998) and Kenward and Molenberghs (1999). Some of these papers address the issue of incomplete longitudinal data for non-continuous outcomes, but many of the important issues are germane to all kinds of outcomes. Most of the contributions to date have avoided the difficulties of specifying a distribution for r, a random vector of 0s and 1s, by considering only one pattern of missing data, namely *drop-out*. In this it is supposed that complete data are observed on an individual up to and including measurement occasion $D - 1$, where $2 \leq D \leq k + 1$, with all subsequent outcomes being missing: $D = k + 1$ indicates that the individual did not drop out. This reduces the modelling problem, as the missing value process has been greatly restricted. While this undoubtedly limits the practical utility of the method, it is an important case and also allows progress in a methodologically challenging area.

Diggle and Kenward (1994) and Diggle (1998) suggest that the missing value process, which can now also be called a drop-out process, can be modelled by

$$\log\left(\frac{\Pr(D = d \mid D \geq d, \boldsymbol{y})}{1 - \Pr(D = d \mid D \geq d, \boldsymbol{y})}\right) = \alpha_d + \sum_{j=0}^{s} \beta_j y_{d-j}, \qquad (12.57)$$

where s is a prespecified integer and for notational convenience we take $y_j = 0$ for $j \leq 0$. This model is not the only one that could be considered, but it is plausible; it assumes that the probability of drop-out at any given stage can depend on the outcomes up to and including that stage, but not on the future of the process. If all the βs are 0 then the process is MCAR, and if $\beta_0 = 0$ the process is MAR. If neither of these simplifications obtains then the log-likelihood for the observed data has an extra term over those in (12.56), which accommodates the way the parameters $\boldsymbol{\beta}$ and $\boldsymbol{\theta}$ jointly determine aspects of the data. This will involve contributions from probabilities in (12.57) but this depends on the unobserved value y_d, so it is necessary to compute an expression for $P(D = d \mid D \geq d, \boldsymbol{y}_o)$ by integrating the probability in (12.57) over the conditional distribution of the unobserved value, $f(y_d \mid \boldsymbol{y}_o)$. By this means valid inferences can be drawn about $\boldsymbol{\theta}$ even when data are missing not at random.

The MCAR, MAR classification of Little and Rubin (1987) is naturally expressed by factorizing $f(\boldsymbol{y}, \boldsymbol{r})$ as $f(\boldsymbol{r} \mid \boldsymbol{y}) f(\boldsymbol{y})$ and then specifying particular forms for the first factor; these are known as *selection models*. Another approach would be to use the alternative factorization, $f(\boldsymbol{y} \mid \boldsymbol{r}) f(\boldsymbol{r})$, which gives rise to *pattern mixture models*, so called because they view the joint distribution as a mixture of different distributions on the outcomes, one distribution for each pattern of missing data. This view, which is extensively discussed in Little (1993), Hogan and Laird (1997), Diggle (1998) and Kenward and Molenberghs (1999), gives an alternative and in many ways complementary approach to the problem. The reliance of the MAR, MCAR classification on the form of $f(\boldsymbol{r} \mid \boldsymbol{y})$ means that the extent to which this classification can be carried over into pattern mixture models is not transparent. Molenberghs *et al.* (1998) have shown that for drop-out, but not for more general patterns of missing data, MAR models can be seen to correspond to certain classes of pattern mixture model.

In order to make valid inferences about $f(\boldsymbol{y}, \boldsymbol{r})$ from incomplete data $(\boldsymbol{y}_o, \boldsymbol{r})$, various models have to be constructed or assumptions made. A fundamental problem is that the observed data do not contain all the information needed to assess these models or test the assumptions. Furthermore, not all the parameters in the models can be estimated from the observed data. These issues are seen particularly clearly in the pattern mixture framework. If the outcomes y have a multivariate normal distribution, then the $f(y|r)$ specify separate such distributions for each pattern of missing data. Problems arise even if the r are restricted to drop-out patterns; parameters relating to the final observation time (such as a mean, a variance and several covariances) cannot be estimated for any group but that with complete data; parameters relating to the final two times cannot be estimated for individuals who dropped out before that stage, and so on. The problem is clearly a general one that does not rely on the assumption of normality. Little (1993) introduces restrictions on the distributions that allow all parameters to be estimated, essentially by forcing certain relationships between identifiable and unidentifiable parameters. These restrictions are similar to those which Molenberghs *et al.* (1998) found corresponded to MAR. The veracity of neither set of restrictions can be decided on the basis of (y_o, r) and this also implies that MAR cannot be verified from the observed data alone.

Although difficult to assess, the effect of using a model for non-random drop-out can be very striking, as is illustrated in the case-study presented in §9.4 of Diggle (1998). This shows observed means from a clinical trial comparing placebo and two drugs, haloperidol and risperidone, for the treatment of chronic schizophrenia. Figure 9.6 in the paper shows fitted curves for the mean response (a score on a rating scale) that are distant from the observed data. This reflects the feature of the model that suggests that those who dropped out had a poor response, so the distance between the fitted and observed means may reflect the bias inherent in the observed values. Despite the plausibility of this explanation, the effect has arisen from an essentially unverifiable model and is very marked. The extent to which any statistician would wish to base inferences on such fitted models is unclear. However, unease about using the results of such a model gives no support whatsoever to naïve methods that ignore why missing values are absent. It may be that this methodology is best seen as a form of sensitivity analysis which gives the statistician the framework in which to assess the sort of impact the missing data might have had on conclusions of interest.

There are two further features of this kind of analysis that deserve comment. The first is that, even if the model for the missing value process were known, matters might not be straightforward. If neither MCAR nor MAR obtained, then inference about θ would be affected by inference about β and inference about β would be affected by the level of missing data. If there are too few values missing, then the precision attached to estimates of β would be poor and this lack of information could, in principle, and rather paradoxically, adversely affect inference about θ.

A second and more important consideration is whether the analyst really does want to make inferences about θ, the parameter governing the outcomes y. The approaches to missing data described above essentially consider missing data to be a nuisance that prevents the investigators from describing the process that would have been observed in the absence of missing data. However, there are many circumstances where this may be quite inappropriate; for example, in a controlled trial comparing a new treatment with placebo, some patients may be unable to tolerate the new treatment and withdraw. They will appear to have dropped out of the study and it may well be that the drop-out process is neither MCAR nor MAR, so it cannot be ignored. However, the analyses that have been described above are likely to be unrealistic, as they would refer to the distribution of outcomes that would have been seen among patients who cannot tolerate the treatment had they persisted with treatment. It is important when implementing the techniques just described for missing data that the analysis proposed addresses questions relevant to the study.

The foregoing description of missing data has concentrated exclusively on problems that arise because of missing responses, rather than missing covariates. Covariates are not immune from the vagaries that lead to missing data, although the problems they present are not as closely tied to longitudinal data as are some issues for missing responses. For these reasons and reasons of space, the important problems and techniques related to missing covariates are not discussed in detail. The interested reader is referred to Little and Rubin (1987), Rubin (1987), Schafer (1997, 1999) and Horton and Laird (1999) (and the other papers in Issue 1 of Volume 8 of *Statistical Methods in Medical Research*).

12.7 **Time series**

Some statistical investigations involve long series of observations on one or more variables, made at successive points of time. Three medical examples are: (i) a series of mortality rates from a certain cause of death, recorded in a particular community over a period of, say, 100 years; (ii) haemodynamic measurements on a pregnant woman, made at intervals of 1 min during a period of 1 h; and (iii) a continuous trace from an electroencephalogram (EEG) over 5 min. The widespread use of automatic analysers and other devices for the automatic recording of clinical measurements has led to an enormous increase in the output of data of this sort—often much more data than can conveniently be analysed and interpreted.

The first purpose of a statistical analysis of time series data is to describe the series by a model which provides an appropriate description of the systematic and random variation. This may be useful merely as a summary description of a large and complex set of data—for example, by identifying any points of time at which changes in the characteristics of the series occurred, or by noting any periodic effects. Or it may be necessary to describe the structure of the series before any valid inferences can be made about the effects of possible explanatory variables. Again, some features revealed by a statistical analysis, such as a periodic effect, or a relation between movements in several time series, may provide insight into biological mechanisms.

Time series analysis may, however, have a more operational role to play. In the monitoring of clinical measurements, one may wish to predict future observations by taking into account recent changes in the series, perhaps taking remedial action to forestall dangerously large changes. Prediction and control are also important in vital statistics—for example, in the monitoring of congenital malformations.

The problem in time series analysis can be regarded as one of regression—the measurement in question being a dependent variable, with time as an explanatory variable—but the methods outlined in Chapters 7 and 11 are unlikely to be very useful. Trends exhibited by long-term series are unlikely to be representable by the simple mathematical functions considered in these chapters and the repeated measurements that comprise the time series will generally be expected to exhibit serial correlation, in the same way as was discussed in §12.6 for longitudinal data.

The techniques discussed in §§12.1, 12.2 and §12.4 can be useful in the analysis of the trends encountered in times series. The serial correlation can be addressed by the methods discussed in §12.6, but in time series analysis the emphasis is usually rather different. In the examples discussed in §12.6 it was expected that serial measurements would be taken on each of several independent units, such as patients or animals, but that the number of measurements on each unit was not substantial, typically between 2 and 20. In time series analysis, there will often be only one series of measurements but the number of measurements in each series will run into the hundreds at least. This provides much more information on the nature of the evolution of the series over time and has given rise to a more elaborate theory, which has developed somewhat separately from that described in §12.6. The details of these methods are too complex to be described at all fully here and we shall only give a brief outline of one or two general approaches. For further details, see Diggle (1990) or Chatfield (1996).

It is convenient to distinguish between analyses in the *time domain* and those in the *frequency domain*. The two approaches are, in fact, mathematically equivalent, in that one form of analysis can be derived from the other. However, they emphasize different features of a time series and can usefully be considered separately. The time domain is concerned with relationships between observations at different times, in particular with serial correlations at different time lags. In the frequency domain, the observations are regarded as being composed of contributions from periodic terms at different frequencies, and the analysis is concerned with the relative amplitudes at different frequencies, as in the spectral decomposition of light.

Before considering these two approaches further, it is worth making one or two elementary points.

1 In the analysis of any time series it is good practice to plot the data before doing any computations. A visual inspection may reveal features of the data, such as heterogeneity of different sections or a grossly non-normal distribution, which should affect the choice of method of analysis (in the latter case, perhaps by suggesting an initial transformation of the data).

2 Look for extreme outliers, and enquire whether there are special reasons for any aberrant readings which may justifiably lead to their exclusion.

3 Many series exhibit an obvious long-term trend. It is often useful to remove this at the outset, either by fitting a linear or other simple curve or by taking differences between successive observations. Time series analysis may then be applied to the residuals from the fitted curve or the successive differences.

The time domain

An important class of models is that of *autoregressive series*. Here the expected value of the dependent variable at any time depends to some extent on the values at previous points of time. In the simplest model of this sort, the *first-order autoregressive* (or *Markov*) scheme, the dependence is only on the immediately preceding observation. If Y_t denotes the deviation from the long-run mean at time t, the first-order process may be expressed by the equation

$$Y_t = \rho Y_{t-1} + \varepsilon_t,$$

where the ε_t are random errors, independently distributed around a mean of zero. If the series is to be stationary, i.e. to retain the same statistical properties throughout time, the coefficient ρ must lie between -1 and $+1$. If the variance of Y_t is σ^2, the variance of ε_t will be $\sigma^2(1 - \rho^2)$. The correlation between adjacent values of Y_t is ρ and that between values separated by a lag of k time units is ρ^k. Thus, values of ρ near $+1$ lead to series in which observations at neighbouring points of time tend to be close together, while longer stretches of the series exhibit wandering characteristics. This type of behaviour illustrates the danger of applying standard statistical methods to different portions of a time series. With a high value of ρ, it would be quite easy to find two sets, each of, say, five adjacent observations, such that there was relatively little variation within each set, but quite a large difference between the two means. A two-sample t test might show a 'significant' difference, but the probability level would have no useful meaning because the assumption of independence which underlies the t test is invalid. This point is particularly important when the two sets differ in some specific feature, such as the occurrence of an intervention of some sort between the two time periods. A 'significant' difference cannot be ascribed to the effect of the intervention, since it may be merely a reflection of the structure of a time series which, in the long run, is stationary. In contrast, values of ρ near -1 show marked oscillation between neighbouring values, as was indicated as a possibility on p. 450.

The first-order process has been suggested by Wilson *et al.* (1981) as a representation of repeated blood pressure measurements taken at 5-min intervals. However, their analysis dealt only with short series, and it is not clear that the model would be appropriate for longer series. More general autoregressive series, with dependence on more than one preceding reading, were used by Marks (1982) in a study of the relations between different hormone levels in rats receiving hormone injections following oophorectomy. This paper illustrates the way in which autoregressive models, in which preceding values act as explanatory variables, can also incorporate other explanatory variables, such as the current or earlier values in other time series.

Another broad class of models is that of *moving-average* schemes. If x_1, x_2, x_3, etc., are independent random variables, the quantities

$$y_2 = \tfrac{1}{3}(x_1 + x_2 + x_3), \quad y_3 = \tfrac{1}{3}(x_2 + x_3 + x_4), \text{etc.},$$

are examples of simple moving averages. Note that y_2 and y_3 are correlated, because of the common terms x_2 and x_3, but y_2 and y_5 are not correlated, because they have no terms in common. The y_t series is a simple example of a moving-average scheme, more general schemes being obtainable by altering the number of xs in each y and also their weights. Although time series are not usually formed explicitly by taking simple moving averages, observed series may nevertheless be found to behave in a similar way, showing positive correlations between a short range of neighbouring observations. A wide variety of different models for time series may be obtained by combining autoregressive and moving-average features. For a discussion of some ways of distinguishing between different models, see Box and Jenkins (1976).

Reference was made earlier to the problem of monitoring time series of clinical and other measurements with a view to the detection of changes in the statistical pattern. Most medical applications have adapted methods derived from industrial quality control, in which observations are usually assumed to vary independently. Thus, Weatherall and Haskey (1976) describe methods for monitoring the incidence of congenital malformations, using quality control charts designed to detect outlying readings, and cumulative sum (cusum) methods designed to detect changes in the mean incidence rate. In this application the random variation may be assumed to follow the Poisson distribution. Rowlands *et al.* (1983) describe the application of similar methods to control data used in routine radioimmunoassays of progesterone. In many situations the assumption of serial independence will not be valid. Smith *et al.* (1983) and Trimble *et al.* (1983) describe a Bayesian approach to the monitoring of plasma creatinine values in individual patients following a kidney transplant. By formulating a specific model for their data, they provide posterior probabilities that, at any stage, the process is in a state of steady evolution, that there has been a change in the level of response, or in the slope, or that the current observation is an outlier.

The frequency domain

In this approach the time series is decomposed into a number of periodic components of a sinusoidal form, as in the periodic regression model of §12.4. Inferences are then made about the amplitudes of waves of different frequencies. The first approach to be discussed here, harmonic analysis, is concerned with periodic fluctuations with predetermined frequencies. The second approach, spectral analysis, allows the whole frequency band to be studied simultaneously.

Harmonic analysis

If k observations are available at equally spaced points of time, the whole set of data can be reproduced exactly in terms of k parameters, namely, one parameter for the general mean and $k - 1$ parameters representing the amplitude and phase of a series of sinusoidal curves. If k is odd, there will be $\frac{1}{2}(k - 1)$ of these components; if k is even, there will be $\frac{1}{2}k$ components, one of which has a predetermined phase. The periods of these components are (in terms of the time interval between observations) $k, k/2, k/3, k/4$, and so on. If the observations are supposed to follow a trend with less than the full set of parameters, and if the random variance is known or can be estimated, the amplitudes of different components can be tested for significance, so that simple models with fewer parameters can be regarded as providing an adequate description of the data.

Example 12.7

Pocock (1974) describes a harmonic analysis of a 5-year series of weekly records of sickness absence in an industrial concern. There were $k = 261$ weekly observations. Periods of $261/j$ will be fractions of a year if j is a multiple of 5 ($j = 5$ being a complete year). Collectively, therefore, these frequencies represent a 'seasonal' trend, repeated in each of the 5 years. Other frequencies with significant amplitudes represent significant departures from the overall seasonal pattern in particular years. Significance tests can be carried out on the plausible assumption that random variation follows a Poisson distribution, the variance of which can be estimated by the overall mean. In Fig. 12.11, the irregular line shows the seasonal trend, composed of 26 frequencies. The smooth curve

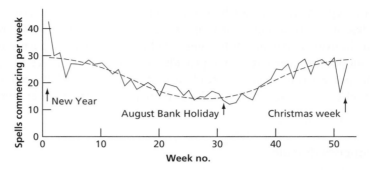

Fig. 12.11 The estimated seasonal trend in weekly spells of sickness absence (1960–64) (reproduced from Pocock, 1974, with permission from the author and publishers).

is a single sinusoidal curve with a period of 1 year. A comparison of the two curves shows that the seasonal trend is nearly sinusoidal, but that there are clear departures from the simple curve, particularly at annual holiday periods.

Spectral analysis

Here the time series is effectively decomposed into an infinite number of periodic components, each of infinitesimal amplitude, so the purpose of the analysis is to estimate the contributions of components in certain ranges of frequency. A spectral analysis may show that contributions to the fluctuations in the time series come from a continuous range of frequencies, and the pattern of spectral densities may suggest a particular time-domain representation. Or the spectral analysis may suggest one or two dominant frequencies, leading to a subsequent harmonic analysis. A further possibility is that the spectrum may be a mixture of discrete and continuous components, as, for example, in a time series in which a harmonic term is combined with an autoregressive error term.

Various features of a spectral decomposition may provide useful summary statistics for a time series. Gevins (1980), for instance, reviews a considerable body of work in which spectral analyses of series of human brain electrical potentials have been used to discriminate between different clinical states or as a basis for various forms of pattern recognition and cluster analysis.

13 Multivariate methods

13.1 General

In multiple regression each individual provides observations simultaneously on several variables; thus the data are *multivariate*. Yet only one of these, the dependent variable, is regarded as a random variable and the purpose of the analysis is to explain as much as possible of the variation in this dependent variable in terms of the multiple predictor variables. Multiple regression is, therefore, an extension of the other methods considered so far in this book and essentially involves no new concepts beyond those introduced in Chapter 7 for a simple linear regression with just one independent variable. The function of the predictor variables in multiple regression is to classify the individual in a way which is rather similar to the qualitative classifications in an experimental design.

Multivariate analysis is a collection of techniques appropriate for the situation in which the random variation in several variables has to be studied simultaneously. The subject is extensive and is treated in several textbooks; there are useful introductory texts by Chatfield and Collins (1980), Krzanowski and Marriott (1994, 1995) and Manly (1994), and a more advanced text by Mardia *et al.* (1979). The subject cannot be explored in detail in the present book, but this chapter contains a brief survey of some methods which have been found useful in medical research.

A general point to note is that tests of significance play a much less important role in multivariate analysis than in univariate analysis. As noted in comment **3** on p. 90, a univariate significance test is often useful as giving an immediate indication of the likely direction of any departure from the null hypothesis. With multivariate data, no such simple interpretation is possible. If, for instance, a significance test shows that two multivariate samples are unlikely to come from the same population, it may not be at all obvious in what respect they differ— whether, for instance, there are clear differences for each of the component variates, or for only some of them. The main emphasis in the methods to be described below is therefore on estimation—that is, on the attempt to describe the nature of the data structure. Nevertheless, significance tests sometimes play a modest role, particularly in preliminary analyses of data before more searching methods are applied, and we shall describe a few of the more useful techniques.

13.2 **Principal components**

Often observations are made on a medium or large number of separate variables on each individual, even though the number of different characteristics it is required to determine of the individuals is much less. For example, on p. 14, part of a questionnaire is given in which six different questions are asked about stress or worry. The purpose of these separate questions may be to obtain information on an individual's overall stress or worry, with no particular interest in what has contributed to the stress. The separate questions are asked only because no single question would be adequate. In some cases sufficient may be known of the field of application to allow a combined variable or score to be calculated; for example, the answers to the six stress questions considered above could be combined by averaging to give a single variable, 'stress'. In other cases some analysis is required to determine which variables might be sensibly combined.

Suppose we have observations on p variables, $x_1, x_2, \ldots, x_p$, made on each of n individuals. We could ask whether it is possible to combine these variables into a small number of other variables which could provide almost all the information about the way in which one individual differed from another. One way of expressing this is to define new variables,

$$
\begin{aligned}
y_1 &= a_{11}x_1 + a_{12}x_2 + \ldots + a_{1p}x_p, \\
y_2 &= a_{21}x_1 + a_{22}x_2 + \ldots + a_{2p}x_p,
\end{aligned}
\tag{13.1}
$$

etc., so that y_1 has the highest possible variance and so represents better than any other linear combination of the xs the general differences between individuals. (If no restrictions are placed on the a_{ij}s, this is a pointless requirement, since larger values will lead to a larger variance of y_1; we therefore standardize their general magnitude by requiring that $\sum_{j=1}^{p} a_{ij}^2 = 1$.) Then we could choose y_2 such that it is uncorrelated with y_1 and has the next largest variance; and so on. If $p = 3$, the individual observations can be visualized as a three-dimensional scatter diagram with n points, perhaps clustered in the shape of an airship. The first *principal component*, y_1, will represent distances along the length of the airship. The second component, y_2, represents distances along the widest direction perpendicular to the length (say, side to side); the third and last component, y_3, will then represent distances from top to bottom of the airship. There are, in general, p principal components, but the variation of all but a few may be quite small. If, in the previous example, the airship were very flat, almost like a disc, y_3 would show very little variation, and an individual's position in the whole diagram would be determined almost exactly by y_1 and y_2.

The method of analysis involves the calculation of *eigenvalues* or *latent roots* of the covariance or correlation matrix. There are p eigenvalues:

$$
\lambda_1 \geq \lambda_2 \geq \lambda_3 \geq \ldots \geq \lambda_p.
$$

With each eigenvalue there is an associated component, y_i, and

$$\lambda_i = \text{var}(y_i).$$

Defining the total variability as the sum of the variances of the x_i,

$$\sum \text{var}(x_i) = \sum \text{var}(y_i) = \sum \lambda_i.$$

An important point is that if the scale of measurement for any variable is changed, even by a multiplying factor, all the results are changed. This problem may be avoided by working with the covariance matrix of the logarithms of the original variables, but it is more usual to standardize each variable initially by dividing by its standard deviation; this is equivalent to working with the correlation matrix. Since the standardized variables each have a variance of unity,

$$\lambda_1 + \lambda_2 + \ldots + \lambda_p = p.$$

The first principal component accounts for a proportion λ_1/p of the total variation, the second for a proportion λ_2/p of the total variation, etc.

The complete set of principal components is a rotation of the original axes and has not introduced any economy in describing the data. This economy is introduced if the first few components account for a high proportion of the total variation and the remaining variation is ignored. Then the data are described in fewer than p components.

The interpretation of any of the components, the jth, say, defined by (13.1) involves consideration of the relative values of the coefficients a_{ij} for that component. If all the coefficients were about equal, then the component could be interpreted as an average of all the variables. If some of the coefficients were small, then the corresponding variables could be ignored and the component interpreted in terms of a subset of the original variables. The application of the method will only have produced a useful reduction in the dimensionality of the data if the components have an interpretation that appears to represent some meaningful characteristics. Thus, interpretation is to some extent subjective and involves knowledge of the field of application.

Since interpretation of the components is in terms of the original variables, it is informative to assess the contribution of each variable to a component in terms of the correlations of the original variables with the component, rather than in terms of the coefficients a_{ij}. For principal components calculated from the correlation matrix these correlations are obtained by multiplying each component by the square root of the corresponding eigenvalue, that is,

$$b_{ij} = a_{ij}\sqrt{\lambda_i}.$$

Then the b_{ij} are termed the *component correlations* or *loadings*, although the latter term is sometimes used for the coefficients of (13.1), and $b_{ij} = \text{correlation}\,(y_i, x_j)$.

High loadings, say, 0·5 or higher, indicate those variables with which a component is correlated and hence are used to guide the interpretation of that component.

Another aspect of the analysis is the choice of the number of components to include. Whilst various methods have been suggested, there is no universally accepted method and the decision is usually made with the interpretation of the components in mind, and the total amount of variability that may be explained. The following criteria may be used:

1   Plot the eigenvalues, λ_i against i; this plot is termed a *scree plot*. The eigenvalues decrease with i, but the shape of the plot may be steep for a few values, which may correspond to useful components, before a more gradual decline as the scree plot tails off.

2   Account for a reasonably high proportion of total variability, say, greater than 50%, but do not choose eigenvalues less than 1 since these account for less than the average of all p values.

3   Select only components that are interpretable in terms of the situation under analysis. It is seldom worth including an extra component if that component cannot be given a meaningful interpretation.

Once a decision has been made on the number of components to include, the data have effectively been reduced to that number of dimensions; for example, if two components are accepted, then the observations are regarded as lying in two-dimensional space and the remaining $p - 2$ dimensions of the original variables are ignored. A point in two-dimensional space is represented by two coordinates with respect to two axes; using the representation (13.1), the point would be (y_1, y_2). There are, however, many ways of constructing the axes. Restricting attention to orthogonal axes, that is, axes at right angles to one another, the pair of axes could be rotated together about the origin and would remain an orthogonal pair of axes. The coordinates of a point would change, to (y'_1, y'_2), say, but the geometrical configuration of the points would be unaltered. Corresponding to (13.1), we should have

$$y'_1 = a'_{11}x_1 + a'_{12}x_2 + \ldots + a'_{1p}x_p,$$
$$y'_2 = a'_{21}x_1 + a'_{22}x_2 + \ldots + a'_{2p}x_p,$$

(13.2)

etc. If a rotation could be found so that the components defined in (13.2) were more readily interpretable than those of (13.1), then the analysis would be improved. Several criteria for choosing a rotation have been suggested but the most widely used is the *varimax* method. In this method the aim is that for each component, the coefficients should divide into two groups, with those in one group as large as possible and those in the other as near zero as possible. That is, each component is expressed in terms of a subset of the original variables with the minimum contamination from variables not in the subset. The rotated components are no longer principal and the relationship between the coefficients of (13.2) and the component correlations is more complicated than for principal components. Provided that the components are scaled to have unit variance before the rotation procedure is applied, then the rotated components are uncorrelated with one another.

Equation (13.1) or (13.2) can be used to assign values to each component for each individual. These values are termed the *component scores* and can be used in further steps of the analysis instead of the full set of x variables. Sometimes, for example, the component scores are used as a reduced set of independent variables in a regression analysis of some other variables not considered in the principal component analysis.

Example 13.1

Cockcroft *et al.* (1982) recorded answers to 20 questions designed to characterize patients with chronic respiratory disability in a clinical trial according to the influence of their illness on everyday living. The answers were recorded by marking a line joining two opposite statements (this is called a *visual analogue scale*) and analysed after a transformation of the proportional distance of the mark from one end of the line. The correlation matrix of the variables is given in Table 13.1; an abbreviated version of the statement at the favourable end of each line is also shown.

The first eigenvalue was 5·97, the second 3·42, followed by 1·99, 1·36, 1·31 and 1·14, and the remaining 14 eigenvalues were all less than 1. The first principal component accounts for 29·9% of the total variation in the 20 variables, the second for 17·1%, the third for 10·0%, the fourth for 6·8%, the fifth for 6·5% and the sixth for 5·7%, whilst the remaining 14 components account for 24% of the total variation. A scree plot of the values is shown in Fig. 13.1. This plot suggests that the first three eigenvalues represent meaningful variation. They account for 57% of the variability and, whilst there are three more

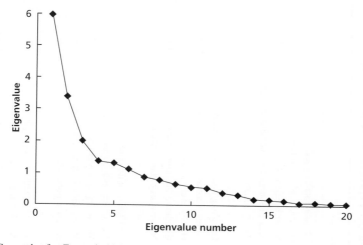

Fig. 13.1 Scree plot for Example 13.1.

Table 13.1 Correlation matrix of 20 variables.

Variable	1	2	3	4	5	6	7	8	9
1 Physical health good									
2 Optimistic about future	0.17								
3 Never breathless	0.44	0.05							
4 Breathlessness does not distress me	0.35	0.14	0.40						
5 Rarely cough	0.45	0.02	0.37	0.36					
6 Coughing does not trouble me	0.35	0.07	0.37	0.42	0.92				
7 Never wheezy	0.44	0.07	0.55	0.42	0.61	0.64			
8 Hardly ever feel ill	0.64	0.23	0.37	0.67	0.55	0.59	0.57		
9 Condition has improved	0.42	-0.13	0.34	0.35	0.70	0.67	0.56	0.45	
10 Never worry about future	-0.06	0.46	0.11	0.42	0.04	0.11	-0.14	0.10	-0.12
11 Confident could cope	0.16	0.33	0.21	0.49	0.27	0.30	0.03	0.29	0.00
12 Health depends on me	0.23	0.31	0.18	0.15	-0.08	0.08	0.27	0.23	-0.17
13 Worth trying anything	0.06	0.23	-0.04	0.13	0.06	0.10	-0.04	0.01	0.11
14 Wife happy with my condition	0.41	-0.06	0.29	0.38	0.44	0.46	0.62	0.37	0.68
15 Feel like going out	-0.09	0.03	-0.38	-0.01	-0.18	-0.10	-0.44	-0.18	-0.17
16 Relaxing with other people	0.10	0.15	0.22	0.09	-0.12	-0.05	-0.06	-0.07	-0.08
17 Support the family	0.38	0.16	0.24	0.28	0.52	0.46	0.38	0.46	0.52
18 Making a useful contribution	0.39	0.33	0.26	0.31	0.13	0.13	0.12	0.48	0.01
19 Accept my condition	0.37	0.36	0.45	0.56	0.08	0.10	0.34	0.46	0.07
20 Feel happy	-0.02	0.61	-0.29	0.02	-0.27	-0.26	-0.22	0.05	-0.32

Table 13.1 (cont.)

Variable	10	11	12	13	14	15	16	17	18	19
1 Physical health good										
2 Optimistic about future										
3 Never breathless										
4 Breathlessness does not distress me										
5 Rarely cough										
6 Coughing does not trouble me										
7 Never wheezy										
8 Hardly ever feel ill										
9 Condition has improved										
10 Never worry about future										
11 Confident could cope	0·71									
12 Health depends on me	0·26	0·46								
13 Worth trying anything	0·32	0·21	−0·02							
14 Wife happy with my condition	0·01	0·11	0·20	−0·11						
15 Feel like going out	0·12	−0·02	−0·20	0·31	−0·29					
16 Relaxing with other people	0·24	0·15	−0·01	0·59	−0·07	0·50				
17 Support the family	0·03	0·04	−0·03	0·03	0·43	−0·13	−0·09			
18 Making a useful contribution	0·21	0·63	0·50	0·09	0·05	−0·18	0·05	0·09		
19 Accept my condition	0·52	0·27	0·17	0·08	0·30	−0·26	0·22	0·25	0·23	
20 Feel happy	0·28	0·18	0·04	−0·03	−0·23	0·20	0·07	−0·11	0·18	0·27

eigenvalues exceeding 1, they lie in the tail of the scree plot. Most importantly, when three components were fitted, there was a clear interpretation, but adding another component did not give a fourth interpretable component. Accordingly, three components were retained.

In Table 13.2 the first three components are given. The variables have been reordered, and component correlations exceeding 0·5 are given in bold type, to show the main features of each component. The first component is correlated more with variables 1, 3, 4, 5, 6, 7, 8, 9, 14 and 17, and may be interpreted as 'physical health'. The second component is correlated with variables 2, 10, 11, 12, 18, 19 and 20, and may be interpreted as 'optimism'. The third component is correlated with variables 13, 15 and 16, and may be interpreted as 'socializing'. The identification of the components in terms of the original variables is clearer for the rotated components. These three components accounted for 57% of the total variation and, since no clear interpretation was made of the next component, attention was restricted to these three.

In the above example the dimensionality of the data was reduced from 20 to 3 by the use of principal component analysis. It would appear that the method was highly effective. However, the original questions were chosen to represent a few characteristics and, before the data were collected, groupings of the questions

Table 13.2 Component correlations (loadings) for the first three principal components.

Variable	Component			Rotated component		
	1	2	3	1	2	3
1 Physical health good	**0·67**	0·02	−0·01	**0·59**	0·32	−0·07
3 Never breathless	**0·63**	−0·02	−0·08	**0·55**	0·28	−0·14
4 Breathlessness does not distress me	**0·69**	0·28	0·10	**0·53**	**0·51**	0·13
5 Rarely cough	**0·76**	−0·31	0·24	**0·86**	0·00	0·04
6 Coughing does not trouble me	**0·77**	−0·23	0·26	**0·84**	0·07	0·08
7 Never wheezy	**0·77**	−0·29	−0·12	**0·77**	0·13	−0·29
8 Hardly ever feel ill	**0·81**	0·08	−0·08	**0·67**	0·45	−0·12
9 Condition has improved	**0·68**	−0·47	0·30	**0·86**	−0·19	0·04
14 Wife happy with my condition	**0·66**	−0·29	−0·04	**0·69**	0·06	−0·21
17 Support the family	**0·59**	−0·19	0·13	**0·63**	0·06	0·00
2 Optimistic about future	0·22	**0·66**	−0·08	−0·07	**0·68**	0·15
10 Never worry about future	0·23	**0·74**	0·14	−0·04	**0·69**	0·38
11 Confident could cope	0·43	**0·64**	−0·04	0·13	**0·75**	0·16
12 Health depends on me	0·29	0·41	−0·47	−0·01	**0·61**	−0·31
18 Making a useful contribution	0·43	0·49	−0·32	0·12	**0·70**	−0·15
19 Accept my condition	**0·52**	0·44	−0·13	0·27	**0·64**	0·10
20 Feel happy	−0·14	**0·61**	−0·15	−0·40	**0·50**	0·00
13 Worth trying anything	0·09	0·37	**0·68**	0·10	0·15	**0·76**
15 Feel like going out	−0·33	0·27	**0·68**	−0·23	−0·12	**0·76**
16 Relaxing with other people	0·01	0·43	**0·64**	0·00	0·18	**0·75**

were perceived that were similar to those of the components extracted. Although it may be argued that the weights, a_{ij}, of the different variables in the components (13.1) are optimum, this may only be so for the particular data set. Quantitatively, the components are not necessarily generalizable outside the data set, even though qualitatively they may be. For the sake of wider generalizability and standardization among research workers it may be preferable to choose equal weights in each component after verifying that the subsets of variables defining each component are reasonable.

Factor analysis

This method has been used extensively by psychologists. It is closely related to principal component analysis, but differs in that it assumes a definite model for the way in which the observed variables, x_i, are influenced by certain hypothetical underlying factors. Suppose the xs are educational tests applied to children and that each test reflects to a differing extent certain factors—for example, general intelligence, verbal facility, arithmetical ability, speed of working, etc. Imagine that each individual has a certain value for each of these common factors, $f_1, f_2, f_3, \ldots$, which are uncorrelated, but that these cannot be measured directly. The factor-analysis model is

$$x_1 = b_{11} f_1 + b_{12} f_2 + b_{13} f_3 + \ldots + \mu_1 + \varepsilon_1,$$
$$x_2 = b_{21} f_1 + b_{22} f_2 + b_{23} f_3 + \ldots + \mu_2 + \varepsilon_2,$$

(13.3)

etc. Here μ_i is the mean of x_i and ε_i is the residual specific to the ith test after taking account of the contributions of the factors. The values of the factors, $f_1, f_2, f_3, \ldots$, vary from one subject to another, but have zero mean and unit variance, and are assumed to be uncorrelated with one another and with the residuals. The quantities b_{ij} are constants, like regression coefficients, indicating how much each test is affected by each factor. The b_{ij} are referred to as the *factor loadings*; where the x_i are standardized to zero mean and unit variance, then the factor loading b_{ij} is the correlation between the ith test and the jth factor. The variance in x_i that is explained by the factor model (13.3) is called the *communality*; for standardized x_i the communality is the proportion of variance explained.

The factor loadings, the communalities and the number of factors required have to be estimated from the data, usually from the sample correlation matrix. Of course, multiple regression methods cannot be used because the values of the fs are unknown. A good general account is that of Lawley and Maxwell (1971). If the basic model can be justified on psychological grounds, a factor analysis may be expected to throw some light on the number of factors apparently affecting the test scores and to show which tests are closely related to particular factors.

The place of factor analysis in other scientific fields is very doubtful. It is often used in situations for which simpler multivariate methods, with fewer assumptions, would be more appropriate. For example, the interpretation placed on the factor loadings is usually very similar to that placed on the coefficients of the first few principal components.

13.3 **Discriminant analysis**

Suppose there are k groups of individuals, with n_i individuals in the ith group, and that on each individual we measure p variables, $x_1, x_2, \ldots, x_p$. A rule is required for discriminating between the groups, so that, for any new individual known to come from one of the groups (the particular group being unknown), the rule could be applied and the individual assigned to the most appropriate group. This situation might arise in taxonomic studies, the xs being physical measurements and the groups being species. The rule would then allocate a new individual to one or other of the species on the basis of its physical characteristics. Another example might arise in differential diagnosis. Observations would be made on patients known to fall into particular diagnostic groups. The object would be to obtain a rule for allotting a new patient to one of these groups by measuring the same variables. In each of these examples, and in all applications of discriminant functions, the original classification into groups must be made independently of the x variables. In the diagnostic situation, for example, the patients' diagnoses may be determined by authoritative but arduous procedures, and one may wish to see how reliably the same diagnoses can be reached by using variables (the xs) which are cheaper or less harrowing for the patient. Alternatively, the correct diagnoses may have become available only after the lapse of time, and one may wish to determine these as far as possible by variables measurable at a much earlier stage of the disease.

Consider first the situation with $k = 2$, denoting the two groups by A and B. We shall approach this problem from three different points of view, all of which we shall find leading to the same solution.

(a) *Fisher's linear discriminant function*

Suppose we look for a linear function

$$z = b_1 x_1 + b_2 x_2 + \ldots + b_p x_p. \tag{13.4}$$

If this is going to discriminate well between the groups we should expect the mean values of z in the two groups to be reasonably far apart in comparison with the variation of z within groups. We could, therefore, try to find values of the bs such that the ratio

$$D^2 = \frac{(\bar{z}_A - \bar{z}_B)^2}{\text{variance of } z \text{ within groups}} \tag{13.5}$$

is as large as possible. The estimated variance of z will, in general, be different in the two groups, but a pooled estimate could be calculated as in the two-sample t test.

The solution of this problem is as follows:

1 Calculate the pooled sums of squares and products of the xs within groups, divide by $n_A + n_B - 2$ to obtain the matrix of within-group variances and covariances, and obtain the inverse matrix with general term c_{ij}. Here, n_A and n_B are the numbers of individuals in groups A and B, respectively.

2 Calculate the bs as follows:

$$b_1 = c_{11}(\bar{x}_{A1} - \bar{x}_{B1}) + c_{12}(\bar{x}_{A2} - \bar{x}_{B2}) + \ldots + c_{1p}(\bar{x}_{Ap} - \bar{x}_{Bp})$$
$$b_2 = c_{21}(\bar{x}_{A1} - \bar{x}_{B1}) + c_{22}(\bar{x}_{A2} - \bar{x}_{B2}) + \ldots + c_{2p}(\bar{x}_{Ap} - \bar{x}_{Bp})$$
$$\cdot$$
$$\cdot \tag{13.6}$$
$$\cdot$$
$$b_p = c_{p1}(\bar{x}_{A1} - \bar{x}_{B1}) + c_{p2}(\bar{x}_{A2} - \bar{x}_{B2}) + \ldots + c_{pp}(\bar{x}_{Ap} - \bar{x}_{Bp}).$$

Here, $\bar{x}_{Ai}$ is the mean of x_i in group A and so on.

To use (13.4) for allocating future individuals to one of the two groups we need an end-point, or cut-point, to discriminate between A and B. A completely symmetrical rule would be to use the mean, z_0, of $\bar{z}_A$ and $\bar{z}_B$. From (13.4),

$$\bar{z}_A = b_1\bar{x}_{A1} + b_2\bar{x}_{A2} + \ldots + b_p\bar{x}_{Ap}$$

and $\tag{13.7}$

$$\bar{z}_B = b_1\bar{x}_{B1} + b_2\bar{x}_{B2} + \ldots + b_p\bar{x}_{Bp},$$

whence

$$z_0 = b_1\left(\frac{\bar{x}_{A1} + \bar{x}_{B1}}{2}\right) + b_2\left(\frac{\bar{x}_{A2} + \bar{x}_{B2}}{2}\right) + \ldots + b_p\left(\frac{\bar{x}_{Ap} + \bar{x}_{Bp}}{2}\right). \tag{13.8}$$

If $\bar{z}_A > \bar{z}_B$ the allocation rule is: allocate an individual to A if $z > z_0$ and to B if $z < z_0$. Many computer programs calculate the value of z for each individual in the two original samples. It is thus possible to count how many individuals in the two groups would have been wrongly classified by the allocation rule. This unfortunately gives an overoptimistic picture, because the allocation rule has been determined to be the best (in a certain sense) for these two particular samples, and it is likely to perform rather less well on the average with subsequent observations from the two groups (see Hills, 1966).

Various methods have been proposed to overcome this problem (Krzanowski & Marriott, 1995, §§9.32–9.44). One method is to split the sample randomly into two subsamples. The first subsample, the *training* sample, is used to estimate the allocation rule, and the misclassification rate is then estimated by applying this rule to the second subsample, the *test* sample. This method is inefficient in the use of the data and is only feasible with large samples. However, the concept behind this method can be exploited through use of the jackknife or bootstrap (§10.7). With the bootstrap method a sample is drawn from the original sample with replacement. The allocation rule is estimated from the bootstrap sample and two misclassification rates are established. The first is the misclassification rate when the allocation rule is applied to the original sample, and the second when the rule is applied to the bootstrap sample. The difference between these two rates is an estimate of the bias through using the same sample to estimate both the allocation rule and the misclassification rate. Repeating this process over B boostrap samples gives an accurate estimate of the bias, and this is then subtracted from the misclassification rate, obtained by applying the allocation rule estimated from the original sample to the original sample, to give a corrected estimate. This is a computer-intensive method, since it involves repeating the whole estimation process sufficient times to estimate the bias accurately.

The allocation rule based on z_0 is intended to get close to minimizing the sum of two probabilities of misclassification—that of allocating an A individual to group B, and that of allocating a B individual to group A. Two situations lead to some modifications. In the first, suppose that the individuals come from a population in which it is known, from past experience, that the proportion in category A, p_A, is different from that in category B, $p_B(= 1 - p_A)$. Then it would be reasonable to take account of this by moving the cut-point to increase the probability of allocation to the group with the higher prior probability. This is a situation where Bayes' theorem (§3.3) may be applied to adjust the prior probabilities, using the observations on an individual to obtain posterior probabilities. If this approach is taken, then the cut-point would be increased by $\ln(p_B/p_A)$, again assuming $\bar{z}_A > \bar{z}_B$ (otherwise the cut-point would be decreased). Secondly, the consequences of misclassification might not be symmetric. In diagnostic screening (see §19.12), for example, the consequences of missing a case of disease (false negative) might be more serious than wrongly classifying a disease-free individual to the disease category (false positive). In the former case, treatment may be delayed by several months and the prognosis be much poorer, whilst in the latter the individual may only experience the inconvenience of attending for more tests before being classified as disease-free. If the consequences of the two types of misclassification can be given a score, then the aim of the discrimination would be to minimize the expected value of this score for each individual. Often the scores are called costs, but this terminology does not imply that the scores need to be expressible in monetary terms. If c_A is the penalty for failing to classify an A individual into group A, and c_B is similarly defined, then the cut-point should be increased by $\ln(c_B/c_A)$. Thus only the ratio of the two penalties is required.

Another way of assessing the effectiveness of the discrimination is to calculate the ratio D^2 from (13.5). Its square root, D, is called the *generalized distance*, or *Mahalanobis distance*, between the two groups. If D is greater than about 4, the situation is like that in two univariate distributions whose means differ by more than 4 standard deviations: the overlap is quite small, and the probabilities of misclassification are correspondingly small. An alternative formula for D^2, equivalent to (13.5), is:

$$D^2 = \sum b_i (\bar{x}_{Ai} - \bar{x}_{Bi}). \tag{13.9}$$

(b) *Likelihood rule*

If there were only one variable, x, following a continuous distribution in each group, it would be natural to allocate an individual to the group which gave the higher probability density for the observed value of x; another way of expressing this is to say that the allocation is to the group with the higher likelihood. If there are several xs, we cannot easily depict the probability density, but given the mathematical form of the distribution of the xs this density, or likelihood, can be calculated. One particular form of distribution is called the *multivariate normal distribution*; it implies, among other things, that each x separately follows a normal distribution and that all regressions of one variable on any set of other variables are linear. If the xs followed multivariate normal distributions with the same variances and correlations for group A as for group B, but with different means, the ratio of the likelihoods of A and B would be found to depend on a linear function

$$z = \beta_1 x_1 + \beta_2 x_2 + \ldots + \beta_p x_p,$$

and the βs would be estimated from the two initial samples precisely by the bs, as calculated in (a). The rule described above, in which the allocation is to A or B according to whether $z > z_0$ or $z < z_0$, is equivalent to asking which of the two groups is estimated to have the higher likelihood.

In practice, of course, multivariate distributions are not normal, and are perhaps less likely to be nearly normal than are univariate distributions. Nevertheless, the discriminant function (13.4) is likely to be a good indication of the relative likelihoods of the two groups.

(c) *Regression with a dummy dependent variable*

Suppose we define a variable y which takes the value 1 in group A and 0 in group B. Putting all the observations into one group, we could do the multiple regression of y on $x_1, x_2, \ldots, x_p$. This would give a linear function of the xs which would predict the observed values of y as well as possible. If the multiple correlation coefficient is reasonably high, the predicted values of y for groups A and B should therefore be rather well separated (clustering near the observed values of 1 and 0). The estimated regression function can be shown to be (apart from a constant factor) the same as the linear discriminant function obtained by method (a). This is a useful identity, since method (c) can be carried out on a computer with a multiple regression program, whereas method (a) requires a special program.

A further advantage of the regression approach is that the usual variance ratio test for the significance of the multiple regression can also be interpreted as a valid test for the discriminant function. The null hypothesis is that, in the two groups from which the samples are drawn, the xs have exactly the same joint distribution; in that case, of course, no discrimination is possible. Furthermore, the usual t tests for the partial regression coefficients give a useful indication of the importance of particular variables in the discrimination.

Although multiple regression provides a useful way of calculating the discriminant function, it is important to realize that the usual model for multiple regression is no longer valid. Usually, in multiple regression, y is a random continuous variable and the xs are arbitrary variables. In the present problem the xs are random variables and y is an arbitrary score characterizing the two groups. A related point is that the average value of y for a particular set of xs should not be interpreted as the probability that an individual with these xs falls in group A rather than in group B; if the regression equation were interpreted in this way, it might lead to some predicted probabilities greater than 1 or less than 0.

The usual analysis of variance of y corresponding to the multiple regression analysis provides a useful method of estimating the generalized distance, D:

$$D^2 = \frac{(n_A + n_B)(n_A + n_B - 2)}{n_A n_B} \times \frac{\text{SSq due to regression}}{\text{SSq about regression}}. \tag{13.10}$$

Computer programs for the whole calculation are widely available and, as for all multivariate methods, the availability of appropriate software is generally essential. However, to illustrate the method, an example with two variables will be worked through.

Example 13.2

The data shown in Table 13.3 relate to 79 infants affected by haemolytic disease of the newborn, of whom 63 survived and 16 died. For each infant there are recorded the cord haemoglobin concentration, x (measured in g/100 ml) and the bilirubin concentration, y (mg/100 ml). It is required to predict by means of these two measurements whether any particular infant is more likely to die or to survive.

Table 13.3 Concentration of haemoglobin and bilirubin for infants with haemolytic disease of the newborn (x, haemoglobin (g/100 ml); y, bilirubin (mg/100 ml)).

Survivals ($n = 63$)

x	y	x	y	x	y	x	y
18·7	2·2	15·8	3·7	14·3	3·3	11·8	4·5
17·8	2·7	15·8	3·0	14·1	3·7	11·6	3·7
17·8	2·5	15·8	1·7	14·0	5·8	10·9	3·5
17·6	4·1	15·6	1·4	13·9	2·9	10·9	4·1
17·6	3·2	15·6	2·0	13·8	3·7	10·9	1·5
17·6	1·0	15·6	1·6	13·6	2·3	10·8	3·3
17·5	1·6	15·4	4·1	13·5	2·1	10·6	3·4
17·4	1·8	15·4	2·2	13·4	2·3	10·5	6·3
17·4	2·4	15·3	2·0	13·3	1·8	10·2	3·3
17·0	0·4	15·1	3·2	12·5	4·5	9·9	4·0
17·0	1·6	14·8	1·8	12·3	5·0	9·8	4·2
16·6	3·6	14·7	3·7	12·2	3·5	9·7	4·9
16·3	4·1	14·7	3·0	12·2	2·4	8·7	5·5
16·1	2·0	14·6	5·0	12·0	2·8	7·4	3·0
16·0	2·6	14·3	3·8	12·0	3·5	5·7	4·6
16·0	0·8	14·3	4·2	11·8	2·3		
						875·5	194·7

Deaths ($n = 16$)

x	y	x	y
15·8	1·8	7·1	5·6
12·3	5·6	6·7	5·9
9·5	3·6	5·7	6·2
9·4	3·8	5·5	4·8
9·2	5·6	5·3	4·8
8·8	5·6	5·3	2·8
7·6	4·7	5·1	5·8
7·4	6·8	3·4	3·9
		124·1	77·3

Sums of squares and products within groups

	S_{xx}	S_{xy}	S_{yy}
Survivals	500·6593	−108·4219	96·6943
Deaths	143·3794	−21·3281	26·9744
Pooled	644·0387	−129·7500	123·6687
Var./cov.	8·3641	−1·6851	1·6061

We follow method (a). The within-groups covariance matrix and its inverse are

$$\begin{pmatrix} 8\cdot3641 & -1\cdot6851 \\ -1\cdot6851 & 1\cdot6061 \end{pmatrix}$$

and

$$\begin{pmatrix} 0\cdot151602 & 0\cdot159057 \\ 0\cdot159057 & 0\cdot789510 \end{pmatrix}.$$

The means, and their differences and means, are

	$\bar{x}$	$\bar{y}$
Survivals (S)	13·897	3·090
Deaths (D)	7·756	4·831
Difference, S − D	6·141	−1·741
Mean, $\frac{1}{2}$(S + D)	10·827	3·961

From (13.6),

$$b_1 = (0\cdot151602)(6\cdot141) + (0\cdot159057)(-1\cdot741) = 0\cdot6541$$

$$b_2 = (0\cdot159057)(6\cdot141) + (0\cdot789510)(-1\cdot741) = -0\cdot3978.$$

The discriminant function is

$$z = 0\cdot6541x - 0\cdot3978y. \tag{13.11}$$

From (13.8),

$$z_0 = (0\cdot6541)(10\cdot827) + (-0\cdot3978)(3\cdot961) = 5\cdot506.$$

The symmetric allocation rule would predict survival if $z > 5\cdot506$ and death if $z < 5\cdot506$.

The position is shown in Fig. 13.2, where the diagonal line represents critical points for which $z = z_0$. It is clear from Fig. 13.2 that discrimination by z is much better than by y alone, but hardly better than by x alone. This is confirmed by a count of the numbers of individuals misclassified by x alone (using a critical value of 10·83), by y alone (critical value 3·96) and by z:

Actual group	Group to which individual is allocated						
	By x		By y		By z		
	S	D	S	D	S	D	Total
S	53	10	47	16	54	9	63
D	2	14	5	11	2	14	16

It seems, therefore, that discrimination between deaths and survivals is improved little, if at all, by the use of bilirubin concentrations in addition to those of haemoglobin.

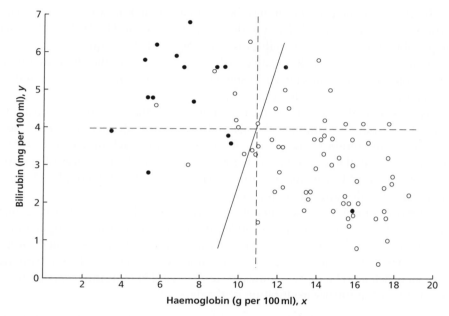

Fig. 13.2 Scatter diagram of haemoglobin and bilirubin values for infants with haemolytic disease (Table 13.3) showing a line of discrimination between deaths (•) and survivals (○).

To calculate D, we find, using (13.9),

$$D^2 = (0{\cdot}6541)(6{\cdot}141) + (-0{\cdot}3978)(-1{\cdot}741) = 4{\cdot}709,$$

and

$$D = \sqrt{4{\cdot}709} = 2{\cdot}17.$$

For two normal distributions with equal variance, separated by 2·17 standard deviations, the proportion of observations misclassified by the mid-point between the means would be the single tail area beyond a normal deviate of 1·085, which is 0·139. As it happens the proportion of misclassification by z is given above as $11/79 = 0{\cdot}139$, but the closeness of the agreement is fortuitous!

The reader with access to a multiple regression program is invited to analyse these data by method (c), using (13.10) as an alternative formula for D^2.

If the proportions of survivors and deaths in the sample were considered typical of the individuals to whom the discrimination rule would be applied in the future, then the cut-point would be increased by ln (16/63), i.e. by $-1{\cdot}371$, to 4·135. This would reduce the number of individuals misclassified in the sample to eight, but four of these would be deaths misclassified as survivors. If it were more important to classify probable deaths correctly, perhaps to give them more intensive care, then the cut-point would be increased and the number of deaths misclassified as survivors would be reduced at the expense of a larger increase in the number of survivors misclassified as deaths.

In the discussion so far it has been assumed that it was known which variables should be included in the discriminant function (13.4). Usually a set of possible discriminatory variables is available, and it is required to find the minimum number of such variables which contribute to the discrimination. Many computer programs include a stepwise procedure, similar to that in multiple regression (see p. 357), to achieve this.

The likelihood rule was derived assuming that the xs had a multivariate normal distribution. Although the method may prove adequate in some cases, when this assumption breaks down an alternative approach may be preferable. In particular, if the xs contain categorical variables, then the use of logistic regression (see §14.2) would be appropriate. The data of Example 13.2 are analysed using this approach on p. 492.

In most examples of discriminant analysis, there will be little point in testing the null hypothesis that the two samples are drawn from identical populations. The important question is *how* the populations differ. There are, though, some studies, particularly those in which two treatments are compared by multivariate data, in which a preliminary significance test is useful in indicating whether there is much point in further exploration of the data.

Multiple testing

Before discussing multivariate significance tests, we consider the problem in terms of multiple testing. Suppose each of the p variables is tested by a univariate method, such as a two-sample t test. Then some variables may differ significantly between groups whilst others may not. A difficulty in interpretation is that p tests have been carried out so that, even if the overall null hypothesis that none of the variables differ between groups is true, the probability of finding at least one significant difference is higher than the nominal significance level adopted. There are similarities with the multiple comparisons problem discussed in §8.4.

The Bonferroni procedure is sometimes used to correct for this. If p independent comparisons are carried out at a significance level of α', then the probability that one or more are significant is $1 - (1 - \alpha')^p$, and when α' is small this is approximately $p\alpha'$. Therefore setting $\alpha' = \alpha/p$ ensures that the probability of finding one or more significant effects does not exceed α. One problem with this method is that it takes no account of the multivariate correlations and it is conservative in the usual multivariate situation when the comparisons are not independent. A modification due to Simes (1986a) is to order the p values such that $P_{(1)} \leq P_{(2)} \leq \ldots \leq P_{(p)}$. Then the null hypothesis is rejected at level α if any $P_{(j)} \leq j\alpha/p$. This modification is more powerful than the Bonferroni procedure whilst still ensuring that the overall significance level does not exceed α for positively correlated variables (Sarkar & Chang, 1997)—that is, the test remains conservative.

The above considerations are in terms of controlling the *error rate per study*. If a set of variables represents an overall latent characteristic, such as a battery of tests designed to assess neuropsychological function, then this may be a reasonable thing to do. In other cases different characteristics may be examined within a single study, which may be regarded as a set of studies which have been combined for convenience and economy. Then it is not desirable to control the error rate of the whole study, since this would reduce the power for each characteristic according to other characteristics.

Hotelling's T² tests

Hotelling's two-sample T² statistic

Usually we are interested in possible differences in the mean values of the variates, and the appropriate test is based on Hotelling's two-sample T^2 statistic. This assumes that the data follow a multivariate normal distribution, but is reasonably robust against departures from normality.

Using the same notation as before, calculate

$$T^2 = \left(\frac{n_A\, n_B}{n_A + n_B}\right) D^2. \tag{13.12}$$

This is the square of the highest possible value of t that could be obtained in a two-sample t test for any linear combination of the p variables. If the null hypothesis is true,

$$\frac{(n_A + n_B - p - 1)}{(n_A + n_B - 2)p} T^2 \tag{13.13}$$

follows the F distribution on p and $n_A + n_B - p - 1$ degrees of freedom (DF). If $p = 1$, (13.13) reduces to the square of the usual t statistic.

In Example 13.2, there is no real point in carrying out a significance test, since Fig. 13.2 shows clearly that the two bivariate distributions differ significantly. However, as an illustration of the calculations, we have

$$T^2 = \left(\frac{63 \times 16}{79}\right) \times 4.709 = 60.08$$

and, since $p = 2$, $76T^2/(77 \times 2) = 29.65$ is referred to the F distribution on 2 and 76 DF, giving $P < 0.001$. The difference is highly significant, as expected. In most applications of Hotelling's T^2 test, it is useful to explore further any significant result by calculating the discriminant function to show the best way in which the variates combine to reveal the difference between the groups.

Paired data: Hotelling's one-sample T^2 statistics

In most problems of discrimination, particularly where the object is to obtain allocation rules, the individuals from the two populations will not be paired or matched in any way. However, in the related situations discussed earlier, where treatments are compared on multivariate data, the individual observations might well be paired. For example, two treatments might be administered on different occasions and several clinical responses observed for each treatment application, or, with a single treatment, observations might be made before and after the administration.

In studies of this type it is natural to work with the differences, either between two treatments or between the readings before and after treatment. Each subject will provide a multivariate set of differences, $d_1, d_2, \ldots, d_p$, and the natural questions to ask are: (i) is there any evidence that the expected values of the differences are other than zero? and (ii) if so, what is the nature of these effects?

The procedure is a simple variant on the two-sample methods described above. Suppose there are n subjects, each providing a multivariate set of p differences, d_i. The corrected sums of squares and products of the ds are calculated in the usual way, and the estimated variances and covariances are obtained by dividing by $n - 1$. The inverse matrix is obtained, with general term c_{ij}. The coefficients b_i in the discriminant function are calculated as in (13.6), but with the terms $\bar{x}_{Ai} - \bar{x}_{Bi}$ in (13.6) replaced by the mean differences $\bar{d}_i$. The test statistic is then obtained as

$$T^2 = n \sum b_i \bar{d}_i. \tag{13.14}$$

Finally, if the null hypothesis is true,

$$\frac{(n-p)T^2}{p(n-1)} \tag{13.15}$$

follows the F distribution on p and $n - p$ DF. If the result is significant, the coefficients in the discriminant function will indicate the way in which the variates combine to yield the most significant effect.

Example 13.3

Table 13.4 shows selected data from a small pilot trial to compare the efficacy and safety of various treatments to prevent anaemia in premature infants during the first few months of life. The table refers to 10 infants receiving one particular treatment, and presents measurements on four variables made when the infants were aged about 25 and 50 days. Haemoglobin is a measure of the efficacy of treatment, while the three other variables are recorded for monitoring the safety of the treatment.

Measurements at younger ages show clear trends in some of these and other physiological measurements, but between 25 and 50 days the position seems more stable.

Table 13.4 Efficacy and safety measurements for 10 premature infants receiving treatment for the prevention of anaemia.

Age (days):	Haemoglobin (g/dl)		Platelets ($\times 10^9$/l)		Leucocytes ($\times 10^9$/l)		Systolic blood pressure (mmHg)	
	25	50	25	50	25	50	25	50
Patient number								
1	10·5	10·5	700	596	8·0	9·8	71	65
2	10·4	11·4	363	370	16·0	7·6	54	68
3	10·4	10·2	456	645	10·9	16·1	67	69
4	15·6	13·3	260	301	8·6	8·0	77	82
5	16·3	13·9	387	385	8·4	11·1	60	60
6	11·2	10·2	375	431	13·1	12·6	65	75
7	11·8	10·3	472	337	15·0	10·4	71	69
8	12·8	12·8	469	244	16·2	9·9	61	63
9	10·3	9·1	381	505	16·3	13·0	72	70
10	8·9	11·2	526	539	11·8	8·7	57	65

Changes from day 25 to day 50

	Haemoglobin d_1	Platelets $\times 10^{-2}$ d_2	log Leucocytes $\times 10, d_3$	Systolic BP d_4
1	0·0	−1·0	0·9	−6
2	1·0	0·1	−3·2	14
3	−0·2	1·9	1·7	2
4	−2·3	0·4	−0·3	5
5	−2·4	0·0	1·2	0
6	−1·0	0·6	−0·2	10
7	−1·5	−1·4	−1·6	−2
8	0·0	−2·2	−2·1	2
9	−1·2	1·2	−1·0	−2
10	2·3	0·1	−1·3	8

The purpose of the present analysis is to ask whether there is clear evidence of change during this later period, and if so to identify its nature.

The lower part of Table 13.4 shows the changes, d_i, in the variables from 25 to 50 days. The log transformation for leucocytes was carried out because this variable (particularly in other data sets) shows positive skewness (see §§2.5 and 10.8). The multiplying factors for d_2 and d_3 were introduced, for convenience, to avoid too great a disparity in the ranges of magnitude of the four measures of change; this scaling does not influence the value of T^2 in (13.14), or the contributions ($b_i \bar{d}_i$) of each variable to it.

As a preliminary step we note the means and standard errors of the four differences, together with the results of t tests for the hypotheses that the population mean of each difference is zero:

	Mean ± SE (mean)	t	P
d_1	-0.53 ± 0.46	-1.15	0.28
d_2	-0.03 ± 0.39	-0.08	0.94
d_3	-0.59 ± 0.49	-1.20	0.26
d_4	3.10 ± 1.95	1.59	0.15

None of the mean differences is individually significant, but three exceed their standard errors, and in view of possible correlations between the four differences it seems worth pursuing a multivariate test.

The matrix of covariances between the d_i is

$$\begin{pmatrix} 2.1401 & -0.1188 & -0.8941 & 3.5922 \\ -0.1188 & 1.4868 & 0.7914 & 1.8811 \\ -0.8941 & 0.7914 & 2.4099 & -4.6011 \\ 3.5922 & 1.8811 & -4.6011 & 37.8778 \end{pmatrix}$$

and its inverse is

$$\begin{pmatrix} 0.59389 & 0.03210 & 0.12918 & -0.04223 \\ 0.03210 & 1.20462 & -0.65584 & -0.14254 \\ 0.12918 & -0.65584 & 0.93359 & 0.13373 \\ -0.04223 & -0.14254 & 0.13373 & 0.05373 \end{pmatrix}.$$

Both matrices are obtained by standard computer programs.

The coefficients b_i in the discriminant function are obtained by cross-multiplying the rows of the inverse matrix by the column of means, giving $(-0.5228, -0.1081, -0.1851, 0.1143)$. From (13.14), with $n = 10$,

$$T^2 = 7.439,$$

and, with $p = 4$ in (13.15), the test statistic is

$$6 \times 7.439/36 = 1.24.$$

For $F = 1.24$ on 4 and 6 DF, $P = 0.39$. There is thus no strong evidence of departures from zero in the set of four mean differences.

Note that the main contributions to the test statistic come from the variables d_1 and d_4, which are positively correlated but have means with opposite signs. If the analysis is performed with these two variables alone, the test statistic (as F on 2 and 8 DF) becomes 2.80, with $P = 0.12$. However, the enhanced significance is misleading, since these variables were selected, only after the first analysis had been performed, as being likely to be the most sensitive pair.

Classification trees

The discussion of discrimination, or classification, so far has been in terms of finding a function and allocating individuals into one or other of the two groups according to their values of this function. A different approach, which has been developed over the last 20 years, is the construction of a binary decision tree. This is a computer-intensive method. The method is more similar to diagnostic clinical decision-making than is the construction of a discriminant function.

The basis of the method is that at the first stage, termed a *node*, the individuals are divided into two sets, the *branches*, according to the value of one of the x variables. This variable is chosen from the full set so that the subdivision maximizes the separation of individuals in the groups between the two branches. Also, if the variable is not already dichotomous, then it is converted to binary form to achieve the same maximization. Each branch leads to a new node (Fig. 13.3) and the same procedure is carried out, using the remaining x variables, and noting that the variable used for subdivision at each of the two nodes will most probably be different. Some branches end at a *terminal* node, when the individuals at that node are homogenous with respect to group, and the whole process continues until all branches have terminated.

The choice of the final decision tree is a balance between its quality, defined in terms of homogeneity of the terminal nodes, and a penalty for complexity. This penalty is used to control making the tree unnecessarily complex whilst achieving only minor improvements.

For a fuller description of the method of classification and regression trees, $CART^{TM}$, see Zhang *et al.* (1998).

Discrimination with more than two groups: MANOVA

The linear discriminant function can be generalized to the situation where there are $k(>2)$ groups in two different ways. The first approach leads to what are known as *canonical variates*. We saw from (13.5) that when $k = 2$ the linear discriminant function maximizes the ratio of the difference in means *between* the groups to the standard deviation *within* groups. A natural generalization of this criterion is to maximize the ratio of the sum of squares (SSq) between groups to the SSq within groups. This requirement is found to lead to a standard technique of matrix algebra—the calculation of *eigenvalues* or *latent roots* of a matrix. The appropriate equation, in fact, has several solutions. One solution, corresponding to the highest latent root, gives the coefficient in the linear function which maximizes the ratio of SSqs. This is called the first *canonical variate*, W_1. If one wanted as good discrimination as possible from one linear function, this would be the one to choose. The second canonical variate, W_2, is the function with the highest ratio of SSqs, subject to the condition that it is uncorrelated with W_1 both between and within groups. Similarly, W_3 gives the highest ratio subject to being uncorrelated with W_1 and W_2. The number of canonical variates is the smaller of p or $k - 1$. Thus, the linear discriminant function (13.4) is for $k = 2$ the first and only canonical variate.

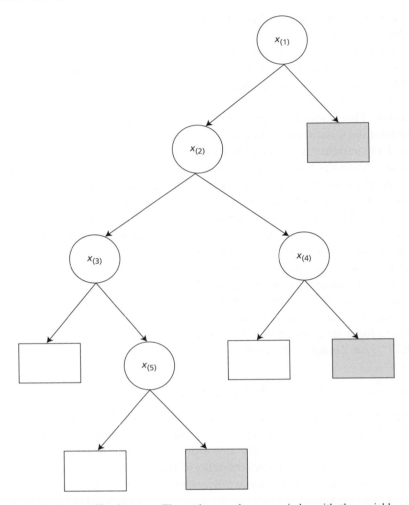

Fig. 13.3 A binary classification tree. The nodes are shown as circles with the variable used to determine the branches below. Terminating nodes are shown as rectangles, where the shaded rectangles indicate classification into one of the groups and the open rectangles into the other. Note that the variables have been renumbered in the order in which they are used in the branching process.

If most of the variation between groups is explained by W_1 and W_2, the ratios of SSqs corresponding to the later canonical variates will be relatively small. It is then convenient to plot the data as a scatter diagram, with W_1 and W_2 as the two axes. This will give a clear picture of any tendency of the groups to form clusters. It may also be interesting to see which of the original variables are strongly represented in each canonical variate. The magnitudes of the coefficients depend on the scales of measurement, so their relative sizes are of no great interest, although it should be noted that the method is scale-invariant. Some computer programs print the correlations between each canonical variate and each x_i, a feature which helps to give some insight into the structure of the canonical variates. Discrimination takes place in the two-dimensional space defined by W_1 and W_2 and an individual is allocated to the group for which the distance between the individual's data point and the group mean is least.

As in the two-group situation, the identification of canonical variates is usually more important than a significance test of the null hypothesis that the populations are identical. Nevertheless, such a test may be useful, particularly as an initial screening step. The appropriate method for testing changes in means of multivariate normal data is the *multivariate analysis of variance* (MANOVA). We shall not describe this in detail here; books such as Krzanowski and Marriott (1994, Chapter 7) give fuller descriptions. In contrast to the two-sample Hotelling's T^2, there are in the general case $(k > 2)$ several alternative test statistics, which fortunately usually lead to similar conclusions. MANOVA can, like the univariate analysis of variance, be used for more complex data structures, such as factorial designs, and can be extended to allow for covariates, as a generalization of the analysis of covariance. Computer programs usually give details of the significance tests for the various factors, and also identify the relevant canonical variates. For an example of the use of MANOVA in the analysis of data from dental clinical trials, see Geary *et al.* (1992).

Returning to the problem of discrimination, a second generalization of the linear discriminant function is to use approach (b) of p. 467 and allocate an individual to the group with highest likelihood. This is equivalent to forming the likelihood ratio of every pair of groups. There are $\frac{1}{2}k(k-1)$ pairs of groups, but only $k-1$ likelihood ratios are needed. For example, if L_j is the log likelihood for the jth group, we could take

$$Z_1 = L_1 - L_2$$
$$Z_2 = L_2 - L_3$$
$$.$$
$$.$$
$$.$$
$$Z_{k-1} = L_{k-1} - L_k,$$

and any difference between pairs of L_js (which is, of course, the log of the corresponding likelihood ratio) can be expressed in terms of the Zs. This could be done by calculating linear discriminant functions by the methods given earlier, for each of the $k-1$ pairs of groups. The only modification is to calculate pooled within-group variances and covariances from all k groups, and to use the inverse of this pooled matrix in the calculation of each discriminant function. The procedure can be simplified by calculating a discriminant score for each group. This score is the log likelihood, omitting any terms common to all groups.

Allocation is then to the group with the highest score. The method is also equivalent to allocating an individual to the group with the nearest mean, in the sense of generalized distance. Computer programs exist for the whole procedure.

This likelihood ratio approach is more appropriate than that of canonical variates if the main purpose is to form an allocation rule. If the purpose is to gain insight into the way in which groups differ, using as few dimensions as possible, then canonical variates are the more appropriate method.

Although the two methods do not usually give identical results, there is a close relationship between them. Using the first canonical variate gives the same discrimination as the likelihood method if the group means are collinear in p-dimensional space. Thus, as noted earlier, the two methods are identical for $k = 2$ because the two group means may be regarded as collinear. If, for example, $k = 3$ and $p > 1$, there will be $k - 1 = 2$ canonical variates, W_1 and W_2, and two independent likelihood ratio discriminators, say $Z_1 = L_1 - L_2$ and $Z_2 = L_2 - L_3$. (Note that $L_3 - L_1 = -(Z_1 + Z_2)$.) If the observations are plotted (i) with W_1 and W_2 as axes, and (ii) with Z_1 and Z_2 as axes, it will be found that the scatter diagrams are essentially similar, differing only in the orientation and scaling of the axes. Thus, the use of both canonical variates is equivalent to the likelihood approach. In general, using $k - 1$ canonical variates gives the same discrimination as the likelihood approach. However, the idea behind using canonical variates is to reduce the dimensionality, and the only advantage of this approach is if it is possible to use just a few variates without any material loss in discriminating ability. For further discussion of this point, see Marriott (1974).

Scoring systems, using canonical variates

Suppose that a variable is measured on a p-point scale from 1 to p. For example, a patient's response to treatment may be graded in categories ranging from 'much worse' (scored 1) to 'much better' (scored p). This sequence of equidistant integers may not be the best scale on which to analyse the data. The best method of scoring will depend on the criterion we wish to optimize. Suppose, for example, that patients were classified into k treatment groups. It might be reasonable to choose a system of scoring which maximized differences between treatments as compared with those within treatments. For this purpose consider a set of p dummy variables, $x_1, x_2, \ldots, x_p$, such that, for a patient in category j, the value of x_j is 1 and that of the other x_is is 0. Now choose the first canonical variate of the xs, say,

$$g = l_1 x_1 + l_2 x_2 + \ldots + l_p x_p.$$

Then g will take the value l_j in category j, and will define the system which maximizes the ratio of the Between-Groups SSq to the Within-Groups SSq. There is, however, no guarantee that the scores follow in magnitude the natural order of the categories. Bradley *et al.* (1962) have shown how the ratio of SSq can be maximized subject to there being no reversals of the natural order.

The investigator might want a scoring system which was as closely correlated as possible with some other variable. For instance, in dose–response experiments in serology, a reaction may be classified as $--$, $-$, 0, $+$ or $++$, and it may be useful to replace these categories by a score which forms a good linear regression on the log dose of some reagent. The approach is similar to that in the previous problem, the ratio of SSq to be maximized being that of the SSq due to regression to the Total SSq (for an example, see Ipsen, 1955).

13.4 **Cluster analysis**

Component analysis and factor analysis are 'internal' methods of analysis, in that the individuals are not classified by any criteria other than the variables used in the analysis. In some problems, no initial grouping is imposed on the data, but the object of the analysis is to see whether the individuals can be formed into any natural system of groups. The number of groups may not be specified in advance. The individuals could, of course, be grouped in an entirely arbitrary way, but the investigator seeks a system such that the individuals within a group resemble each other (in the values taken by the variables) more than do individuals in different groups. This specification is rather vague, and there are several ways of defining groups to make it more explicit. In addition to chapters in Chatfield and Collins (1980, Chapter 11) and Krzanowski and Marriott (1995, Chapter 10), an introductory text is Everitt (1980), whilst a more mathematical treatment is in Mardia *et al.* (1979, Chapter 13).

Two broad approaches may be distinguished. The first is to do a principal component analysis of all the data. If most of the variation is explained by the first two or three components, the essential features of the multidimensional scatter can be seen by a two-dimensional scatter diagram, or perhaps a two-dimensional representation of a three-dimensional model. Any clustering of the individuals into groups would then become apparent—at least in its main features—although the precise definitions of the groups might be open to question. If the scatter is not largely represented by the first two or three components, the method will be very much less useful.

A closely related approach is that of *correspondence analysis* (extensively developed in France under the title '*analyse des correspondences*'). Here the variables are categorical, and can be represented by dummy, or indicator, variables, as on p. 349. Linear functions of the indicator variables are chosen in such a way that the multidimensional scatter is most closely approximated by a diagram in a small number of dimensions (normally two). The individuals in a particular response category can be represented by a point in this diagram, and it may then be possible to identify interesting clusters of individuals. A very full account is given by Greenacre (1984), who lists (pp. 317, 318) some references to medical applications.

The second approach, that of *numerical taxonomy*, is discussed in detail by Sneath and Sokal (1973). The idea here is to calculate an index of similarity or dissimilarity for each pair of individuals. The precise definition of this index will depend on the nature of the variables. If all the variables are recorded on a continuous scale, a suitable index of dissimilarity might be the distance in multi-dimensional space between the two points whose coordinates are the values of the variables of two individuals; this index is the Euclidean distance. If, as in some clinical applications, the variables are dichotomies (expressing the presence or absence of some feature), a suitable similarity index might be the proportion of variables for which the two individuals show the same response. Alternative measures are discussed fully by Sneath and Sokal. When the similarity indices have been calculated, some form of sorting is carried out so that pairs of individuals with high values of the index are sorted into the same group. These procedures can be effected by a computer once a method of forming clusters has been chosen.

A medical application which suggests itself is the definition of a system of related diseases. Hayhoe *et al.* (1964), for instance, studied the classification of the acute leukaemias from this point of view. Whether the methods are really useful will depend largely on whether the classifications subsequently perform any useful function. For example, in the definition of disease categories, one would hope that any system suggested might lead to suggestions about aetiology, recommendations about future treatment, or at the very least a useful system for tabulating vital statistics. One of the problems in medical applications is how to define generally any groups that may have been formed by a clustering procedure. Lists of particular individuals placed in the groups in any one study are, of course, of insufficient general interest, and some more general definitions are required.

Cluster analysis may also be used to cluster variables rather than individuals, that is, to arrange the variables into groups such that the variables in each group measure a similar or closely related feature of the individuals whilst the separate groups represent different features. This objective is similar to that of principal component analysis and, where the variables are measured on a continuous scale, principal component analysis is probably to be preferred. For example, if cluster analysis is applied to the data of Example 13.1, the arrangements of variables into clusters is very similar to the groups extracted using principal components.

The different methods of defining clusters will generally give different results when applied to the same data. The most appropriate method in a particular case depends on the structure in the data, which is often unknown. In effect, each method imposes implicit assumptions on the type of clustering expected, and if these assumptions are invalid the results may be meaningless. For this reason we suggest that cluster analysis should only be used in circumstances where other multivariate methods are inappropriate, and the results must be interpreted with a great deal of caution.

Finally, the method of cluster analysis should not be confused with the problem of determining whether cases of disease occur in clusters in time, space or families. This problem gives rise to different methods discussed in §19.13.

Multidimensional scaling

Suppose data are available on a set of individuals and it is possible to derive an index of similarity, or dissimilarity, between every pair of individuals. This index would be of the same type as those considered in the discussion of cluster analysis. Then multidimensional scaling is a method of arranging the individuals in a space of a few dimensions so that the distances between the points in this space are nearly the same as the measures of dissimilarity. In particular, if two dimensions provide an adequate representation, then it is possible to plot the individuals on a two-dimensional graph, and examination of how the individuals are arranged on this graph might lead to some useful interpretation. For example, the individuals might occur in clusters.

The method is, like many multivariate methods, an attempt to reduce dimensionality. If the dissimilarities are measured using a set of continuous variables, then the method of principal components has a similar aim.

For more details on this method, see Chatfield and Collins (1980) and Cox and Cox (2001).

13.5 **Concluding remarks**

All the multivariate methods rely on a large amount of computation and have only been widely applicable in the last three decades following the development of computer statistical software. The ease of performing the calculations leads to a risk that multivariate methods may be applied blindly in circumstances different from those for which they were designed, and that incorrect conclusions may be drawn from them.

The majority of data sets are multivariate and therefore multivariate analysis of some sort is often required. In choosing an approach, it is essential to keep uppermost in mind the objective of the research and only to use a method of analysis if it is appropriate for that objective. In many cases, the objective is to examine the relationship between an outcome variable and a number of possible explanatory variables. In this case, the method of multiple regression (§11.6) is appropriate. If the outcome variable is binary, then the conceptually similar method of multiple logistic regression (§14.2) would be required. Discriminant analysis is often used in the latter case but would only be the most appropriate method if there were some reason to classify future individuals.

Of the methods discussed in this chapter the most widely used in medical research are principal components, factor analysis and discriminant analysis. Some of the other methods we have mentioned briefly not because we think they have wide applicability in medical research, but to provide readers with some indication of their characteristics since their use is sometimes reported in the literature. There is overlap in the aims of several of the methods, and the temptation of trying several methods in the hope that something 'of interest' might emerge should be resisted.

14 Modelling categorical data

14.1 **Introduction**

In §11.6 we considered multiple linear regression and noted that in this method the mean value of the dependent variable is expressed as a linear function of a set of explanatory variables, and that for an observed value of the dependent variable there would be an error term (11.38). The classical method applies to the case where the error terms are independently and normally distributed, with zero mean and constant variance. Thus, the method is not strictly applicable to the case where the dependent variable is qualitative. Yet the concept of a relationship between the distribution of a dependent variable and a number of explanatory variables is just as valid when the dependent variable is qualitative as when it is continuous. For example, consider a binomial variable representing presence or absence of disease. For a homogeneous group of individuals, the number with disease would be distributed according to the binomial distribution with a constant probability of disease (§3.6). Often the individuals will not come from a homogeneous group but will differ on a number of variables associated with the probability of having the disease. That is, there would be a relationship between probability of disease and a set of explanatory variables. This relationship would not usually be linear, since a straight-line relationship would imply probabilities outside the legitimate range of 0 to 1 for some values of the explanatory variables. In order to fit the relationship into the framework of linear regression it is necessary to apply a transformation, and this leads to the methods of *logistic regression* and *probit analysis* discussed below. A second example is when the dependent variable is distributed according to the Poisson distribution (§3.7), and the expectation of the Poisson process is related to a number of explanatory variables. Although regression methods to analyse qualitative variables have been known for over 50 years—for example, the first edition of Finney's book *Probit Analysis* was published in 1947—it is only in the last three decades that the methods have been used widely in a variety of situations. An important paper by Nelder and Wedderburn (1972) developed the concept of *generalized linear models*, which placed all the commonly used models into a unified framework. This in turn led to the introduction of computer software such as GLIM (Healy, 1988) and the glm function in S-PLUS.

485

In this chapter we consider some of the properties of generalized linear models and illustrate their application with examples. Readers interested in a more detailed exposition are referred to the books by McCullagh and Nelder (1989) and Dobson (1990). Cox and Snell (1989), Hosmer and Lemeshow (1989) and Kleinbaum (1994) give details of logistic regression.

General theory

Consider a random variable y distributed according to the probability density $f(y; \mu)$, where μ is the expected value of y; that is,

$$E(y) = \mu. \tag{14.1}$$

Suppose that for each observation y there is a set of explanatory variables $x_1, x_2, \ldots, x_p$, and that μ depends on the values of these variables. Suppose further that, after some transformation of $\mu, g(\mu)$, the relationship is linear; that is,

$$\eta = g(\mu) = \beta_0 + \beta_1 x_1 + \beta_2 x_2 + \ldots + \beta_p x_p. \tag{14.2}$$

Then the relationship between y and the explanatory variables is a *generalized linear model*. The transformation, $g(\mu)$, is termed the *link function*, since it provides the link between the linear part of the model, η, and the random part represented by μ. The linear function, η, is termed the *linear predictor* and the distribution of $y, f(y; \mu)$, is the *error distribution*.

When the error distribution is normal, the classic linear regression model is

$$E(y) = \beta_0 + \beta_1 x_1 + \beta_2 x_2 + \ldots + \beta_p x_p.$$

Thus from (14.1) and (14.2), $\eta = \mu$, and the link function is the identity, $g(\mu) = \mu$. Thus, the familiar multiple linear regression is a member of the family of generalized linear models.

When the basic observations are proportions, then the basic form of random variation might be expected to be binomial. Such data give rise to many of the difficulties described in §10.8. Regression curves are unlikely to be linear, because the scale of the proportion is limited by the values 0 and 1 and changes in any relevant explanatory variable at the extreme ends of its scale are unlikely to produce much change in the proportion. A *sigmoid* regression curve as in Fig. 14.1(a) is, in fact, likely to be found. An appropriate transformation may convert this to a linear relationship. In the context of the reasons for transformations discussed in §10.8, this is a linearizing transformation. The variance of an observed proportion depends on the expected proportion, as well as on the denominator of the fraction (see (3.16)). Finally, the binomial distribution of random error is likely to be skew in opposite directions as the proportion approaches 0 or 1.

Since the linear predictor of (14.2) covers an unlimited range, the link function should transform μ, the binomial probability, from the range 0 to 1 to $-\infty$ to ∞. Two commonly used transformations that achieve this are the probit transformation and the logit transformation. They have very similar effects, and instances in which one is clearly superior to the other are rare.

Probit transformation

For any proportion p, suppose y' is the *normal equivalent deviate* (NED) such that a proportion p of the standard normal distribution falls to the left of y'. That is, if Φ is the cumulative distribution function of a standardized normal variable (§§3.4 and 3.8), so that $\Phi(y') = p$, then

$$y' = \Phi^{-1}(p). \tag{14.3}$$

The *probit* of p is defined as

$$y = 5 + y'. \tag{14.4}$$

The addition of 5 was included in the original definition to avoid negative probits in hand calculations, but (14.3) is also often referred to as the probit transformation. Probits may be obtained from any table of the normal distribution, such as Table A1, using (14.3), and Table IX of Fisher and Yates (1963) uses probits directly rather than NEDs.

The range of the probit scale is infinite, and there is an obvious problem if the data contain some observations with $p = 0$ or $p = 1$, since the corresponding values of y, $-\infty$ and ∞, cannot conveniently be used in standard methods of analysis. In approximate solutions and graphical studies a useful device is to calculate y from an adjusted value of p derived by assuming that $\frac{1}{2}$ (rather than 0) positive or negative response occurred. That is, if $p = r/n$,

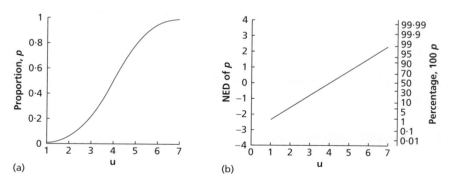

Fig. 14.1 Hypothetical response curve plotted (a) with an arithmetic scale for the ordinate, p; (b) with an arithmetic scale for the NED of p.

calculate $p' = 1/(2n)$ when $r = 0$ and $p' = (2n - 1)/2n$ when $r = n$, and obtain y from p'.

A further point is that the probit transformation does not stabilize variances, even for observations with constant n. Some form of weighting is therefore desirable in any analysis. A rigorous approach is provided by the method called *probit analysis* (Finney, 1971; see also §20.4).

The effect of the probit transformation in linearizing a relationship is shown in Fig. 14.1. In Figure 14.1(b) the vertical axis on the left is the NED of p, and the scale on the right is the probability scale, in which the distances between points on the vertical scale are proportional to the corresponding distances on the probit or NED scale.

Logit transformation

The *logit* of p is defined as

$$y = \ln \frac{p}{1 - p}. \tag{14.5}$$

Occasionally (Fisher & Yates, 1963; Finney, 1978) the definition incorporates a factor $\frac{1}{2}$ so that $y = \frac{1}{2}\ln[p/(1 - p)]$; this has the effect of making the values rather similar to those of the NED (i.e. probit $- 5$).

The effect of the logit (or *logistic*) transformation is very similar indeed to that of the probit transformation.

The probit transformation is reasonable on biological grounds in some circumstances; for example, in a quantal assay of insecticides applied under different controlled conditions, a known number of flies might be exposed at a number of different doses and a count made of the number killed. In this type of study, individual tolerances or their logs may be assumed to have a normal distribution, and this leads directly to the probit model (§20.4).

The logit transformation is more arbitrary, but has important advantages. First, it is easier to calculate, since it requires only the log function rather than the inverse normal distribution function. Secondly, and more importantly, the logit is the logarithm of the odds, and logit differences are logarithms of odds ratios (see (4.22)). The odds ratio is important in the analysis of epidemiological studies, and logistic regression can be used for a variety of epidemiological study designs (§19.4) to provide estimates of relative risk (§19.5).

14.2 **Logistic regression**

The logit transformation gives the method of *logistic regression*:

$$\ln\left(\frac{\mu}{1 - \mu}\right) = \beta_0 + \beta_1 x_1 + \beta_2 x_2 + \ldots \beta_p x_p. \tag{14.6}$$

Fitting a model

Two approaches are possible: first, an approximate method using *empirical weights* and, secondly, the theoretically more satisfactory *maximum likelihood* solution. The former method is a weighted regression analysis (p. 344), where each value of the logit is weighted by the reciprocal of its approximate variance. This method is not exact—first, because the ys are not normally distributed about their population values and, secondly, because the weights are not exactly in inverse proportion to the variances, being expressed in terms of the estimated proportion p. For this reason the weights are often called *empirical*. Although this method is adequate if most of the sample sizes are reasonably large and few of the ps are close to 0 or 1 (Example 14.1 was analysed using this method in earlier editions of this book), the ease of using the more satisfactory maximum likelihood method with statistical software means it is no longer recommended. If the observed proportions p are based on $n = 1$ observation only, their values will be either 0 or 1, and the empirical method cannot be used. This situation occurs in the analysis of prognostic data, where an individual patient is classified as 'success' or 'failure', several explanatory variables x_j are observed, and the object is to predict the probability of success in terms of the xs.

Maximum likelihood

The method of estimation by maximum likelihood, introduced in §4.1, has certain desirable theoretical properties and can be applied to fit logistic regression and other generalized linear models. The likelihood of the data is proportional to the probability of obtaining the data (§3.3). For data of known distributional form, and where the mean value is given in terms of a generalized linear model, the probability of the observed data can be written down using the appropriate probability distributions. For example, with logistic regression the probability for each group or individual can be calculated using the binomial probability from (14.6) in (3.12) and the likelihood of the whole data is the product of these probabilities over all groups or individuals. This likelihood depends on the values of the regression coefficients, and the maximum likelihood estimates of these regression coefficients are those values that maximize the likelihood—that is, the values for which the data are most likely to occur. For theoretical reasons, and also for practical convenience, it is preferable to work in terms of the logarithm of the likelihood. Thus it is the log-likelihood, L, that is maximized. The method also gives standard errors of the estimated regression coefficients and significance tests of specific hypotheses.

By analogy with the analysis of variance for a continuous variable, the *analysis of deviance* is used in generalized linear models. The *deviance* is defined as twice the difference between the log-likelihood of a perfectly fitting model and that of the current model, and has associated degrees of freedom (DF) equal to the difference in the number of parameters between these two models. Where the error distribution is completely defined by the link between the random and linear parts of the model—and this will be the case for binomial and Poisson variables but not for a normal variable, for which the size of the variance is also required—then deviances follow approximately the χ^2 distribution and can be used for the testing of significance. In particular, reductions in deviance due to adding extra terms into the model can be used to assess whether the inclusion of the extra terms had resulted in a significant improvement to the model. This is analogous to the analysis of variance test for deletion of variables described in §11.6 for a continuous variable.

The significance of an effect on a single degree of freedom may be tested by the ratio of its estimate to its standard error (SE), assessed as a standardized normal deviate. This is known as the *Wald* test, and its square as the *Wald* χ^2.

Another test is the *score* test which is based on the first derivative of the log-likelihood with respect to a parameter and its variance (see Agresti, 1996, §4.5.2). Both are evaluated at the null value of the parameter and conditionally on the other terms in the model. This statistic is less readily available from statistical software except in simple situations.

The procedure for fitting a model using the maximum likelihood method usually involves iteration—that is, repeating a sequence of calculations until a stable solution is reached. Fitted weights are used and, since these depend on the parameter estimates, they change from cycle to cycle of the iteration. The approximate solution using empirical weights could be the first cycle in this iterative procedure, and the whole procedure is sometimes called *iterative weighted least squares*. The technical details of the procedure will not be given since the process is obviously rather tedious, and the computations require appropriate statistical software (for example, PROC LOGISTIC in SAS (2000), LOGISTIC REGRESSION in SPSS (1999), or GLIM (Healy, 1988). For further details of the maximum likelihood method see, for example, Wetherill (1981).

Example 14.1

Table 14.1 shows some data reported by Lombard and Doering (1947) from a survey of knowledge about cancer. These data have been used by several other authors (Dyke & Patterson, 1952; Naylor, 1964). Each line of the table corresponds to a particular combination of factors in a 2^4 factorial arrangement, n being the number of individuals in this category and r the number who gave a good score in response to questions about cancer knowledge. The four factors are: A, newspaper reading; B, listening to radio; C, solid reading; D, attendance at lectures.

Table 14.1 A 2^4 factorial set of proportions (Lombard & Doering, 1947). The fitted proportions from a logistic regression analysis are shown in column (4).

Factor combination	(1) Number of individuals n	(2) Number with good score r	(3) Observed proportion (2)/(1) p	(4) Fitted proportion
(1)	477	84	0·176	0·188
(a)	231	75	0·325	0·308
(b)	63	13	0·206	0·240
(ab)	94	35	0·372	0·377
(c)	150	67	0·447	0·382
(ac)	378	201	0·532	0·542
(bc)	32	16	0·500	0·458
(abc)	169	102	0·604	0·618
(d)	12	2	0·167	0·261
(ad)	13	7	0·538	0·404
(bd)	7	4	0·571	0·325
(abd)	12	8	0·667	0·480
(cd)	11	3	0·273	0·485
(acd)	45	27	0·600	0·643
(bcd)	4	1	0·250	0·562
(abcd)	31	23	0·742	0·711

Although the data were obtained from a survey rather than from a randomized experiment, we can usefully study the effect on cancer knowledge of the four main effects and their interactions. The main effects and interactions will not be orthogonal but can be estimated.

There are 16 groups of individuals and a model containing all main effects and all interactions would fit the data perfectly. Thus by definition it would have a deviance of zero and serves as the reference point in assessing the fit of simpler models.

The first logistic regression model fitted was that containing only the main effects. This gave a model in which the logit of the probability of a good score was estimated as

$$-1 \cdot 4604 + 0 \cdot 6498A + 0 \cdot 3101B + 0 \cdot 9806C + 0 \cdot 4204D$$

SE:	0·1154	0·1222	0·1107	0·1910
z:	5·63	2·54	8·86	2·20
P:	<0·001	0·011	<0·001	0·028

Here the terms involving A, B, C and D are included when these factors are present and omitted otherwise.

The significance of the main effects have been tested by Wald's test—that is, the ratio of an estimate to its standard error assessed as a standardized normal deviate. Alternatively, the significance may be established by analysis of deviance. For example, fitting the model containing only the main effects of B, C and D, gives a deviance of 45·47 with 12

DF. Adding the main effect of A to the model reduces the deviance to 13·59 with 11 DF, so that the deviance test for the effect of A, after allowing for B, C and D, is $45·47 - 13·59 = 31·88$ as an approximate $\chi^2_{(1)}$. This test is numerically similar to Wald's test, since $\sqrt{31·88} = 5·65$, but in general such close agreement would not be expected. Although the deviance tests of main effects are not necessary here, in general they are needed. For example, if a factor with more than two levels were fitted, using dummy variables (§11.7), a deviance test with the appropriate degrees of freedom would be required.

The deviance associated with the model including all the main effects is 13·59 with 11 DF, and this represents the 11 interactions not included in the model. Taking the deviance as a $\chi^2_{(11)}$, there is no evidence that the interactions are significant and the model with just main effects is a good fit. However, there is still scope for one of the two-factor interactions to be significant and it is prudent to try including each of the six two-factor interactions in turn to the model. As an example, when the interaction of the two kinds of reading, AC, is included, the deviance reduces to 10·72 with 10 DF. Thus, this interaction has an approximate $\chi^2_{(1)}$ of 2·87, which is not significant ($P = 0·091$). Similarly, none of the other interactions is significant.

The adequacy of the fit can be visualized by comparing the observed and fitted proportions over the 16 cells. The fitted proportions are shown in column (4) of Table 14.1 and seem in reasonable agreement with the observed values in column (3). A formal test may be constructed by calculating the expected frequencies, $E(r)$ and $E(n - r)$, for each factor combination and calculating the Pearson's χ^2 statistic (8.28). This has the value 13·61 with 11 DF ($16 - 5$, since five parameters have been fitted). This test statistic is very similar to the deviance in this example, and the model with just the main effects is evidently a good fit.

The data of Example 13.2 could be analysed using logistic regression. In this case the observed proportions are each based on one observation only. As a model we could suppose that the logit of the population probability of survival, Y, was related to haemoglobin, x_1, and bilirubin, x_2 by the linear logistic regression formula (14.6)

$$Y = \beta_0 + \beta_1 x_1 + \beta_2 x_2.$$

Application of the maximum likelihood method gave the following estimates of β_0, β_1, and β_2 with their standard errors:

$$\hat{\beta}_0 = -2·354 \quad \pm 2·416$$
$$\hat{\beta}_1 = \quad 0·5324 \pm 0·1487 \quad\quad (14.7)$$
$$\hat{\beta}_2 = -0·4892 \pm 0·3448.$$

The picture is similar to that presented by the discriminant analysis of Example 13.2. Haemoglobin is an important predictor; bilirubin is not. An interesting point is that, if the distributions of the xs are multivariate normal, with the same variances and covariances for both successes and failures (the basic model for discriminant analysis), the discriminant function (13.4) can also be used to predict Y. The formula is:

$$Y = \beta_0' + \beta_1' x_1 + \beta_2' x_2 + \ldots + \beta_p' x_p,$$

where

$$\beta_j' = b_j$$

and

$$\beta_0' = -\tfrac{1}{2}[\beta_1'(\bar{x}_{A1} + \bar{x}_{B1}) + \ldots + \beta_p'(\bar{x}_{Ap} + \bar{x}_{Bp})] + \ln(n_A/n_B). \qquad (14.8)$$

In Example 13.2, using the discriminant function coefficients b_1 and b_2 given there, we find

$$\beta_0' = -4\cdot135,$$
$$\beta_1' = 0\cdot6541,$$
$$\beta_2' = -0\cdot3978,$$

which lead to values of Y not differing greatly from those obtained from (14.7), except for extreme values of x_1 and x_2.

An example of the use of the linear discriminant function to predict the probability of coronary heart disease is given by Truett *et al.* (1967). The point should be emphasized that, in situations in which the distributions of xs are far from multivariate normal, this method may be unreliable, and the maximum likelihood solution will be preferable.

To test the adequacy of the logistic regression model (14.6), after fitting by maximum likelihood, an approximate χ^2 test statistic is given by the deviance. This was the approach in Example 14.1, where the deviance after fitting the four main effects was 13·59 with 11 DF (since four main effects and a constant term had been estimated from 16 groups). The fit is clearly adequate, suggesting that there is no need to postulate interactions, although, as was done in the example, a further refinement to testing the goodness of fit is to try interactions, since a single effect with 1 DF could be undetected when tested with other effects contributing 10 DF.

In general terms, the adequacy of the model can be assessed by including terms such as x_i^2, to test for linearity in x_i, and $x_i x_j$, to test for an interaction between x_i and x_j.

The approximation to the distribution of the deviance by χ^2 is unreliable for sparse data—that is, if a high proportion of the observed counts are small. The extreme case of sparse data is where all values of n are 1. Differences between deviances can still be used to test for the inclusion of extra terms in the model. For sparse data, tests based on the differences in deviances are superior to the corresponding Wald test (Hauck & Donner, 1977). Goodness-of-fit tests should be carried out after forming groups of individuals with the same covariate patterns. Even for a case of individual data, it may be that the final model results in a smaller number of distinct covariate patterns; this is particularly likely to be the case if the covariates are categorical variables with just a few levels. The value of the deviance is unaltered by grouping into covariate patterns, but the degrees of freedom are equal to the number of covariate patterns less the number of parameters fitted.

For individual data that do not reduce to a smaller number of covariate patterns, tests based on grouping the data may be constructed. For a logistic regression, grouping could be by the estimated probabilities and a χ^2 test produced by comparing observed and expected frequencies (Lemeshow & Hosmer, 1982; Hosmer & Lemeshow, 1989, §5.2.2). In this test the individuals are ranked in terms of the size of the estimated probability, P, obtained from the fitted logistic regression model. The individuals are then divided into g groups; often $g = 10$. One way of doing this is to have the groups of equal size—that is, the first 10% of subjects are in the first group, etc. Another way is to define the groups in terms of the estimated probabilities so that the first group contains those with estimated probabilities less than 0·1, the second 0·1 to 0·2, etc. A $g \times 2$ table is then formed, in which the columns represent the two categories of the dichotomous outcome variable, containing the observed and expected numbers in each cell. The expected numbers for each group are the sum of the estimated probabilities, P, and the sum of $1 - P$, for all the individuals in that group. A χ^2 goodness-of-fit statistic is then calculated (11.73). Based on simulations, Hosmer and Lemeshow (1980) showed that this test statistic is distributed approximately as a χ^2 with $g - 2$ degrees of freedom. This test can be modified when some individuals have the same covariate pattern (Hosmer & Lemeshow, 1989, §5.2.2), provided that the total number of covariate patterns is not too different from the total number of individuals.

Diagnostic methods based on residuals similar to those used in classical regression (§11.9) can be applied. If the data are already grouped, as in Example 14.1, then standardized residuals can be produced and assessed, where each residual is standardized by its estimated standard error. In logistic regression the standardized residual is

$$\frac{r - n\hat{\mu}}{\sqrt{[n\hat{\mu}(1 - \hat{\mu})]}},$$

where there are r events out of n. For individual data the residual may be defined using the above expression, with r either 0 or 1, but the individual residuals are of little use since they are not distributed normally and cannot be assessed individually. For example, if $\hat{\mu} = 0·01$, the only possible values of the standardized residual are 9·9 and $-0·1$; the occurrence of the larger residual does not necessarily indicate an outlying point, and if accompanied by 99 of the smaller residuals the fit would be perfect. It is, therefore, necessary to group the residuals, defining groups as individuals with similar values of the x_i.

Alternative definitions of the residual include correcting for the leverage of the point in the space of the explanatory variables to produce a residual equivalent to the Studentized residual (11.67). Another definition is the *deviance residual*, defined as the square root of the contribution of the point to the deviance. Cox and Snell (1989; §2.7) give a good description of the use of residuals in logistic regression.

The use of influence diagnostics is discussed in Cox and Snell (1989) and by Hosmer and Lemeshow (1989, §5.3). There are some differences in leverage between logistic regression and classical multiple regression. In the latter (see p. 366) the points furthest from the mean of the x variables have the highest leverages. In logistic regression the leverage is modified by the weight of each observation and points with low or high expected probabilities have small weight. As such probabilities are usually associated with distant points, this reduces the leverage of these points. The balance between position of an observation in the x variable space and weight suggests that the points with highest leverage are those with fitted probabilities of about 0·2 or 0·8 (Hosmer & Lemeshow, 1989, §5.3). The concept of Cook's distance can be used in logistic regression and (11.72) applies, using the modified leverage as just discussed, although in this case only approximately (Pregibon, 1981).

In some cases the best-fitting model may not be a good fit, but all attempts to improve it through adding in other or transformed x variables fail to give any worthwhile improvement. This may be because of overdispersion due to some extra source of variability. Unless this variability can be explained by some extension to the model, the overdispersion can be taken into account in tests of significance and the construction of confidence intervals by the use of a scaling factor. Denoting this factor by ϕ, any χ^2 statistics are divided by ϕ and standard errors are multiplied by $\sqrt{\phi}$. ϕ may be estimated from a goodness-of-fit test. For non-sparse data this could be the residual deviance divided by its degrees of freedom. For sparse data it is difficult to identify and estimate overdispersion. For a more detailed discussion, see McCullagh and Nelder (1989, §4.5).

The model might be inadequate because of an inappropriate choice of the link function. An approach to this problem is to extend the link function into a family indexed by one or more parameters. Tests can then be derived to determine if there is evidence against the particular member of the family originally used (Pregibon, 1980; Brown, 1982; McCullagh & Nelder, 1989).

The strength of fit, or the extent to which the fitted regression discriminates between observed and predicted, is provided by the concordance/discordance of pairs of responses. These measures are constructed as follows:

1 Define all pairs of observations in which one member of the pair has the characteristic under analysis and the other does not.
2 Find the fitted probabilities of each member of the pair, p_+ and p_-.
3 Then,

if $p_+ > p_-$ the pair is concordant;

if $p_+ < p_-$ the pair is discordant;

if $p_+ = p_-$ the pair is tied.

4 Over all pairs find the percentages in the three classes, concordant, discordant and tied.

These three percentages may be combined into a single summary measure in various ways. A particularly useful summary measure is

$$c = (\% \text{ concordant} + 0 \cdot 5\% \text{ tied})/100.$$

A value of c of $0 \cdot 5$ indicates no discrimination and $1 \cdot 0$ perfect discrimination. (c is also the area under the receiver operating characteristic (ROC) curve (see §19.9).)

For small data sets the methods discussed above will be inadequate, because the approximations of the test statistics to the χ^2 distribution will be unsatisfactory, or a convergent maximum likelihood solution may not be obtained with standard statistical software. Exact methods for logistic regression may be applied (Mehta & Patel, 1995) using the LogXact software.

It was mentioned earlier that an important advantage of logistic regression is that it can be applied to data from a variety of epidemiological designs, including cohort studies and case–control studies (§19.4). In a matched case–control study, controls are chosen to match their corresponding case for some variables. Logistic regression can be applied to estimate the effects of variables not included in the matching, but the analysis is conditional within the case–control sets; the method is then referred to as *conditional logistic regression* (§19.5).

14.3 Polytomous regression

Some procedures for the analysis of ordered categorical data are described in of Chapter 15. These procedures are limited in two respects: they are appropriate for relatively simple data structures, where the factors to be studied are few in number; and the emphasis is mainly on significance tests, with little discussion of the need to describe the nature of any associations revealed by the tests. Both of these limitations are overcome by generalized linear models, which relate the distribution of the ordered categorical response to a number of explanatory variables. Because response variables of this type have more than two categories, they are often referred to as *polytomous responses* and the corresponding procedures as *polytomous regression*.

Three approaches are described very briefly here. The first two are generalizations of logistic regression, and the third is related to comparisons of mean scores (see (15.8)).

The cumulative logits model

Denote the polytomous response variable by Y, and a particular category of Y by j. The set of explanatory variables, $x_1, x_2, \ldots, x_p$, will be denoted by the vector $\boldsymbol{x}$. Let

$$F_j(\boldsymbol{x}) = \mathrm{P}(Y \leq j, \text{given } \boldsymbol{x})$$

and

$$L_j = \mathrm{logit}\ F_j(\boldsymbol{x})$$
$$= \ln\left[\frac{F_j(\boldsymbol{x})}{1 - F_j(\boldsymbol{x})}\right].$$

The model is described by the equation

$$L_j(\boldsymbol{x}) = \alpha_j - \boldsymbol{\beta}'\boldsymbol{x}, \tag{14.9}$$

where $\boldsymbol{\beta}'\boldsymbol{x}$ represents the usual linear function of the explanatory variables, $\beta_1 x_1 + \beta_2 x_2 + \ldots + \beta_p x_p$.

This model effectively gives a logistic regression, as in (14.6), for each of the binary variables produced by drawing boundaries between two adjacent categories. For instance, if there are four categories numbered 1 to 4, there are three binary variables representing the splits between 1 and 2–4, 1–2 and 3–4, and 1–3 and 4. Moreover, the regression coefficients $\boldsymbol{\beta}$ for the explanatory variables are the same for all the splits, although the intercept term α_j varies with the split.

Although a standard logistic regression could be carried out for any one of the splits, a rather more complex analysis is needed to take account of the interrelations between the data for different splits. Computer programs are available (for instance, in SAS) to estimate the coefficients in the model and their precision, either by maximum likelihood (as in SAS LOGIST) or weighted least squares (as in SAS CATMOD), the latter being less reliable when many of the frequencies in the original data are low.

The adjacent categories model

Here we define logits in terms of the probabilities for adjacent categories. Define

$$L_j = \ln\left(\frac{\pi_j}{\pi_{j+1}}\right),$$

where π_j is the probability of falling into the jth response category. The model is described by the equation

$$L_j = \alpha_j - \boldsymbol{\beta}'\boldsymbol{x}. \tag{14.10}$$

When there are only two response categories, (14.9) and (14.10) are entirely equivalent, and both the cumulative logits model and the adjacent categories model reduce to ordinary logistic regression. In the more general case, with more than two categories, computer programs are available for estimation of the coefficients. For example, SAS CATMOD uses weighted least squares.

The mean response model

Suppose that scores x are assigned to the categories, as in §15.2, and denote by $M(x)$ the mean score for individuals with explanatory variables x. The model specifies the same linear relation as in multiple regression

$$M(x) = \alpha + \beta'x. \tag{14.11}$$

The approach is thus a generalization of that underlying the comparison of mean scores by (15.8) in the simple two-group case. In the general case the regression coefficients cannot be estimated accurately by standard multiple regression methods, because there may be large departures from normality and disparities in variance. Nor can exact variances such as (15.5) be easily exploited.

Choice of model

The choice between the models described briefly above, or any others, is largely empirical: which is the most convenient to use, and which best describes the data? There is no universally best choice. The two logistic models attempt to describe the relative frequencies of observations in the various categories, and their adequacy for any particular data set may be checked by comparing observed and expected frequencies. The mean response model is less searching, since it aims to describe only the mean values. It may, therefore, be a little more flexible in fitting data, and particularly appropriate where there is a natural underlying continuous response variate or scoring system, but less appropriate when the fine structure of the categorical response is under study.

Further descriptions of these models are given in Agresti (1990, Chapter 9), and an application to repeated measures data is described in Agresti (1989). An example relating alcohol consumption in eight ordered categories to biochemical and haematological variables was discussed by Ashby *et al.* (1986). These authors also discussed a test of goodness of fit, which is essentially an extension of the Hosmer–Lemeshow test, and a method of allocating an individual to one of the groups.

Example 14.2

Bishop (2000) followed up 207 patients admitted to hospital following injury and recorded functional outcome after 3 months using a modified Glasgow Outcome Score (GOS). This score had five ordered categories—full recovery, mild disability, moderate disability, severe disability, and dead or vegetative state.

The relationship between functional outcome and a number of variables relating to the patient and the injury was analysed using the cumulative logits model (14.9) of polytomous regression. The final model included seven βs indicating the relationship between outcome and seven variables, which included age, whether the patient was transferred from a peripheral hospital, three variables representing injury severity, two interaction terms, and four αs representing the splits between the five categories of GOS.

The model fitted well and was assessed in terms of ability to predict GOS for each patient. For 88 patients there was exact agreement between observed and predicted GOS scores compared with 52·4 expected by chance if the model had no predicting ability, and there were three patients who differed by three or four categories on the GOS scale compared with 23·3 expected. As discussed in §13.3, this is likely to be overoptimistic as far as the ability of the model to predict the categories of future patients is concerned.

14.4 **Poisson regression**

Poisson distribution

The expectation of a Poisson variable is positive and so limited to the range 0 to ∞. A link function is required to transform this to the unlimited range $-\infty$ to ∞. The usual transformation is the logarithmic transformation

$$g(\mu) = \ln \mu,$$

leading to the log-linear model

$$\ln \mu = \beta_0 + \beta_1 x_1 + \beta_2 x_2 + \ldots + \beta_p x_p. \tag{14.12}$$

Example 14.3

Table 14.2 shows the number of cerebrovascular accidents experienced during a certain period by 41 men, each of whom had recovered from a previous cerebrovascular accident and was hypertensive. Sixteen of these men received treatment with hypotensive drugs and 25 formed a control group without such treatment. The data are shown in the form of a frequency distribution, as the number of accidents takes only the values 0, 1, 2 and 3. This was not a controlled trial with random allocation, but it was nevertheless useful to enquire whether the difference in the mean numbers of accidents for the two groups was significant, and since the age distributions of the two groups were markedly different it was thought that an allowance for age might be important.

The data consist of 41 men, classified by three age groups and two treatment groups, and the variable to be analysed is the number of cerebrovascular accidents, which takes integral values. If the number of accidents is taken as having a Poisson distribution with

Table 14.2 Distribution of numbers of cerebrovascular accidents experienced by males in hypotensive-treated and control groups, subdivided by age.

| | Number of accidents | Age (years) | | |
		40–	50–	60–
		Number of men	Number of men	Number of men
Control group	0	0	3	4
	1	1	3	8
	2	0	4	1
	3	0	1	0
		1	11	13
Treated group	0	4	7	1
	1	0	4	0
		4	11	1

expectation dependent on age and treatment group, then a log-linear model (14.12) would be appropriate.

Several log-linear models have been fitted and the following analysis of deviance has been constructed:

Analysis of deviance

Fitting	Deviance	DF	Effect	Deviance difference	DF
Constant term	40·54	40			
Treatment, T	31·54	39	T (unadj.)	9·00	1
Age, A	37·63	38	A (unadj.)	2·91	2
T + A	28·84	37	T (adj.)	8·79	1
			A (adj.)	2·70	2
T + A + T × A	27·04	35	T × A	1·80	2

The test of the treatment effect after allowing for age is obtained from the deviance difference after adding in a treatment effect to a model already containing age; that is, $37·63 - 28·84 = 8·79$ (1 DF). Similarly, the effect of age adjusted for treatment has a test statistic of 2·70 (2 DF). There is no evidence of an interaction between treatment and age, or of a main effect of age.

The log-linear model fitting just treatment is

$$\ln \mu = 0·00 - 1·386 \text{ (treated group)},$$

$$\text{SE}: 0·536,$$

giving fitted expectations of $\exp(0 \cdot 00) = 1 \cdot 00$ for the control group and $\exp(-1 \cdot 386) = 0 \cdot 25$ for the treated group. These values are identical with the observed values—25 accidents in 25 men in the control group and four accidents in 16 men in the treated group—although if it had proved necessary to adjust for age this would not have been so.

The deviance of $27 \cdot 04$ with 35 DF after fitting all effects is a measure of how well the Poisson model fits the data. However, it would not be valid to assess this deviance as an approximate χ^2 because of the low counts on which it is based. Note that this restriction does not apply to the tests of main effects and interactions, since these comparisons are based on amalgamated data, as illustrated above for the effect of treatment.

We conclude our discussion of Poisson regression with an example of a log-linear model applied to Poisson counts.

Example 14.4

Table 14.3 gives data on the number of incident cases of cancer in a large group of ex-servicemen, who had been followed up over a 20-year period. The servicemen are in two groups according to whether they served in a combat zone (veterans) or not, and the experience of each serviceman is classified into subject-years at risk in 5-year age groups. The study is described in Australian Institute of Health and Welfare (1992), where the analysis also controlled for calendar year. Each serviceman passed through several of these groups during the period of follow-up. The study was carried out in order to assess if there was a difference in cancer risk between veterans and non-veterans. The model used was a variant on (14.12). If y_{ij} is the number of cases of cancer in group i and age group j, and N_{ij} is the corresponding number of subject-years, then y_{ij}/N_{ij} is the incidence rate.

Table 14.3 Number of incident cases of cancer and subject-years at risk in a group of ex-servicemen (reproduced by permission of the Australian Institute of Health and Welfare).

Age	Veterans		Non-veterans	
	Number of cancers	Subject-years	Number of cancers	Subject-years
–24	6	60 840	18	208 487
25–29	21	157 175	60	303 832
30–34	54	176 134	122	325 421
35–39	118	186 514	191	312 242
40–44	97	135 475	108	165 597
45–49	58	42 620	74	54 396
50–54	56	25 001	88	40 716
55–59	54	13 710	120	33 801
60–64	34	6 163	141	26 618
65–69	9	1 575	108	17 404
70–	2	273	99	14 146
Total	509	805 480	1129	1 502 660

The log-linear model states that the logarithm of incidence will follow a linear model on variables representing the group and age. Thus if μ_{ij} is the expectation of y_{ij}, then

$$\ln \mu_{ij} = \ln N_{ij} + \alpha + \beta_i x_i + \gamma_j z_j, \tag{14.13}$$

where x_i and z_j are dummy variables representing the veteran groups and the age groups, respectively (the dummy variables were defined as in §11.7, with $x_1 = 1$ for the veterans group, and $z_1, z_2, \ldots, z_{10} = 1$ for age groups 25–29, 30–34, …, 70–; no dummy variable was required for the non-veterans or the youngest age group as their effects are included within the coefficient α). This model differs from (14.12) in the inclusion of the first term on the right-hand side, which ensures that the number of years at risk is taken into account (see (19.38)).

The model was fitted by maximum likelihood using GLIM with $\ln N_{ij}$ included as an OFFSET. The estimates of the regression coefficients were:

	Estimate	SE
a	−9·324	
b_1 (veterans)	−0·0035	0·0555
c_1 (25–29)	0·679	0·232
c_2 (30–34)	1·371	0·218
c_3 (35–39)	1·940	0·212
c_4 (40–44)	2·034	0·216
c_5 (45–49)	2·727	0·222
c_6 (50–54)	3·203	0·221
c_7 (55–59)	3·716	0·218
c_8 (60–64)	4·093	0·218
c_9 (65–69)	4·236	0·224
c_{10} (70–)	4·364	0·227

The estimate of the veterans effect is not significant, Wald $z = -0·0035/0·0555 = 0·06 (P = 0·95)$. Converting back from the log scale, the estimate of the relative risk of cancer in veterans compared with non-veterans, after controlling for age, is $\exp(-0·0035) = 1·00$. The 95% confidence limits are $\exp(-0·0035 \pm 1·96 \times 0·0555) = 0·89$ and $1·11$.

15 Empirical methods for categorical data

15.1 **Introduction**

Categorical data show the frequencies with which observations fall into various categories or combinations of categories. Some of the basic methods of handling this type of data have been discussed in earlier sections of the book, particularly §§3.6, 3.7, 4.4, 4.5, 5.2, 8.5, 8.6 and 8.8. In the present chapter we gather together a number of more advanced techniques for handling categorical data.

Many of the techniques described in these sections make use of the χ^2 distributions, which have been used extensively in earlier chapters. These χ^2 methods are, however, almost exclusively designed for significance testing. In many problems involving categorical data, the estimation of relevant parameters which describe the nature of possible associations between variables is much more important than the performance of significance tests of null hypotheses. Chapter 14 is devoted to a general approach to modelling the relationships between variables, of which some particular cases are relevant to categorical data.

It is useful at this stage to make a distinction between three different types of classification into categories, according to the types of variable described in §2.3.

1 *Nominal* variables, in which no ordering is implied.
2 *Ordinal* variables, in which the categories assume a natural ordering although they are not necessarily associated with a quantitative measurement.
3 *Quantitative* variables, in which the categories are ordered by their association with a quantitative measurement.

It is often useful to consider both ordinal and quantitative variables as *ordered*, and to distinguish particularly between nominal and ordered data. But data can sometimes be considered from more than one point of view. For instance, quantitative data might be regarded as merely ordinal if it seemed important to take account of the ordering but not to rely too closely on the specific underlying variable. Ordered data might be regarded as purely nominal if there seemed to be differences between the effects of different categories which were not related to their natural order. We need, therefore, methods which can be adapted to a wide range of situations.

Many of the χ^2 tests introduced earlier have involved test statistics distributed as χ^2 on several degrees of freedom. In each instance the test was sensitive to departures from a null hypothesis, which could occur in various ways. In a $2 \times k$

contingency table, for instance, the null hypothesis postulates equality between the expected proportions of individuals in each column which fall into the first row. There are k of these proportions, and the null hypothesis can be falsified if any one of them differs from the others. These tests may be thought of as 'portmanteau' techniques, able to serve many different purposes. If, however, we were particularly interested in a certain form of departure from the null hypothesis, it might be possible to formulate a test which was particularly sensitive to this situation, although perhaps less effective than the portmanteau χ^2 test in detecting other forms of departure. Sometimes these specially directed tests can be achieved by subdividing the total χ^2 statistic into portions which follow χ^2 distributions on reduced numbers of degrees of freedom (DF).

The situation is very similar to that encountered in the analysis of variance, where a sum of squares (SSq) can sometimes be subdivided into portions, on reduced numbers of DF, which represent specific contrasts between groups (§8.4).

In §§15.2 and 15.3 we describe methods for detecting trends in the probabilities with which observations fall into a series of ordered categories. In §15.4 a similar method is described for a single series of counts. In §15.5 two other situations are described, in which the χ^2 statistic calculated for a contingency table is subdivided to shed light on specific ways in which categorical variables may be associated. In §§15.6 and 15.7 some of the methods described earlier are generalized for situations in which the data are stratified (i.e. divided into subgroups), so that trends can be examined within strata and finally pooled. Finally, in §15.8 we discuss exact tests for some of the situations considered in the earlier sections.

More comprehensive treatments of the analysis of categorical data are contained in the monographs by Fienberg (1980), Fleiss (1981), Cox and Snell (1989) and Agresti (1990, 1996).

15.2 **Trends in proportions**

Suppose that, in a $2 \times k$ contingency table of the type discussed in §8.5, the k groups have a natural order. They may correspond to different values, or groups of values, of a quantitative variable like age; or they may correspond to qualitative categories, such as severity of a disease, which can be ordered but not readily assigned a numerical value. The usual $\chi^2_{(k-1)}$ test is designed to detect differences between the k proportions of observations falling into the first row. More specifically, one might ask whether there is a significant trend in these proportions from group 1 to group k.

For convenience of exposition we shall assign the groups to the rows of the table, which now becomes $k \times 2$ rather than $2 \times k$. Let us assign a quantitative variable, x, to the k groups. If the definition of groups uses such a variable, this can be chosen to be x. If the definition is qualitative, x can take integer values from 1 to k. The notation is as follows:

Group	Variable x	Frequency		Total	Proportion positive
		Positive	Negative		
1	x_1	r_1	$n_1 - r_1$	n_1	p_1
2	x_2	r_2	$n_2 - r_2$	n_2	p_2
$\vdots$					
i	x_i	r_i	$n_i - r_i$	n_i	p_i
$\vdots$					
k	x_k	r_k	$n_k - r_k$	n_k	p_k
All groups combined		R	$N - R$	N	$P(= R/N)$

The numerator of the $\chi^2_{(k-1)}$ statistic, X^2, is, from (8.29),

$$\sum n_i (p_i - P)^2,$$

a weighted sum of squares of the p_i about the (weighted) mean P (see discussion after (8.30)). It also turns out to be a straightforward sum of squares, between groups, of a variable y taking the value 1 for each positive individual and 0 for each negative. This SSq can be divided (as in §11.1) into an SSq due to regression of y on x and an SSq due to departures from linear regression. If there is a trend of p_i with x_i, we might find the first of these two portions to be greater than would be expected by chance. Dividing this portion by PQ, the denominator of (8.29), gives us a $\chi^2_{(1)}$ statistic, X_1^2, which forms part of X^2 and is particularly sensitive to trend.

A little algebraic manipulation (Armitage, 1955) gives

$$X_1^2 = \frac{N(N \sum r_i x_i - R \sum n_i x_i)^2}{R(N - R)[N \sum n_i x_i^2 - (\sum n_i x_i)^2]}, \tag{15.1}$$

often referred to as the Cochran–Armitage test of trend. The difference between the two statistics,

$$X_2^2 = X^2 - X_1^2, \tag{15.2}$$

may be regarded as a $\chi^2_{(k-2)}$ statistic testing departures from linear regression of p_i on x_i. As usual, both of these tests are approximate, but the approximation (15.2) is likely to be adequate if only a small proportion of the expected frequencies are less than about 5. The trend test (15.1) is adequate in these conditions but also more widely, since it is based on a linear function of the frequencies, and is likely to be satisfactory provided that only a small proportion of expected frequencies are less than about 2 and that these do not occur in adjacent rows. If appropriate statistical software is available, an exact test can be constructed (§15.8).

Example 15.1

In the analysis of the data summarized in Table 15.1, it would be reasonable to ask whether the proportion of patients accepting their general practitioner's invitation to attend screening mammography tends to decrease as the time since their last consultation increases. The first step is to decide on scores representing the four time-period categories. It would be possible to use the mid-points of the time intervals, 3 months, 9 months, etc., but the last interval, being open, would be awkward. Instead, we shall use equally spaced integer scores, as shown in the table.

From (15.1),

$$X_1^2 = \frac{(278)[(278)(49) - (86)(236)]^2}{(86)(192)[(278)(530) - (236)^2]}$$

$$= (1\cdot2383 \times 10^{10})/(0\cdot15132 \times 10^{10})$$

$$= 8\cdot18,$$

which, as a $\chi^2_{(1)}$ variate, is highly significant ($P = 0\cdot004$).

The overall $\chi^2_{(3)}$ statistic, from (8.28) or (8.30), is calculated as

$$X^2 = 8\cdot92.$$

The test for departures from a linear trend (15.2) thus gives

$$X_2^2 = 8\cdot92 - 8\cdot18 = 0\cdot74$$

as a $\chi^2_{(2)}$ variate, which is clearly non-significant. There is thus a definite trend which may well result in approximately equal decreases in the proportion of attenders as we change successively to the categories representing longer times since the last consultation.

A number of other formulae are equivalent or nearly equivalent to (15.1). The regression coefficient of y on x, measuring the rate at which the proportion p_i changes with the score x_i, is estimated by the expression

Table 15.1 Numbers of patients attending or not attending screening mammography, classified by time since last visit to the general practitioner (Irwig *et al.*, 1990).

Time since last visit	Score x	Attendance		Total	Proportion attending
		Yes	No		
<6 months	0	59	97	156	0·378
6–12 months	1	10	31	41	0·244
1–2 years	2	12	36	48	0·250
>2 years	3	5	28	33	0·152
		86	192	278	

$$b = \frac{NT}{N \sum n_i x_i^2 - (\sum n_i x_i)^2},$$ (15.3)

where

$$T = \sum r_i x_i - \frac{R \sum n_i x_i}{N} = \sum x_i (r_i - e_i),$$ (15.4)

the cross-product of the scores x_i and the discrepancies $r_i - e_i$ in the contingency table between the frequencies in the first column (i.e. of positives) and their expected values from the margins of the table. Here r_i and e_i correspond to the O and E of (8.28), e_i being calculated as Rn_i/N. On the null hypothesis of no association between rows and columns, for fixed values of the marginal totals, the exact variance of T is

$$\mathrm{var}(T) = \frac{R(N - R)[N \sum n_i x_i^2 - (\sum n_i x_i)^2]}{N^2(N - 1)}.$$ (15.5)

A $\chi^2_{(1)}$ test for the trend in proportions is therefore provided by the statistic

$$X^2_{1a} = \frac{T^2}{\mathrm{var}(T)} = \frac{(N - 1)[\sum x_i(r_i - e_i)]^2}{(N - R)[\sum e_i x_i^2 - (\sum e_i x_i)^2/R]}.$$ (15.6)

In fact, $X^2_{1a} = (N - 1)X^2_1/N$, so the two tests are very nearly equivalent. The distinction is unimportant in most analyses, when N is fairly large, but (15.6) should be used when N is rather small. In particular, it is preferable in situations to be considered in §15.7, where data are subdivided into strata, some of which may be small.

If the null hypothesis is untrue, (15.5) overestimates $\mathrm{var}(T)$, since it makes use of the total variation of y rather than the variation about regression on x. For the regression of a binary variable y on x, an analysis of variance could be calculated, as in Table 11.1. In this analysis the sum of squares about regression turns out to be $R(N - R)(N - X^2_1)/N$, and, using (7.16), $\mathrm{var}(b)$ may be calculated as

$$\mathrm{var}(b) = \frac{R(N - R)(N - X^2_1)}{N(N - 2)[N \sum n_i x_i^2 - (\sum n_i x_i)^2]}.$$ (15.7)

For the calculation of confidence limits for the slope, therefore, the formula after (7.18) may be used, with the percentile of the t distribution on $N - 2$ DF (which in most applications will be close to the standardized normal value), and with $\mathrm{SE}(b) = \sqrt{\mathrm{var}(b)}$.

By analogy with the situation for simple regression (see the paragraph after (7.19)), the test for association based on the regression of y on x, as in (15.1) and (15.6), should give the same significance level as that based on the regression of x on y. Since y is a binary variable, the latter regression is essentially determined by the difference between the mean values of x at the two levels of y. In many problems, particularly where y is clearly the dependent variable, this difference is of no interest. In other situations—for example when the columns of the table represent different treatments and the rows are ordered categories of a response to treatment—this is a natural way of approaching the data. The standard method for comparing two means is, of course, the two-sample t test. The method now under discussion provides an alternative, which may be preferable for categorical responses since the data are usually far from normal.

The difference between the mean scores for the positive and negative responses is

$$d = \frac{NT}{R(N-R)}, \tag{15.8}$$

where T is given by (15.4). Since $d^2/\text{var}(d) = X_{1a}^2$, as given by (15.6), it can easily be checked that

$$\text{var}(d) = \sigma_x^2 \left(\frac{1}{R} + \frac{1}{N-R} \right), \tag{15.9}$$

where σ_x^2 is the variance of x, given by

$$\sigma_x^2 = \frac{\sum n_i x_i^2 - \dfrac{\left(\sum n_i x_i \right)^2}{N}}{N-1}. \tag{15.10}$$

Note that (15.10) is the variance of x for the complete data, not the variance within the separate columns. If the null hypothesis is not true, (15.9) will overestimate the variance of d, and confidence limits for the difference in means calculated from (15.9) will tend to be somewhat too wide.

The test for the difference in means described above is closely related to the Wilcoxon and Mann–Whitney distribution-free tests described in §10.3.

In the previous chapter it was noted that logistic regression is a powerful method of analysing dichotomous data. Logistic regression can be used to test for a trend in proportions by fitting a model on x. If this is done, then one of the test statistics, the score statistic (p. 490), is identical to (15.1).

Example 15.1, continued

Applying (15.3) and (15.7) to the data of Table 15.1 gives:

$b = -0\cdot0728$, SE$(b) = 0\cdot0252$, with 95% confidence limits $(-0\cdot122, -0\cdot023)$.

Note that $b^2/\text{var}(b) = 8\cdot37$, a little higher than X_1^2, as would be expected.

Fitting a logistic regression gives a regression coefficient on x of:

$b' = -0\cdot375$, SE$(b') = 0\cdot133$, with 95% confidence limits $(-0\cdot637, -0\cdot114)$.

Of course, b and b' are different because the former is a regression of the proportion and the latter of the logit transform of proportion. Interpretation of b' is facilitated by taking the exponential, which gives a reduction in odds of proportion of attenders by a factor of 0·69 (95% confidence interval 0·53 to 0·89) per category of time since the last consultation. The χ^2 test statistics of the trend are 8·67 for the deviance test, 7·90 for Wald's test, and 8·18 for the score test, this last value being identical to the value obtained earlier from (15.1).

15.3 **Trends in larger contingency tables**

Tests for trend can also be applied to contingency tables larger than the $k \times 2$ table considered in §15.2. The extension to more than two columns of frequencies gives rise to two possibilities: the columns may be nominal (i.e. unordered) or ordered. In the first case, we might wish to test for differences in the mean row scores between the different columns; this would be an alternative to the one-way analysis of variance, just as the χ^2 test based on (15.8) and (15.9) is an alternative to the two-sample t test. In the second case, of ordered column categories, the problem might be to test the regression of one set of scores on the other, or equivalently the correlation between the row and column scores. Both situations are illustrated by an example, the methods of analysis following closely those described by Yates (1948).

Example 15.2

Sixty-six mothers who had suffered the death of a newborn baby were studied to assess the relationship between their state of grief and degree of support (Tudehope *et al.*, 1986). Grief was recorded on a qualitative ordered scale with four categories and degree of support on an ordered scale with three categories (Table 15.2). The overall test statistic (8.28) is 9·96 (6 DF), which is clearly not significant. Nevertheless, examination of the contingency table suggests that those with good support experienced less grief than those with poor support, whilst those with adequate support were intermediate, and that this effect is being missed by the overall test. The aim of the trend test is to produce a more sensitive test on this specific aspect.

We first ignore the ordering of the columns, regarding them as three different categories of a nominal variable. The calculations proceed as follows.

1 Assign scores to rows (x) and columns (y): integer values starting from 1 have been used. Denote the row totals by R_i, $i = 1$ to r, the column totals by C_j, $j = 1$ to c, and the total number of subjects by N.
2 For each column calculate the sum of the row scores, X_j, and the mean row score $\bar{x}_j$. For the first column,

$$X_1 = (17 \times 1) + (6 \times 2) + (3 \times 3) + (1 \times 4) = 42,$$
$$\bar{x}_1 = 42/27 = 1\cdot56.$$

This calculation is also carried out for the column of row totals to give 126, which serves as a check on the values of X_j, which sum over columns to this value. This total is the sum of the row scores for all the mothers, i.e. $\sum x = 126$.

Table 15.2 Numbers of mothers by state of grief and degree of support (data of Tudehope *et al.*, 1986).

Grief state	Row score x_i	Good	Adequate	Poor	Total R_i	Sum of column scores Y_i
I	1	17	9	8	34	59
II	2	6	5	1	12	19
III	3	3	5	4	12	25
IV	4	1	2	5	8	20
Total, C_j		27	21	18	66	123
Col. score, y_j		1	2	3		
Sum of row scores, X_j		42	42	42	126	
Mean score, $\bar{x}_j$		1·56	2·00	2·33		

3   Calculate the sum of squares of row scores for all the mothers,

$$\sum x^2 = (34 \times 1) + (12 \times 4) + (12 \times 9) + (8 \times 16) = 318.$$

Correct this sum of squares for the mean.

$$S_{xx} = 318 - 126^2/66 = 77 \cdot 455.$$

4   A test of the equality of the mean scores $\bar{x}_j$ may now be carried out. The test statistic is

$$X^2 = (N-1)[\sum(X_j^2/C_j) - (\sum x)^2/N]/S_{xx}$$

$$= \frac{65}{77 \cdot 455}\left(\frac{42^2}{27} + \frac{42^2}{21} + \frac{42^2}{18} - \frac{126^2}{66}\right) \tag{15.11}$$

$$= 5 \cdot 70.$$

This may be regarded as a $\chi^2_{(c-1)}$, i.e. a $\chi^2_{(2)}$ statistic. This is not quite significant at the 5% level ($P = 0 \cdot 058$), but is sufficiently close to allow the possibility that a test for the apparent trend in the column means, $\bar{x}_j$, may be significant. We now, therefore, make use of the column scores, y_j.

5   Repeat steps **2** and **3**, working across rows instead of down columns; it is not necessary to calculate the mean scores.

$$\sum y = 123, \sum y^2 = 273, S_{yy} = 273 - 123^2/66 = 43 \cdot 773.$$

6   Calculate the sum of products of the sum of row scores, X_j, and the corresponding column scores, y_j.

$$\sum X_j y_j = (42 \times 1) + (42 \times 2) + (42 \times 3) = 252.$$

This total is $\sum xy$ over all mothers and correcting for the means

$$S_{xy} = 252 - (123 \times 126)/66 = 17 \cdot 182.$$

7 The test statistic for the trend in the mean scores, $\bar{x}_j$, is

$$
\begin{aligned}
X^2 &= (N-1)S_{xy}^2/(S_{xx}S_{yy}) \\
&= 65 \times 17 \cdot 182^2/(77 \cdot 455 \times 43 \cdot 773) \\
&= 5 \cdot 66.
\end{aligned}
\tag{15.12}
$$

This is approximately a $\chi^2_{(1)}$ statistic and is significant ($P = 0 \cdot 017$). In this example most of the difference between column means lies in the trend. This is clear from examination of the column means, and the corresponding result for the test statistics is that the overall test statistic of 5·70 (2 DF) for equality of column means may be subdivided into 5·66 (1 DF) for linear trend and, by subtraction, 0·04 (1 DF) for departures from the trend.

Note that the test statistic (15.12) is $N - 1$ times the square of the correlation coefficient between the row and column scores, and this may be a convenient way of calculating it on a computer. When $r = 2$, (15.11) tests the equality of c proportions, and is identical with (8.30) except for a multiplying factor of $(N - 1)/N$; (15.12) tests the trend in the proportions and is identical with (15.6).

Both (15.11) and (15.12) are included in the SAS program PROC FREQ, the former as the 'ANOVA statistic' and the latter as the 'Mantel–Haenszel chi-square'.

15.4 **Trends in counts**

In many problems of the type considered in §15.3, the proportions under consideration are very small. If, for instance, the frequencies in the 'positive' column of the table on p. 505 are much smaller than those in the 'negative' column, almost all the contribution to the test statistic comes from the positives. In the limit, as the p_i become very small and the n_i become very large, both (15.1) and (15.6) take the form

$$
X_{1P}^2 = \frac{\left[\sum x_i(r_i - e_i)\right]^2}{\left[\sum e_i x_i^2 - \left(\sum e_i x_i\right)^2/R\right]}.
\tag{15.13}
$$

The subscript P is used for this test statistic because in this limiting situation the observed frequencies r_i can be regarded as Poisson variates with means (under the null hypothesis) e_i, the expected values. In some applications the expected values are proportional to subject-years of observation for individuals in each category (see §19.7).

Example 15.3

In the data shown in Table 15.3, the observed deaths and person-years of observation weighted by time since exposure are shown. If there were no association between the death

Table 15.3 Mortality due to pleural mesothelioma in asbestos factory workers according to an ordered category of amount of exposure (Berry *et al.*, 2000).

Category of exposure, x_i	Observed deaths, r_i	Person-years, P_i	Expected, e_i
1	11	23 522	15·482
2	18	34 269	22·556
3	7	7 075	4·657
4	16	14 138	9·306
Totals	52	79 004	52·001

rate and category of exposure, then the expected frequencies of deaths would be in proportion to the person-years of observation in the different exposure categories, so as to add to the observed total of 52. The total $\chi^2_{(3)}$ statistic, calculated as $\sum (r_i - e_i)^2$, is 8·21, which is significant ($P = 0\cdot042$). There is a suggestion that the association consists of a deficit of deaths in the low-exposure categories and an excess with the higher exposures. Application of (15.13) gives $X^2_{1P} = 7\cdot27$ ($P = 0\cdot007$). There is clearly evidence for a gradual increase in the rate of deaths due to pleural mesothelioma with increasing exposure in this study.

In Example 15.3, the observed number of deaths is a Poisson variable and, therefore, the method of Poisson regression (§14.4) may be applied, but with an additional term in (14.12) to incorporate the fact that the expected number of deaths is proportional to the number of person-years of observation modified by the regression model. The rationale is similar to that used in Example 14.4 leading to (14.13).

Example 15.3, continued

Poisson regression models (§14.4) have been fitted to the data of Table 15.3. The offset was the logarithm of the number of years of observation. The first model fitted was a null model just containing an intercept and this gave a deviance of 7·41 (3 DF). Then the score for category of exposure, x, was added to give a deviance of 0·59 (2 DF). Thus, the deviance test of the trend of mortality with category of exposure was 6·82 which, as an approximate $\chi^2_{(1)}$, gives $P = 0\cdot009$. The regression coefficient of x was 0·3295 with standard error 0·1240, giving a Wald χ^2 of 7·06 ($P = 0\cdot008$). These test statistics and significance levels are in reasonable agreement with the value of 7·27 ($P = 0\cdot007$) found for the trend test.

15.5 **Other components of χ^2**

Most of the χ^2 statistics described earlier in this chapter can be regarded as components of the total χ^2 statistic for a contingency table. Two further examples of the subdivision of χ^2 statistics are given below.

Hierarchical classification

In §15.2, the numerator of the $\chi^2_{(k-1)}$ statistic (8.29) was regarded as the SSq between groups of a dummy variable y, taking the values 0 and 1. We proceeded to subdivide this in a standard way. Other types of subdivision encountered in Chapters 8 and 9 may equally be used if they are relevant to the data under study. For example, if the k groups form a factorial arrangement, and if the n_i are equal or are proportional to marginal totals for the separate factors, the usual techniques could be used to separate SSq and hence components of the $\chi^2_{(k-1)}$ statistic, representing main effects and interactions.

Another situation, in which no conditions need be imposed on the n_i, is that in which the groups form a hierarchical arrangement.

Example 15.4

Table 15.4 shows proportions of houseflies killed by two different insecticides. There are two batches of each insecticide, and each of the four batches is subjected to two tests. The overall $\chi^2_{(7)}$ test gives

$$X^2_7 = (2^2/51 + \ldots + 9^2/48 - 45^2/391)/(0 \cdot 8849)(0 \cdot 1151)$$
$$= 1 \cdot 6628/0 \cdot 1019 = 16 \cdot 32 \text{ on } 7 \text{ DF},$$

which is significant $(P = 0 \cdot 022)$. This can be subdivided as follows.
Between tests (4 DF):

$$X^2_{(4)} = \frac{(2^2/51 + 5^2/48 - 7^2/99) + \ldots + (11^2/50 + 9^2/48 - 20^2/98)}{0 \cdot 1019}$$
$$= 2 \cdot 75 \quad (P = 0 \cdot 60);$$

Table 15.4 Proportion of houseflies killed in experiments with two insecticides.

Insecticide:	A					B					
Batch:	A1		A2		Total	B1		B2		Total	Total
Test:	1	2	1	2	A	1	2	1	2	B	A + B
Flies:											
Killed	49	43	43	48	183	41	44	39	39	163	346
Surviving	2	5	4	1	12	5	8	11	9	33	45
Total	51	48	47	49	195	46	52	50	48	196	391
Proportion killed					0·9385					0·8316	0·8849

Between batches (2 DF):

$$X^2_{(2)} = \frac{(7^2/99 + 5^2/96 - 12^2/195) + (13^2/98 + 20^2/98 - 33^2/196)}{0 \cdot 1019}$$

$$= 2 \cdot 62 \quad (P = 0 \cdot 27).$$

Between insecticides (1 DF):

$$X^2_{(1)} = \frac{(12^2/195 + 33^2/196 - 45^2/391)}{0 \cdot 1019}$$
$$= 10 \cdot 95 \quad (P < 0 \cdot 001).$$

As a check, $X^2_{(1)} + X^2_{(2)} + X^2_{(4)} = 16 \cdot 32$, agreeing with $X^2_{(7)}$. There is thus clear evidence of a difference in toxicity of the two insecticides, but no evidence of differences between batches or between tests.

A few remarks about this analysis follow.

1 Since a difference between A and B has been established it would be logical, in calculating $X^2_{(2)}$ and $X^2_{(4)}$, to use separate denominators for the contributions from the two insecticides. Thus, in calculating $X^2_{(2)}$ the first term in the numerator would have a denominator $(0 \cdot 9385)(0 \cdot 0615) = 0 \cdot 0577$, and the second term would have a denominator $(0 \cdot 8316)(0 \cdot 1684) = 0 \cdot 1400$. The effect of this correction is usually small. If it is made, the various χ^2 indices no longer add exactly to the total.

2 In entomological experiments it is common to find significant differences between replicate tests, perhaps because the response is sensitive to small changes in the environment and all the flies used in one test share the same environment (for example, being often kept in the same box). In such cases comparisons between treatments must take account of the random variation between tests. It is useful, therefore, to have adequate replication. The analysis can often be done satisfactorily by measuring the proportion of deaths at each test and analysing these proportions with or without one of the standard transformations.

3 An experiment of the size of that shown in Table 15.4 is not really big enough to detect variation between batches and tests. Although the numbers of flies are quite large, more replication both of tests and of batches is desirable.

Larger contingency tables

The hierarchical principle can be applied to larger contingency tables (§8.6). In an $r \times c$ table, the total χ^2 statistic, X^2, can be calculated from (8.28). It has $(r - 1)(c - 1)$ DF, and represents departures of the cell frequencies from those expected by proportionality to row and column totals. It may be relevant to ask whether proportionality holds in some segment of the whole table; then in a second segment chosen after collapsing either rows or columns in the first segment; then in a third segment; and so on. If, in performing these successive χ^2 calculations, one uses expected frequencies derived from the whole table, the various χ^2 statistics can be added in a natural way. If, however, the expected frequencies are derived separately for each subtable, the various components of

χ^2 will not add exactly to the total. The discrepancy is unlikely to be important in practice.

Example 15.5

Table 15.5, taken from Example 11.10.2 of Snedecor and Cochran (1989), shows data from a study of the relationship between blood groups and disease. The small number of AB patients have been omitted from the analysis. The overall $\chi^2_{(4)}$ test for the whole table gives $X^2 = 40 \cdot 54$, a value which is highly significant. A study of the proportions in the three blood groups, for each group of subjects, suggests that there is little difference between the controls and the patients with gastric cancer, or between the relative proportions in groups A and B, but that patients with peptic ulcer show an excess of group O. These comparisons can be examined by a subdivision of the 3×3 table into a hierarchical series of 2×2 tables, as shown in Fig. 15.1(a–d). The sequence is deliberately chosen so as to reveal the possible association between group O and peptic ulcer in the subtable (d). The arrows indicate a move to an enlarged table by amalgamation of the rows or columns of the previous table.

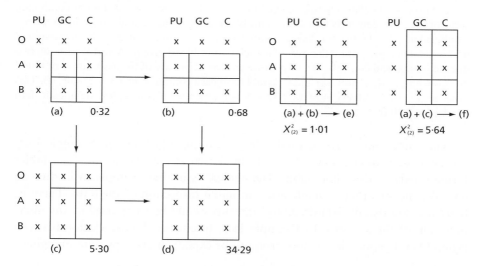

Fig. 15.1 Subdivision of $\chi^2_{(4)}$ statistic for Table 15.5. Tables (a)–(d) show one possible partition into separate $\chi^2_{(1)}$ statistics. Tables (e) and (f) show two ways of combining contrasts.

The corresponding values of $X^2_{(1)}$ are shown in the diagram and are reproduced here:

Row comparison	Column comparison	$X^2_{(1)}$
(a) A vs. B	GC vs. C	0·32
(b) A vs. B	PU vs. (GC, C)	0·68
(c) O vs. (A, B)	GC vs. C	5·30
(d) O vs. (A, B)	PU vs. (GC, C)	34·29
		40·59

Table 15.5 Frequencies (and percentages) of ABO blood groups in patients with peptic ulcer, patients with gastric cancer and controls (Snedecor & Cochran, 1989, Ex. 11.10.2).

Blood group	Peptic ulcer	(%)	Gastric cancer	(%)	Controls	(%)	Total
O	983	(55)	383	(43)	2892	(48)	4258
A	679	(38)	416	(47)	2625	(43)	3720
B	134	(7)	84	(10)	570	(9)	788
Total	1796	(100)	883	(100)	6087	(100)	8766

As noted earlier, the total of the X_1^2 statistics is a little different from the X_4^2 value of 40·54 for the whole table, but the discrepancy is slight. The value of X_1^2 for (c) gives $P = 0·021$, giving rise to some doubt about the lack of association of blood groups and gastric cancer. The outstanding contrast is that between the proportions of group O in the peptic ulcer patients and in the other subjects.

The process of collapsing rows and columns could have been speeded up by combining some of the 1 DF contrasts into 2 DF contrasts. For example, (a) and (b) could have been combined in a 2×3 table, (e). This gives an $X_{(2)}^2$ of 1·01, scarcely different from the sum of 0·32 and 0·68, representing the overall association of blood groups A and B with the two disease groups and controls. Or, to provide an overall picture of the association of blood groups with gastric cancer, (a) and (c) could have been combined in a 3×2 table, (f). This gives an $X_{(2)}^2$ of 5·64 (very close to $0·32 + 5·30$), which is, of course, less significant than the $X_{(1)}^2$ of 5·30 from (c).

There are many ways of subdividing a contingency table. In Example 15.5, the elementary table (a) could have been chosen as any one of the 2×2 tables forming part of the whole table. The choice, as in that example, will often be data-dependent—that is, made after an initial inspection of the data. There is, therefore, the risk of data-dredging, and this should be recognized in any interpretation of the analysis. In Example 15.5, of course, the association between group O and peptic ulcer is too strong to be explained away by data-dredging.

15.6 Combination of 2 × 2 tables

Sometimes a number of 2×2 tables, all bearing on the same question, are available, and it seems natural to combine the evidence for an association between the row and column factors. For example, there may be a number of retrospective studies, each providing evidence about a possible association between a certain disease and a certain environmental factor. Or, in a multicentre clinical trial, each centre may provide evidence about a possible difference between the proportions of patients whose condition is improved with treatment A and treatment B. These are examples of *stratification*. In the clinical trial, for example, the data are *stratified* by centre, and the aim is to study the effect of treatment on the patients' improvement *within the strata*.

How should such data be combined? The first point to make is that it may be quite misleading to pool the frequencies in the various tables and examine the association suggested by the table of pooled frequencies. An extreme illustration is provided by the following hypothetical data.

Example 15.6

The frequencies in the lower left-hand corner of Table 15.6 are supposed to have been obtained in a retrospective survey in which 1000 patients with a certain disease are compared with 1000 control subjects. The proportion with a certain characteristic A is very slightly higher in the control group than in the disease group. If anything, therefore, the data suggest a negative association between the disease and factor A, although, of course, the difference would be far from significant. However, suppose the two groups had not been matched for sex, and that the data for the two sexes separately were as shown in the upper left part of the table. For each sex there is a positive association between the disease and factor A, as may be seen by comparing the observed frequencies on the left with the expected frequencies on the right. The latter are calculated in the usual way, separately for each sex; for example, $144 = (240)(600)/1000$. What has happened here is that the control group contains a higher proportion of females than the disease group, and females have a higher prevalence of factor A than do males. The association suggested by the pooled frequencies is in the opposite direction from that suggested in each of the component tables. This phenomenon is often called *Simpson's paradox*. A variable like sex in this example, related both to the presence of disease and to a factor of interest, is called a *confounding variable*.

Table 15.6 Retrospective survey to study the association between a disease and an aetiological factor; data subdivided by sex.

		Observed frequencies			Expected frequencies	
		Disease	Control	Total	Disease	Control
Male	A	160	80	240	144	96
	Not A	440	320	760	456	304
		600	400	1000	600	400
Female	A	240	330	570	228	342
	Not A	160	270	430	172	258
		400	600	1000	400	600
Male	A	400	410	810	(372)	(438)
+ female	Not A	600	590	1190	(628)	(562)
		1000	1000	2000		

How should the evidence from separate tables be pooled? There is no unique answer. The procedure to be adopted will depend on whether the object is primarily to test the significance of a tendency for rows and columns to be associated in one direction throughout the data, or whether the association is to be measured, and if so in what way.

In some situations it is natural or convenient to study the association in each table by looking at the difference between two proportions. Suppose that, in the ith table, we are interested in a comparison between the proportion of individuals classified as 'positive' in each of two categories A and B, and that the frequencies in this table are as follows:

	A	B	Total A + B
Positive	r_{Ai}	r_{Bi}	$r_{.i}$
Negative	$n_{Ai} - r_{Ai}$	$n_{Bi} - r_{Bi}$	$n_{.i} - r_{.i}$
Total	n_{Ai}	n_{Bi}	$n_{.i}$
Proportion +ve	$p_{Ai} = r_{Ai}/n_{Ai}$	$p_{Bi} = r_{Bi}/n_{Bi}$	$p_{0i} = r_{.i}/n_{.i}$
			$q_{0i} = 1 - p_{0i}$

The differences that interest us are

$$d_i = p_{Ai} - p_{Bi}. \qquad (15.14)$$

These differences could be pooled in a weighted mean

$$\bar{d} = \sum_i w_i d_i / \sum_i w_i. \qquad (15.15)$$

Cochran (1954) suggested the use of the weights defined as:

$$w_i = \frac{n_{Ai}\, n_{Bi}}{n_{Ai} + n_{Bi}}. \qquad (15.16)$$

These have the property that, in general, more weight is given to tables with larger numbers provided they are reasonably balanced between categories A and B. It can be shown that this system of weights is the best for detecting small systematic differences between p_{Ai} and p_{Bi} of such a magnitude that the difference between their logits (14.5) is constant. This is a plausible requirement because a differential effect between A and B is likely to produce a larger d_i when the ps are near $\frac{1}{2}$ than when they are nearer 0 or 1.

Using the usual formula (§4.5) appropriate to the null hypothesis:

$$\text{var}(d_i) = p_{0i}q_{0i}(n_{Ai} + n_{Bi})/n_{Ai}n_{Bi}, \qquad (15.17)$$

we find

$$\text{var}(\bar{d}) = \sum_i w_i p_{0i} q_{0i} / \left(\sum w_i\right)^2,$$

$$\mathrm{SE}(\bar{d}) = \sqrt{\mathrm{var}(\bar{d})},$$

and, on the null hypothesis, $\bar{d}/\mathrm{SE}(\bar{d})$ can be taken as approximately a standardized normal deviate; or its square, $\bar{d}^2/\mathrm{var}(\bar{d})$, as a $\chi^2_{(1)}$ variate. An equivalent formula for the normal deviate is

$$\sum w_i d_i / \sqrt{\left(\sum w_i p_{0i} q_{0i}\right)}.$$

Example 15.7

Table 15.7 shows some results taken from a trial to compare the mortality from tetanus in patients receiving antitoxin and in those not receiving antitoxin. The treatments were allocated at random, but by chance a higher proportion of patients in the 'No antitoxin' group had a more severe category of disease (as defined in terms of incubation period and period of onset of spasms). The third category (unknown severity) is clearly numerically unimportant, but may as well be included in the calculations. The overall results favour the use of antitoxin, but this may be due partly to the more favourable distribution of cases.

Cochran's test proceeds as follows:

Group	p_{0i}	d_i	$p_{0i}q_{0i}$	w_i
I	$37/47 = 0.7872$	0.1319	0.1675	11.62
II	$10/29 = 0.3448$	0.3233	0.2259	6.83
III	$2/3\ \ \ = 0.6667$	0.5000	0.2222	0.67
				19.12

$$\bar{d} = 4.0758/19.12 = 0.2132,$$
$$\mathrm{SE}(\bar{d}) = (\sqrt{3.6381})/19.12 = 0.0997,$$
$$\bar{d}/\mathrm{SE}(\bar{d}) = 2.14,$$

beyond the 5% level of significance ($P = 0.032$).

Table 15.7 Mortality from tetanus in a clinical trial to compare the effects of using and not using antitoxin, with classification of patients by severity of disease (from Brown *et al.*, 1960).

Severity group	No antitoxin		Antitoxin	
	Deaths/ total	Proportion deaths	Deaths/ total	Proportion deaths
I (most severe)	22/26	0.8462	15/21	0.7143
II (least severe)	6/11	0.5455	4/18	0.2222
III (unknown)	1/1	1.0000	1/2	0.5000

Another approach to the problem of combining 2×2 tables is known as the Mantel–Haenszel method (Mantel & Haenszel, 1959). The number of positive individuals in group A in the ith table, r_{Ai}, may be compared with its expected frequency

$$e_{Ai} = r_{.i}n_{Ai}/n_{.i}.$$

The variance of the discrepancy between observed and expected frequencies is

$$\text{var}(r_{Ai} - e_{Ai}) = \frac{n_{Ai}n_{Bi}r_{.i}(n_{.i} - r_{.i})}{n_{.i}^2(n_{.i} - 1)}. \tag{15.18}$$

A test for the association in the ith table is given by the $\chi^2_{(1)}$ statistic

$$X^2_{MH} = \frac{(r_{Ai} - e_{Ai})^2}{\text{var}(r_{Ai} - e_{Ai})}, \tag{15.19}$$

which is, in fact, equal to (4.32) and to the usual χ^2 statistic (4.31) multiplied by the factor $(n_{.i} - 1)/n_{.i}$, which is near to unity for large sample sizes. If desired, a continuity correction analogous to (4.34) can be obtained by subtracting $\frac{1}{2}$ from the absolute value of the discrepancy before squaring the numerator of (15.19).

To test the association in the set of tables combined we merely add the discrepancies and their variances, to obtain the combined statistic

$$X^2_{MH} = \frac{[\sum(r_{Ai} - e_{Ai})]^2}{\sum \text{var}(r_{Ai} - e_{Ai})}, \tag{15.20}$$

which is distributed approximately as a χ^2 with 1 DF. Were it not for the multiplying factors $(n_{.i} - 1)/n_{.i}$, this formula would agree exactly with the expression $\bar{d}^2/\text{var}(\bar{d})$ in Cochran's method (Radhakrishna, 1965). For this reason the present approach is often called the Cochran–Mantel–Haenszel method.

Example 15.7, continued

For the data in Table 15.7 the calculations of the Mantel–Haenszel test proceed as follows:

Group	r_{Ai}	e_{Ai}	$r_{Ai} - e_{Ai}$	$\text{var}(r_{Ai} - e_{Ai})$
I	22	20·468	1·532	1·988
II	6	3·793	2·207	1·598
III	1	0·667	0·333	0·222
	29	24·928	4·072	3·808

$$X^2_{MH} = (4 \cdot 072)^2 / 3 \cdot 808 = 4 \cdot 35,$$
$$X_{MH} = 2 \cdot 09,$$

a little less significant ($P = 0 \cdot 037$) than the standardized deviate of $2 \cdot 14$ ($P = 0 \cdot 032$) given earlier by the Cochran method, the change being due to the multiplying factors used in the variance calculations. With the continuity correction,

$$X^2_{MHc} = 3 \cdot 35, X_{MHc} = 1 \cdot 83 \ (P = 0 \cdot 067).$$

Again this analysis may be performed using logistic regression. The strata are allowed for by including dummy variables (§11.7).

Example 15.7, continued

For the data in Table 15.7 a logistic regression is fitted of the logit of the proportion of deaths on two dummy variables representing the severity groups and a dichotomous variable representing the antitoxin treatment. The test statistics for the treatment effect, after allowing for severity, are $4 \cdot 56$ for the deviance test and $4 \cdot 36$ for Wald's χ^2, giving significance levels of $0 \cdot 033$ and $0 \cdot 037$, respectively.

The score statistic is not available using SAS PROC LOGISTIC but is known to be identical to the value given by (15.20) (see Agresti, 1996, §5.4.4).

The Mantel–Haenszel test is valid even when some or all of the strata have small total frequencies. A particular case is when each stratum consists of a matched pair. Then (15.20) is equivalent to McNemar's test (4.18). The test is likely to be valid provided that $\sum e_{Ai}$ and the corresponding totals in the other three cells all exceed 5. When this is not the case an exact treatment is possible (§15.8).

15.7 **Combination of larger tables**

The sort of problem considered in §15.6 can arise with larger tables. The investigator may be interested in the association between two categorical factors, with r and c categories, respectively, and data may be available for k subgroups or strata, thus forming k separate tables. We can distinguish between: (i) row and column factors both nominal; (ii) one factor (say, columns) nominal, and the other ordinal; and (iii) rows and columns both ordinal. In each case the Mantel–Haenszel method provides a useful approach. The general idea is to obtain discrepancies between observed frequencies and those expected if there were no association between rows and columns within strata. For a fuller account, see Kuritz *et al.* (1988).

When both factors are nominal, the question is whether there is an association between rows and columns, forming a reasonably consistent pattern across the different strata. A natural approach is to obtain expected frequencies from the margins of each table by (8.27), to add these over the k strata, and to compare the observed and expected total frequencies in the rc row–column combinations. One is tempted to do an ordinary χ^2 test on these pooled frequencies, using (8.28). However, this is not quite correct, since the expected frequencies have not been obtained directly from the pooled marginal frequencies. The simple statistic, X^2 from (8.28), does not follow the χ^2 distribution with $(r-1)(c-1)$ DF: the correct DF should be somewhat lower, making high values of X^2 more significant than would at first be thought. The effect is likely to be small, and it will often be adequate to use this as a convenient, although conservative, approximation, realizing that effects are somewhat more significant than they appear.

A correct χ^2 test involves matrix algebra, and is described, for instance, by Kuritz *et al.* (1988) and for tables with $r = 2$ rows by Breslow and Day (1980, §4.5). The test is implemented by various computer programs, e.g. as the 'general association' statistic in the SAS program PROC FREQ. With only one stratum the test statistic is $(N-1)/N$ times the usual statistic (8.28). For $r = c = 2$, so that a series of 2×2 tables are being combined, the test statistic is identical with the Mantel–Haenszel statistic (15.20).

For the second case, of ordinal rows and nominal columns, we need a generalization of the $\chi^2_{(c-1)}$ test for equality of mean scores $\bar{x}_j$ given by (15.11). One solution is the 'ANOVA statistic' in the SAS program PROC FREQ. The case with $c = 2$ is of particular interest, being the stratified version of the test for trends in proportions dealt with in §15.2 (Mantel, 1963). Using the index h to denote a particular stratum, the quantities T_h and $\mathrm{var}(T_h)$ are calculated from (15.4) and (15.5), and the overall trend is tested by the statistic

$$X^2 = \frac{\left(\sum_h T_h\right)^2}{\sum_h \mathrm{var}(T_h)}, \tag{15.21}$$

approximately distributed as $\chi^2_{(1)}$.

Example 15.8

Table 15.8 gives some data from a study by Cockcroft *et al.* (1981). Staff who worked in an operating theatre were tested for antibodies to humidifier antigens. The objective was to establish if there was a relationship between the prevalence of antibodies and the length of time worked in the theatre. Age was related to length of exposure and to antibodies, and it was required to test the association of interest after taking account of age. The calculations are shown in Table 15.8. The test statistic is

$$X^2 = (7 \cdot 92)^2/8 \cdot 45 = 7 \cdot 42 \ (1\,\mathrm{DF}).$$

Thus, there was evidence of an association after allowing for age ($P = 0 \cdot 006$); if age had been ignored the association would have appeared stronger ($X^2_{1a} = 9 \cdot 53$ using (15.6)) but its validity would have been in doubt because of the confounding effect of age.

Table 15.8 Combination of trends in proportions of operating theatre staff with antibodies to humidifier fever antigens.

Length of exposure (years)	Score x	Age (years)							
		$-34 \ (h=1)$		$35–44 \ (h=2)$		$45 – \ (h=3)$		Total	
		Antibodies							
		$+$	$-$	$+$	$-$	$+$	$-$	$+$	$-$
< 1	0	0	9	2	5	0	3	2	17
1–5	1	3	7	2	2	6	1	11	10
> 5	2	3	0	4	2	5	6	12	8
		6	16	8	9	11	10	25	35
$\sum x_{ih} r_{ih}$		9		10		16		35	
$\sum x_{ih} e_{ih}$		4·36		7·53		15·19		27·08	
T_h		4·64		2·47		0·81		7·92	
$\mathrm{var}(T_h)$		2·15		3·43		2·87		8·45	

Again, logistic regression may be used.

Example 15.8, continued

A logistic regression is fitted of the logit of the proportion with antibodies on two dummy variables representing the three age groups and x, the score variable with values 0, 1 and 2 for the three length-of-exposure groups. The test statistics for the trend with length of exposure, after allowing for age, are 8·07 for the deviance test and 7·11 for Wald's χ^2. Assessing these as $\chi^2_{(1)}$ statistics gives significance levels of 0·005 and 0·008, respectively.

The third case, of two ordinal factors, leads (Mantel, 1963) to a generalization of the correlation-type statistic (15.12) distributed approximately as $\chi^2_{(1)}$:

$$X^2 = \frac{(\sum_h S_{xyh})^2}{\sum_h [S_{xxh} S_{yyh}/(N_h - 1)]}. \tag{15.22}$$

Finally, it is useful to note the stratified version of the test for trends in counts given in §15.4. Again using the subscript h to denote a particular stratum, the $\chi^2_{(1)}$ statistic is

$$X^2_{1P} = \frac{\{\sum_h [\sum_i x_{hi}(r_{hi} - e_{hi})]\}^2}{\sum_h [\sum_i e_{hi} x^2_{hi} - (\sum_i e_{hi} x_{hi})^2 / R_h]}. \tag{15.23}$$

This formula is derived from (15.13) by summing over the strata before the numerator is squared, and by summing also in the denominator. Extensive use is made of this statistic by Darby and Reissland (1981) in comparing the numbers of deaths from various causes among workers exposed to different doses of radiation (the x variable) with the numbers expected from the person-years at risk in the different categories (see §19.7). The strata were defined by various personal characteristics, including age and length of time since start of employment.

Several of the examples in this chapter that were analysed using a χ^2 test were also analysed using logistic regression, leading to similar conclusions. The question arises, therefore, of which method is preferable. It was noted in §15.1 that the regression methods give estimates of the size of effects, not just significance tests. Another advantage of logistic regression occurs when there are many variables to be taken account of. For example, the Cochran–Mantel–Haenszel method for combining 2×2 tables (§15.6) can only be applied after stratifying for all these variables simultaneously. This would lead to a large number of strata and possibly few subjects in each, and the stratification would result in loss of information on the association being analysed. Note in particular that if a stratum contained only one subject it would contribute no information, or if it contained two or three subjects, say, but they all occurred in one row, or in one column, there would be no information on the association. Therefore, in situations where there are several variables to consider, stratification will usually lead to a lower power than a logistic regression.

Another point is that the methods discussed in this chapter require that all variables be categorical, whereas in logistic regression variables may be either continuous or categorical.

To summarize, the methods discussed in this chapter are adequate to provide significance tests for an association between two categorical variables where it is required to take account of a third categorical variable. Logistic regression and Poisson regression are much more flexible methods, which can deal with more complex situations.

15.8 **Exact tests for contingency tables**

Fisher's exact test for a single 2×2 table was discussed in §4.5 and the extension of this test to an $r \times c$ table, with unordered rows and columns, in §8.6. The basis of the test is a conditional argument within the constraints of fixing the marginal totals of the table, which provide no information on the association between the row and column factors. In principle all possible tables satisfying the fixed marginal totals may be enumerated and the probability of each table, under the null hypothesis, calculated. The significance level is then obtained by considering where the observed table fits in the distribution of probabilities. Thus, for an $r \times c$ table, the probability level is the sum of probabilities less than or equal to the probability of the observed table. Exact tests are permutation tests, as considered in §10.6.

In the above the probabilities of the tables have been used in two ways: first, as a measure of discrepancy from the null hypothesis and, secondly, to calculate the probability level by summing the probabilities of those tables that are at least as discrepant as the observed table. The second use is the basis of an exact test, but other measures of discrepancy are possible. One possibility is the usual X^2 statistic (8.28) and another is the likelihood ratio.

It was stated above that all possible tables could be enumerated in principle. Except for a 2×2 table, this may be impossible in practice. For an $r \times c$ table the number of possible tables increases rapidly with r and c, even for modest values of the total frequency, to millions and billions, and it is infeasible to enumerate them all. The need to do this may be avoided by two means. The first is the use of network algorithms, in which the possible tables are represented by paths through a network of nodes. For each arc joining a pair of nodes, there are contributions to the discrepancy measure and to the probability. For some paths it is possible to determine at an intermediate node that all successive paths are either less discrepant than, or at least as discrepant as the observed table. Since the probability of reaching the intermediate node may be calculated, it is then possible to exclude, or include, all the tables emanating from that pathway to the node without enumerating these tables separately. Further discussion is beyond the scope of this book and interested readers are referred to Mehta and Patel (1983) and Mehta (1994).

Many problems will be infeasible even with an efficient network algorithm, and the second way of avoiding enumerating all tables is to use a Monte Carlo method. This method has been discussed in §10.6 and essentially involves sampling from the distribution of possible tables, with probability of selection for any table equal to its probability under the null hypothesis. The estimate of the probability value for the test is then the proportion of samples that are at least as discrepant as the observed table. The total number of samples may be set to give a specified precision for this estimate, as discussed in §10.6. The Monte Carlo sampling may be made more efficient by the use of network-based sampling and importance sampling. Again, the details are beyond the scope of this book and interested readers are referred to Mehta et al. (1988).

These methods are clearly computer-intensive and require appropriate statistical software. The software package StatXact (Cytel, 1995) has been developed in parallel with the theoretical developments.

A review of exact tests is given by Mehta and Patel (1998). We now consider some particular cases.

Trends in proportions

An exact trend test may be constructed for the situation discussed in §15.2 instead of using the approximate $\chi^2_{(1)}$ statistic (15.1) or (15.6). Conditional on the marginal totals, the test involves evaluation of the probability that $\sum r_i x_i$ is at least as large as the observed value (Agresti, 1990, §4.8.2). The exact method involves a large amount of calculation and is only feasible with appropriate statistical software, such as StatXact.

The exact test may be extended to cover the testing of a trend when there is a stratifying variable to take into account (§15.7). The χ^2 test for this situation is (15.21). An exact test is based on the probability of obtaining a value of $\sum_h T_h$ at least as large as that observed and, from (15.4), this is equivalent to basing the test on the sum of $\sum r_i x_i$ over the h strata. Conditioning is on the marginal totals in all the strata.

Example 15.9

In Table 15.8 there are several low counts and so there might be some doubt as to the accuracy of the analysis shown in Example 15.8. Using StatXact the test of trend is as follows.

The sum of $\sum r_i x_i$ over the three strata is 35. The exact probability that this sum would be greater than or equal to 35 if there were no effect of length of exposure, and subject to the marginal totals in each of the three age groups, is 0·0050 from StatXact. The corresponding one-sided probability using the $\chi^2_{(1)}$ of 7·42 in Example 15.8 is 0·0032. However, this is based on a test without a continuity correction and is, therefore, equivalent to a mid-P test (see §4.4), whereas the exact value is the usual P value.

If the test statistic in Example 15.8 had been corrected for continuity, then its value would have been $7·24^2/8·45 = 6·52$, giving a one-sided P value of 0·0054 very similar to the exact value of 0·0050.

Conversely, since from StatXact the probability that $\sum r_i x_i$ over the three strata is exactly 35 is 0·0033, the exact one-sided mid-P value is $0·0050 - \frac{1}{2}(0·0033) = 0·0034$, very near to the value from the uncorrected χ^2 of 0·0032.

The tests have been compared on the basis of their one-sided values since, with the exact test, there can be ambiguity on how to obtain a two-sided value (see discussion in Example 4.13). The two-sided levels using the χ^2 are, of course, simply double the one-sided levels, giving 0·0065 and 0·011 for the uncorrected and corrected values. One option of obtaining a two-sided exact level, which we advocated, is to double the one-sided level, giving 0·0067 and 0·010 for the mid-P and P values, respectively.

So, in this example, even though the frequencies are not large, the tests based on χ^2 statistics proved very satisfactory approximations to the exact tests.

Combination of 2 × 2 tables

This is an extension of the exact test in a single 2 × 2 table (§4.5). The one-tailed significance level is the probability that $\sum r_{Ai}$ is equal to or greater than its observed value, where for any value of $\sum r_{Ai}$ the probability is calculated by considering all the possible combinations of tables, with the same marginal totals, over the strata that produce this total (Mehta *et al.*, 1985; Hirji *et al.*, 1988; Agresti, 1990, §7.4.4).

Example 15.10

In Example 15.7 (Table 15.7) the exact test gives the following results.

The sum of $\sum r_{Ai}$ over the three strata is 29. The exact probability that this sum would be greater than or equal to 29 if there were no association between mortality and treatment, subject to the marginal totals in each of the three age groups, is 0·0327 from StatXact. The probability that $\sum r_{Ai} = 29$ is 0·0237, so that the exact one-sided mid-P value is $0\cdot0327 - \frac{1}{2}(0\cdot0237) = 0\cdot0208$. The two-sided tests, based on doubling the one-sided values, are 0·042 and 0·065 for the mid-P and P values, respectively. From Example 15.7, using X_{MH} and X_{MHc}, the corresponding levels are 0·037 and 0·067.

The tests based on χ^2 statistics proved acceptable approximations to the exact values. This is in accord with the earlier comment that the Mantel–Haenszel test is likely to be valid if the smallest of the expected cell frequencies summed over strata is at least 5. In this example, the smallest such expected cell frequency is 13.1.

Exact tests have been discussed above as significance tests. However, the methodology may be used to estimate a confidence interval for a parameter. For example, the odds ratio (4.25) is often used as a measure of association in a 2×2 table in epidemiological studies and an estimate may be obtained of the common odds ratio after combining over strata (§19.5). Exact limits for this estimate follow the rationale illustrated, for a simpler situation, in Fig. 4.8. The exact limits are conservative, due to the discreteness of the data, and mid-P limits are more satisfactory (§4.4); StatXact produces mid-P limits.

16 Further Bayesian methods

16.1 **Background**

In Chapter 6 the basic ideas behind the Bayesian approach to statistical inference were discussed, as were some straightforward methods of analysis for means and proportions. This chapter discusses some of the developments that have allowed Bayesian methods to be extended to the analysis of more complicated situations.

There are substantial philosophical differences between the Bayesian and frequentist approaches to statistical analyses and for many years discussion of Bayesian methods was dominated by these differences. Although these issues are of undoubted importance, they may have arisen in part because comparisons between the schools at a more practical level were seldom encountered. Implementation of Bayesian methods at that time presented insuperable technical challenges in all but straightforward cases, such as those in Chapter 6. In recent years there have been major advances in the technicalities required by Bayesian methodology and it can now be applied widely—perhaps more widely than frequentist methods.

Antagonism between the two schools is largely a thing of the past and, for the present at least, many statisticians accept that both traditions have something to offer. Whether this continues to be the case once wider experience of the practical, rather than philosophical, differences has been gained remains to be seen.

This chapter gives a brief and necessarily incomplete discussion of some of the innovations that have transformed the feasibility of practical Bayesian analysis. Much more complete treatments can be found in many excellent texts: examples with an emphasis on practical matter are Gelman *et al.* (1995), Gilks *et al.* (1996) and Carlin and Louis (2000), whereas Bernardo and Smith (1994) and O'Hagan (1994) give more emphasis to theoretical matters. Applications of Bayesian methods to medical examples can be found in, for example, Breslow (1990) and in the special issue of the journal *Statistical Methods in Medical Research* (1996, volume 5, no. 4). A wide-ranging and valuable discussion can be found in Lindley (2000).

16.2 **Prior and posterior distributions**

As was noted in Chapter 6, Bayesian methods are driven by the prior and posterior distributions and it is necessary to consider some aspects of these quantities in greater detail.

In this chapter it will be useful to have a general notation for these distributions, even if it is convenient to depart slightly from this when discussing specific examples. We shall use $\boldsymbol{\theta}$ to denote a parameter which, in general, will be a k-dimensional vector, with individual elements θ_i, and $\boldsymbol{x}$ denotes the data. For most general discussions it will suffice to think of the parameters and data having continuous distributions: amendments for discrete distributions usually involve changing integrals to sums. The density of the prior distribution is $p(\boldsymbol{\theta})$, and that of the posterior distribution is $p(\boldsymbol{\theta}|\boldsymbol{x})$. It is in keeping with this notation to use $p(\boldsymbol{x}|\boldsymbol{\theta})$ for the density for the data, supposing that the parameters have the given value, which is simply the likelihood for the data. Occasionally we shall refer to the joint distribution of the parameters and data, which is written $p(\boldsymbol{x}, \boldsymbol{\theta})$.

Posterior distributions

The posterior distribution is the key quantity in Bayesian inference. It amalgamates the relevant information from the data and the prior distribution and, once data $\boldsymbol{x}$ have been collected, statements about $\boldsymbol{\theta}$ should be based on $p(\boldsymbol{\theta}|\boldsymbol{x})$. So, for example, the mean of $\boldsymbol{\theta}$ is calculated as:

$$\int_{-\infty}^{\infty} \boldsymbol{\theta} p(\boldsymbol{\theta}|\boldsymbol{x}) \, d\boldsymbol{\theta}.$$

In order to evaluate this we need an expression for the posterior density and this is found by applying Bayes' theorem (§3.3), so:

$$p(\boldsymbol{\theta}|\boldsymbol{x}) = C p(\boldsymbol{x}|\boldsymbol{\theta}) p(\boldsymbol{\theta})$$

where $C = C(\boldsymbol{x})$ is chosen to ensure that the posterior is a genuine distribution (often referred to in this context as a *proper distribution*)—that is, its integral over the possible values of $\boldsymbol{\theta}$ is 1—so

$$C^{-1} = C(\boldsymbol{x})^{-1} = \int p(\boldsymbol{x}|\boldsymbol{\theta}) p(\boldsymbol{\theta}) \, d\boldsymbol{\theta}. \tag{16.1}$$

Determining this value has been the major obstacle to the practical use of Bayesian methods. The integral cannot be evaluated analytically except in one or two special circumstances, such as when conjugate distributions are used (see §6.2). Numerical methods focused on evaluating C directly have been proposed (e.g. Naylor & Smith, 1982) and these can be useful if there are not too many parameters, but if k is larger than about 5 this approach is usually unworkable.

Analytical approximations based on Laplace's method for integrals have also been suggested (see Tierney & Kadane, 1986, and subsequent papers including these authors). However, recent progress has focused on methods that allow the user to describe $p(\boldsymbol{\theta}|\boldsymbol{x})$ without needing to know the value of C.

Indeed, the problem is not confined simply to evaluating C. Useful description of the posterior distribution can require the computation of posterior moments, especially means, variances and covariances. Also, descriptions of individual parameters will focus on the *marginal* distributions, namely, the distribution of just a single element of $\boldsymbol{\theta}$. If $\boldsymbol{\theta} = (\theta_i, \boldsymbol{\theta}_{-i})$, where $\boldsymbol{\theta}_{-i}$ is $\boldsymbol{\theta}$ with θ_i omitted, then the posterior distribution of θ_i is

$$p(\theta_i|\boldsymbol{x}) = \int p(\theta_i, \boldsymbol{\theta}_{-i}|\boldsymbol{x}) \, \mathrm{d}\boldsymbol{\theta}_{-i}.$$

Exact analytical evaluation of this is likely to be impossible, in which case alternative, approximate, methods are needed.

Although the posterior distribution is the key to Bayesian inference, it is, in general, a cumbersome quantity and more succinct and manageable summaries are needed. Graphical summaries of the distribution of each element of $\boldsymbol{\theta}$ can be very informative. Occasionally it is helpful to have some form of pictorial summary of the joint distribution of pairs of elements, such as a contour diagram of the bivariate density. Numerical summaries of each parameter are usually needed, such as their posterior means. If the posterior has a single mode and is sufficiently symmetric for it to be reasonably close to a normal distribution, then it may be helpful to know the posterior variances and covariances of $\boldsymbol{\theta}$. The quantiles of the posterior, such as the median and quartiles, and perhaps descriptors of the tails of the distribution, such as 5th and 95th centiles, may also be important.

From time to time interest may focus on a function of the elements of $\boldsymbol{\theta}$; an example would be the ratio θ_1/θ_2. In a frequentist setting this could be slightly awkward, with inferences having to be made on the basis of approximations, such as the delta method (§5.3). The Bayesian approach is, in principle, more satisfactory: the parameters in $\boldsymbol{\theta}$ can be transformed so that one of them is the ratio, or any other derived parameter of interest, and then inferences can be made using the appropriate marginal of the posterior distribution.

Interval estimates play an important role in Bayesian analysis: a $100\alpha\%$ interval estimate for, say, θ_1 is any pair $(\theta_{1L}, \theta_{1U})$, where

$$\alpha = \int_{\theta_{1L}}^{\theta_{1U}} p(\theta_1, \boldsymbol{\theta}_{-1}|\boldsymbol{x}) \, \mathrm{d}\theta_1 \, \mathrm{d}\boldsymbol{\theta}_{-1}. \tag{16.2}$$

Thus, there is a probability α that θ_1 lies between θ_{1L} and θ_{1U}—a much more natural definition than that for a frequentist confidence interval (see §4.1). Equation (16.2) does not determine a unique interval and several types of interval are encountered in Bayesian analyses. An intuitively appealing choice of interval estimator is the *highest posterior density* (HPD) or *most credible interval*. This comprises a set of values of θ_1 which has probability α under the posterior distribution and such that the posterior density is larger at any point within the set than for any point outside the set. This has the appealing property that the total length of this set is shorter than for any other set that has the same posterior probability. However, there are difficulties with such intervals: (i) they are not invariant under transformation so, for example, the HPD for $\log \theta_1$ may not be straightforwardly related to that for θ_1; (ii) they can be difficult to compute; and (iii) if the posterior is not unimodal the set may not be an interval of the form $(\theta_{1L}, \theta_{1U})$. In view of these difficulties, it is quite common to opt for the *equal tail interval*, which is determined by requiring that the probability of being below θ_{1L} is the same as that of being above θ_{1U}. For posterior distributions that are unimodal and approximately symmetric, equal tail and HPD intervals are likely to be very similar. If the posterior is markedly skew, then the two kinds of interval could be quite different: see Fig. 2.3 of Carlin and Louis (2000).

It might be possible to calculate analytically the summaries of $p(\boldsymbol{\theta}|\boldsymbol{x})$ which have just been discussed, but in most applications this will not be the case. Many of the recently developed techniques for exploring the posterior distribution do so by allowing the analyst to sample from the posterior distribution. This means that the analyst can choose to generate any number of realizations of a variable, say $\boldsymbol{\theta}_1, \boldsymbol{\theta}_2, \ldots, \boldsymbol{\theta}_N$, each of which is drawn from a distribution with density $p(\boldsymbol{\theta}|\boldsymbol{x})$. In these circumstances the summaries are generally found by computing appropriate sample analogues. For example, an estimate of the posterior mean would be

$$\frac{1}{N} \sum_{\ell=1}^{N} \boldsymbol{\theta}_\ell.$$

While this way of summarizing a distribution may seem somewhat inexact, the approach is actually very flexible. For example, the probability that a component, say, θ_1, is less than c is estimated by the proportion of simulated values, θ_{1i}, that are less than c. It is occasionally useful to write this as

$$\frac{1}{N} \sum_{\ell=1}^{N} I(\theta_{1\ell} < c),$$

where $I(\theta < c)$ is 1 if $\theta < c$ and 0 otherwise. More complicated summaries can also be found easily: for example, an estimate of $\mathrm{P}\,(\theta_1 < c_1 | \theta_2 < c_2)$ is computed as the proportion of those simulations that have $\theta_2 < c_2$ which also have $\theta_1 < c_1$. Statements about posterior properties of functions of the elements of $\boldsymbol{\theta}$, such as θ_1/θ_2, can also be made in the obvious way. In principle, the statistician can control the precision of the summaries by appropriate choice of N, although for complicated models the computational burden imposed by choosing large values can be substantial.

Graphical summaries of the distributions of individual components of $\boldsymbol{\theta}$ can be simple histograms, although kernel density estimation will produce smoother estimates (see, for example, Silverman, 1986). However, special techniques may be more appropriate in certain circumstances (see Gelfand & Smith, 1990). For graphical summaries in two dimensions, algorithms for estimating contour diagrams from data are available in several statistical packages.

The values drawn from $p(\boldsymbol{\theta}|\boldsymbol{x})$, namely $\boldsymbol{\theta}_1, \boldsymbol{\theta}_2, \ldots, \boldsymbol{\theta}_N$, are necessarily identically distributed but they are not necessarily independent: whether or not they are independent depends on which algorithm has been used. Many of the common summaries are unaffected by the dependence structure: for example, the expectations of

$$\frac{1}{N} \sum_{\ell=1}^{N} \boldsymbol{\theta}_\ell \text{ and } \frac{1}{N} \sum_{\ell=1}^{N} I(\theta_{1\ell} < c),$$

are, respectively, the posterior mean and the posterior probability that $\theta_1 < c_1$, regardless of the presence of dependence between the $\boldsymbol{\theta}_1, \boldsymbol{\theta}_2, \ldots, \boldsymbol{\theta}_N$.

However, for some quantities more care is needed. The natural estimator of the posterior variance of, for example, θ_1, is

$$\frac{1}{N-1} \sum_{\ell=1}^{N} (\theta_{1\ell} - \bar{\theta}_1)^2 = \frac{1}{N-1} \left[\sum_{\ell=1}^{N} \theta_{1\ell}^2 - N\bar{\theta}_1^2 \right].$$

Provided the simulations are independent the expectation of this is the posterior variance, σ^2. In general, the expectation is $\sigma^2(1 - \bar{\rho})$, where $\bar{\rho}$ is the mean of the $\frac{1}{2}N(N-1)$ correlations between $\theta_{11}, \theta_{12}, \ldots, \theta_{1N}$. Even when the simulations from the posterior are dependent, the mean correlation is often sufficiently small for the correction factor $1 - \bar{\rho}$ to be ignored. However, this is not always the case. If the analyst wishes to know how good the mean of the sample of θ_1 is as an estimate of the posterior mean, then the usual measure of this, the standard error of the mean, can be noticeably affected by correlation between successive values. The variance of

$$\frac{1}{N} \sum_{\ell=1}^{N} \theta_{1\ell}$$

is

$$\frac{\sigma^2}{N} [1 + (N-1)\bar{\rho}],$$

and the correction factor $1 + (N-1)\bar{\rho}$ can deviate substantially from 1, in which case a correction needs to be applied. Brief details will be mentioned in §16.4.

Prior distributions

A Bayesian analysis starts from a prior distribution, $p(\boldsymbol{\theta})$, which is a numerical description of the beliefs the analyst has about the parameters in the model $p(\boldsymbol{x}|\boldsymbol{\theta})$ before any data, $\boldsymbol{x}$, have been collected. Consequently, a prior distribution must be specified before any Bayesian analysis can proceed.

Before discussing the various types of prior distributions that are used, it is helpful to make a few general points, which echo some of the remarks made in Chapter 6.

1 Since $p(\boldsymbol{\theta}|\boldsymbol{x}) = Cp(\boldsymbol{x}|\boldsymbol{\theta})p(\boldsymbol{\theta})$, any value of $\boldsymbol{\theta}$ that has zero prior probability will, necessarily, have zero posterior probability. Consequently, it is important when specifying a prior distribution not to be too prescriptive about impossible parameter values. In practice, zero values for the prior distribution usually arise because of permissible ranges being imposed on certain parameters. If such ranges are necessary, it is important to be careful that they are not too tightly specified.

2 The prior distribution is meant to summarize the analyst's beliefs about $\boldsymbol{\theta}$ before data have been collected. Of course, others assessing the analysis may have different views, which would be expressed through different priors. It has been mooted (Spiegelhalter *et al.*, 1994) that it would be valuable for the results of analyses to be reported in such a way that each reader could see how their own prior was affected by the collected data. Whether or not this is desirable, practical constraints have largely prevented progress on this matter. However, it is important that the effect the prior distribution has had on the analysis is made transparent. Sensitivity analyses, in which the posterior distributions resulting from a variety of prior distributions are compared, would seem to be an essential adjunct to any Bayesian analysis.

3 Unless the sample is small or the prior distribution highly concentrated about a few values, the posterior distribution will, in practice, be more dependent on the likelihood than on the prior distribution. In these circumstances the precise nature of the prior distribution may be unimportant. However, the converse is that, if the data set is small, then the analyst may need to make it clear that posterior inferences largely reflect prior beliefs, rather than any information obtained from data.

The prior distribution can itself depend on parameters, $\boldsymbol{\eta}$, for its specification, and in this case is more fully written as $p(\boldsymbol{\theta}|\boldsymbol{\eta})$. In order to distinguish these parameters from those that are directly involved in the specification of the model, the $\boldsymbol{\eta}$ are often referred to as *hyperparameters*. The values of the hyperparameters can be chosen by the analyst so that $p(\boldsymbol{\theta}|\boldsymbol{\eta})$ adequately describes the prior beliefs. The distribution of the data will depend on $\boldsymbol{\eta}$ because

$$p(\boldsymbol{x}|\boldsymbol{\eta}) = \int p(\boldsymbol{x}|\boldsymbol{\theta})p(\boldsymbol{\theta}|\boldsymbol{\eta})\,\mathrm{d}\boldsymbol{\theta}.$$

One approach to the choice of $\boldsymbol{\eta}$ is to find the values for which $p(x|\boldsymbol{\eta})$ best fits the data. This is the empirical Bayes approach outlined in §6.5. There are two criticisms of this approach, one practical and one philosophical. The practical problem is that there will be uncertainty in the estimates of $\boldsymbol{\eta}$ but they will be used as though they were exact, thereby overestimating the precision of any subsequent analysis: typically, interval estimates will be too narrow. Methods for addressing this are available: see §3.5 of Carlin and Louis (2000). The philosophical problem is that a prior distribution should be specified before the data, or even the form of the data, are known and simply reflect the prior beliefs about $\boldsymbol{\theta}$. Although it can be very useful in some circumstances, we shall not discuss the empirical Bayes approach further in this chapter.

A fully Bayesian approach to the problem of uncertainty in the hyperparameters is to place a distribution on them—a *hyperprior distribution*. This is discussed in, for example, Gelman *et al.* (1995, Chapter 5). In this chapter we shall avoid this level of complexity and assume that, where present, hyperparameters are given values a priori that define the prior uncertainty.

In practice, prior distributions take one of two forms, either *informative* or *non-informative* (sometimes referred to as *vague*). In the former case, the analyst is making a deliberate attempt to describe prior beliefs numerically. On the other hand, if a non-informative prior is used, then there is no such intention. There can be various motivations for using a vague prior. There may genuinely be no prior information. Alternatively there may be a wish to use a prior that is 'objective', in the sense that the corresponding posterior inferences might be claimed to be based solely on the data.

Informative priors

In principle, anyone can construct a prior which represents their beliefs and then form a posterior distribution to observe how those beliefs are modified in the light of the data. However, in a scientific investigation, it is important that the prior should represent beliefs to which the scientific community will give some credence. The view of an expert in the field, or of a panel of experts, can be elicited and put into quantitative form. This is one of the crucial steps for the practical implementation of Bayesian methods. While there is widespread acknowledgement that prior information exists before many scientific investigations commence, it is less easy to reach agreement on appropriate and convincing ways of capturing this knowledge numerically.

Methods for eliciting prior knowledge from experts have been reported using questionnaires (Parmar *et al.*, 1994) or special computer programs (Chaloner *et al.*, 1993). Kadane and Wolfson (1998) point out that, while there has been some work on elicitation methods that can be applied to a general class of problems and models (such as time series or linear models), many applications are likely to demand special approaches that may not be useful in any other context. Nevertheless, Kadane and Wolfson (1998) point out that there is some agreement in the literature on prior elicitation about some aspects of how the process should be conducted. These include:

1 Experts should be asked only to assess observable quantities, perhaps conditioning on observable covariates.

2 Experts might be asked to estimate means, but not other moments of distributions. Rather, they should be asked to describe distributions in terms of percentiles.

3 Frequent feedback should be given to the expert(s) during the process.

The motivation behind these principles stems from the perception that the statistical model used to describe the data and, in particular, the meanings of some of the parameters involved in that model are unlikely to be sufficiently well appreciated by the experts for direct specification to be desirable.

A broader interpretation of the meaning of the prior distribution is that it encapsulates the state of knowledge about an issue as it existed before the data in question were collected. As such, it could be formed on the basis of overviews of existing research. In recent years, the availability of these has increased substantially, particularly as applied to clinical trials (see §18.10). Of course, many of the issues that surround meta-analyses, such as the quality of the studies included and the completeness of the overview, would need to be considered carefully before the meta-analysis could be used as the basis of an overview. Moreover, if the prior in a Bayesian analysis is based on a meta-analysis, then the posterior could essentially mix historical and current data on the same basis. This might sometimes be appropriate, but it will often be undesirable, and the analyst should give careful consideration to this aspect of the analysis.

A possible concern about the use of Bayesian analyses is that the choice of prior might, in some way, 'build in' some prejudice about some aspect of the study. This issue is especially pertinent for regulatory authorities when they are assessing clinical trials of a new product. There may be a suspicion that the prior chosen might automatically confer an advantage on the applicant's own product. Similar concerns may affect other kinds of trial where the investigators may be seen to have some other kind of interest in the success of one of the trial treatments.

A response to this is to use a so-called *sceptical prior*. Spiegelhalter *et al.* (1994) suggest that a plausible interpretation of scepticism is that those planning the trial had been overoptimistic. If the trial has an outcome that is normally distributed and had been planned to give good power to detect a mean difference of μ_A, then a sceptical prior would ensure that $P(\mu > \mu_A)$ was small. Priors that are sceptical about a treatment might be useful, as they will only give rise to posteriors that favour that treatment if the evidence for this from the data is very strong. Of course, such priors may place too great a handicap on a treatment, resulting in useful treatments being discarded. Spiegelhalter *et al.* (1994) also discuss several other kinds of priors that might be used in clinical trials. Spiegelhalter *et al.* (1999) give a more recent perspective on these issues.

Non-informative priors

If it is decided to eschew specific prior knowledge, then a non-informative or vague prior must be adopted. This is often the approach taken when the desire is to have an 'objective' Bayesian analysis in which the prior specification has minimal effect. Many authors argue that the notion of vague prior knowledge is unsatisfactory (see, for example, Bernardo & Smith, 1994, §5.4), for, while the notion of an objective analysis might be superficially attractive, it is inherently flawed. Attempts to reconcile these two views have led to the development of *reference priors*, which attempt to be minimally informative in some well-defined sense; a full discussion of this topic is beyond the scope of this chapter and the interested reader is referred to §5.4 of Bernardo and Smith (1994) and to Bernardo and Ramón (1998). Despite its shortcomings, several approaches to the definition of vague priors are widely used and the rationale behind some of these will be discussed below. An interesting account of the historical background to this topic can be found in §5.6 of Bernardo and Smith (1994).

One of the most practical ways to represent prior ignorance is to choose a prior distribution that is very diffuse. Typically, a prior distribution defined in terms of parameters, $\boldsymbol{\eta}$, is used and the elements of $\boldsymbol{\eta}$ that determine the dispersion of the prior are chosen to be large. If possible, it will usually be convenient to try to arrange for the prior to be conjugate (see §6.2) to the likelihood of the data. For example, in a study of blood pressure, a normal prior with a standard deviation of 1000 mmHg will convey virtually no useful information about the location of the mean. With this standard deviation, it hardly matters what value is ascribed to the prior mean.

Crudely speaking, a normal distribution becomes 'flatter' as its standard deviation increases. A natural limit to this is to take the standard deviation to be infinite. This results in a prior that is flat and, as such, can be thought of as representing an extreme version of prior ignorance, all values being equally likely. Such a limit cannot be taken too literally, as the constant value achieved is zero. Nevertheless, if the posterior is taken to be proportional to the likelihood, i.e. $p(\boldsymbol{\theta}|\boldsymbol{x}) = Cp(\boldsymbol{x}|\boldsymbol{\theta})$, then the prior has effectively been taken to be a constant. Of course, a prior that is constant over the whole real line is not a genuine probability distribution, because it does not integrate to 1, and is known as an *improper prior*. Whether or not the posterior is improper depends on whether or not the integral of the likelihood with respect to $\boldsymbol{\theta}$ is finite; in many cases it is, so a proper posterior can emerge from an improper prior and this approach is widely used. However, the analyst must be vigilant because, if an improper prior is used, there is no guarantee that a proper posterior distribution will result.

Another way to model ignorance is to use a uniform distribution over a finite range. The finite range means that the value of $p(\theta)$ can be chosen so that the distribution integrates to one. The improper prior, mentioned above, can be obtained as the limit as the range tends to infinity. The uniformity of the distribution means that no one value is preferred over any other, which might seem as good an implementation of ignorance as one might expect. However, the use of a uniform distribution to model ignorance is not as satisfactory as it might at first appear. Suppose θ is a scalar. If there is ignorance about the value of θ, then surely there is equal ignorance about any function of θ, such as θ^2 or $\exp(-\theta)$. However, a uniform distribution for θ implies a non-uniform distribution for these (and most other) functions of θ.

A similar problem applies when the range of the parameter is infinite. The discussion of improper priors given above tacitly assumed that the range of the parameters is the whole real line. However, for many parameters, this is not true; for example, a standard deviation, σ, is necessarily positive. However, $\log \sigma$ can take any value and an improper prior for this quantity that is constant on the whole real line transforms to a prior $p(\sigma) = 1/\sigma$ for the standard deviation. This form of improper prior is widely used for parameters that are necessarily positive.

A way to define prior distributions that express ignorance and are invariant under transformations of the parameters was proposed by Jeffreys (1961, p. 181). For scalar θ the *Jeffreys prior* is taken to be proportional to the square root of the Fisher information, i.e.

$$p(\theta) \propto \left[-\int \left\{ \frac{\partial^2}{\partial \theta^2} \log p(x|\theta) \right\} p(x|\theta) \, dx \right]^{1/2}. \tag{16.3}$$

When θ is a vector, the Jeffreys prior is, strictly speaking, proportional to the square root of the determinant of the matrix whose (i, j)th element is

$$-\int \left\{ \frac{\partial^2}{\partial \theta_i \partial \theta_j} \log p(x|\theta) \right\} p(x|\theta) \, dx.$$

The expression for vector θ is often cumbersome and it is quite common to form the Jeffreys prior separately for each component of θ using (16.3) and then use the product of these as the prior for θ. The argument here is that, broadly speaking, ignorance is consistent with independence, so forming the joint prior in this way is reasonable.

Jeffreys priors can lead to some slightly unusual results. If the data have a univariate normal distribution, with mean μ and standard deviation σ, then the following can be obtained:

(i) the prior for μ from (16.3) is $p(\mu) = 1$;
(ii) the prior for σ from (16.3) is $p(\sigma) = 1/\sigma$;
(iii) the joint prior for μ and σ from the matrix expression is $p(\mu, \sigma) = 1/\sigma^2$.

In other words the prior from (iii) is not the simple product of those derived in (i) and (ii). However, in practice such differences are unlikely to be important as the differences between the effects of such diffuse priors will tend not to be noticeable in the posterior density unless the data set is small.

16.3 **The Bayesian linear model**

The variation in many variables encountered in medical research can be modelled by a normal distribution. If the outcome has a normal distribution with mean μ and variance σ^2, and if μ is assumed to have a normal prior distribution with mean μ_0 and variance σ_0^2, then the analysis in Chapter 6 shows that the posterior distribution for μ is also normal. The mean and variance of this distribution are most succinctly described in terms of *precision*, the reciprocal of the variance. The posterior mean is a weighted mean of the sample mean and the prior mean, with weights proportional to their respective precisions, and the posterior precision is the sum of the precisions of the sample mean and prior mean (see §6.2 for details).

Linear model with known variance

As has been seen in Chapters 7, 8 and 11, there is a great deal to be gained by extending the simple normal model so that the mean can vary with covariates, as in multiple regression and analyses of variance. A Bayesian analysis, which is closely analogous to that just outlined for the simple case, is possible for the extended case. It is easiest to explain the extension in suitable generality if the matrix representation of the linear model explained in §11·6 is adopted.

The usual linear model (11.47) can be written in terms of the $n \times 1$ vector of outcomes y as

$$y \,|\, \boldsymbol{\beta} \sim \mathrm{N}(X\boldsymbol{\beta}, \sigma^2 I_n),$$

meaning that, given a value for $\boldsymbol{\beta}$, the outcome vector has mean $X\boldsymbol{\beta}$ and the outcomes are uncorrelated, each with constant variance σ^2. In the following the assumption that the dispersion of y given $\boldsymbol{\beta}$ has this particular form will be used because it is the form encountered most commonly and will adequately illustrate the Bayesian approach to the linear model. However, if it is inappropriate, it can easily be amended.

The mean is now defined by a vector $\boldsymbol{\beta}$ and a multivariate prior distribution is required for this quantity. A natural choice, and one which is conjugate (see §6.1) to the likelihood, is a multivariate normal distribution, with mean $\boldsymbol{\beta}_0$ and dispersion matrix $\boldsymbol{D}$. The posterior distribution of $\boldsymbol{\beta}$ is multivariate normal, with dispersion $\boldsymbol{M}^{-1}$ and mean

$$\boldsymbol{M}^{-1}(\sigma^{-2}\boldsymbol{X}^{\mathrm{T}}\boldsymbol{y} + \boldsymbol{D}^{-1}\boldsymbol{\beta}_0), \tag{16.4}$$

where

$$\boldsymbol{M} = \sigma^{-2}\boldsymbol{X}^{\mathrm{T}}\boldsymbol{X} + \boldsymbol{D}^{-1}. \tag{16.5}$$

Notice that these formulae are multivariate analogues of the univariate version, where the posterior mean was derived as a sum weighted by precisions. The term $\sigma^{-2}\boldsymbol{X}^{\mathrm{T}}\boldsymbol{X}$ in (16.5), being the inverse of (11.51), can be thought of as the multivariate precision of the parameter, and the second term is the prior precision. The analogue of the sample mean is $\boldsymbol{b}$, defined by (11.49), and from this it follows that $\boldsymbol{X}^{\mathrm{T}}\boldsymbol{y} = (\boldsymbol{X}^{\mathrm{T}}\boldsymbol{X})\boldsymbol{b}$. Substituting this in (16.4) clearly demonstrates that the posterior mean has the form of a weighted sum, analogous to the univariate case. The situation where no prior information is available could be modelled by using an improper prior in which, formally, $\boldsymbol{D}^{-1} = 0$. Consequently, from (16.4) and (16.5), the posterior mean and variance reduce to the quantities (11.49) and (11.51), which are familiar from frequentist analysis. Of course, as $\boldsymbol{\beta}$ is now considered to be a random variable, there would be subtle differences in the way the uncertainty in the estimate of the regression coefficients would be expressed.

This result, and for that matter the simpler univariate version adduced in Chapter 6, is not, in itself, very useful because it supposes σ^2 is known and has not been included as a random quantity in the Bayesian analysis. How to include this parameter will now be discussed but, as will be seen, realistic approaches lead to complications.

Conjugate and related analyses of normal samples with unknown variance

The analysis in §6.2 is sufficiently realistic and elegant for it to be natural to attempt to extend the use of conjugacy arguments to accommodate unknown variance. When conjugate informative priors are sought for this problem some difficulties arise, and these will be described below. However, some insight into the form of distribution that will be required can be gained from the case where an improper uninformative prior is used. From §16.2, the uninformative prior for (μ, σ^2) is $p(\mu, \sigma^2) = 1/\sigma^2$ and from this it follows that the posterior is

$$p(\mu, \sigma^2 \mid \boldsymbol{y}) \propto \sigma^{-n-2} \exp\left\{ -\frac{1}{2\sigma^2}[(n-1)s^2 + n(\bar{y} - \mu)^2] \right\}, \tag{16.6}$$

where $\bar{y}$ is the mean of a sample of size n which has variance s^2.

From (16.6) various results can be obtained. The posterior distribution of μ alone (i.e. the *marginal* posterior distribution) is found by integrating $p(\mu, \sigma^2 | y)$ with respect to σ^2 and this gives

$$p(\mu|y) \propto \left[1 + \frac{n(\mu - \bar{y})^2}{(n-1)s^2}\right]^{-n/2}.$$

This is a form of t distribution which includes a location and scale parameter as well as the usual degrees of freedom. Details can be found in Appendix A of Gelman *et al.* (1995), but a simpler description is that the marginal posterior distribution of the mean is the same as that of $\bar{y} + Ts/\sqrt{n}$, where T has a standard t distribution with $n-1$ degrees of freedom.

The marginal posterior for σ^2 is similarly found by integrating (16.6). The integral with respect to μ is essentially the integral of a normal density and this quickly leads to the form

$$p(\sigma^2|y) \propto (\sigma^2)^{-(n+1)/2} \exp\left[-\frac{(n-1)s^2}{2\sigma^2}\right].$$

This form of density is reminiscent of a gamma or χ^2 density and in fact it is closely related to these: it is the scaled inverse-χ^2 density with scale factor s^2 and $n-1$ degrees of freedom. The scaled inverse-χ^2 distribution is an important distribution for describing the variance in Bayesian analyses of the normal distribution. In general, if X is a random variable with a χ^2 distribution with v degrees of freedom, then $s^2 v/X$ has a scaled inverse-χ^2 distribution with v degrees of freedom and scale factor s^2. Crudely speaking, as X has mean v, then a scaled inverse-χ^2 distribution would be expected to have values located around the scale factor. More precisely, the mean is $vs^2/(v-2)$, and the variance is $2/(v-4)$ times the square of the mean. The distribution is positively skewed, with a heavy tail.

The analysis based on the improper prior $1/\sigma^2$ has led to results that are very familiar from a frequentist analysis, where $(\bar{y} - \mu)\sqrt{n}/s$ has a t distribution with $n-1$ degrees of freedom and s^2/σ^2 has a χ^2 distribution with the same degrees of freedom. Moreover, if the degrees of freedom, $n-1$, do not exceed 4, the marginal posterior distribution for σ^2 has infinite variance and for degrees of freedom ≤ 2 it has infinite mean. This illustrates that, for small data sets, improper priors can lead to posteriors which, while not improper, lack some of the attributes that many statisticians would consider important for data description.

Extending this analysis to one with an informative and conjugate prior requires the definition of a composite distribution, the normal-inverse-χ^2 (NIC) distribution. The prior for σ^2 is an inverse-χ^2 with v_0 degrees of freedom and scale factor σ_0^2. The prior for μ is a normal distribution with mean μ_0 and variance

σ^2/m_0. Note that the prior distribution for μ depends on σ^2; in other words, the joint prior distribution $p(\mu, \sigma^2)$ has been defined in terms of the marginal prior distribution for σ^2 and the conditional distribution of μ given σ^2, i.e. through $p(\mu, \sigma^2) = p(\sigma^2)p(\mu|\sigma^2)$. The four parameters of the NIC distribution are: (i) the degrees of freedom, ν_0, which determine the dispersion of σ^2 about its location, with smaller values corresponding to greater dispersion; (ii) the scale factor σ_0^2, which essentially measures the location of σ^2; (iii) μ_0, the prior expectation for the mean; and (iv) the effective sample size, m_0. Expressing the prior variance of the mean as σ^2/m_0 allows the prior information about μ to be notionally thought of as the information that would come from a sample of size m_0.

The NIC is the conjugate distribution for a normal variable. If a sample of size n has mean $\bar{y}$ and variance s^2, then the posterior distribution $p(\mu, \sigma^2|y)$ is also an NIC distribution and the amended values of the four parameters are:

(i) New degrees of freedom $= n + \nu_0$.

(ii) New scale factor $= (n + \nu_0)^{-1}\left[\nu_0\sigma_0^2 + (n-1)s^2 + \dfrac{m_0 n}{m_0 + n}(\bar{y} - \mu_0)^2\right]$.

(iii) New expectation for $\mu = \dfrac{m_0}{m_0 + n}\mu_0 + \dfrac{n}{m_0 + n}\bar{y}$.

(iv) New effective sample size $= n + m_0$.

The marginal posterior distribution for σ^2 is a scaled inverse-χ^2 distribution with degrees of freedom and scale factor given by (i) and (ii). The marginal posterior distribution for μ is again that of a random variable $\mu_n + kT$, where μ_n is given by (iii), k is the ratio of (ii) to (iv) and T has a standard t distribution with degrees of freedom given by (i).

A similar distribution is available for the regression setting, where the mean is given by $X\beta$. The distribution for the residual variance σ^2 is exactly the same as in the above, whereas the distribution for β conditional on σ^2 is a multivariate normal distribution. The updating of the parameters in the light of the data follows from expressions analogous to those in (i) to (iv), but using appropriate vector and matrix terms: details can be found in §9.10 of O'Hagan (1994).

Although the convenience of this approach makes it superficially attractive, it has a drawback. Conditional on σ^2, the prior variance of μ is σ^2/m_0, so the prior uncertainty on μ is necessarily larger the larger the value of σ^2. In many circumstances, particularly when there is little prior information about either parameter, this linkage between the two may be of little consequence (indeed, in the limit as m_0 and ν_0 tend to 0, which gives the uninformative prior $1/\sigma^2$, the two parameters become independent, albeit in a rather ill-defined sense). However, it is possible that there may be useful prior information about the mean but that there is substantial prior uncertainty about the value of the variance. In this circumstance, prior dependence between the parameters seems less satisfactory.

A straightforward way of circumventing this problem is to take the prior for μ to be a normal distribution with mean μ_0 and prior variance ω_0^2, which now does not depend on σ^2. The prior for σ^2 is a scaled inverse-χ^2 distribution with parameters ν_0 and σ_0^2 independent of μ. Unfortunately, this prior is no longer conjugate to the likelihood and the resulting posterior distribution does not have a standard form. However, some of the conjugacy structure remains: the posterior distribution of μ conditional on σ^2 is simply the normal distribution described in §6.2, where a known value of σ^2 was assumed. This is an example of conditional conjugacy, which is more fully explained in §§9.45–9.49 of O'Hagan (1994) and which can be used to effect important simplifications in analyses using this model. The model can extended to the regression setting, with the prior on $\boldsymbol{\beta}$ being the multivariate normal form described above. The independent prior for σ^2 is, again, a scaled inverse-χ^2 distribution with hyperparameters ν_0 and σ_0^2.

Several approaches to the analysis of this model are available and two will be described briefly. As the posterior distribution does not have a standard form, analytical descriptions of its properties will not be available and both approaches provide descriptions of the posterior by allowing the analyst to simulate samples, of any desired size, from the posterior.

Suppose a sample, $\boldsymbol{y}$, of size n with mean $\bar{y}$ and variance s^2, has been observed from a normal distribution with mean μ and variance σ^2, which have independent prior distributions of the form described above, and it is desired to describe the posterior distribution, $p(\mu, \sigma^2 | \boldsymbol{y})$. The first analysis proceeds by noting that the conditional posterior $p(\mu | \sigma^2, \boldsymbol{y})$ is known to be a normal distribution with mean

$$\mu_n = \frac{\omega_0^{-2}\mu_0 + n\sigma^{-2}\bar{y}}{\omega_0^{-2} + n\sigma^{-2}}, \tag{16.7}$$

and variance

$$\omega_n^2 = (\omega_0^{-2} + n\sigma^{-2})^{-1}. \tag{16.8}$$

A pair of values could be simulated from $p(\mu, \sigma^2 | \boldsymbol{y}) = p(\mu | \sigma^2, \boldsymbol{y}) \, p(\sigma^2 | \boldsymbol{y})$ by first drawing a value of σ^2 from its marginal posterior distribution. This value of σ^2 is then used in (16.7) and (16.8) to define the conditional distribution $p(\mu | \sigma^2, \boldsymbol{y})$ from which a value of μ can be drawn.

There remains the difficulty of drawing a value from $p(\sigma^2 | \boldsymbol{y})$, as this has a non-standard form. A useful device that can be used is to note that Bayes' theorem gives:

$$p(\sigma^2 \mid \boldsymbol{y}) = \frac{p(\mu, \sigma^2 | \boldsymbol{y})}{p(\mu | \sigma^2, \boldsymbol{y})}.$$

The numerator is proportional to the product of n normal densities (for the data) and of the prior density. The denominator is the normal distribution defined by

(16.7) and (16.8). The density of the marginal posterior for σ^2 is proportional to the following rather unappealing expression,

$$q(\sigma^2) = p(\sigma^2)\sigma^{-n} \exp\left[-\frac{(n-1)s^2}{2\sigma^2}\right] \sqrt{\left(\frac{\omega_n^2}{\omega_0^2}\right)} \exp\left[-\frac{1}{2}\left(\frac{n\bar{y}^2}{\sigma^2} - \frac{\mu_n^2}{\omega_n^2}\right)\right]. \qquad (16.9)$$

Several things should be noted about this density.

1 It must be remembered that ω_n^2 and μ_n both depend on σ^2.
2 The expression does not correspond to any standard density function.
3 If a non-informative prior is used for μ, with $\mu_0 = 0$ and $\omega_0 \to \infty$, then the final exponentiated factor in (16.9) reduces to unity and the factor $\sqrt{(\omega_n^2/\omega_0^2)}$ essentially adds a further factor of σ to the density. The resulting expression is a scaled inverse-χ^2 distribution, so, if $p(\sigma^2)$ is also a scaled inverse-χ^2 distribution, conjugancy is restored.
4 Sampling from the density proportional to (16.9) requires numerical methods. A simple approach is to compute a discrete approximation at a fine grid of points, say, $\sigma_1, \sigma_2, \ldots, \sigma_M$, with the probability that σ is less than or equal to the ith of these being given by

$$P(\sigma \le \sigma_i) = \frac{\sum\limits_{j=1}^{i} q(\sigma_j)}{\sum\limits_{j=1}^{M} q(\sigma_j)}. \qquad (16.10)$$

The posterior density is $q(\sigma)/\int q(\sigma)\, d\sigma$, but the integral would be impossible to evaluate analytically. The discrete approximation has the advantage that a valid distribution function can be formed knowing only the *un-normalized* density $q(.)$. Samples that are approximated from the marginal posterior density can be obtained from the *inverse cumulative distribution function* (*CDF*) method described in Gelman *et al.* (1995, §10.2), with the approximation (16.10) used for the cumulative distribution function.

The method can readily be extended to the linear regression case, albeit at the expense of some notational complexity. However, an elegant alternative approach is possible. It will be seen that the method has severe practical drawbacks but can be useful when the number of parameters is small, say, fewer than four or five. This method relies on a general method for sampling from distributions that are awkward to handle and this must first be described.

Rejection sampling

Although we shall use it for sampling from a posterior distribution, this technique can be used to generate samples from a wide range of distributions and at the start of this subsection our notation will reflect this generality. Suppose that the aim is to generate from a distribution which has density $kf(x)$, where x may be a vector or a scalar. It is supposed that $f(x)$ is known but that the constant k may be unknown. This formulation is useful because in Bayesian analyses the posterior density is proportional to $p(\theta)p(y \mid \theta)$ and this is usually known, even though the constant required to ensure that the integral of the posterior is unity may be elusive. The method requires the analyst to identify a known probability density $g(x)$ from which samples can readily be drawn, together with a constant K such that for all x, $f(x) < Kg(x)$. The rejection sampling algorithm is as follows.

1   Draw a trial value X_T from $g(x)$.
2   Draw a value U that is uniformly distributed on the interval $(0, 1)$.
3   If $KUg(X_T) < f(X_T)$, then accept the trial value as the next element of the sample; otherwise reject the value and return to **1** to try again.

The retained values can be shown to be a sample from the density $kf(x)$ (see Devroye, 1986, pp. 40–2). It is intuitively clear that the bounding density $g(x)$ should be chosen so that $Kg(x)$ 'only just' bounds $f(x)$, for otherwise too many trial values will be rejected and the algorithm will be inefficient. The probability that a trial value is accepted can be evaluated: conditional on the value X_T, the probability of acceptance is simply $f(X_T)/[Kg(X_T)]$, so the unconditional probability of acceptance is:

$$\int \{f(u)/[Kg(u)]\}g(u)\ \mathrm{d}u = 1/(kK).$$

Unfortunately, this depends on k which, in many instances, will be unknown.

If the aim is to sample from a posterior distribution, it will usually be convenient to take $f(x)$ to be $p(y \mid \theta)p(\theta)$. If $\hat{\theta}$ is the maximum likelihood estimator of θ, then for all $\theta, p(y \mid \theta) \leq p(y \mid \hat{\theta}) = L_{\max}$, say. Consequently, we can satisfy the requirements of the rejection algorithm by taking $g(x)$ to be the prior distribution, $p(\theta)$, and $K = L_{\max}$. It will usually be the case that a proper prior distribution will be sufficiently standard for sampling from it to be reasonably straightforward. This method is intuitively attractive because a trial value, θ_T, say, is accepted with probability

$$\frac{f(X_T)}{Kg(X_T)} = \frac{p(\theta_T)p(y \mid \theta_T)}{p(\theta_T)L_{\max}} = \frac{p(y \mid \theta_T)}{L_{\max}},$$

which is the likelihood at the trial value as a proportion of the maximum likelihood. In other words, θ is generated from the prior distribution but only has a good chance of being retained if it is supported by the data.

Although intuitively attractive and, in most instances, computationally straightforward, the method is, in fact, only useful in low-dimensional problems with priors that are simple to sample from, as illustrated in Example 16.1. In all but low-dimensional problems, the acceptance probability is generally too small to be practical. Unfortunately, problems that have many parameters are common in practice and other methods for generating samples from complex posterior distributions must be sought. Some recent developments are discussed in §16.3.

Example 16.1

In Example 7.1, for each of 32 babies the change in weight between the 70th and 100th day of life, expressed as a percentage of the birth weight, y, was related to the birth weight x (in oz.): the data are given in Table 7.1. A Bayesian analysis of these data will now be presented. The model for the data is:

$$y_i = \alpha + \beta(x_i - \bar{x}) + \varepsilon_i,$$

where, given the parameters α and β, the residual terms are independent normal variables, with mean zero and constant variance σ^2. Note that the birth-weight variable has been centred about its sample mean, as this can improve numerical aspects of the analysis.

A full Bayesian analysis will estimate the joint posterior distribution of the intercept, slope and variance parameters, $p(\alpha, \beta, \sigma^2 \mid \mathbf{y})$. It is thought unlikely that knowledge of the parameters governing the mean percentage change in weight will be related to knowledge of the residual variation, so the prior distribution $p(\alpha, \beta, \sigma^2)$ is taken to be of the form $p(\alpha, \beta)p(\sigma^2)$. The prior for α and β is taken to be a bivariate normal distribution and the prior for the residual variance is a scale inverse-χ^2 distribution. In a complete analysis the parameters for the prior distributions might be elicited using an appropriate procedure, such as that discussed in Kadane and Wolfson (1998). In this example, analyses using four priors will be illustrated, although there is no implication that any is based on expert prior knowledge. There are seven hyperparameters to be specified in each joint prior distribution and those for each prior are shown in Table 16.1. The values for α and β obtained in Example 7.1 were 71·28 ($\bar{y}$) and $-0·8643$, with standard errors of 3·15 and 0·1757, respectively. The estimate of σ^2 was 316·74.

The motivation behind the choice of priors is as follows. Prior I uses values that are very close to the results obtained in the analysis presented in Example 7.1: in such a case it is expected that the results of the Bayesian analysis would be similar to those obtained previously. Slightly greater uncertainty than is present in Example 7.1 has been introduced to the prior for the residual variance. Prior II uses the same means for the prior for α, β as Prior I, on the grounds that it may be that an expert would have an idea of these values

Table 16.1 Priors used in analysis of data on growth rate in relation to birth weight.

	Hyperparameters in $p(\alpha, \beta)$					Hyperparameters in $p(\sigma^2)$	
Prior	Mean α	Mean β	SD α	SD β	Correlation α, β	Scale	DF
Prior I	70·0	−0·85	3·0	0·2	0·0	300·0	10·0
Prior II	70·0	−0·85	100·0	100·0	0·0	300·0	1·0
Prior III	0·0	0·00	100·0	100·0	0·0	1000·0	0·2
Prior IV	70·0	1·0	10·0	0·2	0·0	300·0	1·0

but may wish to acknowledge the uncertainty in these values by ascribing large prior standard deviations to these values. The expert may also have some idea of the residual variance, so the scale factor is in line with that obtained in Example 7.1, but the degrees of freedom have been reduced to 1, again to reflect uncertainty in the specified value. Prior II therefore contains elements of both an informative and an uninformative prior. Prior III is a more conventional uninformative prior, with large values set for the standard deviations and the scale parameter, and a small value for its degrees of freedom. Prior IV is informative but a positive mean has been ascribed to the slope parameter, i.e. the analyst has decided that the change in weight from the 70th to the 100th day of life will be greater for babies who were heavier at birth. This is somewhat implausible, as it is smaller babies who generally exhibit faster growth in the early days of life, perhaps trying to 'catch up' with their heavier peers. Nevertheless, Prior IV is a proper prior and might well represent the genuine beliefs of some investigator.

The likelihood, $p(y \mid \alpha, \beta, \sigma^2)$ can be written most conveniently as

$$\log p(y|\alpha, \beta, \sigma^2) = -\frac{1}{2} n \log \sigma^2 - \frac{1}{2\sigma^2} \sum_{i=1}^{n} [y_i - \alpha - \beta(x_i - \bar{x})]^2 = -\frac{1}{2} n \log \sigma^2 - \frac{Q}{2\sigma^2}$$

(ignoring constants that are immaterial), where here $n = 32$. At the maximum likelihood estimator of α, β, σ^2 this has value

$$\log p(y|\hat{\alpha}, \hat{\beta}, \hat{\sigma}^2) = -\frac{1}{2} n \log \hat{\sigma}^2 - \frac{1}{2} n,$$

where here $\hat{\sigma}^2$ is the residual sum of squares divided by n, rather than by the residual degrees of freedom.

The algorithm described above draws samples from the posterior distribution by drawing a tentative value $\alpha_T, \beta_T, \sigma_T^2$ from the prior and then retaining this value if

$$U < \frac{p(y|\alpha_T, \beta_T, \sigma_T^2)}{p(y|\hat{\alpha}, \hat{\beta}, \hat{\sigma}^2)},$$

where U is a random variable drawn from a uniform distribution on the interval $[0, 1]$. In fact, as this procedure is likely to be repeated many times when performing the simulation, it is useful to try to be as numerically efficient as possible. If it is noted that $E = -\log U$ has an exponential distribution with mean 1, then the above test is equivalent to retaining $\alpha_T, \beta_T, \sigma_T^2$ if

$$E > \frac{1}{2} \log \frac{\hat{\sigma}^2}{\sigma_T^2} + \frac{1}{2} n - \frac{Q_T}{2\sigma_T^2},$$

where Q_T is the value of Q evaluated at α_T, β_T.

It was intended to draw samples of 1000 from the posterior corresponding to each of the priors given above. For Prior I this required 4815 tentative samples to be drawn from the prior. As Prior I was chosen to be well supported by the data, this number represents a very efficient implementation for this method of sampling from the posterior. This is emphasized by the more diffuse priors: for Prior II 123 850 252 samples from the prior were required to yield 1000 from the posterior, and for Prior III this value rose to 414 395 959. As the priors used here are simple to sample from, these values are feasible.

Table 16.2 Estimated summary quantities for posterior distributions for each of Priors I–III.

Prior	Slope β			Residual variance σ^2		
	Mean	Median	Interval	Mean	Median	Interval
I	−0·863	−0·862	−1·139, −0·602	321·3	311·5	200·3, 500·2
II	−0·867	−0·866	−1·232, −0·489	341·0	327·6	203·0, 568·3
III	−0·851	−0·850	−1·218, −0·472	348·9	331·7	207·7, 571·7

However, none of the first 100 000 000 tentative values drawn from Prior IV was retained. This prior is concentrated around values of the slope that are simply not supported by the data and in these cases this method is likely to be very inefficient. However, a Bayesian analysis when the prior and data are so disparate is unlikely to be of much practical value. At this point the analysis based on Prior IV was abandoned and only the results for Priors I to III are reported.

The mean and median of the posterior are estimated from the sample mean and median of the 1000 values. Posterior 95% intervals can be estimated as the interval from the 25th to 975th largest values in the sample. These summaries are shown in Table 16.2 for the slope β and the residual variance σ^2. These compare with point estimates from the frequentist analysis of −0·864 for β and 316·7 for σ^2. The corresponding 95% confidence intervals are (−1·223, −0·506) and (202·3, 565·9). There is relatively little difference between the results for Priors II and III, and each is similar to the frequentist analysis. The interval estimates from Prior I are shorter than for the other priors, reflecting the relatively informative nature of this distribution.

Graphical summaries of the posterior distributions can be produced by applying kernel density estimation (cf. §12.2 or Silverman, 1986) to the samples. These are shown in Fig. 16.1 for β and σ^2. As might be anticipated, the posterior corresponding to Prior I is rather more concentrated than that for the other priors. However, the distributions are broadly similar, illustrating the limited effect that a prior distribution has, even with a data set comprising only 32 points. The distribution of the variance is noticeably more skewed than that for the slope.

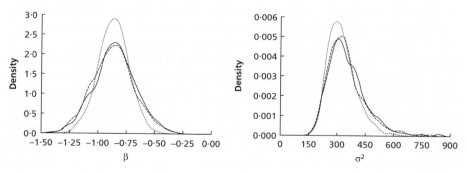

Fig. 16.1 Density estimates for β and σ^2 based on Prior I (- - - -), Prior II (– – –) and Prior III (———).

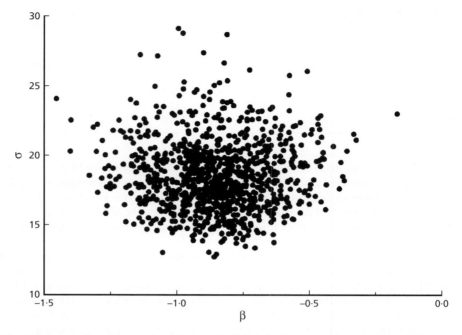

Fig. 16.2 Scatter plot of slope and residual standard deviation from posterior corresponding to Prior III.

Other aspects of the posterior can be investigated similarly. For example, the joint distribution of the residual standard deviation and the slope can be assessed by a simple scatter plot, as shown in Fig. 16.2 for Prior III. These are uncorrelated, with sample correlation -0.0105.

16.4 **Markov chain Monte Carlo methods**

Many of the recent developments in Bayesian methodology have focused on methods for sampling from the posterior distribution; properties of this distribution can then be described through the analyses of samples, as described in §16.2. As the sample size is determined by the analyst, sampling variation can be controlled by drawing sufficiently large samples. This is straightforward when the posterior has a standard form, such as a normal or gamma distribution, but in many applications this will not be the case. Example 16.1 demonstrates that some algorithms for sampling from non-standard posterior distributions can be very time-consuming, even when used for a very simple model. The rejection method described in §16.3 would not be a practical proposition if the application called for a more elaborate model, perhaps with a larger data set, than was encountered in Example 16.1. The need for more efficient methods of sampling from the posterior distribution is transparent and a class of methods known as

Markov chain Monte Carlo methods, or *MCMC methods*, has proved to be of great value.

The 'Monte Carlo' part of MCMC arises because the method is essentially based on the generation of random samples—a similar use to that encountered in the context of permutation tests (see §10.6). The 'Markov chain' element of MCMC refers to the theoretical underpinning of the method and this will be explained very briefly later. However, before this, the Gibbs sampler, perhaps the most intuitively accessible MCMC method, will be described.

MCMC methods are currently the subject of intensive research and all aspects of the subject, theoretical, practical and computational, are developing very rapidly. The present description is at a very naïve level and the reader interested in deeper explanations should consult the current literature: Besag *et al.* (1995) Gilks *et al.* (1996) and Brooks (1998) are good starting-points in a literature that is already large and likely to expand much further in the next few years.

The Gibbs sampler

The Gibbs sampler is perhaps the most widely used MCMC method. In the form most commonly used today it was introduced by Geman and Geman (1984) in a specialized context to do with image analysis using distributions known as *Gibbs distributions*. This explains what is an unfortunate aspect of the nomenclature, because the method can be applied to a much wider range of distributions. It is also a special case of methods that were introduced much earlier by Metropolis *et al.* (1953) and Hastings (1970), which will be explained later.

The problem is how to draw samples from a distribution, $p(\theta|y)$ whose argument is a k-dimensional vector, and which will often be of a non-standard form. The Gibbs sampler uses the k so-called *full conditional distributions*, which are the conditional distributions

$$p(\theta_1|\boldsymbol{\theta}_{-1}, \boldsymbol{y})$$
$$p(\theta_2|\boldsymbol{\theta}_{-2}, \boldsymbol{y})$$
$$\vdots$$
$$p(\theta_k|\boldsymbol{\theta}_{-k}, \boldsymbol{y}).$$

The distributions are *full* conditionals because all the parameters other than the argument are included in the conditioning event. If the problem were specified in terms of three parameters, $\theta_1, \theta_2, \theta_3$ then $p(\theta_1|\theta_2, \theta_3, \boldsymbol{y})$ is a full conditional whereas $p(\theta_1|\theta_2, \boldsymbol{y})$ is not.

The analyst must start the Gibbs sampler by providing an arbitrary starting vector $\boldsymbol{\theta}^{(0)}$. The sampler then proceeds to generate a sequence of vectors $\boldsymbol{\theta}^{(1)}, \boldsymbol{\theta}^{(2)}, \boldsymbol{\theta}^{(3)}, \ldots, \boldsymbol{\theta}^{(N)}$ where N is under the control of the analyst (although in practice computational constraints may mean that the analyst must settle for a smaller value of N than might be ideal).

The first element of $\boldsymbol{\theta}^{(1)}, \theta_1^{(1)}$, is the result of drawing a value from the distribution

$$p(\theta_1 | \theta_2^{(0)}, \theta_3^{(0)}, \ldots, \theta_N^{(0)}, \boldsymbol{y}),$$

i.e. from the full conditional for θ_1, with the other elements of $\boldsymbol{\theta}$ taking the values they have in $\boldsymbol{\theta}^{(0)}$. The second element, $\theta_2^{(1)}$, is the result of a draw from the full conditional for θ_2,

$$p(\theta_2 | \theta_1^{(1)}, \theta_3^{(0)}, \ldots, \theta_N^{(0)}, \boldsymbol{y}).$$

Notice that the conditioning value for θ_1 is the first element of $\boldsymbol{\theta}^{(1)}$, which was generated in the previous step, rather than the first element of $\boldsymbol{\theta}^{(0)}$. The remaining elements of $\boldsymbol{\theta}^{(1)}$ are generated using the remaining full conditional distributions. At each stage, the values of the elements of $\boldsymbol{\theta}^{(1)}$ that are available by that stage are used in the conditioning, with the other elements taking the values they were ascribed in $\boldsymbol{\theta}^{(0)}$. The generation of $\boldsymbol{\theta}^{(2)}$ proceeds analogously; initially all the conditioning values are from $\boldsymbol{\theta}^{(1)}$ and as the algorithm proceeds they are successively replaced by the newly generated elements of $\boldsymbol{\theta}^{(2)}$.

In its simplest form, each full conditional distribution is a distribution of a scalar quantity. The practical value of the algorithm is that it will often be feasible to generate from these k distributions, whereas generating directly from the joint distribution is impossible. Even if it is possible to generate directly from the joint distribution, generating via the Gibbs sampler may be much easier or more efficient. There may be circumstances where each full conditional is a distribution of standard form when the joint distribution is not. Even if some of the conditionals are not of standard form, the method remains useful. It might be much easier to find efficient bounding densities for these full conditionals, so that rejection sampling might be employed at different stages of the algorithm, than to attempt to find a single, efficient, bounding density for the joint distribution. A valuable extension to standard rejection sampling, namely *adaptive rejection sampling*, was introduced by Gilks and Wild (1992) and is now widely used in conjunction with Gibbs sampling.

Several questions about the Gibbs sampler arise almost immediately. The first is that, if you have all the full conditional distributions, will these determine the joint distribution? If two different joint distributions gave rise to the same set of full conditional distributions, then an algorithm which only uses the full conditional distributions could not hope to generate, unambiguously, samples from the desired joint distribution. Fortunately this is not the case and, as Brook (1964) and Besag (1974) show, the complete collection of full conditional distributions characterizes the joint distribution.

The second problem centres on the choice of $\boldsymbol{\theta}^{(0)}$. How important is the choice of this value? Must it come from the required joint distribution? Clearly an affirmative answer to the last question would be problematic, as the use of the algorithm is only being entertained because drawing values from $p(\boldsymbol{\theta}|\boldsymbol{y})$ is so difficult. In fact, in a strict sense, no element of the sequence can be guaranteed to come from $p(\boldsymbol{\theta}|\boldsymbol{y})$. The underlying theory only guarantees that the distributions of the successive values in the sequence $\boldsymbol{\theta}^{(1)}, \boldsymbol{\theta}^{(2)}, \boldsymbol{\theta}^{(3)}, \ldots, \boldsymbol{\theta}^{(N)}$ get closer to $p(\boldsymbol{\theta}|\boldsymbol{y})$ as N becomes larger, i.e. the distribution of the $\boldsymbol{\theta}^{(i)}$ *converges* to $p(\boldsymbol{\theta}|\boldsymbol{y})$. In practice, this aspect is dealt with by discarding the first part of the sequence, the so-called *burn-in* period, and basing inferences on the remainder of the sample. It is hoped that in this way the precise choice of $\boldsymbol{\theta}^{(0)}$ will have minimal influence. However, the choice of starting value, the length of burn-in required and more general assessments of convergence are difficult matters which are the subject of active research.

A third issue concerns the independence of the successive values, $\boldsymbol{\theta}^{(1)}, \boldsymbol{\theta}^{(2)}, \boldsymbol{\theta}^{(3)}, \ldots, \boldsymbol{\theta}^{(N)}$, in the sample. Most simple data-analytic procedures require that the data points be *independent*—that is, the value of one point does not affect, nor is affected by, other points in the sample. However, from the method of construction of the sequence, it is clear that successive values from the Gibbs sampler will not be independent. As the final inferences made about $p(\boldsymbol{\theta}|\boldsymbol{y})$ will generally be obtained by applying standard data-analytic techniques to the sequence obtained from the Gibbs sampler, the extent to which these conclusions remain valid in the face of this dependence is an important question. Crudely speaking, averages across the sequences remain valid, but assessment of the precision of the estimates obtained requires more refined methods than simply computing naïve standard errors (see Geyer, 1992).

An obvious further concern is the calculation of the full conditional distributions. How readily can these be computed? For problems specified in terms of a few parameters, conventional methods will usually suffice. In the present context, where properties of densities are determined by sampling from them, it is often possible to make progress if the density is only specified up to a constant. Determining full conditional distributions only up to proportionality allows for considerable simplification. For example, repeated applications of Bayes' theorem (§3.3) shows that the full conditional distribution $p(\theta_1|\boldsymbol{\theta}_{-1}, \boldsymbol{y})$ can be written as

$$p(\theta_1|\boldsymbol{\theta}_{-1}, \boldsymbol{y}) = \frac{p(\theta_1, \boldsymbol{\theta}_{-1}|\boldsymbol{y})}{p(\boldsymbol{\theta}_{-1}|\boldsymbol{y})} = \frac{p(\boldsymbol{\theta}, \boldsymbol{y})}{p(\boldsymbol{\theta}_{-1}, \boldsymbol{y})}. \tag{16.11}$$

The final denominator in (16.11) is simply

$$p(\boldsymbol{\theta}_{-1}, \boldsymbol{y}) = \int p(\theta_1, \boldsymbol{\theta}_{-1}, \boldsymbol{y}) \, d\theta_1,$$

which does not depend on θ_1, so $p(\theta_1|\boldsymbol{\theta}_{-1}, \boldsymbol{y}) \propto p(\boldsymbol{\theta}, \boldsymbol{y})$. If needed, the exact full conditional density can be found as

$$\frac{p(\boldsymbol{\theta}, \boldsymbol{y})}{\int p(\boldsymbol{\theta}, \boldsymbol{y}) \, d\theta_1} = \frac{p(\boldsymbol{\theta}, \boldsymbol{y})}{\int p(\theta_1, \boldsymbol{\theta}_{-1}, \boldsymbol{y}) \, d\theta_1}, \tag{16.12}$$

although knowing $p(\theta_1|\boldsymbol{\theta}_{-1}, \boldsymbol{y})$ up to proportionality will often suffice.

In practice the joint distribution of the parameters and data, $p(\boldsymbol{\theta}, \boldsymbol{y})$, usually comprises the product of several factors. For the purpose of deriving $p(\theta_1|\boldsymbol{\theta}_{-1}, \boldsymbol{y})$ any of these factors which do not contain θ_1 can be ignored, as they would appear in both the numerator and denominator of (16.12). In the analysis of complicated systems, realistic models often give rise to joint distributions $p(\boldsymbol{\theta}, \boldsymbol{y})$ that have many factors, and devices, such as that just outlined, which simplify the calculation of full conditional distributions are important.

An important way in which the structure of $p(\boldsymbol{\theta}, \boldsymbol{y})$ can be helpfully organized is through the representation of the model, and in particular the structure of the dependence between the elements of $\boldsymbol{\theta}$ and $\boldsymbol{y}$, using a graph, or more precisely a *directed acyclic graph*. Here, graph is being used in the sense employed in graph theory, where a graph is a collection of nodes and connecting edges, rather than a plot such as a histogram or scatter plot. It turns out that representing the random quantities in the analysis, parameters and data, by nodes in the graph, and the dependence structure by connections between the nodes, allows the dependence structure of the data to become apparent. In particular, it means that it is relatively straightforward to decide which parts of $p(\boldsymbol{\theta}, \boldsymbol{y})$ can be ignored when deriving each full conditional distribution. The use of these types of graphical methods for statistical modelling is fully exploited in the computer package WinBUGS (Spiegelhalter *et al.*, 2000, available at http://www.mrc-bsu.cam. ac.uk/bugs/). A more detailed description of this kind of modelling is beyond the scope of the present discussion. The reader interested in the use of graphs to represent properties of statistical models can consult Whittaker (1990), Cox and Wermuth (1996) and Lauritzen (1996). Illuminating descriptions of particular applications can be found in Spiegelhalter *et al.* (1993, 1996). A more general discussion of full conditional distributions can be found in Gilks (1996).

Example 16.1, continued

An alternative approach to simulating from $p(\alpha, \beta, \sigma^2|\boldsymbol{y})$ is to use the Gibbs sampler. For the form of prior, namely $p(\alpha, \beta, \sigma^2) = p(\alpha, \beta)p(\sigma^2)$, the joint distribution of the data and parameters is

$$p(\boldsymbol{y}|\alpha, \beta, \sigma^2)p(\alpha, \beta)p(\sigma^2).$$

The prior for the variance is a scaled inverse-χ^2 distribution and that for the slope and intercept is a bivariate normal distribution. Using the notation introduced previously,

$$p(y|\alpha, \beta, \sigma^2) \propto \sigma^{-n} \exp\left(-\frac{Q}{2\sigma^2}\right), \tag{16.13}$$

where $Q = Q(\alpha, \beta)$ is the residual sum of squares for the given slope and intercept.

In order to implement the Gibbs sampler, it is necessary to be able to simulate from each of the full conditional distributions of the posterior, namely, from $p(\sigma^2|\alpha, \beta, y)$, $p(\alpha|\sigma^2, \beta, y)$ and $p(\beta|\alpha, \sigma^2, y)$. Using the method outlined above, the first of these is easily found from (16.13) by picking out the factors which depend on σ^2. Therefore,

$$p(\sigma^2|\alpha, \beta, y) \propto \sigma^{-n} \exp\left(-\frac{Q}{2\sigma^2}\right)p(\sigma^2),$$

and substituting the prior scaled inverse-χ^2 distribution with ν_0 degrees of freedom and scale factor s_0^2 for $p(\sigma^2)$, it emerges that $p(\sigma^2|\alpha, \beta, y)$ is a scaled inverse-χ^2 distribution with degrees of freedom $n + \nu_0$ and scale factor $[Q(\alpha, \beta) + \nu_0 s_0^2]/(n + \nu_0)$.

A similar approach allows the remaining full conditional distributions to be found. In this application all the prior distributions used assume that the slope and intercept are uncorrelated. For a more general bivariate normal prior on the slope and intercept, it would be helpful to derive the full conditionals in two stages, namely, first to derive $p(\alpha, \beta|\sigma^2, y)$ and then to proceed to the full conditionals. The posterior $p(\alpha, \beta|\sigma^2, y)$ is essentially the same as the posterior for a linear model with known variance, which is a bivariate normal distribution with mean and variance given by (16.4) and (16.5), respectively. As the prior correlation is zero and the x variables have been centred, matrix (16.5) is diagonal, so under the posterior distribution α and β are independent. Consequently, the full conditional $p(\alpha|\beta, \sigma^2, y)$ is a normal distribution with mean $(\sigma_\alpha^{-2} + n\sigma^{-2})^{-1} \times (\sigma_\alpha^{-2}\mu_\alpha + n\sigma^{-2}\hat{\alpha})$ and variance $(\sigma_\alpha^{-2} + n\sigma^{-2})^{-1}$, where μ_α and σ_α^2 are the prior mean and variance for α, and $\hat{\alpha}$ is the usual estimate of intercept, as calculated, for example, in Example 7.1. The distribution $p(\beta|\alpha, \sigma^2, y)$ is also normal, with mean $(\sigma_\beta^{-2} + S_{XX}\sigma^{-2})^{-1}(\sigma_\beta^{-2}\mu_\beta + S_{XX}\sigma^{-2}\hat{\beta})$ and variance $(\sigma_\beta^{-2} + S_{XX}\sigma^{-2})^{-1}$, with definitions for $\mu_\beta, \sigma_\beta^2$ and $\hat{\beta}$ that are analogous to those for α, and S_{XX} is the sum of squares of the x_i about their mean.

As all the full conditional distributions are, in this application, standard distributions, it is straightforward to run the Gibbs sampler efficiently. Generating 10 000 samples from the posterior and discarding the first 1000 (to allow for possible non-convergence) can be done far more quickly than was possible with the rejection method used previously. For Priors I and III, the results are shown in Table 16.3 and can be seen to be similar to those obtained using rejection sampling. The results shown are for Gibbs samplers that were

Table 16.3 Estimated summary quantities for posterior distributions using output from the Gibbs sampler, for each of Priors I and III.

Prior	Slope β			Residual variance σ^2		
	Mean	Median	Interval	Mean	Median	Interval
I	−0·858	−0·860	−1·112, −0·599	322·8	312·7	209·8, 493·3
III	−0·861	−0·861	−1·228, −0·491	345·9	329·9	206·2, 574·6

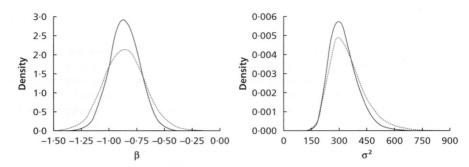

Fig. 16.3 Density estimates for β and σ^2 based on Prior I (- - -) and Prior III (————) from 9000 draws obtained using a Gibbs sampler.

started at the means of the prior distributions: samplers started at other values gave very similar results.

The kernel density estimates for the distributions of β and σ^2 are shown in Fig. 16.3. They are smoother than those obtained using the output from the rejection sampler because the latter were based on only 1000 values, as opposed to the 9000 values that could be efficiently obtained with the Gibbs sampler.

Markov chains

This is a rather theoretical topic to appear as a heading in a book which emphasizes the practical aspects of medical statistics. However, MCMC methods are already widespread and likely to become more so in the future. Moreover, while their theoretical underpinnings might be challenging, these methods have resulted in many applications being subjected to more realistic analyses than might have been possible with more conventional methods. In this sense, MCMC methodology is a practical advance of the highest importance. Consequently, an appreciation of the basis of MCMC methods, albeit in very rudimentary and heuristic terms, is becoming of importance for even the most practical statistician. The following is a very loose and elementary description of an area that admits much more rigorous analysis. Readers interested in a more formal exposition can consult texts such as Taylor and Karlin (1984) or Grimmett and Stirzacker (1992).

A *stochastic process* can be thought of as an evolving sequence of random variables, $X_1, X_2, \ldots, X_n, \ldots$. A Markov chain is an important example of a stochastic process, which imposes certain conditions on how the process evolves. The subscripts on the variables can be thought of as representing time—in other words, time is thought of as being discrete. Markov chains can be defined in continuous time but this is an elaboration that we shall not need and it will be assumed that all processes described herein evolve through discrete time. More vividly, the process could be thought of as evolving a day at a time, with only one change of stage allowed each day.

The *state space* of the process is the set of values that each X_i might take. The simplest form of Markov chain occurs when the X_i are scalars which can take only a finite number of discrete values. This is the form in which Markov chains are usually first encountered in textbooks.

The fundamental property that makes a stochastic process a Markov chain is that the probability distribution of the states the process might be in tomorrow depends on the state it is in today, but it does not depend on where the chain was yesterday. So, for a Markov chain with a state space that has just K states, there is a separate distribution for each state. For example, associated with state 1 there will K probabilities (summing to 1) describing the chances of being in each of the other states tomorrow, given that you are in state 1 today. A similar set of probabilities will be associated with each of the other states in the state space. These probabilities are usually written as the rows of a $K \times K$ matrix, P, which is known as the *transition matrix* of the process. The matrix P describes how the next element in the evolution can be generated from the present realization.

Many Markov chains will have a *stationary distribution* and this property is fundamental to the value of MCMC methods. If a chain possessing a stationary distribution is allowed to evolve over a long period, the distribution of the states will eventually settle down to the stationary distribution of the chain. In the application of MCMC methods, the aim is to construct a Markov chain which has the required posterior distribution as its stationary distribution.

Slightly more precision can be given to this explanation as follows. Suppose that the distribution of the chain at time n is summarized by w_n, a row vector of length K whose ith element is the probability of being in state i at time n. The corresponding quantity for time $n + 1$, w_{n+1}, is found from the matrix multiplication $w_{n+1} = w_n P$. Similarly, the distribution at time $n + 2$ is given by $w_{n+1} P$. The stationary distribution is a vector of probabilities π such that $\pi P = \pi$, i.e. a distribution that is unchanged by an evolution of one step in the process. If at any stage the distribution $w_n = \pi$, then the distribution at the next time is $w_{n+1} = w_n P = \pi P = \pi$, i.e. in probabilistic terms the chain has stopped evolving and become *stationary*. For many chains the distributions w_n will eventually become close to π even if one of the w_n has never actually coincided with π.

It has been explained that MCMC methods depend for their success on the existence of stationary distributions and that most chains have such. Clearly, it is important to know if a chain being used for an MCMC analysis possesses a stationary distribution. This is not a straightforward matter but some of the attributes of a Markov chain that are of importance can be described, albeit crudely. For a chain to converge to a stationary distribution, it must be *irreducible, aperiodic* and *positive recurrent*. Irreducibility is essentially a condition that ensures that the chain can get to all parts of the state space and positive recurrence is a property that ensures that the chain can keep getting to all parts of the space. Aperiodicity stops the chain from cycling within a subset of the state space. See Roberts and Smith (1994) and Roberts (1996) for more precise and thorough discussions.

In an application of MCMC methods, the elements of the chain, X_i, will usually correspond to the parameters in the model—in other words, the X_i will be vectors. Moreover, most of the parameters will be real numbers so the state space of the Markov chain will not be the simple finite set discussed so far, but a suitable subset of k-dimensional space. At the very informal level of the fore-going discussion, there is little difference between Markov chains with discrete or continuous state spaces. At deeper levels, the technicalities of general state spaces are more demanding, and some of the concepts need to be amended; see Tierney (1996) for an illuminating introduction.

From a practical point of view, MCMC is useful only if the output from the Markov chain can be used to estimate useful summaries of the posterior dis-tribution. Many estimators can be written in the form

$$\frac{1}{N}\sum_{\ell=1}^{N}f(\boldsymbol{\theta}^{(\ell)}),\tag{16.14}$$

where $\boldsymbol{\theta}^{(1)}, \boldsymbol{\theta}^{(2)}, \boldsymbol{\theta}^{(3)}, \ldots, \boldsymbol{\theta}^{(N)}$ denotes the output from an MCMC procedure and $f(\cdot)$ is an appropriately chosen function. For example, if the intention were to estimate the marginal posterior mean of the first element of $\boldsymbol{\theta}$, then f would be defined by $f(\boldsymbol{\theta}) = \theta_1$. If $f(\boldsymbol{\theta}) = 1$ if $\theta_2 < c$ and 0 otherwise, then (16.14) would be used to estimate the posterior probability that $\theta_2 < c$.

While it is well known that means of the form (16.14) will be good estimators of the posterior expectation of $f(\boldsymbol{\theta})$ in straightforward circumstances—for ex-ample, when the $\boldsymbol{\theta}^{(1)}, \boldsymbol{\theta}^{(2)}, \boldsymbol{\theta}^{(3)}, \ldots, \boldsymbol{\theta}^{(N)}$ are independent and come from the same distribution—this will not be the case for MCMC output. There will be dependence between the different elements of the sequence and the elements will not share a common distribution. However, as N gets larger, the later elements of the sequence will all come close to having the stationary distribution and, if the stationary distribution is the required posterior distribution, it can be shown that (16.14) does provide a valid estimate of the posterior expectation of $f(\boldsymbol{\theta})$.

Many MCMC practitioners would replace (16.14) by

$$\frac{1}{N-M}\sum_{\ell=M+1}^{N}f(\boldsymbol{\theta}^{(\ell)}).\tag{16.15}$$

They would omit the information from the first M draws from the Markov chain on the grounds that at those times the chain had not been running for sufficiently long for it to be reasonable to assume that the draws would have distributions close to the stationary distribution. The length, M, of this burn-in period is chosen in the belief that the distribution of the later draws from the chain will be close to the stationary distribution and we can consider that, for all practical purposes, the chain has *converged* by time M. The length of the chain that is used to explore the posterior distribution, $N - M$, should be controlled by choosing N so that the precision of the estimate obtained from (16.15) is adequate.

There are practical difficulties in assessing the adequacy of (16.15), because of the dependence between the $\theta^{(i)}$, and time series methods (see §12.7) are often used (see Geyer, 1992). Even once a Markov chain has, for all practical purposes, converged, it may be slow to *mix*. This means that the chain evolves slowly and takes many iterations to move round the state space. This can occur when the correlation between successive outputs from the chain are highly correlated. Unless such chains are run for very long periods, they will give results that have poor precision. The parameterization chosen for the model can lead to problems with mixing, and reparameterization can be a useful remedy. This and other ways to improve the practical performance of MCMC methods are discussed in Gilks and Roberts (1996).

Metropolis–Hastings algorithms

Starting from arbitrary initial values, the Gibbs sampler indicates how to simulate the next draw from the posterior, $\theta^{(i+1)}$, from the present draw $\theta^{(i)}$. In the simple form described above, each element of $\theta^{(i+1)}$ is updated by taking a sample from the appropriate full conditional distribution. The Gibbs sampler is, in fact, a special case of a more general algorithm for producing MCMC samples. This algorithm was originally due to Metropolis *et al.* (1953) and extended by Hastings (1970)—it is now generally referred to as the Metropolis—Hastings algorithm.

The algorithm has aspects which are reminiscent of the method of rejection sampling discussed in §16.3, in that the generation of $\theta^{(i+1)}$ requires the specification of a *proposal distribution* from which to draw a *candidate value*, θ_C. The algorithm ensures the correct distribution for $\theta^{(i+1)}$ by accepting θ_C (i.e. setting $\theta^{(i+1)} = \theta_C$) with an astutely chosen probability. However, unlike the rejection sampling method, multiple draws are not needed in order to determine $\theta^{(i+1)}$—if θ_C is not accepted, then $\theta^{(i+1)} = \theta^{(i)}$.

The results will be valid for any proposal distribution, although the closer the proposal distribution approximates the posterior, the more efficient will be the method. The posterior is $p(\theta|y)$ and the proposal distribution must have a density which is a function of a vector of the same dimension as $\theta, q(\theta|\theta^{(i)})$, which can depend on both y and $\theta^{(i)}$, although dependence on y has been suppressed in the notation. The candidate value, θ_C, is drawn from this distribution and is accepted as $\theta^{(i+1)}$ with probability

$$\alpha = \min\left\{1, \frac{p(\boldsymbol{\theta}_C|\boldsymbol{y})q(\boldsymbol{\theta}^{(i)}|\boldsymbol{\theta}_C)}{p(\boldsymbol{\theta}^{(i)}|\boldsymbol{y})q(\boldsymbol{\theta}_C|\boldsymbol{\theta}^{(i)})}\right\}.$$

This gives a very general class of methods for generating Markov chains that converge to a given posterior distribution. The efficient use of these methods depends, to a certain extent, on the analyst's ability to determine an appropriate proposal distribution. A very wide class of proposal distributions will yield a valid chain that eventually converges to the correct distribution. However, it is clear that if q results in values for α that are generally rather small, then the candidate $\boldsymbol{\theta}_C$ will seldom be accepted and the chain will stick on particular values for long periods. This is an example of slow mixing, and sequences generated from slow-mixing chains will take a very long time to visit all important regions of the state space.

Some practical matters

MCMC methods provide a powerful way to obtain samples from a posterior distribution. They allow samples to be drawn from distributions that at first sight might seem impossibly complicated and intractable. However, this power is obtained at the expense of using a method whose practical implementation is not entirely straightforward or free from danger. Some relevant issues are listed here, but few details are given: this is an area of very active research and it is, as yet, unclear what general recommendations can be given. A fuller discussion, together with more references, can be found in various articles in Gilks *et al.* (1996) and in Brooks (1998).

Convergence and 'burn-in'

The output from an MCMC is not a sequence from the posterior distribution that the investigator wishes to explore; rather, the distribution of members of the sequence will get closer to the required posterior distribution as the length of the sequence increases. To be useful there must come a point beyond which the distribution of the elements of the sequence can be taken, for all practical purposes, to correspond to the required posterior distribution. Samples generated before this point was reached can be discarded and inference based on the remaining values. How can the analyst know when such a point has been reached? Theoretical calculations about rates of convergence have been contemplated but are generally too difficult to be helpful. In practice it is necessary to try to decide on convergence by examining the output from the chain itself; important early references are Gelman and Rubin (1992) and Raftery and Lewis (1992). Raftery and Lewis (1996) provide an approach based on the analysis of eigenvalues of the transition matrix $\boldsymbol{P}$ for a reduced chain with two states.

An important idea, although not one that is universally accepted, is to run more than one chain. The advantages of many chains over one much longer chain have been discussed widely (see Gelman & Rubin, 1992, and associated following discussion). In any given application the issue may be resolved by practical considerations of the computational equipment available. However, multiple chains clearly allow the possibility of starting chains from a variety of values and assessing how long the influence of the starting value appears to persist. Gelman (1996) argues that methods which try to assess convergence on the basis of a single sequence from an MCMC method often fail to detect non-convergence.

Inference

Once the length of the 'burn-in' period has been determined, it remains to decide how many further samples should be used to make inferences about the posterior distribution. Essentially this is just a problem in estimation for which standard sample-size calculations might be contemplated. If the aim is to estimate the posterior mean of some scalar function, $f(\boldsymbol{\theta})$, of the parameter, then generating enough values from the posterior to ensure that the standard error of this quantity is below a specified value might be a sensible approach. If an estimate of the standard deviation, σ, of $f(\boldsymbol{\theta})$ is available, then, assuming that the values obtained from the chain are independent, the usual formula for the standard error, $\sigma/\sqrt{n}$ can be used to estimate the number, n, of simulations required.

However, it will often be inappropriate to assume that the values obtained from the chain are independent and time series methods can be applied. For example, a first-order autoregression (see §12.7) can be fitted to the successive values of $f(\boldsymbol{\theta})$ obtained from the chain. If this approach is followed then the appropriate formula for the standard error becomes

$$\frac{\sigma}{\sqrt{n}}\sqrt{\left(\frac{1+\rho}{1-\rho}\right)},$$

where ρ is the autocorrelation coefficient. It can be appreciated from this formula that, if there is substantial autocorrelation in the series, so that ρ is close to 1, a very large value of n may be needed to ensure that the standard error is below the required value. A valuable discussion of related issues can be found in Geyer (1992). See also Raftery and Lewis (1992).

If it is necessary to use a very long chain to obtain adequate estimates of relevant quantities, then problems can arise with the amount of computer storage required. If the successive values are highly correlated (and, as just seen, very long runs are likely to be required in just this circumstance), perhaps little will be lost by keeping only every Lth value of $\boldsymbol{\theta}$ obtained from the chain. Applying this device, which is known as *thinning*, may well result in a set of values which exhibit substantially smaller autocorrelation, and an apparently smaller value will be needed for n. However, as the series can only be obtained by discarding $L - 1$ out of every L values, there is no saving in the amount of computation needed. Gelman (1996) points out that there is no inferential advantage to using the thinned series, even when there is high correlation, and the only arguments for thinning are computational.

Blocking and related matters

The description of the Gibbs sampler given at the start of this section supposes that the aim is to draw samples from a posterior distribution on the k-dimensional vector $\boldsymbol{\theta}$ via the k full conditional distributions, $p(\theta_i|\boldsymbol{\theta}_{-i})$, $i = 1, \ldots, k$. In other words, each of the full conditional distributions is a distribution on a scalar quantity. However, this is not necessary. An alternative, which may be helpful in some circumstances, is to divide the vector $\boldsymbol{\theta}$ into h components, with $1 \le h < k$. This means that at least some of the full conditional distributions will be distributions on vector variables. This idea of *blocking* can also be used with more general Metropolis–Hastings algorithms. In this instance the extreme case $h = 1$ might be useful, as judicious choice of a proposal distribution may allow the analyst to sample directly from the full posterior. A Gibbs sampler with $h = 1$ amounts to an instruction to sample directly from the full posterior distribution, and if this were feasible MCMC methods need not have been contemplated in the first place.

The choice of blocks is another issue that calls for experience and judgement on the part of the analyst. Generally, the components will be scalars or low-dimensional vectors. Occasionally it may be sensible to combine highly correlated components. Another area where blocking may be natural is for random effects. If the full conditional distributions on higher-dimensional components of $\boldsymbol{\theta}$ are not of standard form, finding efficient proposal distributions can be challenging.

Another feature of the way the Gibbs sampler was introduced that is not strictly necessary is the way the various components, whether vectors or scalars, are updated. The descriptions hitherto have assumed that all components are updated at each cycle of the algorithm and that samples are drawn from the full conditional distributions in a fixed order. Neither is necessary. The components can be updated in random order. It might also be beneficial to update some components more frequently than others. For example, it might improve the mixing of a chain if highly correlated components were updated more frequently.

16.5 **Model assessment and model choice**

Chapter 6 and §16.2 have addressed the issues of how inferences are made in a Bayesian setting and how a posterior distribution can be described. The details of implementing these ideas for the linear model have been outlined in §16.3. More sophisticated simulation-based methods have been presented in §16.4, and these allow more complicated models, such as log-linear models and generalized linear models (see §§14.2–14.4), to be fitted (see also Dellaportas & Smith, 1993).

Issues that are, perhaps, less fundamental but of undoubted practical importance, such as how to choose and assess a model, have been discussed in a frequentist setting (see §11.9). This section discusses some of these more practical issues from a Bayesian viewpoint.

Model assessment

Most exercises in statistical modelling will start with a sample of outcomes, y_i, and associated covariates x_i on individual $i, i = 1, \ldots, n$. While the statistician may postulate a model, $p(y_i|x_i, \theta)$, defined in terms of unknown parameters θ, for various purposes, such as summarization and explanation of the data, in reality the model remains an unobserved artefact of the analysis. It is useful only in so far as it suits the purposes of the analysis and fits the data. Consequently, one approach to assessing the fit of the model to the data that is possible in a Bayesian setting is to focus on the outcomes that the model implies will be associated with the observed covariates. This can be done through the *marginal* distribution of the outcomes. Given that θ has a specified value, then the distribution of the outcome, y, for a unit with covariates x, is given by the density associated with the model, $p(y|x, \theta)$. However, we will not generally know the value of θ. In the frequentist setting the way round this problem is to substitute an estimate, such as the maximum likelihood estimate, $\hat{\theta}$, for θ. This procedure often works well in practice but the procedure does use $\hat{\theta}$ as if it were the known value of θ and ignores the uncertainty in the estimate. The principles of Bayesian statistics offer a way around this rather *ad hoc* procedure. As the parameters are unknown, they can be removed from the procedure by integrating with respect to their prior distribution, $p(\theta)$, that is, the density of y is

$$p(y|x) = \int p(y|\theta, x)p(\theta) \, d\theta,$$

which is the marginal distribution of the outcome. This function could be evaluated for each outcome in the data set. Isolated small values for this function might cast doubt on the values for these points, i.e. they may be outliers (see §11.9) whose values need further investigation. If many of the data points give small values, then doubt is cast on the model itself.

There are problems with using the marginal distribution of the outcome for model checking. Deciding on what is an implausibly small value for the function and deciding when there are too many of these are difficult judgements. A more serious practical problem is that the marginal distribution will not be a genuine distribution if the prior is improper. This is easily seen from the following (here the inessential dependence on a covariate is suppressed in the notation):

$$p(y) = \int p(y|\boldsymbol{\theta})p(\boldsymbol{\theta})\, d\boldsymbol{\theta},$$

and, if this is a proper distribution, integrating it with respect to y should give 1. However, performing this integration and interchanging the order of the integrations with respect to data and parameters gives

$$\int p(y)\, dy = \int\int p(y|\boldsymbol{\theta})p(\boldsymbol{\theta})\, d\boldsymbol{\theta}\, dy = \int p(\boldsymbol{\theta})\left(\int p(y|\boldsymbol{\theta})\, dy\right) d\boldsymbol{\theta} = \int p(\boldsymbol{\theta})\, d\boldsymbol{\theta},$$

and this is infinite for improper priors (the integration in parentheses has used the fact that, for a given $\boldsymbol{\theta}, p(y|\boldsymbol{\theta})$ is a genuine density for y). Experience has shown that the apparently fanciful notion of an improper prior distribution for parameters can usefully be sustained, provided it leads to a proper posterior distribution. However, the data clearly must have a proper distribution, so the marginal distribution is not a sensible quantity to consider when it has been decided to use an improper prior distribution.

In fact, the problem with the marginal distribution of the outcomes arises because this form of analysis uses the prior distribution for the parameters rather than the posterior. In other words, it does not allow the information from the data to inform what weights are given to the various values of $\boldsymbol{\theta}$ when values of $p(y|\boldsymbol{x}, \boldsymbol{\theta})$ are aggregated to form the distribution of the outcome given the data. A solution to this is to use a *predictive* density.

Suppose that data $\boldsymbol{y}$ have been observed, a model, $p(\boldsymbol{y}|\boldsymbol{\theta})$, has been postulated for these data and a prior $p(\boldsymbol{\theta})$ specified for the parameters in the model. What can now be said about the distribution of a future outcome, y_f, say? If there are covariates $\boldsymbol{x}_f$ associated with y_f then the distribution of y_f, for a given $\boldsymbol{\theta}$ is described by $p(y_f|\boldsymbol{x}_f, \boldsymbol{\theta})$ and, in the light of the data, we believe that $\boldsymbol{\theta}$ follows the posterior distribution, $p(\boldsymbol{\theta}|\boldsymbol{y})$. Consequently, the predictive distribution of y_f is given by

$$p(y_f|\boldsymbol{x}_f, \boldsymbol{y}) = \int p(y_f|\boldsymbol{x}_f, \boldsymbol{\theta})p(\boldsymbol{\theta}|\boldsymbol{y})\, d\boldsymbol{\theta}. \tag{16.16}$$

This distribution has wide uses outside model assessment, as it is the basis of making predictions in a Bayesian framework. However, it does play a substantial role in model assessment. Rubin (1984) and also Gelman *et al.* (1995) have advocated *posterior predictive* model checks. In a sense, if the model is correct, then data sampled from (16.16) should 'look the same' as the observed data. The interested reader should consult Gelman *et al.* (1995, §6.2) or Carlin and Louis (2000, §2.4).

In a frequentist setting, perhaps the most important quantities in the assessment of a model are the residuals. The frequentist version was defined in §11.9 as

$y_i - Y_i$, where y_i is the ith data point and Y_i is the fitted value for the ith data point. A natural way to approach the definition of analogous quantities in a Bayesian framework is to use the posterior predictive distribution to obtain a prediction of y_i from the model. The expected value of the outcome for a variable which has covariate x_f under (16.16) is

$$\int y_f p(y_f | x_f, y) \, \mathrm{d}y_f = \int\int y_f p(y_f | x_f, \theta) p(\theta | y) \, \mathrm{d}y_f \, \mathrm{d}\theta$$
$$= \int \mathrm{E}(y_f | \theta, x_f) p(\theta | y) \, \mathrm{d}\theta,$$

(16.17)

so the predicted value for y_f is the expectation of $\mathrm{E}(y_f | \theta, x_f)$ over the posterior distribution of θ. For a linear model, $\mathrm{E}(y_f | \theta, x_f)$ is simply $x_f^\mathrm{T}\beta$, where, for consistency with previous usage, β has been used for the vector of parameters of the linear model. Consequently, the predicted value for y_f, Y_f, is $x_f^\mathrm{T}\bar{\beta}$, where $\bar{\beta}$ is the posterior mean of β. If the posterior has been computed by sampling, a value for $\bar{\beta}$ can be found from the means of the sampled parameters. These values are substituted in $x_f^\mathrm{T}\bar{\beta}$ to yield Y_f.

If x_f is taken, successively, as x_i, the covariates in the data, y, then the discrepancies $y_i - Y_i$ will be the Bayesian analogues of frequentist residuals and can be used in broadly similar ways. Indeed, there are broadly similar concerns with the definition. Ideally, the residuals would be defined in the above terms, but with posterior distribution $p(\theta | z)$, where z is a 'training' data set, which is quite separate from the data y being used to assess the fit of the model. This is because it is likely that assessments based on the same data that were used to determine the posterior distribution would be overoptimistic, because, to a certain extent, the data are being used to predict themselves. This is the same concern that attaches to frequentist residuals, because the residual for ith data point involves an estimate for the parameter which was, in part, based on y_i. In a frequentist setting a solution is to use jackknife residuals (see §11.9), and there is a similar resolution in the Bayesian setting. Rather than base the predicted value of y at x_i on the predictive distribution, which uses all the observed data y, a jackknife version is used, namely,

$$p(y_i | x_i, y_{-i}) = \int p(y_i | x_i, \theta) p(\theta | y_{-i}) \, \mathrm{d}\theta,$$

where y_{-i} is y without the ith data value.

Assessing the influence of the prior distribution

One aspect of Bayesian model assessment which is necessarily absent from frequentist analysis is determining the extent to which inferences are dependent on the prior distribution assumed for the parameters. In strictly Bayesian terms the sensitivity of the posterior to the prior is, perhaps, unimportant. The prior should be chosen carefully so that it represents the genuine beliefs of the analyst; the associated posterior will then faithfully describe how these beliefs are modified by the data. The extent to which substantially different posterior inferences arise from plausible changes to the prior distribution does not matter, as the changed prior is not relevant to the analyst. The fact that another analyst, starting with a different prior distribution, may legitimately arrive at quite different conclusions simply reflects the subjective nature of the Bayesian method.

However philosophically cogent the Bayesian approach might be, many find this potential volatility in statistical inferences rather disturbing. Consequently the practical analyst will wish not only to adduce the posterior corresponding to the chosen prior but to demonstrate that posterior inferences are broadly similar for a range of plausible prior distributions. This is not a forlorn hope: when the data are extensive the likelihood will usually dominate the prior in the formation of the posterior distribution, so for larger data sets the effect of the prior may be limited (unless the prior is very concentrated).

It is therefore useful to perform a sensitivity analysis, in which the posterior distribution, or at least a relevant summary of it, is computed for a range of prior distributions. However, a systematic approach to this can be computationally onerous. A simple sensitivity analysis might proceed by replacing the prior location of each element of $\boldsymbol{\theta}$ with a mean or median that is larger or smaller than that originally envisaged. However, combining all these leads to 3^k analyses. If the posterior is estimated via a sample, perhaps generated using an MCMC method, then a determination of one posterior can be time-consuming and estimating 3^k posterior distributions can be impractical.

Rather than limiting the scope of the sensitivity analysis, a technique known as *importance sampling* (Hammersley & Handscomb, 1964, pp. 57–9; Carlin & Louis, 2000, pp. 131–2) can be used to obtain estimates for posterior expectations corresponding to a perturbed prior from the sample generated using the unperturbed version. Suppose that the posterior distribution $p(\boldsymbol{\theta}|\boldsymbol{y})$ corresponds to a prior distribution $p(\boldsymbol{\theta})$ and an alternative posterior, $p_a(\boldsymbol{\theta}|\boldsymbol{y})$, corresponds to a perturbed prior, $p_a(\boldsymbol{\theta})$. A sample, $\boldsymbol{\theta}_1, \boldsymbol{\theta}_2, \ldots, \boldsymbol{\theta}_N$, generated from $p(\boldsymbol{\theta}|\boldsymbol{y})$ is available and it is desired to evaluate the expectation of some relevant summary with respect to the alternative posterior. The summary might be a mean, a variance or a percentile and, for generality, is written here as $h(\boldsymbol{\theta})$. In this context importance sampling notes that the expectation of $h(\boldsymbol{\theta})$ with respect to $p_a(\boldsymbol{\theta}|\boldsymbol{y})$ can be written

$$\int h(\boldsymbol{\theta}) p_a(\boldsymbol{\theta}|\boldsymbol{y}) \, d\boldsymbol{\theta} = \frac{\int h(\boldsymbol{\theta}) p(\boldsymbol{y}|\boldsymbol{\theta}) p_a(\boldsymbol{\theta}) \, d\boldsymbol{\theta}}{\int p(\boldsymbol{y}|\boldsymbol{\theta}) p_a(\boldsymbol{\theta}) \, d\boldsymbol{\theta}} = \frac{\int h(\boldsymbol{\theta}) g(\boldsymbol{\theta}) p(\boldsymbol{\theta}|\boldsymbol{y}) \, d\boldsymbol{\theta}}{\int g(\boldsymbol{\theta}) p(\boldsymbol{\theta}|\boldsymbol{y}) \, d\boldsymbol{\theta}},$$

where $g(\boldsymbol{\theta}) = p_a(\boldsymbol{\theta})/p(\boldsymbol{\theta})$. However, the right-hand integral is simply the ratio of the posterior expectation of $h(\boldsymbol{\theta})g(\boldsymbol{\theta})$ to the posterior expectation of $g(\boldsymbol{\theta})$, using the unperturbed posterior distribution. Consequently, the perturbed expectation of $h(\boldsymbol{\theta})$ can be approximated by

$$\frac{\sum_{j=1}^{N} h(\boldsymbol{\theta}_j)g(\boldsymbol{\theta}_j)}{\sum_{j=1}^{N} g(\boldsymbol{\theta}_j)}.$$

This approximation is better the closer $g(\boldsymbol{\theta})$ remains to 1, so it may be questionable if the alternative prior differs markedly from the original prior, but it provides a valuable saving in computational effort if the perturbations to the prior remain modest.

Model choice

Choosing which statistical model to use in the analysis of a data set is an exercise which calls on the technical expertise, scientific judgement and common sense of the statistician. Formal methods for comparing the goodness of fit of nested models are well developed (see §11.6), those for non-nested models perhaps less so (Royston & Thompson, 1995). Nevertheless, in the frequentist setting, the whole procedure is difficult to formalise.

The rather richer probabilistic modelling inherent in the Bayesian method affords the opportunity to take a more formal approach to the comparison of models. Suppose that there are two models, M_1 and M_2, which are being considered for the data y; for example, M_1 may fit a linear and M_2 a quadratic function to the data. The incorporation of the model into the Bayesian analysis introduces another level to the hierarchy, which starts by ascribing prior probabilities to the models themselves. As it is supposed that one of the models will be used to fit the data, this amounts to ascribing a value to the probability that model M_1 is the correct model, which we write $p(M_1)$. Consequently $p(M_2) = 1 - p(M_1)$. Each model might be specified in terms of different parameters, say, $\boldsymbol{\theta}_i$ for model M_i and, given that model M_i is to be used, prior probabilities must be ascribed to $\boldsymbol{\theta}_i$, say, $p(\boldsymbol{\theta}_i|M_i)$. The likelihood under model i is conveniently written as $p(y|\boldsymbol{\theta}_i, M_i)$.

Prior views on which model is correct are incorporated in the value of $p(M_1)$ and the analyst is likely to be interested in how this view should be modified once the data have been included in the analysis. That is, the values of the posterior probabilities of the models, $p(M_1|y)$ and $p(M_2|y) = 1 - p(M_1|y)$ are important in helping the analyst to decide which model should be used. These posterior probabilities can be found by applying the usual methods, i.e. the joint probability of the data and model M_1 is

$$p(\mathbf{y}, M_1) = \int p(\mathbf{y}|\mathbf{\theta}_1, M_1) p(\mathbf{\theta}_1 | M_1) p(M_1) \, d\mathbf{\theta}_1. \tag{16.18}$$

There is a similar expression for $p(\mathbf{y}, M_2)$, so Bayes' theorem (§3.3) immediately gives $p(M_1|\mathbf{y}) = p(M_1, \mathbf{y})/[p(M_1, \mathbf{y}) + p(M_2, \mathbf{y})]$.

The usual way to express these quantities is through the ratio of the posterior odds to the prior odds of model M_1, a quantity known as the *Bayes factor, BF* (§3.3); that is,

$$BF = \frac{p(M_1|\mathbf{y})/p(M_2|\mathbf{y})}{p(M_1)/p(M_2)}$$

This kind of analysis can readily be extended to consider m competing models, $M_1, \ldots, M_m$. Bayes factors can then be used to make pairwise comparisons between models. Alternatively, interest may be focused on the models with the largest posterior probabilities.

There are some difficulties with the Bayes factor for comparing two models. The first concerns the practicalities of computing BF via (16.18), as this involves the specification of prior distributions for the parameters in each of the models. If the priors have to be established using an elicitation procedure, then having to accommodate several possible models can make the elicitation procedure much more cumbersome and complicated. An approach which avoids the need to specify prior distributions was developed by Schwarz (1978), who showed that for samples of size n, with n large,

$$-2 \log BF \approx -2 \log LR - (k_2 - k_1) \log n, \tag{16.19}$$

where k_i is the number of parameters in model M_i and LR is the usual (frequentist) likelihood ratio between the models, i.e. $LR = p(\mathbf{y}|\hat{\mathbf{\theta}}_1)/p(\mathbf{y}|\hat{\mathbf{\theta}}_2)$, where $\hat{\mathbf{\theta}}_i$ is the maximum likelihood estimator for model M_i. The quantity in (16.19) is sometimes referred to as the *Bayesian information criterion*, (BIC).

It might be asked to what extent it is possible to approximate a quantity such as the Bayes factor, which depends on prior distributions, using a quantity which does not depend on any priors at all. However, the approximation in (16.19) is valid only for large n, and for large n (and priors that are not too concentrated) the likelihood plays a more important role in determining quantities such as (16.18) than does the prior.

It might have been thought that an alternative to avoiding the specification of the priors was to use non-informative priors. This would be possible if the non-informative priors are proper but is not possible for improper priors. This is because (16.18) does not define a proper distribution if the prior for the parameters of the model is not proper. This occurs for exactly the same reason as was encountered when attempting to use the marginal distribution of y for model checking. Various methods for overcoming this difficulty have been discussed (see, for example, O'Hagan, 1994, Chapter 7), but all involve some degree of arbitrariness.

Suppose the result of the model comparisons is to decide that model M_1 should be used to describe the data. It would then be natural to base inferences on the posterior distribution corresponding to that model. However, in the notation of the present discussion, this amounts to basing inferences on $p(\boldsymbol{\theta}_1|y, M_1)$. This approach takes the model to be fixed and ignores the uncertainty encountered in the choice of the model. This is a Bayesian analogue of the problem that was illustrated in Fig. 12.8. There, two estimates of an asymptote were found from two non-linear regression equations. The two estimates differed by much more than their standard errors under each model. The standard errors had taken no account of the uncertainty in choosing the model and the high precisions ascribed to each estimate arose because in each case the underlying model was taken as correct. In Bayesian terms this amounts to basing inferences on $p(\boldsymbol{\theta}_1|y, M_1)$.

The more formal framework provided by the Bayesian approach appears to allow a resolution of this problem. Suppose that m models are available for the data and each contains a parameter, τ, about which inferences must be made. If appropriate priors for the parameters in each model are specified, then the marginal posterior distribution for τ under model i can be determined as $p(\tau|y, M_1)$ and the posterior distribution of τ, unconditional on any model, can be estimated by

$$p(\tau|y) = \sum_{j=1}^{m} p(\tau|y, M_j)p(M_j|y). \tag{16.20}$$

This technique is sometimes referred to as *Bayesian model averaging*. In a formal sense it overcomes the problem of overstating the precision of estimators because uncertainty in model selection has been overlooked. It also has implications for model choice, in so far as the use of (16.20) for inference avoids the need to decide on which model to use. Draper (1995) discusses many of these issues.

The procedure has a number of drawbacks. It can be difficult to decide on an appropriate family of models, $M_1, \ldots, M_m$, on which to base the model averaging. On a purely technical level, if m is large (and basing the family of models on all main-effects regressions for 10 covariates would give $m = 2^{10}$), the computation of (16.20) can be demanding. However, more fundamentally, the utility of divorcing an inference from the underlying model will also be questionable in many circumstances. Although superficially attractive, the practical utility of many formal techniques for assessing model uncertainty has yet to find universal acceptance; see, for example, the contributions of Cox and Tukey to the discussion of Draper (1995).

17 Survival analysis

17.1 Introduction

In many studies the variable of direct interest is the length of time that elapses before some event occurs. This event may be death, or death due to a particular disease, and for this reason the analysis of such data is often referred to as *survival analysis*.

An example of such a study is a clinical trial for the treatment of a malignant tumour where the prognosis is poor; death or remission of the tumour would be the end-point. Such studies usually include individuals for whom the event has not occurred at the time of the analysis. Although the time to the event for such a patient is unknown, there is some information on its value since it is known that it must exceed the current survival time; an observation of this type is referred to as a *censored* value. Methods of analysis must be able to cope with censored values. Often a number of variables are observed at the commencement of a trial, and survival is related to the values of these variables; that is, the variables are prognostic. Methods of analysis must be able to take account of the distribution of prognostic variables in the groups under study.

The number of studies of the above type has increased during the last three decades and statistical methods have been developed to analyse them; many of these methods were developed during the 1970s. Some of the methods will be described in this chapter; readers interested in more details are referred to a review by Andersen and Keiding (1998), to the books by Kalbfleisch and Prentice (1980), Lawless (1982), Cox and Oakes (1984), Collett (1994), Marubini and Valsecchi (1995), Parmar and Machin (1995), Kleinbaum (1996) and Klein and Moeschberger (1997), and to the two papers by Peto *et al.* (1976, 1977). Software for performing the computations are reviewed by Goldstein and Harrell (1998).

A second situation where survival analysis has been used occurs in the study of occupational mortality where it is required to assess if a group of workers who are exposed to a pollutant are experiencing excess mortality. Subjects enter the study when healthy and, for this reason, a common method of analysis has been the comparison of observed mortality, both in timing and cause, with what would be expected if the study group were subject to a similar mortality to that of the population of which it is a part. Discussion of this situation is deferred until §19.7.

Many of the methods of analysis are based on a life-table approach and in the next section the life-table is described.

17.2 **Life-tables**

The *life-table*, first developed adequately by E. Halley (1656–1742), is one of the basic tools of vital statistics and actuarial science. Standardization is introduced in §19.3 as a method of summarizing a set of age-specific death rates, thus providing a composite measure of the mortality experience of a community at all ages and permitting useful comparison with the experience of other groups of people. The life-table is an alternative summarizing procedure with rather similar attributes. Its purpose is to exhibit the pattern of survival of a group of individuals subject, throughout life, to the age-specific rates in question.

There are two distinct ways in which a life-table may be constructed from mortality data for a large community; the two forms are usually called the *current life-table* and the *cohort* or *generation life-table*. The current life-table describes the survival pattern of a group of individuals, subject throughout life to the age-specific death rates currently observed in a particular community. This group is necessarily hypothetical. A group of individuals now aged 60 years will next year experience approximately the current mortality rate specific to ages 60–61; but those who survive another 10 years will, in the 11th year, experience not the *current* rate for ages 70–71 but the rate prevailing 10 years hence. The current life-table, then, is a convenient summary of current mortality rather than a description of the actual mortality experience of any group.

The method of constructing the current life-tables published in national sources of vital statistics or in those used in life assurance offices is rather complex (Chiang, 1984). A simplified approach is described by Hill and Hill (1991). The main features of the life-table can be seen from Table 17.1, the left side of which summarizes the English Life Table No. 10 based on the mortality of males in England and Wales in 1930–32. The second column gives q_x, the probability that an individual, alive at age x years exactly, will die before his or her next birthday. The third column shows l_x, the number of individuals out of an arbitrary 1000 born alive who would survive to their xth birthday. To survive for this period an individual must survive the first year, then the second, and so on. Consequently.

$$l_x = l_0 \, p_0 \, p_1 \ldots p_{x-1}, \tag{17.1}$$

where $p_x = 1 - q_x$. This formula can be checked from Table 17.1 for $x = 1$, but not subsequently because values of q_x are given here only for selected values of x; such a table is called an *abridged life-table*.

Table 17.1 Current and cohort abridged life-tables for men in England and Wales born around 1931.

Age (years)	Current life-tables 1930–32			Cohort life-table, 1931 cohort
	Probability of death between age x and $x+1$	Life-table survivors	Expectation of life	Life-table survivors
x	q_x	l_x	$\overset{\circ}{e}_x$	l_x
0	0·0719	1000	58·7	1000
1	0·0153	928·1	62·2	927·8
5	0·0034	900·7	60·1	903·6
10	0·0015	890·2	55·8	894·8
20	0·0032	872·4	46·8	884·2
30	0·0034	844·2	38·2	874·1
40	0·0056	809·4	29·6	861·8
50	0·0113	747·9	21·6	829·7
60	0·0242	636·2	14·4	—
70	0·0604	433·6	8·6	—
80	0·1450	162·0	4·7	—

The fourth column shows $\overset{\circ}{e}_x$, the expectation of life at age x. This is the mean length of additional life beyond age x of all the l_x people alive at age x. In a complete table $\overset{\circ}{e}_x$ can be calculated approximately as

$$\overset{\circ}{e}_x = (l_{x+1} + l_{x+2} + \ldots)/l_x + \frac{1}{2}, \tag{17.2}$$

since the term in parentheses is the total number of years lived beyond age x by the l_x individuals if those dying between age y and age $y + 1$ did so immediately after their yth birthday, and the $\frac{1}{2}$ is a correction to allow for the fact that deaths take place throughout each year of age, which very roughly adds half a year to the mean survival time.

The cohort life-table describes the actual survival experience of a group, or 'cohort', of individuals born at about the same time. Those born in 1900, for instance, are subject during their first year to the mortality under 1 year of age prevailing in 1900–01; if they survive to 10 years of age they are subject to the mortality at that age in 1910–11; and so on. Cohort life-tables summarize the mortality at different ages at the times when the cohort would have been at these ages. The right-hand side of Table 17.1 summarizes the l_x column from the cohort life-table for men in England and Wales born in the 5 years centred around 1931. As would be expected, the values of l_1 in the two life-tables are very similar, being dependent on infant mortality in about the same calendar years. At higher ages the values of l_x are greater for the cohort table because this is based on mortality rates at the higher ages which were experienced since 1931 and which are lower than the 1931 rates.

Both forms of life-table are useful for vital statistical and epidemiological studies. Current life-tables summarize current mortality and may be used as an alternative to methods of standardization for comparisons between the mortality patterns of different communities. Cohort life-tables are particularly useful in studies of occupational mortality, where a group may be followed up over a long period of time (§19.7).

17.3 **Follow-up studies**

Many medical investigations are concerned with the survival pattern of special groups of patients—for example, those suffering from a particular form of malignant disease. Survival may be on average much shorter than for members of the general population. Since age is likely to be a less important factor than the progress of the disease, it is natural to measure survival from a particular stage in the history of the disease, such as the date when symptoms were first reported or the date on which a particular operation took place.

The application of life-table methods to data from follow-up studies of this kind will now be considered in some detail. In principle the methods are applicable to situations in which the critical end-point is not death, but some non-fatal event, such as the recurrence of symptoms and signs after a remission, although it may not be possible to determine the precise time of recurrence, whereas the time of death can usually be determined accurately. Indeed, the event may be favourable rather than unfavourable; the disappearance of symptoms after the start of treatment is an example. The discussion below is in terms of survival after an operation.

At the time of analysis of such a follow-up study patients are likely to have been observed for varying lengths of time, some having had the operation a long time before, others having been operated on recently. Some patients will have died, at times which can usually be ascertained relatively accurately; others are known to be alive at the time of analysis; others may have been lost to follow-up for various reasons between one examination and the next; others may have had to be withdrawn from the study for medical reasons—perhaps by the intervention of some other disease or an accidental death.

If there were no complications like those just referred to, and if every patient were followed until the time of death, the construction of a life-table in terms of time after operation would be a simple matter. The life-table survival rate, l_x, is l_0 times the proportion of survival times greater than x. The problem would be merely that of obtaining the distribution of survival time—a very elementary task. To overcome the complications of incomplete data, a table like Table 17.2 is constructed.

This table is adapted from that given by Berkson and Gage (1950) in one of the first papers describing the method. In the original data, the time intervals

Table 17.2 Life-table calculations for patients with a particular form of malignant disease, adapted from Berkson and Gage (1950).

(1) Interval since operation (years) x to $x+1$	(2) and (3) Last reported during this interval		(4) Living at start of interval n_x	(5) Adjusted number at risk n_x'	(6) Estimated probability of death q_x	(7) Estimated probability of survival p_x	(8) Percentage of survivors after x years l_x
	Died d_x	Withdrawn w_x					
0–1	90	0	374	374·0	0·2406	0·7594	100·0
1–2	76	0	284	284·0	0·2676	0·7324	75·9
2–3	51	0	208	208·0	0·2452	0·7548	55·6
3–4	25	12	157	151·0	0·1656	0·8344	42·0
4–5	20	5	120	117·5	0·1702	0·8298	35·0
5–6	7	9	95	90·5	0·0773	0·9227	29·1
6–7	4	9	79	74·5	0·0537	0·9463	26·8
7–8	1	3	66	64·5	0·0155	0·9845	25·4
8–9	3	5	62	59·5	0·0504	0·9496	25·0
9–10	2	5	54	51·5	0·0388	0·9612	23·7
10–	21	26	47	—	—	—	22·8

were measured from the time of hospital discharge, but for purposes of exposition we have changed these to intervals following operation. The columns (1)–(8) are formed as follows.

(1) The choice of time intervals will depend on the nature of the data. In the present study estimates were needed of survival rates for integral numbers of years, to 10, after operation. If survival after 10 years had been of particular interest, the intervals could easily have been extended beyond 10 years. In that case, to avoid the table becoming too cumbersome it might have been useful to use 2-year intervals for at least some of the groups. Unequal intervals cause no problem; for an example, see Merrell and Shulman (1955).

(2) and (3) The patients in the study are now classified according to the time interval during which their condition was last reported. If the report was of a death, the patient is counted in column (2); patients who were alive at the last report are counted in column (3). The term 'withdrawn' thus includes patients recently reported as alive, who would continue to be observed at future follow-up examinations, and those who have been lost to follow-up for some reason.

(4) The numbers of patients living at the start of the intervals are obtained by cumulating columns (2) and (3) from the foot. Thus, the number alive at 10 years is $21 + 26 = 47$. The number alive at 9 years includes these 47 and also the $2 + 5 = 7$ died or withdrawn in the interval 9–10 years; the entry is therefore $47 + 7 = 54$.

(5) The adjusted number at risk during the interval x to $x + 1$ is

$$n'_x = n_x - \tfrac{1}{2} w_x.$$ (17.3)

The purpose of this formula is to provide a denominator for the next column. The rationale is discussed below.

(6) The estimated probability of death during the interval x to $x + 1$ is

$$q_x = d_x / n'_x.$$ (17.4)

For example, in the first line,

$$q_0 = 90/374{\cdot}0 = 0{\cdot}2406.$$

The adjustment from n_x to n'_x is needed because the w_x withdrawals are necessarily at risk for only part of the interval. It is possible to make rather more sophisticated allowance for the withdrawals, particularly if the point of withdrawal during the interval is known. However, it is usually quite adequate to assume that the withdrawals have the same effect as if half of them were at risk for the whole period; hence the adjustment (17.3). An alternative argument is that, if the w_x patients had *not* withdrawn, we might have expected about $\tfrac{1}{2} q_x w_x$ extra deaths. The total number of deaths would then have been $d_x + \tfrac{1}{2} q_x w_x$ and we should have had an estimated death rate

$$q_x = \frac{d_x + \tfrac{1}{2} q_x w_x}{n_x}.$$ (17.5)

(17.5) is equivalent to (17.3) and (17.4).

(7) $p_x = 1 - q_x$.

(8) The estimated probability of survival to, say, 3 years after the operation is $p_0 \, p_1 \, p_2$. The entries in the last column, often called the *life-table survival rates*, are thus obtained by successive multiplication of those in column (7), with an arbitrary multiplier $l_0 = 100$. Formally,

$$l_x = l_0 \, p_0 \, p_1 \ldots p_{x-1},$$ (17.6)

as in (17.1).

Two important assumptions underlie these calculations. First, it is assumed that the withdrawals are subject to the same probabilities of death as the non-withdrawals. This is a reasonable assumption for withdrawals who are still in the study and will be available for future follow-up. It may be a dangerous assumption for patients who were lost to follow-up, since failure to examine a patient for any reason may be related to the patient's health. Secondly, the various values of p_x are obtained from patients who entered the study at different points of time. It must be assumed that these probabilities remain reasonably constant over time;

otherwise the life-table calculations represent quantities with no simple interpretation.

In Table 17.2 the calculations could have been continued beyond 10 years. Suppose, however, that d_{10} and w_{10} had both been zero, as they would have been if no patients had been observed for more than 10 years. Then n_{10} would have been zero, no values of q_{10} and p_{10} could have been calculated and, in general, no value of l_{11} would have been available unless l_{10} were zero (as it would be if any one of $p_0, p_1, \ldots, p_9$ were zero), in which case l_{11} would also be zero. This point can be put more obviously by saying that no survival information is available for periods of follow-up longer than the maximum observed in the study. This means that the expectation of life (which implies an indefinitely long follow-up) cannot be calculated from follow-up studies unless the period of follow-up, at least for some patients, is sufficiently long to cover virtually the complete span of survival. For this reason the life-table survival rate (column (8) of Table 17.2) is a more generally useful measure of survival. Note that the value of x for which $l_x = 50\%$ is the *median* survival time; for a symmetric distribution this would be equal to the expectation of life.

For further discussion of life-table methods in follow-up studies, see Berkson and Gage (1950), Merrell and Shulman (1955), Cutler and Ederer (1958) and Newell *et al.* (1961).

17.4 **Sampling errors in the life-table**

Each of the values of p_x in a life-table calculation is subject to sampling variation. Were it not for the withdrawals the variation could be regarded as binomial, with a sample size n_x. The effect of withdrawals is approximately the same as that of reducing the sample size to n_x'. The variance of l_x is given approximately by the following formula due to Greenwood (1926), which can be obtained by taking logarithms in (17.6) and using an extension of (5.20).

$$\mathrm{var}(l_x) = l_x^2 \sum_{i=0}^{x-1} \frac{d_i}{n_i'(n_i'-d_i)}. \tag{17.7}$$

In Table 17.2, for instance, where $l_4 = 35{\cdot}0\%$,

$$\mathrm{var}(l_4) = (35{\cdot}0)^2 \left[\frac{90}{(374)(284)} + \frac{76}{(284)(208)} + \frac{51}{(208)(157)} + \frac{25}{(151)(126)} \right]$$
$$= 6{\cdot}14$$

so that $\mathrm{SE}(l_4) = \sqrt{6{\cdot}14} = 2{\cdot}48$, and approximate 95% confidence limits for l_4 are

$$35{\cdot}0 \pm (1{\cdot}96)(2{\cdot}48) = 30{\cdot}1 \text{ and } 39{\cdot}9.$$

Application of (17.7) can lead to impossible values for confidence limits outside the range 0 to 100%. An alternative that avoids this is to apply the double-log transformation, $\ln(-\ln l_x)$, to (17.6), with $l_0 = 1$, so that l_x is a proportion with permissible range 0 to 1 (Kalbfleisch & Prentice, 1980). Then Greenwood's formula is modified to give 95% confidence limits for l_x of

$$l_x^{\exp(\pm\,1\cdot96s)}, \tag{17.8}$$

where

$$s = \text{SE}(l_x)/(-l_x \ln l_x).$$

For the above example, $l_4 = 0\cdot35, \text{SE}(l_4) = 0\cdot0248, s = 0\cdot0675, \exp(1\cdot96s) = 1\cdot14, \exp(-1\cdot96s) = 0\cdot876$, and the limits are $0\cdot35^{1\cdot14}$ and $0\cdot35^{0\cdot876}$, which equal $0\cdot302$ and $0\cdot399$. In this case, where the limits using (17.7) are not near either end of the permissible range, (17.8) gives almost identical values to (17.7).

Peto *et al.* (1977) give a formula for $\text{SE}(l_x)$ that is easier to calculate than (17.7):

$$\text{SE}(l_x) = l_x \sqrt{[(1 - l_x)/n_x']}. \tag{17.9}$$

As in (17.8), it is essential to work with l_x as a proportion. In the example, (17.9) gives $\text{SE}(l_4) = 0\cdot0258$. Formula (17.9) is conservative but may be more appropriate for the period of increasing uncertainty at the end of life-tables when there are few survivors still being followed.

Methods for calculating the sampling variance of the various entries in the life-table, including the expectation of life, are given by Chiang (1984, Chapter 8).

17.5 The Kaplan–Meier estimator

The estimated life-table given in Table 17.2 was calculated after dividing the period of follow-up into time intervals. In some cases the data may only be available in group form and often it is convenient to summarize the data into groups. Forming groups does, however, involve an arbitrary choice of time intervals and this can be avoided by using a method due to Kaplan and Meier (1958). In this method the data are, effectively, regarded as grouped into a large number of short time intervals, with each interval as short as the accuracy of recording permits. Thus, if survival is recorded to an accuracy of 1 day then time intervals of 1-day width would be used. Suppose that at time t_j there are d_j deaths and that just before the deaths occurred there were n_j' subjects surviving. Then the estimated probability of death at time t_j is

$$q_{t_j} = d_j/n'_j. \tag{17.10}$$

This is equivalent to (17.4). By convention, if any subjects are censored at time t_j, then they are considered to have survived for longer than the deaths at time t_j and adjustments of the form of (17.3) are not applied. For most of the time intervals $d_j = 0$ and hence $q_{t_j} = 0$ and the survival probability $p_{t_j}(= 1 - q_{t_j}) = 1$. These intervals may be ignored in calculating the life-table survival using (17.6). The survival at time t, l_t, is then estimated by

$$l_t = \prod_j p_{t_j} = \prod_j \frac{n'_j - d_j}{n'_j}, \tag{17.11}$$

where the product is taken over all time intervals in which a death occurred, up to and including t. This estimator is termed the *product-limit* estimator because it is the limiting form of the product in (17.6) as the time intervals are reduced towards zero. The estimator is also the maximum likelihood estimator. The estimates obtained are invariably expressed in graphical form. The survival curve consists of horizontal lines with vertical steps each time a death occurred (see Fig. 17.1 on p. 580). The calculations are illustrated in Table 17.4 (p. 579).

17.6 **The logrank test**

The test described in this section is used for the comparison of two or more groups of survival data. The first step is to arrange the survival times, both observed and censored, in rank order. Suppose, for illustration, that there are two groups, A and B. If at time t_j there were d_j deaths and there were n'_{jA} and n'_{jB} subjects alive just before t_j in groups A and B, respectively, then the data can be arranged in a 2×2 table:

	Died	Survived	Total
Group A	d_{jA}	$n'_{jA} - d_{jA}$	n'_{jA}
Group B	d_{jB}	$n'_{jB} - d_{jB}$	n'_{jB}
Total	d_j	$n'_j - d_j$	n'_j

Except for tied survival times, $d_j = 1$ and each of d_{jA} and d_{jB} is 0 or 1. Note also that if a subject is censored at t_j then that subject is considered at risk at that time and so included in n'_j.

On the null hypothesis that the risk of death is the same in the two groups, then we would expect the number of deaths at any time to be distributed between the two groups in proportion to the numbers at risk. That is,

$$E(d_{jA}) = n'_{jA}d_j/n'_j,$$
$$\text{var}(d_{jA}) = \frac{d_j(n'_j - d_j)n'_{jA}n'_{jB}}{n'^2_j(n'_j - 1)}. \tag{17.12}$$

In the case of $d_j = 1$, (17.12) simplifies to

$$E(d_{jA}) = p'_{jA},$$
$$\text{var}(d_{jA}) = p'_{jA}(1 - p'_{jA}),$$

where $p'_{jA} = n'_{jA}/n'_j$, the proportion of survivors who are in group A.

The difference between d_{jA} and $E(d_{jA})$ is evidence against the null hypothesis. The logrank test is the combination of these differences over all the times at which deaths occurred. It is analogous to the Mantel–Haenszel test for combining data over strata (see §15.6) and was first introduced in this way (Mantel, 1966).

Summing over all times of death, t_j, gives

$$O_A = \sum d_{jA}$$
$$E_A = \sum E(d_{jA})$$
$$V_A = \sum \text{var}(d_{jA}) \tag{17.13}$$

Similar sums can be obtained for group B and it follows from (17.12) that $E_A + E_B = O_A + O_B$.

E_A may be referred to as the 'expected' number of deaths in group A but since, in some circumstances, E_A may exceed the number of individuals starting in the group, a more accurate description is the *extent of exposure to risk of death* (Peto *et al.*, 1977). A test statistic for the equivalence of the death rates in the two groups is

$$X^2_1 = \frac{(O_A - E_A)^2}{V_A}, \tag{17.14}$$

which is approximately a $\chi^2_{(1)}$. An alternative and simpler test statistic, which does not require the calculation of the variance terms, is

$$X^2_2 = \frac{(O_A - E_A)^2}{E_A} + \frac{(O_B - E_B)^2}{E_B}. \tag{17.15}$$

This statistic is also approximately a $\chi^2_{(1)}$. In practice (17.15) is usually adequate, but it errs on the conservative side (Peto & Pike, 1973).

The logrank test may be generalized to more than two groups. The extension of (17.14) involves the inverse of the variance–covariance matrix of the $O - E$ over the groups (Peto & Pike, 1973), but the extension of (17.15) is straightforward. The summation in (17.15) is extended to cover all the groups, with the quantities in (17.13) calculated for each group in the same way as for two groups. The test statistic would have $k - 1$ degrees of freedom (DF) if there were k groups.

The ratios O_A/E_A and O_B/E_B are referred to as the relative death rates and estimate the ratio of the death rate in each group to the death rate among both groups combined. The ratio of these two relative rates estimates the death rate in Group A relative to that in Group B, sometimes referred to as the *hazard ratio*. The hazard ratio and sampling variability are given by

$$\left. \begin{aligned} h &= \frac{O_A/E_A}{O_B/E_B} \\ \mathrm{SE}[\ln(h)] &= \sqrt{\left(\frac{1}{E_A} + \frac{1}{E_B}\right)} \end{aligned} \right\}. \tag{17.16}$$

An alternative estimate is

$$\left. \begin{aligned} h &= \exp\left(\frac{O_A - E_A}{V_A}\right) \\ \mathrm{SE}[\ln(h)] &= \sqrt{\frac{1}{V_A}} \end{aligned} \right\} \tag{17.17}$$

(Machin & Gardner, 1989). Formula (17.17) is similar to (4.33). Both (17.16) and (17.17) are biased, and confidence intervals based on the standard errors (SE) will have less than the nominal coverage, when the hazard ratio is not close to unity. Formula (17.16) is less biased and is adequate for h less than 3, but for larger hazard ratios an adjusted standard error may be calculated (Berry *et al.*, 1991) or a more complex analysis might be advisable (§17.8).

Example 17.1

In Table 17.3 data are given of the survival of patients with diffuse histiocytic lymphoma according to stage of tumour. Survival is measured in days after entry to a clinical trial. There was little difference in survival between the two treatment groups, which are not considered in this example.

The calculations of the product-limit estimate of the life-table are given in Table 17.4 for the stage 3 group and the comparison of the survival for the two stages is shown in Fig. 17.1. It is apparent that survival is longer, on average, for patients with a stage 3 tumour than for those with stage 4. This difference may be formally tested using the logrank test.

The basic calculations necessary for the logrank test are given in Table 17.5. For brevity, only deaths occurring at the beginning and end of the observation period are shown. The two groups are indicated by subscripts 3 and 4, instead of A and B used in the general description.

Table 17.3 Survival of patients with diffuse hystiocytic lymphoma according to stage of tumour (data abstracted from McKelvey *et al.*, 1976).

	Survival (days)							
Stage 3	6	19	32	42	42	43*	94	126*
	169*	207	211*	227*	253	255*	270*	310*
	316*	335*	346*					
Stage 4	4	6	10	11	11	11	13	17
	20	20	21	22	24	24	29	30
	30	31	33	34	35	39	40	41*
	43*	45	46	50	56	61*	61*	63
	68	82	85	88	89	90	93	104
	110	134	137	160*	169	171	173	175
	184	201	222	235*	247*	260*	284*	290*
	291*	302*	304*	341*	345*			

*Still alive (censored value).

Table 17.4 Calculation of product-limit estimate of life-table for stage 3 tumour data of Table 17.3.

Time (days) t_j	Died d_j	Living at start of day n'_j	Estimated probability of:		Percentage of survivors at end of day l_{t_j}
			Death q_{t_j}	Survival p_{t_j}	
0	—	19	—	—	100·0
6	1	19	0·0526	0·9474	94·7
19	1	18	0·0556	0·9444	89·5
32	1	17	0·0588	0·9412	84·2
42	2	16	0·1250	0·8750	73·7
94	1	13	0·0769	0·9231	68·0
207	1	10	0·1000	0·9000	61·2
253	1	7	0·1429	0·8571	52·5

Applying (17.14) gives

$$X_1^2 = (8 - 16·6870)^2/11·2471$$
$$= 8·6870^2/11·2471$$
$$= 6·71 \quad (P = 0·010).$$

To calculate (17.15) we first calculate E_4, using the relationship $O_3 + O_4 = E_3 + E_4$. Thus $E_4 = 37·3130$ and

$$X_2^2 = 8·6870^2(1/16·6870 + 1/37·3130)$$
$$= 6·54 \quad (P = 0·010).$$

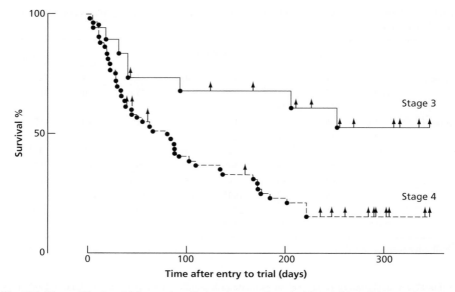

Fig. 17.1 Plots of Kaplan–Meier product-limit estimates of survival for patients with stage 3 or stage 4 lymphoma. ● times of death. ↟ censored times of survivors.

Table 17.5 Calculation of logrank test (data of Table 17.3) to compare survival of patients with tumours of stages 3 and 4.

Days when deaths occurred	Numbers at risk		Deaths			
	n'_3	n'_4	d_3	d_4	$E(d_3)$	$var(d_3)$
4	19	61	0	1	0·2375	0·1811
6	19	60	1	1	0·4810	0·3606
10	18	59	0	1	0·2338	0·1791
11	18	58	0	3	0·7105	0·5278
13	18	55	0	1	0·2466	0·1858
17	18	54	0	1	0·2500	0·1875
19	18	53	1	0	0·2535	0·1892
20	17	53	0	2	0·4857	0·3624
⋮						
201	10	12	0	1	0·4545	0·2479
207	10	11	1	0	0·4762	0·2494
222	8	11	0	1	0·4211	0·2438
253	7	8	1	0	0·4667	0·2489
Total			8	46	16·6870	11·2471
			O_3	O_4	E_3	V_3

Thus it is demonstrated that the difference shown in Fig. 17.1 is unlikely to be due to chance.

The relative death rates are $8/16\cdot6870 = 0\cdot48$ for the stage 3 group and $46/37\cdot3130 = 1\cdot23$ for the stage 4 group. The ratio of these rates estimates the death rate of stage 4 relative to that of stage 3 as $1\cdot23/0\cdot48 = 2\cdot57$. Using (17.16), $\mathrm{SE}[\ln(h)] = 0\cdot2945$ and the 95% confidence interval for the hazard ratio is $\exp[\ln(2\cdot57) \pm 1\cdot96 \times 0\cdot2945] = 1\cdot44$ to $4\cdot58$. Using (17.17), the hazard ratio is $2\cdot16$ (95% confidence interval $1\cdot21$ to $3\cdot88$).

The logrank test can be extended to take account of a covariate that divides the total group into strata. The rationale is similar to that discussed in §§15.6 and 15.7 (see (15.20) to (15.23)). That is, the quantities in (17.13) are summed over the strata before applying (17.14) or (17.15). Thus, denoting the strata by h, (17.14) becomes

$$X_1^2 = \frac{(\sum_h O_A - \sum_h E_A)^2}{\sum_h V_A}. \tag{17.18}$$

As in analogous situations in Chapter 15 (see discussion after (15.23)), stratification is usually only an option when the covariate structure can be represented by just a few strata. When there are several variables to take into account, or a continuous variable which it is not convenient to categorize, then methods based on stratification become cumbersome and inefficient, and it is much preferable to use regression methods (§17.8).

The logrank test is a non-parametric test. Other tests can be obtained by modifying Wilcoxon's rank sum test (§10.3) so that it can be applied to compare survival times for two groups in the case where some survival times are censored (Cox & Oakes, 1984, p. 124). The generalized Wilcoxon test was originally proposed by Gehan (1965) and is constructed by using weights in the summations of (17.13). Gehan's proposal was that the weight is the total number of survivors in each group. These weights are dependent on the censoring and an alternative avoiding this is to use an estimator of the combined survivor function (Prentice, 1978). If none of the observations were censored, then this test is identical to the Wilcoxon rank sum test. The logrank test is unweighted—that is, the weights are the same for every death. Consequently the logrank test puts more weight on deaths towards the end of follow-up when few individuals are surviving, and the generalized Wilcoxon test tends to be more sensitive than the logrank test in situations where the ratio of hazards is higher at early survival times than at late ones. The logrank test is optimal under the proportional-hazards assumption, that is, where the ratio of hazards is constant at all survival times (§17.8). Intermediate systems of weights have been proposed, in particular that the weight is a power, ξ, between 0 and 1, of the number of survivors or the combined survivor function. For the generalized Wilcoxon test $\xi = 1$, for the logrank test $\xi = 0$, and the square root, $\xi = \frac{1}{2}$, is intermediate (Tarone & Ware, 1977).

17.7 **Parametric methods**

In mortality studies the variable of interest is the survival time. A possible approach to the analysis is to postulate a distribution for survival time and to estimate the parameters of this distribution from the data. This approach is usually applied by starting with a model for the death rate and determining the form of the resulting survival time distribution.

The death rate will usually vary with time since entry to the study, t, and will be denoted by $\lambda(t)$; sometimes $\lambda(t)$ is referred to as the *hazard function*. Suppose the probability density of survival time is $f(t)$ and the corresponding distribution function is $F(t)$. Then, since the death rate is the rate at which deaths occur divided by the proportion of the population surviving, we have

$$\left.\begin{array}{l} \lambda(t) = \dfrac{f(t)}{1 - F(t)} \\[2mm] = f(t)/S(t) \end{array}\right\}, \tag{17.19}$$

where $S(t) = 1 - F(t)$ is the proportion surviving and is referred to as the *survivor function*.

Equation (17.19) enables $f(t)$ and $S(t)$ to be specified in terms of $\lambda(t)$. The general solution is obtained by integrating (17.19) with respect to t and noting that $f(t)$ is the derivative of $F(t)$ (§3.4). We shall consider certain cases. The simplest form is that the death rate is a constant, i.e. $\lambda(t) = \lambda$ for all t. Then

$$\lambda t = -\ln[S(t)]. \tag{17.20}$$

That is,

$$S(t) = \exp(-\lambda t).$$

The survival time has an exponential distribution with mean $1/\lambda$. If this distribution is appropriate, then, from (17.20), a plot of the logarithm of the survivor function against time should give a straight line through the origin.

Data from a group of subjects consist of a number of deaths with known survival times and a number of survivors for whom the censored length of survival is known. These data can be used to estimate λ, using the method of maximum likelihood (§14.2). For a particular value of λ, the likelihood consists of the product of terms $f(t)$ for the deaths and $S(t)$ for the survivors. The maximum likelihood estimate of λ, the standard error of the estimate and a significance test against any hypothesized value are obtained, using the general method of maximum likelihood, although, in this simple case, the solution can be obtained directly without iteration.

The main restriction of the exponential model is the assumption that the death rate is independent of time. It would usually be unreasonable to expect this assumption to hold except over short time intervals. One way of overcoming this restriction is to divide the period of follow-up into a number of shorter intervals, and assume that the hazard rate is constant within each interval but that it is different for the different intervals (Holford, 1976).

Another method of avoiding the assumption that the hazard is constant is to use a different parametric model of the hazard rate. One model is the *Weibull*, defined by

$$\lambda(t) = \alpha\gamma t^{\gamma-1}, \tag{17.21}$$

where γ is greater than 1. This model has proved applicable to the incidence of cancer by age in humans (Cook *et al.*, 1969) and by time after exposure to a carcinogen in animal experiments (Pike, 1966). A third model is that the hazard increases exponentially with age, that is,

$$\lambda(t) = \alpha \exp(\beta t). \tag{17.22}$$

This is the *Gompertz* hazard and describes the death rate from all causes in adults fairly well. A model in which the times of death are log-normally distributed has also been used but has the disadvantage that the associated hazard rate starts to decrease at some time.

17.8 **Regression and proportional-hazards models**

It would be unusual to analyse a single group of homogeneous subjects but the basic method may be extended to cope with more realistic situations by modelling the hazard rate to represent dependence on variables recorded for each subject as well as on time. For example, in a clinical trial it would be postulated that the hazard rate was dependent on treatment, which could be represented by one or more dummy variables (§11.7). Again, if a number of prognostic variables were known, then the hazard rate could be expressed as a function of these variables. In general, the hazard rate could be written as a function of both time and the covariates, that is, as $\lambda(t, x)$, where x represents the set of covariates $(x_1, x_2, \ldots, x_p)$.

Zippin and Armitage (1966) considered one prognostic variable, x, the logarithm of white blood count, and an exponential survival distribution, with

$$\lambda(t, x) = (\alpha + \beta x)^{-1}; \tag{17.23}$$

the mean survival time was thus linear in x. Analysis consisted of the estimation of α and β. A disadvantage of this representation is that the hazard rate becomes negative for high values of x (since β was negative). An alternative model avoiding this disadvantage, proposed by Glasser (1967), is

$$\lambda(t, x) = \alpha \exp(\beta x); \tag{17.24}$$

the logarithm of the mean survival time was thus linear in x.

Both (17.23) and (17.24) involve the assumption that the death rate is independent of time. Generally the hazard would depend on time and a family of models may be written as

$$\lambda(t, \boldsymbol{x}) = \lambda_0(t) \exp(\boldsymbol{\beta}^{\mathrm{T}} \boldsymbol{x}), \tag{17.25}$$

where $\boldsymbol{\beta}^{\mathrm{T}} \boldsymbol{x}$ is the matrix representation of the regression function, $\beta_1 x_1 + \beta_2 x_2 + \ldots + \beta_p x_p$ and $\lambda_0(t)$ is the time-dependent part of the hazard. The term $\lambda_0(t)$ could represent any of the models considered in the previous section or other parametric functions of t. Equation (17.25) is a regression model in terms of the covariates. It is also referred to as a *proportional-hazards* model since the hazards for different sets of covariates remain in the same proportion for all t. Data can be analysed parametrically using (17.25) provided that some particular form of $\lambda_0(t)$ is assumed. The parameters of $\lambda_0(t)$ and also the regression coefficients, $\boldsymbol{\beta}$, would be estimated. Inference would be in terms of the estimate b of $\boldsymbol{\beta}$, and the parameters of $\lambda_0(t)$ would have no direct interest.

Another way of representing the effect of the covariates is to suppose that the distribution of survival time is changed by multiplying the time-scale by $\exp(\boldsymbol{\beta}_a^{\mathrm{T}} \boldsymbol{x})$, that is, that the logarithm of survival time is increased by $\boldsymbol{\beta}_a^{\mathrm{T}} \boldsymbol{x}$. The hazard could then be written

$$\lambda(t, \boldsymbol{x}) = \lambda_0[t \exp(-\boldsymbol{\beta}_a^{\mathrm{T}} \boldsymbol{x})] \exp(-\boldsymbol{\beta}_a^{\mathrm{T}} \boldsymbol{x}). \tag{17.26}$$

This is referred to as an *accelerated failure time* model. For the exponential distribution, $\lambda_0(t) = \lambda$, (17.25) and (17.26) are equivalent, with $\boldsymbol{\beta}_a = -\boldsymbol{\beta}$, so the accelerated failure time model is also a proportional-hazards model. The same is true for the Weibull (17.21), with $\boldsymbol{\beta}_a = -\boldsymbol{\beta}/\gamma$, but, in general, the accelerated failure time model would not be a proportional-hazards model. However, it may be difficult to determine whether a proportional-hazards or an accelerated failure time model is the more appropriate (§17.9), but then the two models may give similar inferences of the effects of the covariates (Solomon, 1984).

Procedures for fitting models of the type discussed above are available in a number of statistical computing packages; for example, a range of parametric models, including the exponential, Weibull and log-normal, may be fitted using PROC LIFEREG in the SAS program.

Cox's proportional-hazards model

Since often an appropriate parametric form of $\lambda_0(t)$ is unknown and, in any case, not of primary interest, it would be more convenient if it were unnecessary to substitute any particular form for $\lambda_0(t)$ in (17.25). This was the approach introduced by Cox (1972). The model is then non-parametric with respect to time but parametric in terms of the covariates. Estimation of $\boldsymbol{\beta}$ and inferences are developed by considering the information supplied at each time that a death occurred. Consider a death occurring at time t_j, and suppose that there were n'_j subjects alive just before t_j, that the values of $\boldsymbol{x}$ for these subjects are $\boldsymbol{x}_1, \boldsymbol{x}_2, \ldots, \boldsymbol{x}_{n'_j}$, and that the subject that died is denoted, with no loss of generality, by the subscript 1. The set of n'_j subjects at risk is referred to as the *risk set*. The risk of death at time t_j for each subject in the risk set is given by (17.25). This does not supply absolute measures of risk, but does supply the relative risks for each subject, since, although $\lambda_0(t)$ is unknown, it is the same for each subject. Thus, the probability that the death observed at t_j was of the subject who did die at that time is

$$p_j = \exp(\boldsymbol{\beta}^\mathrm{T}\boldsymbol{x}_1)/\sum \exp(\boldsymbol{\beta}^\mathrm{T}\boldsymbol{x}_i), \qquad (17.27)$$

where summation is over all members of the risk set. Similar terms are derived for each time that a death occurred and are combined to form a likelihood. Technically this is called a *partial likelihood*, since the component terms are derived conditionally on the times that deaths occurred and the composition of the risk sets at these times. The actual times at which deaths occurred are not used but the order of the times of death and of censoring—that is, the ranks—determine the risk sets. Thus, the method has, as far as the treatment of time is concerned, similarities with non-parametric rank tests (Chapter 10). It also has similarities with the logrank test, which is also conditional on the risk sets.

As time is used non-parametrically, the occurrence of ties, either of times of death or involving a time of death and a time of censoring, causes some complications. As with the non-parametric tests discussed in Chapter 10, this is not a serious problem unless ties are extensive. The simplest procedure is to use the full risk set, of all the individuals alive just before the tied time, for all the tied individuals (Breslow, 1974).

The model is fitted by the method of maximum likelihood and this is usually done using specific statistical software, such as **PROC PHREG** in the **SAS** program. In Example 17.2 some of the steps in the fitting process are detailed to illustrate the rationale of the method.

Example 17.2

The data given in Table 17.3 and Example 17.1 may be analysed using Cox's approach. Define a dummy variable that takes the value zero for stage 3 and unity for stage 4. Then the death rates, from (17.25), are $\lambda_0(t)$ for stage 3 and $\lambda_0(t)\exp(\beta)$ for stage 4, and $\exp(\beta)$ is the death rate of stage 4 relative to stage 3. The first death occurred after 4 days (Table 17.5) when the risk set consisted of 19 stage 3 subjects and 61 stage 4 subjects. The death was of a stage 4 subject and the probability that the one death known to occur at this time was the particular stage 4 subject who did die is, from (17.27),

$$p_1 = \exp(\beta)/[19 + 61 \ \exp(\beta)].$$

The second time when deaths occurred was at 6 days. There were two deaths on this day and this tie is handled approximately by assuming that they occurred simultaneously so that the same risk set, 19 stage 3 and 60 stage 4 subjects, applied for each death. The probability that a particular stage 3 subject died is $1/[19 + 60 \ \exp(\beta)]$ and that a particular stage 4 subject died is $\exp(\beta)/[19 + 60 \ \exp(\beta)]$ and these two probabilities are combined, using the multiplication rule, to give the probability that the two deaths consist of the one subject from each stage,

$$p_2 = \exp(\beta)/[19 + 60 \ \exp(\beta)]^2.$$

Strictly this expression should contain a binomial factor of 2 (§3.6) but, since a constant factor does not influence the estimation of β, it is convenient to omit it. Working through Table 17.5, similar terms can be written down and the log-likelihood is equal to the sum of the logarithms of the p_j. Using a computer, the maximum likelihood estimate of β, b, is obtained with its standard error:

$$b = 0\cdot9610,$$
$$\text{SE}(b) = 0\cdot3856.$$

To test the hypothesis that $\beta = 0$, that is, $\exp(\beta) = 1$, we have the following as an approximate standardized normal deviate:

$$z = 0\cdot9610/0\cdot3856 = 2\cdot49 \ (P = 0\cdot013).$$

Approximate 95% confidence limits for b are

$$0\cdot9610 \pm 1\cdot96 \times 0\cdot3856$$

$$= 0\cdot2052 \text{ and } 1\cdot7168.$$

Taking exponentials gives, as an estimate of the death rate of stage 4 relative to stage 3, 2·61 with 95% confidence limits of 1·23 and 5·57.

The estimate and the statistical significance of the relative death rate using Cox's approach (Example 17.2) are similar to those obtained using the logrank test (Example 17.1). The confidence interval is wider in accord with the earlier remark that the confidence interval calculated using (17.16) has less than the required coverage when the hazard ratio is not near to unity. In general, when both the logrank test and Cox's proportional hazards regression model are fitted to the same data, the score test (§14.2) from the regression approach is identical to the logrank test (similar identities were noted in Chapter 15 in relation to logistic regression and Mantel–Haenszel type tests for combining strata).

The full power of the proportional-hazards model comes into play when there are several covariates and (17.25) represents a multiple regression model. For example, Kalbfleisch and Prentice (1980, pp. 89–98) discuss data from a trial of treatment of tumours of any of four sites in the head and neck. There were many covariates that might be expected to relate to survival. Four of these were shown to be prognostic: sex, the patient's general condition, extent of primary tumour (T classification), and extent of lymph-node metastasis (N classification). All of these were related to survival in a multivariate model (17.25). Terms for treatment were also included but, unfortunately, the treatment effects were not statistically significant.

With multiple covariates the rationale for selecting the variables to include in the regression is similar to that employed in multiple regression of a normally distributed response variable (§11.6). Corresponding to the analysis of variance test for the deletion of a set of variables is the *Wald test*, which gives a statistic approximately distributed as χ^2 on q DF, to test the deletion of q covariates. For $q = 1$, the Wald χ^2 on 1 DF is equivalent to a standardized normal deviate as used in Example 17.2.

If the values of some of the covariates for an individual are not constant throughout the period of follow-up, then the method needs to be adjusted to take account of this. In principle, this causes no problem when using Cox's regression model, although the complexity of setting up the calculations is increased. For each time of death the appropriate values of the covariates are used in (17.27).

Cox's semi-parametric model avoids the choice of a particular distributional form. Inferences on the effects of the covariates will be similar with the Cox model to those with an appropriate distributional form (Kay, 1977; Byar, 1983), although the use of an appropriate distributional form will tend to give slightly more precise estimates of the regression coefficients.

Extensions to more complicated situations

In some situations the time of failure may not be known precisely. For example, individuals may be examined at intervals, say, a year apart, and it is observed that the event has occurred between examinations but there is no information on when the change occurred within the interval. Such observations are referred to as *interval-censored*. If the lengths of interval are short compared with the total length of the study it would be adequate to analyse the data as if each event occurred at the mid-point of its interval, but otherwise a more stringent analysis is necessary. The survival function can be estimated using an iterative method (Turnbull, 1976; Klein and Moeschberger, 1997, §5.2). A proportional-hazards model can also be fitted (Finkelstein, 1986).

McGilchrist and Aisbett (1991) considered recurrence times to infection in patients on kidney dialysis. Following an infection a patient is treated and, when the infection is cleared, put back on dialysis. Thus a patient may have more than one infection so the events are not independent; some patients may be more likely to have an infection than others and, in general, it is useful to consider that, in addition to the covariates that may influence the hazard rate, each individual has an unknown tendency to become infected, referred to as the *frailty*. The concept of frailty may be extended to any situation where observations on survival may not be independent. For example, individuals in families may share a tendency for long or short survival because of their common genes, or household members because of a common environment. Subjects in the same family or the same environment would have a common value for their frailty. The proportional hazards model (17.25) is modified to

$$\lambda(t, \boldsymbol{x}_{ik}) = \lambda_0(t)\exp(\boldsymbol{\beta}^{\mathrm{T}}\boldsymbol{x}_{ik})\exp(\sigma f_i)$$

or, equivalently, to

$$\lambda(t, \boldsymbol{x}_{ik}) = \lambda_0(t)\exp(\boldsymbol{\beta}^{\mathrm{T}}\boldsymbol{x}_{ik} + \sigma f_i), \tag{17.28}$$

where i represents a group sharing a common value of the frailty, f_i, and k a subject within the group. The parameter σ expresses the strength of the frailty effect on the hazard function. Of course, the frailties, f_i, are unobservable and there will usually be insufficient data within each group to estimate the frailties for each group separately. The situation is akin to that discussed in §12.5 and the approach is to model the frailties as a set of random effects, in terms of a distributional form. The whole data set can then be used to estimate the parameters of this distribution as well as the regression coefficients for the covariates. McGilchrist and Aisbett (1991) fitted a log-normal distribution to the frailties but other distributional forms may be used. For a fuller discussion, see Klein and Moeschberger (1997, Chapter 13). The situation is similar to those where empirical Bayesian methods may be employed (§6.5) and the frailty estimates are shrunk towards the mean. This approach is similar to that given by Clayton and Cuzick (1985), and Clayton (1991) discusses the problem in terms of Bayesian inference.

17.9 **Diagnostic methods**

Plots of the survival against time, usually with some transformation of one or both of these items, are useful for checking on the distribution of the hazard. The *integrated* or *cumulative hazard*, defined as

$$H(t) = \int_0^t \lambda(u) \, \mathrm{d}u = -\ln S(t), \tag{17.29}$$

is often used for this purpose. The integrated hazard may be obtained from the Kaplan–Meier estimate of $S(t)$ using (17.29), or from the cumulative hazard, evaluated as the sum of the estimated discrete hazards at all the event times up to t. A plot of $\ln H(t)$ against $\ln t$ is linear with a slope of γ for the Weibull (17.21), or a slope of 1 for the exponential (17.20).

For a more general model (17.25), the plot of $\ln H(t)$ against $\ln t$ has no specified form but plots made for different subgroups of individuals—for example, defined by categories of a qualitative covariate or stratified ranges of a continuous covariate—may give guidance on whether a proportional-hazards or accelerated failure time model is the more appropriate choice for the effect of the covariates. For a proportional-hazards model the curves are separated by constant vertical distances, and for an accelerated failure time model by constant horizontal distances. Both of these conditions are met if the plots are linear, reflecting the fact that the Weibull and exponential are both proportional-hazards and accelerated failure time models. Otherwise it may be difficult to distinguish between the two possibilities against the background of chance variability, but then the two models may give similar inferences (Solomon, 1984).

The graphical approach to checking the proportional-hazards assumption does not provide a formal diagnostic test. Such a test may be constructed by including an interaction term between a covariate and time in the model. In an analysis with one explanatory variable x, suppose that a time-dependent variable z is defined as $x \ln (t)$, and that in a regression of the log hazard on x and z the regression coefficients are, respectively, β and γ. Then the relative hazard for an increase of 1 unit in x is $t^{\gamma} \exp(\beta)$. The proportional-hazards assumption holds if $\gamma = 0$, whilst the relative hazard increases or decreases with time if $\gamma > 0$ or $\gamma < 0$, respectively. A test of proportional hazards is, therefore, provided by the test of the regression coefficient γ against the null hypothesis that $\gamma = 0$.

As discussed in §11.9, residual plots are often useful as a check on the assumptions of the model and for determining if extra covariates should be included. With survival data it is not as clear as for a continuous outcome variable what is meant by a residual. A generalized residual (Cox & Snell, 1968) for a Cox proportional-hazards model is defined for the ith individual as

$$r_i = \hat{H}_0(t) \exp(\boldsymbol{b}^{\mathrm{T}} \boldsymbol{x}_i), \tag{17.30}$$

where $\boldsymbol{b}$ is the estimate of $\boldsymbol{\beta}$, and $\hat{H}_0(t)$ is the fitted cumulative hazard corresponding to the time-dependent part of the hazard, $\lambda_0(t)$ in (17.25), which may be estimated as a step function with increment $1/\exp(\boldsymbol{b}^{\mathrm{T}} \boldsymbol{x}_j)$ for each death. These residuals should be equivalent to a censored sample from an exponential distribution with mean 1, and, if the r_i are ordered and plotted against the estimated cumulative hazard rate of the r_i, then the plot should be a straight line through the origin with a slope of 1.

The *martingale residual* is defined in terms of the outcome and the cumulative hazard up to either the occurrence of the event or censoring; for an event the martingale residual is $1 - r_i$, and for a censored individual the residual is $-r_i$. These residuals have approximately zero mean and unit standard deviation but are distributed asymmetrically, with large negative values for long-term survivors and a maximum of 1 for a short-term survivor. This skewness makes these residuals difficult to interpret.

An alternative is the *deviance residual* (Therneau *et al.*, 1990). These residuals are defined as the square root of the contribution to the deviance (§14.2) between a model maximizing the contribution of the point in question to the likelihood and the fitted model. They have approximately a standard normal distribution and are available in SAS program PROC PHREG.

Chen and Wang (1991) discuss some diagnostic plots that are useful for assessing the effect of adding a covariate, detecting non-linearity or influential points in Cox's proportional-hazards model. Aitkin and Clayton (1980) give an example of residual plotting to check the assumption that a Weibull model is appropriate and Gore *et al.* (1984) gave an example in which the proportional-hazards assumption was invalid due to the waning of the effect of covariates over time in a long term follow-up of breast cancer survival.

This brief description of diagnostic methods may be supplemented by Marubini and Valsecchi (1995, Chapter 7) and Klein and Moeschberger (1997, Chapter 11).

18 Clinical trials

18.1 Introduction

Clinical trials are controlled experiments to compare the efficacy and safety, for human subjects, of different medical interventions. Strictly, the term *clinical* implies that the subjects are patients suffering from some specific illness, and indeed many, or most, clinical trials are conducted with the participation of patients and compare treatments intended to improve their condition. However, the term *clinical trial* is often used in a rather wider sense to include controlled trials of prophylactic agents such as vaccines on individuals who do not yet suffer from the disease under study, and for trials of administrative aspects of medical care, such as the choice of home or hospital care for a particular type of patient. Cochrane (1972), writing particularly about the latter category, used the term *randomized controlled trial* (RCT).

Since a clinical trial is an experiment, it is subject to the basic principles of experimentation (§9.1), such as randomization, replication and control of variability. However, the fact that the experimental units are human subjects calls for special consideration and gives rise to many unique problems. First, in clinical trials patients are normally recruited over a period of time and the relevant observations accrue gradually. This fact limits the opportunity to exploit the more complex forms of experimental design in which factors are balanced by systems of blocking; the designs used in trials are therefore relatively simple. Secondly, there are greater potentialities for bias in assessing the response to treatment than is true, for instance, of most laboratory experiments; we consider some of these problems in §18.5. Thirdly, and perhaps most importantly, any proposal for a clinical trial must be carefully scrutinized from an ethical point of view, for no doctor will allow a patient under his or her care to be given a treatment believed to be clearly inferior, unless the condition being treated is extremely mild. There are many situations, though, where the relative merits of treatments are by no means clear. Doctors may then agree to random allocation, at least until the issue is resolved. The possibility that the gradual accumulation of data may modify the investigator's ethical stance may lead to the adoption of a *sequential* design (§18.7).

Trials intended as authoritative research studies, with random assignment, are referred to as *Phase III*. Most of this chapter is concerned with Phase III trials. In drug development, *Phase I* studies are early dose-ranging projects, often with healthy volunteers. *Phase II* trials are small screening studies on patients, designed to select agents sufficiently promising to warrant the setting up of larger Phase III trials. The design of Phase I and II trials is discussed more fully in §18.2. *Phase IV* studies are concerned with postmarketing surveillance, and may take the form of surveys (§19.2) rather than comparative trials.

The organization of a clinical trial requires careful advance planning. This is particularly so for multicentre trials, which have become increasingly common in the study of chronic diseases, where large numbers of patients are often required, and of other conditions occurring too rarely for one centre to provide enough cases. Vaccine trials, in particular, need large numbers of subjects, who will normally be drawn from many centres.

The aims and methods of the trial should be described in some detail, in a document usually called a *protocol*. This will contain many medical or administrative details specific to the problem under study. It should include clear statements about the purpose of the trial, the types of patients to be admitted and the therapeutic measures to be used. The number of patients, the intended duration of the recruitment period and (where appropriate) the length of follow-up should be stated; some relevant methods have been described in §4.6.

In the following sections of this chapter we discuss a variety of aspects of the design, execution and analysis of clinical trials. The emphasis is mainly on trials in therapeutic medicine, particularly for the assessment of drugs, but most of the discussion is equally applicable in the context of trials in preventive medicine or medical care. For further details reference may be made to the many specialized books on the subject, such as Schwartz *et al.* (1980), Pocock (1983), Shapiro and Louis (1983), Buyse *et al.* (1984), Meinert (1986), Piantadosi (1997), Friedman *et al.* (1998) and Matthews (2000). Many of the pioneering collaborative trials organized by the (British) Medical Research Council are reported in Hill (1962); see also Hill and Hill (1991, Chapter 23).

18.2 **Phase I and Phase II trials**

The use of a new drug on human beings is always preceded by a great deal of research and development, including pharmacological and toxicological studies on animals, which may enable the investigators to predict the type and extent of toxicity to be expected when specified doses are administered to human subjects. Phase I trials are the first studies on humans. They enable clinical pharmacological studies to be performed and toxic effects to be observed so that a safe dosage can be established, at least provisionally.

Phase I studies are often performed on human volunteers, but in the development of drugs for the treatment of certain conditions, such as cancer, it may be necessary to involve patients since their toxic reactions may differ from those of healthy subjects. The basic purpose in designing a Phase I trial is to estimate the dose (the *maximum tolerated dose* (*MTD*)) corresponding to a maximum accept-able level of toxicity. The latter may be defined as the proportion of subjects showing some specific reaction, or as the mean level of a quantitative variable such as white blood-cell count. The number of subjects is likely to be small, perhaps in the range 10–50.

One approach to the design of the study is to start with a very low dose, determined from animal experiments or from human studies with related drugs. Doses, used on very small groups of subjects, are escalated until the target level of toxicity is reached (Storer, 1989). This strategy is similar to the 'up-and-down' method for quantal bioassay (§20.4), but the rules for changing the dose must ensure that the target level is rarely exceeded. This type of design clearly provides only a rough estimate of the MTD, which may need modification when further studies have been completed.

Another approach (O'Quigley *et al.*, 1990) is the *continual reassessment method* (*CRM*), whereby successive doses are applied to individual subjects, and at each stage the MTD is estimated from a statistical model relating the response to the dose. The procedure may start with an estimate based on prior information, perhaps using Bayesian methods. Successive doses are chosen to be close to the estimate of MTD from the previous observations, and will thus tend to cluster around the true value (although again with random error). For a more detailed review of the design and analysis of Phase I studies, see Storer (1998).

In a Phase II trial the emphasis is on efficacy, although safety will never be completely ignored. A trial that incorporates some aspects of dose selection as well as efficacy assessment may be called Phase I/II. Phase II trials are carried out with patients suffering from the disease targeted by the drug. The aim is to see whether the drug is sufficiently promising to warrant a large-scale Phase III trial. In that sense it may be regarded as a screening procedure to select, from a number of candidate drugs, those with the strongest claim to a Phase III trial.

Phase II trials need to be completed relatively quickly, and efficacy must be assessed by a rapid response. In situations, as in cancer therapy, where patient survival is at issue, it will be necessary to use a more rapidly available measure, such as the extent of tumour shrinkage or the remission of symptoms; the use of such *surrogate* measures is discussed further in §18.8.

Although nomenclature is not uniform, it is useful to distinguish between Phases IIA and IIB (Simon & Thall, 1998). In a Phase IIA trial, the object is to see whether the drug produces a minimally acceptable response, so that it can be considered as a plausible candidate for further study. No comparisons with other treatments are involved. The sample size is usually quite small, which unfortu-nately means that error probabilities are rather large. The sample size may be chosen to control the Type I and Type II errors (the probabilities of accepting an ineffective drug and of rejecting a drug with an acceptable level of response). The first type of error would be likely to be redressed in the course of further studies, whereas the second type might lead to the permanent neglect of a worthwhile treatment. Ethical considerations may require that a Phase II trial does not continue too long if the response is clearly inadequate, and this may lead to a *sequential* design, in which patients enter the trial serially, perhaps in small groups, and the trial is terminated early if the cumulative results are too poor.

In a Phase IIB design, explicit comparisons are made between the observed efficacy of the candidate drug and the observed or supposed efficacy of a standard treatment or one or more other candidates. In a comparison with a standard, the question arises whether this should be based on contemporary controls, preferably with random assignment, or whether the performance of the standard can be estimated from previous observations or literature reports. Although randomization is highly desirable in Phase III trials, it is not so clearly indicated for Phase II trials. These have rather small sample sizes, typically of the order of 50–100 patients, and the random sampling error induced by a comparison of results on two groups of size $n/2$ may exceed the combined sampling error of a single group of size n together with the (unknown) bias due to the non-randomized comparison. With larger sample sizes (as in Phase III trials) the balance swings in favour of randomization. In some situations, with a rapid measure of response following treatment, it may be possible for each patient to receive more than one treatment on different occasions, so that the treatment comparisons are subject to intrapatient, rather than the larger interpatient, variability. Such *crossover* designs are described in §18.9.

A randomized Phase II trial may not be easily distinguishable from a small Phase III trial, especially if the latter involves rapid responses, and the term Phase II/III may be used in these circumstances.

For a review of Phase II trials, see Simon and Thall (1998).

18.3 **Planning a Phase III trial**

A Phase III trial may be organized and financed by a pharmaceutical company as the final component in the submission to a regulatory authority for permission to market a new drug. It may, alternatively, be part of a programme of research undertaken by a national medical research organization. It may concern medical procedures other than the use of drugs. In any case, it is likely to be of prime importance in assessing the effectiveness and safety of a new procedure and therefore to require very careful planning and execution.

The purposes of clinical trials have been described in a number of different ways. One approach is to regard a trial as a selection procedure, in which the investigator seeks to choose the better, or best, of a set of possible treatments for a specific condition. This leads to the possible use of decision theory, in which the consequences of selecting or rejecting particular treatments are quantified. This seems too simplistic a view, since the publication of trial results rarely leads to the immediate adoption of the favoured treatment by the medical community, and the consequences of any specific set of results are extremely hard to quantify.

A less ambitious aim is to provide reliable scientific evidence of comparative merits, so that the investigators and other practitioners can make informed choices. A useful distinction has been drawn by Schwartz and Lellouch (1967) between *explanatory* and *pragmatic* attitudes to clinical trials. An explanatory trial is intended to be closely analogous to a laboratory experiment, with carefully defined treatment regimens. A pragmatic trial, in contrast, aims to simulate more closely the less rigid conditions of routine medical practice. The distinction has important consequences for the planning and analysis of trials.

In most Phase III trials the treatments are compared on *parallel groups* of patients, with each patient receiving just one of the treatments under comparison. This is clearly necessary when the treatment and/or the assessment of response requires a long follow-up period. In some trials for the short-term alleviation of chronic disease it may be possible to conduct a crossover study, in which patients receive different treatments on different occasions. As noted in §18.2, these designs are sometimes used in Phase II trials, but they are usually less appropriate for Phase III; see §18.9.

In some clinical studies, called *equivalence trials*, the aim is not to detect possible differences in efficacy, but rather to show that treatments are, within certain narrow limits, equally effective. In Phase I and Phase II studies the question may be whether different formulations of the same active agent produce serum levels that are effectively the same. In a Phase III trial a new drug may be compared with a standard drug, with the hope that its clinical response is similar or at least no worse, and that there are less severe adverse effects. The term *non-inferiority trial* may be used for this type of study. Equivalence trials are discussed further in §18.9.

The protocol

The investigators should draw up, in advance, a detailed plan of the study, to be documented in the protocol. This should cover at least the following topics:
- Purpose of, and motivation for, the trial.
- Summary of the current literature concerning the safety and efficacy of the treatments.
- Categories of patients to be admitted.
- Treatment schedules to be administered.
- Variables to be used for comparisons of safety and efficacy.
- Randomization procedures.

- Proposed number of patients and (if appropriate) length of follow-up.
- Broad outline of proposed analysis.
- Monitoring procedures.
- Case-report forms.
- Arrangements for obtaining patients' informed consent.
- Administrative arrangements, personnel, financial support.
- Arrangements for report writing and publication.

Most of these items involve statistical considerations, many of which are discussed in more detail in this and later sections of this chapter. For a fuller discussion of the contents of the protocol, see Piantadosi (1997, §4.6.3).

Definition of patients

A clinical trial will be concerned with the treatment of patients with some specific medical condition, the broad nature of which will usually be clear at a very early stage of planning. The fine detail may be less clear. Should the sex and age of the patients be restricted? Should the severity of the disease be narrowly defined? These criteria for eligibility must be considered afresh for each trial, but the general point made in §9.1, in connection with replication in experimental design, should be borne in mind. There is a conflict between the wish to achieve homogeneity in the experimental subjects and the wish to cover a wide range of conditions. It is usually wise to lean in the direction of permissiveness in defining the entry criteria. Not only will this increase the number of patients (provided that the resources needed for their inclusion are available), but it will also permit treatment comparisons to be made separately for different categories of patient. The admission of a broad spectrum of patients in no way prevents their division into more homogeneous subgroups for analysis of the results. However, comparisons based on small subgroups are less likely to detect real differences between treatment effects than tests based on the whole set of data. There is, moreover, the danger that, if too many comparisons are made in different subgroups, one or more of the tests may easily give a significant result purely by chance (see the comments on 'data dredging' in §8.4). Any subgroups with an a priori claim to attention should therefore be defined in the protocol and consideration given to them in the planning of the trial.

Definition of treatments

Again, the therapeutic regimes to be compared are usually known in broad terms from the outset. Should they be defined and standardized down to the last detail? In a multicentre trial different centres may wish to adopt minor variants of the same broad regimen or to use different concomitant therapy. It will often be better to allow these variations to enter the study, particularly when they are commonly found in medical practice, rather than to introduce a degree of standardization which may not be widely accepted or adhered to either during the trial or subsequently.

With many therapeutic measures, it is common practice to vary the detailed schedule according to the patient's condition. The dose of a drug, for instance, may depend on therapeutic response or on side-effects. In trials of such treatments there is a strong case for maintaining flexibility; many trials have been criticized after completion on the grounds that the treatment regimens were unduly rigid.

The advice given in this and the previous subsection, that the definitions of patients and treatments should tend towards breadth rather than narrowness, accords with the 'pragmatic' attitude to clinical trials, referred to earlier in this section.

Baseline and response variables

A clinical trial is likely to involve the recording of a large number of measurements for each patient. These fall into two categories.

1 *Baseline variables*. These record demographic and medical characteristics of the patient before the trial treatment starts. They are useful in providing evidence that the groups of patients assigned to different treatments have similar characteristics, so that 'like is compared with like'. More technically, they enable the treatment effects to be related to baseline characteristics by separate analyses for different subgroups or by the use of a technique such as the analysis of covariance. Such analyses reduce the effect of sampling variation and permit the study of possible interactions between baseline and response variables.

2 *Response variables*. These measure the changes in health characteristics during and after the administration of treatment. They may include physiological and biochemical test measurements, clinical signs elicited by the doctor, symptoms reported by the patient and, where appropriate, survival times. In follow-up studies it may be desirable to assess the quality of life by measuring functional ability and general well-being.

The number of variables to be recorded is potentially very high, particularly when patients return for regular follow-up visits. The temptation to record as much as possible, in case it turns out to be useful, must be resisted. An excess of information may waste resources better spent in the recruitment of more patients, it is likely to detract from the accuracy of recording and it may reduce the enthusiasm and performance level of the investigators. A special danger attaches to the recording of too many response variables, since nominally significant treatment effects may arise too readily by chance, as in the danger of data dredging referred to in §8.4.

If the response variable showing the most significant difference is picked out for special attention for that reason only, the multiplicity of possible variables must be taken into account. However, the appropriate adjustment depends in a complex way on the correlation between the variables. In the unlikely event that the variables are independent, the Bonferroni correction (§13.3) is appropriate, whereby the lowest P value, $P_{\min}$, is adjusted to a new value given by $P' = 1 - (1 - P_{\min})^k$, where k is the number of variables considered. If the variables are correlated, this is unduly conservative, i.e. it produces too great a correction.

The danger of data dredging is usually reduced by the specification of one response variable, or perhaps a very small number of variables, as a *primary endpoint*, reflecting the main purpose of the trial. Differences in these variables between treatments are taken at their face value. Other variables are denoted as *secondary endpoints*. Differences in these are regarded as important but less clearly established, perhaps being subjected to a multiplicity correction or providing candidates for exploration in further trials.

Reference was made above to the assessment of quality of life in follow-up studies. The choice of variables to be measured will depend on the sort of impairment expected as a natural consequence of the disease under study or as a possible adverse effect of treatment. It may be possible to identify a range of conditions, all of which should be monitored, and to form a single index by combining the measurements in some way. The purpose of quality of life measurements is to permit a balance to be drawn between the possible benefit of treatment and the possible disbenefit caused by its side-effects. In a trial for treatments of a chronic life-threatening disease, such as a type of cancer, the duration of survival will be a primary endpoint, but a modest extension of life may be unacceptable if it is accompanied by increased disability or pain. In some studies it has been possible to use *quality-adjusted* survival times, whereby each year (or other unit of time) survived is weighted by a measure of the quality of life before standard methods of survival analysis (Chapter 17) are applied. These methods have been adopted for survival analysis in cancer trials, where the relevant measure may be the time without symptoms and toxicity (*TWiST*), leading to the quality-adjusted version, *Q-TWiST* (Gelber *et al.*, 1989; Cole *et al.*, 1995). For general reviews of quality of life assessment, see Cox *et al.* (1992) and Olschewski (1998).

Trial size

The precision of comparisons between treatments is clearly affected by the numbers of patients receiving them. The standard approach is to determine the intended numbers by the considerations described in §4.6. That is, a value δ_1 is chosen for a parameter δ, representing a sufficiently important difference in efficacy for one not to want to miss it. Values are chosen for the significance level α in a test of the null hypothesis that $\delta = 0$, and for the power $1 - \beta$ against the alternative value $\delta = \delta_1$. With some assumptions about the distribution of the estimate of δ, in particular its variance, the sample size is determined by formulae such as (4.41).

As noted in §4.6, sample-size determination is an inexact science, if only because the choice of δ_1, α and β are to an extent arbitrary, and the variability of the test statistic may be difficult to estimate in advance. Nevertheless, the exercise gives the investigators some idea of the sensitivity likely to be achieved by a trial of any specific size. We note here some additional points that may be relevant in a clinical trial.

1   In a chronic disease study the primary response variable may be the incidence over time of some adverse event, such as the relapse of a patient with malignant disease, the reoccurrence of a cardiovascular event or the patient's death. The precision of a treatment comparison is determined largely by the expected number of events in a treatment group, and this can be increased either by enrolling more patients or by lengthening the follow-up time. The latter choice has the advantage of extending the study over a longer portion of the natural course of the disease, but the disadvantage of delaying the end of the trial.

2   Many early trials can now be seen to have been too small, resulting often in the dismissal of new treatments because of non-significant results when the test had too low a power to detect worthwhile effects (Pocock *et al.*, 1978). Yusuf *et al.* (1984) have argued strongly in favour of large, simple trials, on the grounds that large trials are needed in conditions such as cardiovascular disease, where the event rate is low but relatively small reductions would be beneficial and cost-effective. Substantial increases in sample size are made more feasible if protocols are 'simple' and the administrative burdens on the doctors are minimized. However, as Powell-Tuck *et al.* (1986) demonstrate, small trials, efficiently analysed, may sometimes provide evidence sufficiently conclusive to affect medical practice.

3   As noted in §6.4, some of the uncertainties in the determination of sample size may be resolved by a Bayesian approach (Spiegelhalter & Freedman, 1986; Spiegelhalter *et al.*, 1994). In particular, a prior distribution may be introduced for the difference parameter δ, as indicated in §6.4. Investigators are likely to differ in their prior assessments, and a compromise may be necessary. Calculations may be performed with alternative prior distributions, representing different degrees of enthusiasm or scepticism about a possible treatment effect. In a Bayesian approach, inference about the parameter value should be expressed in terms of the posterior distribution. Suppose that a value $\delta_S > 0$ would be regarded as indicating superiority of one of the treatments. The requirement that the posterior probability that $\delta > \delta_S$ should be high will determine a critical value X_S for the relevant test statistic X. The predictive probability that X will exceed X_S may be determined by the

methods of Bayesian prediction outlined in §6.4. These calculations will involve the sample size, and it may be possible to choose this in such a way as to ensure a high predictive probability. However, with a 'sceptical' prior distribution, giving low probability to values of $\delta > \delta_S$, this will not be achievable, and the conclusion will be that the trial, however large, cannot be expected to achieve a positive conclusion in favour of this treatment.

4   An outcome in favour of one treatment or another is desirable, but by no means necessary for the success of a trial. Reliable information is always useful, even when it appears to show little difference between rival treatments. A trial which appears to be inconclusive in isolation may contribute usefully to a meta-analysis showing more clear-cut results (§18.8).

See §18.6 for a note on the effect of non-compliance on the determination of sample size.

18.4 **Treatment assignment**

Randomization

Many investigators in the eighteenth and nineteenth centuries realized that treatments needed to be compared on groups of patients with similar prognostic characteristics, but lacked the technical means of achieving this balance. An excellent survey of this early work is given by Bull (1959); see also the website http://www.rcpe.ac.uk/controlled trials/ sponsored by the Royal College of Physicians of Edinburgh.

During the late nineteenth and early twentieth centuries several trial investigators assigned two treatments to alternate cases in a series. This system has the defect that the assignment for any patient is known in advance, and may lead to bias, either in the assessment of response (§18.5) or in the selection of patients. The latter possibility, of *selection bias*, may arise since a knowledge or suspicion of the treatment to be used for the next patient may affect the investigator's decision whether or not to admit that patient to the trial. A few isolated examples exist of allocation by a physical act of randomization (Peirce & Jastrow, 1885; Theobald, 1937), but the main initiative was taken by A. Bradford Hill (1897–1991), who used strictly random assignment for the trial of streptomycin for the treatment of tuberculosis (Medical Research Council, 1948) and the trial of pertussis vaccines started earlier but published later (Medical Research Council, 1951), and advocated the method widely in his writings. Randomization was, of course, a central feature of the principles of experimental design laid down by R.A. Fisher (see §9.1).

Randomization was originally carried out from tables of random numbers, but nowadays computer routines are normally used, individual assignments being determined only after a patient has entered the trial and been given an identifying number.

Balance

A randomized assignment will ensure that there is no systematic reason for imbalance between treatment groups in any given baseline variable. But, purely by chance, some degree of imbalance must occur, and an extreme degree of imbalance in a baseline variable prognostic for a response variable may lead to a misleadingly significant estimate of treatment effect, even if none really exists. It is therefore desirable to guard in some way against imbalance in known prognostic variables.

This can be done either in the analysis, by analysing the data separately within subgroups defined by prognostic variable, or by a model such as the analysis of covariance; or in the design of the study by modifying the randomization scheme to provide the balance required.

In many early trials, balance was achieved by the method of *restricted randomization*, or *permuted blocks*. Here, strata are defined by prognostic variables or designated combinations of these such as: female, age 30–39 years, duration of symptoms less than 1 year. A randomization scheme is constructed separately for each stratum, so that the numbers allocated to different treatments are equalized at regular intervals, e.g. in blocks of 10. When the intake of patients comes to an end the numbers on different treatments will not be exactly equal, but they are likely to be more nearly so than with simple randomization.

A defect of permuted blocks is that the assignment for a new patient is predetermined if that patient happens to come at the end of a block. Another problem is that, if too many baseline variables are used, many of the strata will be too small to permit adequate balancing of treatments.

It is now more usual to use some form of *minimization* (Taves, 1974; Begg & Iglewitz, 1980). The aim here is to assign patients in such a way as to minimize (in some sense) the current disparity between the groups, taking into account simultaneously a variety of prognostic variables. For further description, see Pocock (1983, pp. 84–6). Minimization can be carried out by computing staff at the trial coordinating centre, so that an assignment can be determined almost immediately when the centre is notified about the values of baseline variables for a new patient. In a multicentre study it is usual to arrange that the clinical centre is one of the factors to be balanced, so that each centre can claim to have satisfactory balance in case a separate analysis is needed for the patients at that centre.

In any of these methods of balancing by the design of the allocation scheme, the groups will tend to be more alike in relevant respects than by simple randomization, and a consequence of this is that the random variability of any test statistic for comparing groups is somewhat reduced. This is a welcome feature, of course, but the extent of the reduction cannot be determined without an analysis taking the balance into account. If the effects of the covariates can be represented by a linear regression model, for example, a standard multiple regression analysis will provide the appropriate estimate of error variance. Unfortunately, this precaution is usually overlooked.

An alternative approach is to assign patients by simple randomization, and adjust for the effects of covariates in the analysis. This will have the dual effect of correcting for any imbalance in baseline variables and reducing the error variance. The variance of the treatment comparison will be somewhat greater than that produced by minimization, because of the initial disparity between mean values in different treatment groups and the greater effect of uncertainty about the appropriate model for the covariate effects. However, the advantage of minimization is likely to be relatively small (Forsythe & Stitt, 1977). Its main advantage is probably psychological, in reassuring investigators in different centres that their contribution of even a small number of patients to a multi-centre study is of value, and in ensuring that the final report of the trial produces convincing evidence of similarity of treatment groups.

Data-dependent allocation

In most clinical trials, patients are assigned in equal proportions to different treatment groups, or in simple ratios, such as 2 : 1, which are retained throughout the trial. In a trial with one control treatment and several new treatments, for instance, it may be useful to assign a higher proportion to the control group.

Ethical considerations will normally mean that, initially, investigators would regard it as proper to give any of the rival treatments to any patient. However, if evidence accumulates during the course of the trial suggesting that one treatment is inferior to one or more of the others, the investigators' ethical 'equipoise' may be weakened. To some extent, this concern is met by the existence of monitoring procedures (§18.7), which permit early termination of the trial on ethical grounds. However, some researchers have argued that, instead of implementing equal assignment proportions to all treatments until a sudden termination occurs, it would be ethically preferable to allow the proportionate assignments to vary throughout the trial in such a way that more patients are gradually assigned to the apparently more successful treatments.

An early proposal for trials with a binary outcome (success or failure) was by Zelen (1969), who advocated a 'play the winner' rule, by which, with two treatments, a success is followed by an assignment of the next patient to the same treatment, but a failure leads to a switch to the other treatment. More complex systems of data-dependent allocation have since been devised (Chernoff & Petkau, 1981; Bather, 1985; Berry & Fristedt, 1985) and active research into the methodology continues.

The consequence of any such scheme is that, if efficacy differences between treatments exist, the number of patients eventually placed on the better treatment will exceed, perhaps very considerably, the number on the inferior treatment(s), even though the evidence for the reality of the effect may be weak. The latter feature follows because a comparison between two groups of very different sizes is less precise than if the two groups had been pooled and divided into groups of equal size. Difficulties may also arise if there is a time trend in the prognostic characteristics of patients during the trial. Patients entered towards the end of the trial, and thus assigned predominantly to the favoured treatment, may have better (or worse) prognoses than those entered early, who were assigned in equal proportions to different treatments. It may be difficult to adjust the results to allow for this effect. A more practical difficulty is that doctors may be unwilling to assign, say, one patient in 10 to an apparently worse treatment, and may prefer a system by which their ethical equipoise is preserved until the evidence for an effect is compelling. See Armitage (1985) for a general discussion.

Data-dependent allocation of this sort should perhaps be called 'outcome-dependent allocation' to distinguish it from schemes such as minimization, discussed in the last subsection. In the latter, the allocation may depend on the values of baseline variables for the patient, but not on the outcome as measured by a response variable, which is the essential feature of the present discussion. The term *adaptive assignment* is also widely used.

Adaptive schemes have rarely been used in practice. A well-known example is the trial of extracorporeal membrane oxygenation (ECMO) for newborn infants with respiratory failure (Bartlett *et al.*, 1985). This followed a so-called *biased coin design* (Wei & Durham, 1978), which is a modified form of play the winner. For two treatments, A and B, assignment is determined by drawing an A or B ball from an urn. Initially, there is one ball of each type. After a success with, say, A, an A ball is added to the urn and, after a failure with A, a B ball is added; and vice versa. A higher proportion of successes with A than with B thus leads to a higher probability of assignment with A. In the event, the first patient was treated with ECMO and was a success. The second patient received the control treatment, which failed. There then followed 10 successive successes on ECMO and the trial stopped. The proportions of successes were thus 11/11 on ECMO and 0/1 on control. The correct method of analysing this result has caused a great deal of controversy in the statistical literature (Ware, 1989; Begg, 1990). Perhaps the most useful comment is that of Cox (1990):

> The design has had the double misfortune of producing data from which it would be hazardous to draw any firm conclusion and yet which presumably makes further investigation ethically difficult. There is an imperative to set minimum sample sizes.

Randomized consent

It is customary to seek the informed consent of each patient before he or she is entered into a clinical trial. If many patients withhold their consent, or if physicians find it difficult to ask patients to agree to their treatment being determined by a random process, it may be difficult to recruit an adequate number of patients into the trial. Zelen (1979) has suggested a procedure which may be useful in some trials in which a new treatment, N, is to be compared with a standard treatment, S.

In Zelen's design, eligible patients are randomized to two groups, **N** and **S**. Patients in **S** are given the treatment S without any enquiry about consent. Patients in **N** are asked whether they consent to receive N; if so, they receive N—if not, they receive S. The avoidance of consent from the **S** group, even though these patients receive standard treatment, has sometimes caused controversy, and the design should not be used without full approval from ethical advisers.

As will be noted in §18.6, a fair comparison may be made by the *intention-to-treat* approach, based on the total groups **N** and **S**, even though not all patients in **N** actually received N. If there is a difference in the effects of the two treatments, it will tend to be underestimated by the difference in mean responses of **N** and **S**, because of the diluting effect of the non-consenters in **N**. It is possible to estimate the true difference among the subgroup of consenters, but this will be rather inefficient if the proportion of consenters is low; for details, see Zelen (1979, 1990). For further comment, see Altman *et al.* (1995).

The ECMO trial described above used this design, although in the event only one patient received the standard treatment. The method was also used in a further trial of ECMO (O'Rourke *et al.*, 1989), the results of which tended to confirm the relative benefit of ECMO.

18.5 **Assessment of response**

Randomization, if properly performed, ensures the absence of bias due to the assignment of patients with different prognostic features to different treatment groups. It is important also to avoid bias that might arise if different standards of recording response were applied for different treatments.

Most trials compare one active treatment against another. It is sometimes desirable to compare a new treatment with its absence, although both treatment groups may receive, simultaneously, a standard therapy. In such a trial the mere knowledge that an additional intervention is made for one group only may produce an apparent benefit, irrespective of the intrinsic merits of that intervention. For this reason, the patients in the control group may be given a *placebo*, an inert form of treatment indistinguishable from the new treatment under test. In a drug trial, for instance, the placebo will be an inert substance formulated in the same tablet or capsule form as the new drug and administered according to the same regimen. In this way, the pharmacological effect of the new drug can be separated from the psychological effect of the knowledge of its use.

The principle of *masking* the identity of a treatment may be extended to trials in which two or more potentially active treatments are compared. The main purpose here is to ensure that the measurement of the response variable is not affected by a knowledge of the specific treatment administered. If the relevant response is survival or death, this is almost certain to be recorded objectively and accurately, and no bias is likely to occur. Any other measure of the progress of disease, such as the reporting of symptoms by the patient, the eliciting of signs by the doctor, the recording of major exacerbations of disease, or even the recording of biomedical test measurements, may be influenced by knowledge of the treatment received. This includes knowledge by the patient or by the physician or other technical staff.

It is important, therefore, to arrange when possible for treatments to be administered by some form of masking. (The term *blinding* is often used, but is perhaps less appropriate, if only because of the ambiguity caused in trials for conditions involving visual defects.) In a *single-masked* (or *single-blind*) trial, the treatment identity is hidden from the patient. In the more common *double-masked* (or *double-blind*) design, the identity is hidden from the physician in charge and from any other staff involved with the assessment of response. In some cases it may be necessary for the physician to be aware of the treatment identity, particularly with a complex intervention, but possible for the assessments of response to be completely masked.

Masking is achieved by ensuring that the relevant treatments are formulated in the same way. If two drugs have to be administered in different ways, for instance by tablet or capsule, it may be possible to use a *double-dummy* technique. To compare drug A by tablet with drug B by capsule, the two groups would receive

Active A tablets, plus placebo B capsules

or

Placebo A tablets, plus active B capsules.

Once the treatment assignment for a patient has been decided, the tablets, capsules, etc., should be packaged and given a label specific to that patient. An alternative system is sometimes used, whereby a particular treatment is given a code letter, such as A, and all packages containing that drug are labelled A. This system has the defect that, if the identity of A becomes known or suspected—for instance, through the recognition of side-effects—the code may be effectively broken for all patients subsequently receiving that treatment.

The use of a placebo may be impracticable, either because a treatment causes easily detectable side-effects, which cannot, or should not, be reproduced with a placebo, or because the nature of the intervention cannot be simulated. The latter situation would, for instance, normally arise in surgery, except perhaps for very minor procedures. Masking devices, therefore, although highly effective in most situations, should not be regarded as a panacea for the avoidance of response bias. It will often be wise to check their effectiveness by enquiring, from supposedly masked patients and physicians, which treatment they thought had been administered, and comparing these guesses with the true situation.

18.6 **Protocol departures**

After randomization, patients should rarely, if ever, be excluded from the trial. The chance of exclusion for a particular patient may depend on the treatment received, and to permit the removal of patients from the trial may impair the effectiveness of randomization and lead to biased comparisons.

A few patients may be discovered to contravene the eligibility criteria after randomization: they should be omitted only if it is quite clear that no bias is involved—for example, when diagnostic tests have been performed before randomization but the results do not become available until later, or when errors in recording the patient's age are discovered after randomization. Omission would be wrong if the eligibility failure arose from a revised diagnosis made after deterioration in the patient's condition, since this condition might have been affected by the choice of treatment.

A more serious source of difficulty is the occurrence of departures from the therapeutic procedures laid down in the protocol. Every attempt should be made to encourage participants to follow the protocol meticulously, and types of patients (such as the very old) who could be identified in advance as liable to cause protocol departures should have been excluded by the eligibility criteria. Nevertheless, some departures are almost inevitable, and they may well include withdrawal of the allotted treatment and substitution of an alternative, or defection of the patient from the investigator's care. The temptation exists to exclude such patients from the groups to which they were assigned, leading to a so-called *per protocol* or (misleadingly) *efficacy* analysis. Such an analysis seeks to follow the explanatory approach (§18.3) by examining the consequences of precisely defined treatment regimens. The problem here is that protocol deviants are almost certain to be atypical of the whole patient population, and some forms of deviation are more likely to arise with one treatment than with another. A comparison of the residual groups of protocol compliers has therefore lost some of the benefit of randomization, and the extent of the consequent bias is unknown. A *per protocol* analysis may be useful as a secondary approach to the analysis of a Phase III trial, or to provide insight in an early-stage trial to be followed by a larger study. It should never form the main body of evidence for a major trial.

It is similarly dangerous to omit from the analysis of a trial any events or other responses occurring during specified periods after the start of treatment. It might, for example, be thought that a drug cannot take effect before at least a week has elapsed, and that therefore any adverse events occurring during the first week can be discounted. These events should be omitted only if the underlying assumption is universally accepted; otherwise, the possibility of bias again arises. Similarly, adverse events (such as accidental deaths) believed to be unrelated to the disease in question should be omitted only if their irrelevance is beyond dispute (and this is rarely so, even for accidental deaths). However, events especially relevant for the disease under study (such as cardiovascular events in a trial for treatments for a cardiovascular disease) should be reported separately and may well form one of the primary endpoints for the trial.

The policy of including in the analysis, where possible, all patients in the groups to which they were randomly assigned, is called the *intent(ion)-to-treat* (ITT) or *as-randomized* approach. It follows the pragmatic approach to trial design (§18.3), in that groups receive treatments based on ideal strategies laid down in the protocol, with the recognition that (as in routine medical practice) rigidly prescribed regimens will not always be followed. In a modified form of ITT it is occasionally thought reasonable to omit a small proportion of patients who opted out of treatment before that treatment had started. In a double-masked drug trial, for instance, it may be clear that the same pressures to opt out apply to all treatment groups. This would not be so, however, in a trial to compare immediate with delayed radiotherapy, since the group assigned delayed treatment would have more opportunity to opt out before the start of radio-therapy.

If a high proportion of patients abandon their prescribed treatment regimen, perhaps switching to an alternative regimen under study, the estimates of differences in efficacy between active agents will be biased, probably towards zero. In a later subsection we discuss whether adjustments can be made to allow for this incomplete compliance.

Withdrawals and missing data

An ITT analysis may be thwarted because response variables, or other relevant information, are missing for some patients. These lacunae can arise for various reasons. The patient may have withdrawn from the investigator's care, either because of dissatisfaction with the medical care or because of removal to another district. In a follow-up study, information may be missing for some prescribed visits, because the patient was unwell. Technical equipment may have failed, leading to loss of test results, or other administrative failures may have occurred.

In such situations it may be possible to retrieve missing information by assiduous enquiry at the medical centre. In trials for which mortality is the primary endpoint, it is possible in some countries (such as the UK) to determine each patient's survival status at any interval after the start of the trial, from a national death registration system.

If the value of a response variable is definitely missing for some patients, the statistical analyst faces the problems discussed at some length in §12.6. It will often be true, and can rarely be discounted, that the missingness is *informative*; that is, the tendency to be missing will be related to the observation that would otherwise have been made, even after relevant predictive variables have been taken into account. For example, in a follow-up study, a patient may fail to appear for one of the scheduled examinations because of a sudden exacerbation of the illness. An analysis comparing results in different treatment groups at this particular time point might be biased because the extent of, and reasons for, missing information might vary from one treatment group to another.

As noted in §12.6, some progress can be made by assuming some model for the relationship between the missingness and the random fluctuation of the missing observation. But such an analysis is somewhat speculative, and should probably be conducted as a sensitivity analysis using different models. In the routine analysis of a clinical trial, as distinct from more prolonged research studies, it is probably best to analyse results omitting the missing data, and to report clearly that this has been done.

A particular pattern of missing data, also discussed in §12.6, is caused by patients who withdraw, or drop out, from a schedule of periodic follow-up visits. The data here might be missing *at random* (if, for instance, the patient moved out of the district for reasons unconnected with the illness), but it is more likely to be informative (indicating deterioration in the patient's condition).

Some models for informative drop-out data are discussed in §12.6. As noted in the discussion there of the case-study presented by Diggle (1998), models are usually unverifiable, and the choice of model can appreciably affect the results of an analysis. Simpler, *ad hoc*, methods are also difficult to validate, but they may be useful in some cases. Suppose the relevant endpoint is a test measurement at the end of a series of tests carried out at regular intervals—for instance, on serum concentrations of some key substance. One common approach is the *last observation carried forward* (*LOCF*) method, whereby each patient contributes the last available record. This is self-evidently flawed if there is a trend in the observations during the follow-up, and if the pattern of drop-outs varies between treatments. It may be a useful device in situations where the readings remain fairly constant during the follow-up, but takes no account of the possibly informative nature of the drop-outs, obscuring the possibility that missing readings might have been substantially different from those observed.

Another approach is to assign some arbitrarily poor score to the missing responses. Brown (1992), for instance, suggests that in a trial to compare an active drug with a placebo, a score equal to the median response in the placebo group could be assigned to a patient who dropped out. In the analysis, a broad categorical response category should then include all patients with that score or worse. Treatment groups are then compared by the Mann–Whitney test (§10.3). Devices of this type may be useful, even unavoidable, if crucial responses are missing, but they involve the sacrifice of information, and estimation may be biased. The best solution is to avoid withdrawals as far as possible by careful advance planning.

Compliance

The term *compliance* may imply adherence to all the protocol requirements. In drug trials it usually refers more specifically to the ingestion of the drug at the prescribed times and in the prescribed quantities.

The effects of *non-compliance* in the broad sense have been discussed throughout this section. They are multifarious and difficult to quantify. Nevertheless, attempts have been made to model non-compliance in some very simple situations, which we describe below. The aim here is to estimate the effect of non-compliance on treatment comparisons, and hence to go beyond an ITT approach to the estimation of treatment effects.

The narrower sense of drug compliance is somewhat more amenable to modelling, since the proportion of the scheduled amount of drug that was actually taken can often be estimated by patient reports, counts of returned tablets, serum concentrations, etc. Models for this situation are described later.

A simple model for non-compliance is described by Sommer and Zeger (1991) and attributed by them to Tarwotjo *et al.* (1987). It relates to a trial of an active treatment against a control, with a binary outcome of success or failure. Non-compliers may form part of each group, but are likely to form different proportions and to be different in prognostic characteristics. The analysis concentrates on the subgroup of compliers in the treatment group. The proportion of successes in this subgroup is observed, and the aim of the analysis is to estimate the proportion of successes that would have been observed *in that subgroup* if those patients had received the control treatment. The key assumption is that this proportion is the same (apart from random error) as the proportion of successes observed in the control group. The calculations are illustrated in Example 18.1.

Example 18.1

Table 18.1 shows results from a trial of vitamin A supplementation to reduce mortality over an 8-month period among preschool children in rural Indonesia, reported by Tarwotjo *et al.* (1987) and discussed by Sommer and Zeger (1991).

Table 18.1 Results from a trial of vitamin A supplementation in Indonesian preschool children (reproduced from Sommer & Zeger, 1991, with permission from the authors and publishers).

	Control group			Treatment group		
	Compliance			Compliance		
	No (1)	Yes (2)	Total (3)	No (4)	Yes (5)	Total (6)
Alive	?(m_{00})	?(m_{01})	11 514 ($m_{0.}$)	2385 (n_{00})	9663 (n_{01})	12 048 ($n_{0.}$)
Dead	?(m_{10})	?(m_{11})	74 ($m_{1.}$)	34 (n_{10})	12 (n_{11})	46 ($n_{1.}$)
Total		?($m_{.1}$)	11 588 (M)		9675 ($n_{.1}$)	12 094 (N)

In Table 18.1, columns (1) and (2) refer to subjects who would have been compliant or non-compliant if they had been in the treatment group and, of course, their numbers are unknown. However, these numbers can be estimated. On the assumption that the proportion of deaths would be the same for the non-compliers in columns (1) and (4), since neither subgroup received treatment, and since the expected proportions of non-compliers should be the same in the treatment and control groups, the entries in column (1) can be estimated as $\hat{m}_{00} = (M/N)n_{00}$ and $\hat{m}_{10} = (M/N)n_{10}$, and those in column (2) by $\hat{m}_{01} = m_{0.} - \hat{m}_{00}$ and $\hat{m}_{11} = m_{1.} - \hat{m}_{10}$. The adjusted proportion of deaths among treatment-compliers in the control group is now estimated as $\hat{p}_C = \hat{m}_{11}/\hat{m}_{.1}$, to compare with the observed proportion in the treatment group, $p_{TC} = n_{11}/n_{.1}$.

In this example, $\hat{p}_C = 41 \cdot 4/9270 \cdot 2 = 0 \cdot 447\%$, and $p_{TC} = 12/9675 = 0 \cdot 124\%$, a reduction of 72%. In the ITT analysis, the overall proportions of deaths are $p_C = 74/11\,588 = 0 \cdot 639\%$ and $p_T = 46/12\,094 = 0 \cdot 380\%$, a reduction of 41%.

Several points should be noted about the analysis illustrated in Example 18.1.

1 The assumption that the non-compliers on the treatment would respond in the same way if allocated to the control group is crucial. It is perhaps defensible in Example 18.1, where the response is survival or death, but would be less self-evident in a trial with a more subjective response. The experience of assignment to, and then rejection of, an active treatment may influence the response, perhaps by causing a behaviour pattern or emotional reaction that would not have been seen if the patient had been assigned to the control group.

2 The model used in Example 18.1 could be adapted for the analysis of a randomized consent trial (§18.4), the act of consenting to treatment in the latter case corresponding to compliance in the former. In practice, an ITT analysis is usually preferred for the randomized consent trial, to avoid the assumption analogous to that described in **1**, namely, that a non-consenter would respond in the same way to either assignment.

3 The results in the two groups in Example 18.1 have been compared by the ratio of the proportions of death. This is reasonable in this example, since the

absolute death rate will depend on the arbitrary duration of follow-up. In other trials it may be preferable to quote the difference in proportions of positive responses.

4 The sampling error of the estimated response proportion $\hat{p}_C$ differs from the usual binomial variance (3.16) appropriate for a direct observation from a random sample of size $\hat{m}_{.1}$. Formulae for the calculation of the variance of the estimated relative risk are given in the Appendix to Sommer and Zeger (1991).

5 In some examples of the use of this model, the control group may also be subdivided, with known numbers of compliers and non-compliers to the control regime. These numbers are not needed for the analysis, since the characteristics of patients who comply with the treatment are likely to differ from those who comply with the control regime. See Zeger (1998) for an example. For this reason, it would be quite wrong to compare success proportions in the two *per protocol* subgroups (compliers to treatment and compliers to control).

The model used in Example 18.1 is *saturated*, in the sense that there are the same number of parameters, four, as random observations. The parameters can be chosen to be θ, the probability that a patient is a treatment-complier; the probabilities of death, π_1 and π_2, for the treatment compliers and non-compliers, respectively, in the control group; and δ, the reduction in the probability of death due to treatment, among the treatment-compliers. The independent observations may be taken as t, the observed proportion of compliers in the treatment group; and p_C, p_{TC} and p_{TNC}, the proportions of deaths in the control group and among the compliers and non-compliers in the treatment group, respectively.

In a saturated model of this kind, the maximum likelihood estimates of the parameters are such that the expected frequencies are identical with those observed, and the parameters may be easily estimated by equating the observed and expected values. The calculations in Example 18.1 follow this approach. Thus, the estimate of the treatment effect δ is

$$\hat{\delta} = \frac{p_C - (1-t)p_{TNC}}{t} - p_{TC}. \tag{18.1}$$

Substituting in (18.1) from Table 18.1, with $t = 9675/12\,094, p_C = 74/11\,588$, $p_{TC} = 12/9675$ and $p_{TNC} = 34/2419$, we find $\hat{\delta} = 0.00323$, in agreement with the estimate $(0.447\% - 0.124\%)$ given earlier in Example 18.1.

Similar models can be constructed for other trial designs with binary responses (Angrist *et al.*, 1996). Suppose, for example, that there are two active treatments, A and B, with three categories of patients: non-compliers who will receive A whatever their assignment, those who will receive B whatever their assignment, and compliers who will follow the assigned treatment. There are now six parameters and six independent observed quantities, so again a simple solution is available. As before, the model involves crucial assumptions. The non-compliers who receive A are assumed to have the same outcome whether they are assigned to A or whether they default from an assignment to B; and similarly with those receiving B. Moreover, the basic assumption that non-compliers merely switch to the other treatment is unrealistic: in practice, a non-complier might take the assigned treatment in a non-prescribed manner, or follow a regimen quite different from either A or B.

In drug trials, a common form of non-compliance occurs when the patient takes the prescribed drug but to an incomplete extent. Compliance can then be measured as a continuous variable—the proportion of the prescribed dose actually taken. The aim will be to compare the responses to different treatment regimens among patients with complete compliance. However, those who comply completely with one treatment, say, A, cannot be assumed to be equivalent in prognostic features to those who comply completely with another treatment, B. The situation differs from that previously considered, in that observations may be available relating the degree of compliance to the response, which need not be binary. Various approaches have been suggested.

Heitjan (1999) describes various analyses for a small data set from a trial comparing a drug and a placebo, with a continuous response variable, in which some patients assigned to the drug switched to the placebo. The methods used are: (i) ITT; (ii) *as treated*, in which the non-compliant patients are transferred to the placebo group; (iii) a *causal* model akin to that described above; and (iv) a *non-ignorable* method. In the latter, it is assumed that the propensity to switch depends on the response that would have been observed if the assigned treatment had been used, and a logistic model is proposed for this relationship. The author points out that the results from the non-ignorable model are 'highly sensitive to assumptions that the data generally cannot address' and suggests that 'it is best to regard such a model only as an adjunct to some more objective analysis'. Efron and Feldman (1991), in a paper followed by a discussion, considered a placebo-controlled drug trial in which measures of compliance were available for all patients in each group. Although the distribution of compliance varies between groups, it is assumed that a given patient would have been similarly ranked for compliance to whichever group he or she was assigned.

Another approach, developed by Goetghebeur and Lapp (1997) and Fischer-Lapp and Goetghebeur (1999), uses a so-called *structural mean model*. In a placebo-controlled drug trial, suppose that compliance measures are available for the drug group but not necessarily for the placebo group. Regressions on baseline covariates are performed for the placebo response, the compliance measure and the treatment response. The difference between the predicted responses on drug and placebo may then be derived as a function of baseline covariates and compliance. A useful step is to include, as a covariate, the compliance observed during a run-in period. This approach involves various assumptions that may not be easily testable. In particular, it is assumed that the regressions of response on compliance for the two groups have the same intercept at zero compliance, so that a non-compliant patient would have the same expected response whatever the assignment (as in the model of Example 18.1). Dunn (1999) discusses the effect of error in the compliance measurement, and concurs with a view expressed earlier by Pocock and Abdalla (1998) that complex models for compliance should not replace ITT analyses, but should be regarded as additional explanatory descriptions.

The journal issue edited by Goetghebeur and van Houwelingen (1998) contains several useful papers on this evolving body of methodology.

We note finally that non-compliance may affect any calculations of sample-size requirements made before the start of a trial. In an ITT analysis, the effect of non-compliance is likely to be to bias the difference in mean response between two treatments towards zero. This will be especially so in a trial to compare a new treatment against a placebo, if non-compliance results in patients assigned to the new treatment switching to the placebo. Suppose the expected difference is reduced by a fraction φ. Then the number of patients required to provide the intended power against this reduced treatment effect must be increased by a multiple $1/(1 - \varphi)^2$. This can be taken into account in the planning of the trial if φ can be estimated reasonably accurately. Unfortunately, this will often not be possible. As we have seen, non-compliance can take many forms and have many consequences, the nature and extent of which will usually be unknown at the outset. It may be possible to estimate the proportion, θ, of non-compliant patients from previous experience of similar trials, but the effects of these protocol departures on the outcomes for the different groups may be less obvious. The best plan may be to make a simple, plausible assumption and err, if at all, in the direction of overstating the required trial size. One such assumption, in a two-treatment trial, might be that the outcome for a non-compliant patient is, on average, the same as that in the non-assigned group. The consequence of that assumption is that $\varphi = \theta$, and hence the intended trial size should be increased by a factor $1/(1 - \theta)^2$ (Donner, 1984).

18.7 **Data monitoring**

In any large trial, the investigators should set up a system of *administrative monitoring*, to check that high standards are maintained in the conduct of the trial. Such a system will check whether the intended recruitment rate is being met, detect violations in entry criteria and monitor the accuracy of the information being recorded. Administrative monitoring may reveal unsatisfactory features of the protocol, leading to its revision. If the rate of recruitment is below expectation, the investigators may seek the cooperation of other medical centres or perhaps liberalize the entry criteria.

Administrative monitoring will normally make no use of the outcome data for patients in the trial. In contrast, *data monitoring* is concerned with the evidence emerging from the accumulating data on the safety and efficacy of the treatments under trial.

Safety will be an important issue in almost every trial. Most medical treatments and procedures produce minor side-effects, which will often have been anticipated from the results of earlier studies and may not cause serious concern. *Serious adverse events* (SAEs), especially when potentially life-threatening, must be carefully monitored (and perhaps reported to a central agency). A high incidence of unexpected SAEs, not clearly balanced by advantages in patient survival, may lead to early termination of the trial, or at least the modification or abandonment of the suspect treatment.

Differences in efficacy may arise during the course of the trial and give rise to ethical concerns. The investigators will probably have started the trial from a position of ethical equipoise, regarding all the rival treatments as potentially acceptable. If the emerging evidence suggests that one treatment is inferior to another, the investigators may feel impelled to stop the trial or at least drop the offending treatment.

The mechanisms for conducting data monitoring are discussed in the following subsections.

The Data Monitoring Committee

The responsibility for early termination or changes in protocol rests with the investigators (who, in a multicentre or other large trial, will normally form a *Steering Committee*). However, in a double-masked trial they will be unaware of the treatment assignments and unable to monitor the results directly. It is usual for the task to be delegated to an independent group, known as the *Data [and Safety] Monitoring Committee* (D[S]MC) or some similar title. The DMC will typically comprise one or more statisticians, some medical specialists in the areas under investigation and perhaps some lay members. It will not normally include investigators or commercial sponsors, although there is some variation of opinion on this point (Harrington *et al.*, 1994; Meinert, 1998).

The DMC should meet at approximately regular intervals, and receive unmasked data summaries presented by the trial statisticians. It will normally report to the Steering Committee, avoiding explicit descriptions of the data but presenting a firm recommendation for or against early termination or protocol modification.

In assessing the evidence, the DMC will need to bear in mind the difficulties arising from the repeated analysis of accumulating data. These are discussed in general terms in the next subsection, which is followed by a more explicit description of methods of analysis.

Sequential analysis

A *sequential* investigation is one in which observations are obtained serially and the conduct, design or decision on termination depend on the data so far observed. We are particularly concerned here with the possibility of early termination. *Sequential analysis* provides methods for analysing data in which the decision whether to terminate at any point depends on the data obtained. It was originally developed in pioneering work by A. Wald (1902–50).

Implicit in any sequential analysis is the concept of a *stopping rule*, defining the way in which the termination decision depends on the results obtained. A simple example arises in *sequential estimation*, where the purpose of an investigation might be to estimate a parameter to a specified level of precision. Suppose that, in a random sample of size n from a distribution with mean μ and variance σ^2, the estimated mean is $\bar{x}_n$ and the estimated standard deviation is s_n (the subscript indicating that these statistics will change randomly as n increases). The estimated standard error of $\bar{x}_n$ is $s_n/\sqrt{n}$ and, although s_n will fluctuate randomly, this standard error will tend to decrease as n increases.

A possible stopping rule for the sequential estimation of μ might therefore be to continue sampling until the standard error falls to some preassigned low value, and then to stop.

Standard methods of analysis, such as those described in the early chapters of this book, have assumed a fixed sample size, n. The question then arises whether these methods are valid for sequential studies in which n is not preassigned but depends on the accumulating data. The question can be answered at two different levels. From a frequentist point of view, the properties of a statistical procedure are affected by sequential sampling, in that the long-run properties have to be calculated for hypothetical repetitions of the data with the same sequential stopping rule rather than with the same sample size. However, for sequential estimation, as in the simple case described above, the effect is rather small. For instance, the probability that a confidence interval based on the estimated standard error covers the parameter value is not greatly affected, particularly in large samples. However, we shall see in the next subsection that other procedures, such as significance tests, may be more seriously affected.

From another standpoint we may wish to make inferences from the likelihood function, or, with a Bayesian interpretation, from the posterior distribution with some appropriate prior distribution. The stopping rule is now irrelevant, since likelihoods for different parameter values assume the same ratios whatever the stopping rule. This important result is called the *strong likelihood principle*.

In the data monitoring of a clinical trial, the case for early termination is likely to arise because there is strong evidence for an effect in favour of, or against, one treatment, and the standard way of examining such evidence in a non-sequential experiment is by means of a significance test. Suppose that a significance test to compare the mean effects of two treatments is carried out repeatedly on the accumulating data, either at the occasional meetings of a DMC or more frequently by the trial statisticians. It is easy to see that the Type I error probability exceeds the nominal level of the significance test, because the investigator has a number of opportunities to find a 'significant' effect purely by chance, if the null hypothesis is true.

This effect is similar to that of multiple comparisons (§8.4), although the two situations are conceptually somewhat different. A hypothetical example will show that the effect of repeated significance tests is not negligible.

Suppose that, in a double-masked cross-over trial (§18.9), each patient receives two analgesic drugs, A and B, in adjacent weeks, in random order. At the end of the 2-week period each patient gives a preference for the drug received in the first week or that received in the second week, on the basis of alleviation of pain. These are then decoded to form a series of preferences for A or B.

It seems reasonable to test the cumulative results at any stage to see whether there is a significant preponderance of preferences in favour of A or B. The appropriate conventional test, at the nth stage, would be that based on the binomial distribution with sample size n and with $\pi = \frac{1}{2}$ (see §4.4). Suppose the tests are carried out at the two-sided 5% significance level. The investigator, proceeding sequentially, might be inclined to stop if at some stage this significance level were reached, and to publish the results claiming a significant difference at the 5% level. Indeed, this is a correct assessment of the evidence *at this particular stage*. The likelihood principle enunciated in the last subsection shows that the relative likelihoods of different parameter values (in this case different values of π, the probability of a preference for A) are unaffected by the stopping rule. However, some selection of evidence has taken place. The investigator had a large number of opportunities to stop at the 5% level. Even if the null hypothesis is true, there is a substantial probability that a 'significant' result will be found in due course, and this probability will clearly increase the longer the trial continues.

In this example, the discrete nature of the binomial distribution means that it is impossible to get a result significant at the two-sided 5% level until $n = 6$ preferences have been recorded, and then the Type I error probability is (again because of the discreteness) less than 5%, namely 0·031. With $n = 50$, the Type I error probability has risen to 0·171, and with $n = 100$ it is 0·227. In fact, it rises continually as n increases, eventually approaching 1.

For repeated t tests on a continuous response variable, assumed to be normally distributed with unknown variance, the effect is even more striking, since the error probabilities are not reduced by discreteness. For $n = 100$, the Type I error probability is 0·39 (McPherson, 1971).

To control the Type I error probability at a low value, such as 5%, a much more stringent significance level (that is, a *lower* probability) is required for assessing the results at any one stage. Suppose that the stopping rule is to stop the trial if the cumulative results at any stage show a significant difference at the nominal two-sided $2\alpha'$ level, or to stop after N stages if the trial has not stopped earlier. To achieve a Type I error probability, 2α, of 5%, what value should be chosen for $2\alpha'$, the significance level at any one stage? The answer clearly depends on N: the larger the value of N, the smaller $2\alpha'$ must be. Some results for binomial responses, and for normally distributed responses with known variance, are shown in Table 18.2.

The choice of N, the maximum sample size in a sequential test, will depend on much the same considerations as those outlined in §4.6. In particular, as in criterion **3** of that section, one may wish to select a sequential plan which not only controls the Type I error probability, but has a specified power, say, $1 - \beta$, of providing a significant result when a certain alternative to the null hypothesis is true. In the binomial test described earlier, a particular alternative hypothesis might specify that the probability of a preference for drug A, which we denote by π, is some value π_1 different from $\frac{1}{2}$. If the sequential plan is symmetrical, it will automatically provide the same power for $\pi = \pi_{-1}(= 1 - \pi_1)$ as for π_1.

Table 18.3 shows the maximum sample sizes, and the significance levels for individual tests, for binomial sequential plans with Type I error probability $2\alpha = 0\cdot05$ and a power $1 - \beta = 0\cdot95$ against various alternative values of π. These are examples of *repeated significance test* (RST) *plans*. More extensive tables are given in Armitage (1975, Tables 3.9–3.12).

Table 18.2 Repeated significance tests on cumulative binomial and normal observations; nominal significance level to be used for individual tests for Type I error probability $2\alpha = 0\cdot05$.

Number of stages, N	Nominal significance level (two-sided), $2\alpha'$, for individual tests	
	Binomial	Normal
1	—	0·050
5	—	0·016
10	0·031	0·010
15	0·023	0·008
20	0·022	0·007
50	0·013	0·005
100	0·008	0·004
150	0·007	0·003

Table 18.3 Maximum sample size, N, and nominal significance levels for individual tests, $2\alpha'$, for binomial RST plans with Type I error probability $2\alpha = 0\cdot05$ and power $1 - \beta = 0\cdot95$ against various values of π differing from the null value of $0\cdot5$.

π_1	$2\alpha'$	N
0·95	0·0313	10
0·90	0·0225	16
0·85	0·0193	25
0·80	0·0147	38
0·75	0·0118	61
0·70	0·0081	100

We have assumed so far that sequential monitoring of the data is carried out continuously, after every new observation. This is very unlikely to be the case in any large-scale trial, where data summaries are normally prepared at intervals, in preparation for meetings of the DMC. However, the effect of periodic monitoring may be much the same as for continuous monitoring, in that, when a periodic review suggests that a termination point may be encountered in the near future, a more intensive review is likely to be conducted for new data arriving in the immediate future. In that case, the trial is likely to be terminated at the same time as if continuous monitoring had been in place.

The book by Armitage (1975) presents plans for continuous monitoring, but is largely superseded by the more comprehensive book by Whitehead (1997). The latter book also concentrates mainly on continuous monitoring, but with a wide range of data types and alternative stopping rules.

The extensive use of DMCs, with interim data analyses at a relatively small number of times, has led to the widespread use of stopping rules based on *group sequential* schemes, whereby only a small number of repeated analyses are considered. We discuss these in the next subsection.

Group sequential schemes

A group sequential plan with specified Type I error probability could be obtained as a particular case of repeated significance tests with a small value of N, with the understanding that each of the N 'observations' is now a statistic derived from a group of individual observations. We need, though, to consider a more general framework. In the schemes for repeated significance tests illustrated in Tables 18.2 and 18.3, the proviso that the nominal significance level is the same for all the individual tests is unnecessarily restrictive. Some wider possibilities are illustrated in Example 18.2.

Example 18.2

In Example 4.14 (p. 140), we determined the sample size required to achieve specified power in a comparison of means of two groups of measurements from a lung-function test. Observations were assumed to be normally distributed with known variance, and, with a two-sided significance level of 0·05, a power of 0·8 was required for an alternative hypothesis that the standardized difference in means was 0·5. (The specified difference was $\delta_1 = 0·251$, and the standard deviation was $\sigma = 0·51$, but for present purposes it is the standardized difference, δ_1/σ, that matters.) The solution was that $n = 63$ individuals were needed in each group, a total of 126. We now consider various alternative group sequential plans that provide the same power.

Table 18.4 gives details of three group sequential plans, achieving the same power requirements. They all require five equally spaced inspections of the data. The table shows the standardized normal deviate (z value), calculated from a comparison of the means of the data so far, which would indicate termination of the trial at each stage. These are plotted in Fig. 18.1, and form sequential boundaries for the z value. Alternative methods of plotting boundaries use either (i) the bounds for the parameter estimate (in this case the difference in means); or (ii) those for a cumulative sum (in this case the difference between the two totals). These are easily obtained from the bounds for z, after n' observations in each group, by multiplying by $\sigma\sqrt{(2/n')}$ and $\sigma\sqrt{(2n')}$, respectively.

The characteristics of the three schemes illustrated in Table 18.4 and Fig. 18.1 are described below.

The *Pocock* boundaries (Pocock, 1977) are based on repeated significance tests at a fixed level, as described earlier. (The z value of 2·41 shown in Table 18.4 corresponds to the two-sided nominal significance level of 0·016 shown in Table 18.2.) The bounds for z determine the Type I error probability, while the power is controlled by the terminal sample size shown in the lower part of Table 18.4. Note that the terminal sample size, 155, exceeds the fixed sample size of 126, but

Table 18.4 Three group sequential schemes for the trial described in Example 18.2. Bounds for the standardized normal deviate (z value) at interim and final inspections. Entries in this table are derived from EaSt for Windows (1999) and Geller and Pocock (1987).

	Pocock	O'Brien–Fleming	Haybittle–Peto
Interim inspection			
1	2·41	4·56	3·29
2	2·41	3·22	3·29
3	2·41	2·63	3·29
4	2·41	2·28	3·29
5	2·41	2·04	1·97
Sample size			
Terminal	155	130	126
Mean on H_0	151	129	126
Mean on H_1	101	103	113

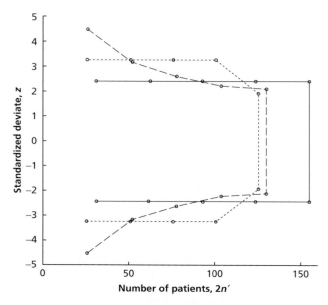

Fig. 18.1 Boundaries for three group sequential schemes with five interim inspections, as detailed in Table 18.4. (——) Pocock; (– – –) O'Brien–Fleming; (- - -) Haybittle–Peto.

if the alternative hypothesis is true (in this case a standardized difference of 0·5) the mean sample size is reduced substantially, to 101. Note also that the terminal bound for z substantially exceeds the fixed sample-size value of 1·96, so, if the trial continued to the fifth stage with a final value of z between 1·96 and 2·41, the interpretation would be difficult to explain. As Piantadosi (1997) remarks, 'this is an uncomfortable position for investigators'.

The other two schemes illustrated in Table 18.4 largely avoid this difficulty. The *O'Brien–Fleming* (OBF) scheme (O'Brien & Fleming, 1979) uses constant bounds for the cumulative sum that are very close to those appropriate for a fixed sample-size test at the final inspection. A consequence is that the bounds for z at the kth inspection ($k = 1, 2, \ldots, K$) are equal to those for the final inspection ($k = K$) multiplied by $\sqrt{(K/k)}; K = 5$ in this example. They are thus initially very wide, as shown in Table 18.4 and Fig. 18.1, and converge to final values close to those appropriate for a non-sequential test. When H_0 is true, trial results will usually lead to termination at the Kth inspection, and, as indicated by Table 18.4, the mean sample size is close to the maximum, lower for the OBF scheme than for the Pocock scheme. When H_1 is true, the two schemes have very similar properties. In some variants of OBF, the excessively wide bounds for $k = 1$ are pulled in to the standardized normal deviate corresponding to the 0·001 level, $z = 3·29$.

Haybittle (1971) and Peto *et al.* (1976) suggested that a constant, but high, value of z should be used for all the interim analyses, which (as in OBF) permits a value close to the fixed sample-size value to be used at the final stage. For a Type I error probability of 0·05, different variants of the *Haybittle–Peto* scheme use 3·29 (as in Table 18.4) or 3·00 for the interim bounds.

In choosing between these three schemes, an informal Bayesian approach may be helpful. The Pocock scheme will lead to earlier termination than the others if the treatment effect is very large. If the initial view is that such large differences are plausible, it may be wise to adopt this scheme. Otherwise, the O'Brien–Fleming or Haybittle–Peto schemes will be preferable, avoiding, as they do, undue reliance on results from a small number of early observations, and removing the ambiguity about the bound for the final inspection. Further general comments about the use of group sequential schemes are contained in the final subsection.

The schemes described so far require the number of inspections to be decided in advance, and their timing to be at equally spaced intervals. These conditions are rarely achievable. Flexibility is provided by the *alpha-spending function* approach (Lan & DeMets, 1983; Kim & DeMets, 1987; DeMets & Lan, 1994), whereby the predetermined Type I error probability can be 'spent' in a flexible way, the schedule being decided for the convenience of the DMC, although independently of the trial results.

We have assumed so far that the observations are normally distributed with known variance. This is, of course, unlikely to be true, but, as in many of the methods described in this book, the normal distribution methodology often provides a useful approximation for a wide range of other situations. However, special methods have been developed for many other data types, including binary observations and survival times. A comprehensive account of group sequential methods is given by Jennison and Turnbull (2000), and other useful surveys are those by Kittleson and Emerson (1999) and Whitehead (1999). Geller and Pocock (1987) tabulate boundaries for various schemes. Useful software is provided by EaSt for Windows (1999) and the PEST system (MPS Research Unit, 2000).

Whitehead (1997) develops a very general system of sequential designs for continuous monitoring, implemented in PEST. For the standard normal model with known variance, they possess boundaries which are linear for the cumulative sum plot. Group sequential designs are handled by providing so-called *Christmas tree corrections* to the continuous boundaries.

Stochastic curtailment

The schemes described above permit early stopping when convincing evidence arises for a difference in efficacy between treatments. The main motivation there is the ethical need to avoid the continued use of an inferior treatment.

A somewhat different situation may arise if the interim results for, say, two treatments are very similar, and when it can be predicted that the final difference would almost certainly be non-significant. Methods for curtailing a trial under these circumstances have been proposed by many authors (Schneiderman & Armitage, 1962; Lan *et al.*, 1982 (using the term *stochastic curtailment*); Ware *et al.*, 1985 (using the term *futility*); Spiegelhalter & Freedman, 1988 (using Bayesian methods)). Boundaries permitting stochastic curtailment can be incorporated into schemes permitting early stopping for efficacy effects and are easily implemented with EaSt or PEST.

Although this approach may be useful in enabling research efforts to be switched to more promising directions, there is a danger in placing too much importance on the predicted results of a final significance test. Data showing non-significant treatment effects may nevertheless be valuable for estimation, especially in contributing to meta-analyses (see §18.10). It may be unwise to terminate such studies prematurely, particularly when there is no treatment difference to provide an ethical reason for stopping.

Other considerations

The methods described in this section have been developed mainly from a non-Bayesian point of view. As indicated earlier, in the Bayesian approach the stopping rule is irrelevant to the inferences to be made at any stage. A trial could reasonably be stopped whenever the posterior distribution suggested strong evidence of a clear advantage for one treatment. This approach to the design, analysis and monitoring of clinical trials has been strongly advocated, for instance, by Berry (1987) and Spiegelhalter *et al.* (1994). Grossman *et al.* (1994) have discussed the design of group sequential trials which preserve Type I error probabilities and yet involve boundaries determined by a Bayesian formulation, the prior distribution representing initial scepticism about the possible treatment effect.

We have assumed, in describing repeated significance tests, that the null hypothesis specifies a lack of difference in efficacy between treatments. It may be useful to base a stopping rule on tests of a specific non-zero difference (Meier, 1975; Freedman *et al.*, 1984; see also §4.6, p. 140, and the discussion of equivalence trials in §18.9). All the sequential methods outlined here can be adapted by basing the boundaries on tests of the required non-zero values.

The rather bewildering variety of methods available for data monitoring can perhaps be put into perspective by the widely held view that all such rules should be treated flexibly, as guidelines rather than rigid prescriptions. Many authors would argue that a DMC should define a stopping rule at the outset, even though its implementation is flexible. Others (Armitage, 1999) have favoured a more open approach, without a formal definition of the stopping rule, but with a realization of the effect of repeated inspections of data on the Type I error. An intermediate attitude is perhaps to use the Haybittle–Peto approach, whereby differences of less than about three times their standard error are generally ignored during the interim analyses.

The reason for this sort of flexibility is that a decision to stop will usually depend on more than the analysis of a single response variable. There may be several primary endpoints, for both efficacy and safety, and, in a follow-up study, these may be measured at various times during follow-up. Effects seen at an early stage of follow-up might not persist over a longer period. Results from other relevant trials may suggest the need to terminate the current trial or amend the protocol. Changes in clinical practice or in evidence from other studies may change the views of the investigators about the importance or otherwise of significant but small effects. No single stopping rule would take account of all these features. Finally, it should be remembered that the decision whether or not to stop rests with the investigators: the DMC will make recommendations, but these need not necessarily be followed by the Steering Committee.

18.8 **Interpretation of trial results**

As noted in §18.3, the results of a clinical trial do not necessarily have an immediate impact on clinical practice. Other practitioners may have stronger prior convictions than the trial investigators, the refutation of which requires stronger evidence than that produced by the trial. Or there may be concern about long-term adverse effects or changes in efficacy. In this section we note a number of issues that affect the acceptability or interpretation of trial results.

Number needed to treat (NNT)

A new treatment may be more expensive or less acceptable to patients than a standard treatment. An important general question is whether the benefit apparently conferred by a new treatment justifies its use on the large number of patients falling into the relevant category. To some extent this should have been taken into account by the trial investigators, in designing the study, and discussed in the published report of the trial. In trials with a binary response variable, such as the incidence of stroke within a 3-year period, a useful index is available to indicate the balance between future usage and benefit.

Suppose that the probabilities of a specified adverse response in patients receiving a new or a control treatment are, respectively, π_T and π_C, estimated from the trial by p_T and p_C. Then, the number of patients needed to be treated to prevent one single adverse outcome (the NNT) is $1/(\pi_C - \pi_T)$, and this is estimated by $1/(p_C - p_T)$. Note that this is the reciprocal of the absolute risk reduction, and is not expressible purely in terms of the relative risk reduction.

A trial showing a large relative risk reduction (i.e. small ratio p_T/p_C) may nevertheless have a large estimated NNT, because both these proportions are small, and therefore be judged to be of limited value. Conversely (as in Example 18.3 below) the relative risk reduction may be small, and yet the NNT may be seen to justify widespread use of the new treatment.

Since the absolute risk reduction will be approximately normally distributed, unless the numbers of events are very small, its reciprocal, the NNT, will have a distribution with very long tails, which cannot be assumed to be approximately normal. Any calculations of sampling error are best performed first for the absolute reduction $p_C - p_T$ and then converted to the reciprocal scale if necessary (Lesaffre & Pledger, 1999). For example, confidence limits for the difference can be calculated by standard methods (§4.5), and their reciprocals used as confidence limits for the NNT.

Example 18.3

The Fourth International Study of Infarct Survival (ISIS-4) Collaborative Group (1995), reporting results of a large-scale trial of treatments for patients with suspected acute myocardial infarction (MI), combined these results with those from other relevant trials (see §18.10). In one such overview, the authors analysed mortality during the first month after onset for patients receiving converting enzyme inhibitors (CEI) and those in a control group. The numbers of deaths and patients treated were 3671/50 496 (7·27%) in the CEI group, and 3903/50 467 (7·73%) in the control group. The proportions of deaths are small but similar, and the relative risk is 0·94, close to unity. The trial population is sufficiently large to ensure that the difference is highly significant ($P = 0·006$).

Here, $p_C - p_T = 0·07734 - 0·07270 = 0·00464$, with a standard error of 0·00166. Hence, the NNT estimate is $1/0·00464 = 216$. The authors comment that 'such treatment saves about 5 lives per 1000 treated'.

The 95% confidence limits for the difference in proportions, using the normal approximation, are:

$$0·00464 \pm (1·96)(0·00166) = 0·00139 \text{ and } 0·00789,$$

with corresponding limits for NNT of

$$1/0·00789 = 127 \text{ and } 1/0·00139 = 719.$$

Note the asymmetry and extent of the confidence interval for the NNT. Even with such a large data set, the NNT cannot be determined at all precisely.

Bayesian considerations

Medical practitioners and others reading the report of a clinical trial may well have had different prior assessments of possible treatment effects from those of the trial investigators, and so, from a Bayesian point of view, their posterior assessments would also be expected to differ. Many authors have advocated that trial results should be reported in terms of the likelihood function, so that readers can arrive at their own posterior probabilities by applying their own prior distributions. Results reported by the usual frequentist methods—for instance, with point estimates and standard errors or confidence limits—can, if necessary, be translated into likelihood statements, at least approximately, by the use of normal approximations.

Some authors have presented a more general, and more sceptical, argument based on the (largely unsubstantiated) premise that most new treatments are really ineffective. It would follow from this that a high proportion of apparently positive findings from clinical trials (i.e. those favouring a new treatment) are false positives, thrown up by the play of chance. Very similar arguments are relevant to the assessment of findings from diagnostic tests, discussed further in §19.9.

The argument can be described by a very simple (and rather unrealistic) model. Suppose that new treatments are categorized as 'effective' or 'ineffective', in comparison with a control, and that trial results are categorized as 'positive' or 'negative', according to whether they show a difference significant at some acceptable level. Suppose further that the proportion of trials with an effective treatment is θ, and that the Type I and Type II error probabilities (averaged over all trials) are, respectively, α and β. Then the overall probability of a positive finding is

$$\theta(1 - \beta) + (1 - \theta)\alpha = \theta(1 - \alpha - \beta) + \alpha,$$

and the probability that, in a trial with a positive finding, the new treatment is really *ineffective* is

$$\frac{(1 - \theta)\alpha}{\theta(1 - \alpha - \beta) + \alpha}, \tag{18.2}$$

which approaches unity as θ approaches zero. Equation (18.2) is a posterior probability in a Bayesian model with prior probabilities θ and $1 - \theta$ and likelihoods α, $1 - \alpha$, β and $1 - \beta$. In the analogous theory of diagnostic tests (§19.9), (18.2) represents 1 minus the *predictive value of a positive test*.

The rather pessimistic conclusion drawn here, for the situation where θ is very small, can be put into context by noting that, if this were the case, the proportion of trials with negative outcomes would be

$$\theta\beta + (1 - \theta)(1 - \alpha) = \theta(\alpha + \beta - 1) + (1 - \alpha),$$

which is approximately $1 - \alpha$ (i.e. nearly 1) when θ is very small. That is, a very high proportion of trials conducted would have negative outcomes. This does not appear to be the case in general, although it may be almost true in some branches of medicine in which improvements in therapy are hard to find.

Publication bias

The dissemination of trial results is sometimes thwarted by failure to publish the report. Unfortunately, failure to publish is more likely if the trial is small and the results are negative (i.e. not showing a difference in efficacy), or if a new treatment seems to be worse than a standard, than if differences are claimed in favour of a new treatment. This *publication bias* is partly due to the diminished enthusiasm of the investigators, and partly to the reluctance of editors to publish negative findings. Publication bias has been studied by Begg and Berlin (1988), Easterbrook *et al.* (1991), Dickersin and Min (1993) and others. The effect is that published information from trials on any specific issue is biased in favour of a non-zero effect.

This effect is particularly important in meta-analysis (§18.10), where results of trials are combined. It is potentially important also for research topics covered by a very small number of published trials. A single trial showing a positive result would be much less convincing if it were known that non-confirmatory evidence was contained in one or more unpublished reports. It is desirable that the results of every Phase III trial should be published, irrespective of the outcome. Investigators should be encouraged to seek publication of negative results, and publishers should be encouraged to find ways of presenting them, if only in abbreviated form. Matthews (2000) reports that *The Lancet* is willing to review draft papers before a trial is conducted, with a guarantee that papers accepted at this stage will be published after completion of the trial, irrespective of outcome.

Methods for detecting, and correcting for, publication bias are summarized briefly in §18.10.

Surrogacy

In trials where the most relevant response measurement requires long follow-up (as with survival time), or is expensive to administer, it is tempting to replace it by a simpler and more immediately available measure. This may be a biological marker, or one based on signs or symptoms. The hope is that inferences about treatment effects on the intermediate response variable may be valid also for the (unobserved) clinical outcome. If this is true, the intermediate response may be regarded as a *surrogate* for the final clinical response.

Unfortunately, this assumption may be untrue. For patients receiving any one treatment, the two responses may be highly correlated. Nevertheless, unless the two are on precisely the same physiological pathway, a change of treatment may affect one and not the other. In the study of patients with human immunodeficiency virus (HIV) disease, the progression of the disease, involving symptoms of acquired immune deficiency syndrome (AIDS), is related to the fall in the CD4 cell count. A trial to assess the effect of treatments on disease progression and survival will inevitably involve long follow-up, and it would be convenient if the assessment period could be shortened by reliance on changes in CD4. Unfortunately, CD4 is not an effective surrogate. The Concorde Coordinating Committee (1994) reported results of a large-scale trial to compare two policies of zidovudine (AZT) treatment for symptom-free persons infected with HIV: immediate versus deferred treatment. The trial showed clear evidence that immediate treatment reduced CD4 counts, but there was little difference in progression rates, and the death rate was somewhat (although not significantly) lower in the group receiving deferred treatment. Fleming *et al.* (1998) quote several other examples of ineffective surrogacy.

   The adequacy of a possible surrogate response can only be studied in a trial in which both the intermediate and clinical responses are measured. If adequacy is thought to have been established in such a trial, comparing treatments A and B, say, the question will arise whether it can be assumed to hold for any other treatment comparisons for the same category of patients. It will be difficult to be confident about this, unless clear biological evidence for the pathways involved is available. It would seem necessary to establish the adequacy for several such treatment comparisons in different trials, before relying on the intermediate response alone.

   Prentice (1989) proposed a general approach to the question whether an intermediate response x is an adequate surrogate for a final response y. It is first necessary that x and y are correlated. Secondly, any treatment effect on y must be mediated through x, in the sense that for a given value of x the treatment effect on y is zero. In practice it may be hard to establish whether these conditions are satisfied. Effectively, they imply that an analysis of covariance of y on x will show no treatment effect. In any one trial, there will be random error, partly due to biological variation and partly to measurement error, and the treatment effect corrected for the covariance may have a large sampling error. There may also be uncertainty about the appropriate model for the relationship between x and y. However, this type of analysis may rule out the possibility of surrogacy (if there is a clear treatment effect after the covariance adjustment), or, if the corrected effect is small or non-significant, it may suggest the need for confirmatory studies from other trials.

18.9 **Special designs**

Cross-over trials

Almost all the earlier discussions have concerned parallel-group trials, in which subjects are allocated to one, and only one, treatment group. On the general principles of experimental design (§9.1), one would expect that treatments could be compared with greater precision if more than one could be administered on different occasions to the same individual. Treatments would then be assessed against within-subject random error, which would be expected to be less than between-subject error. An additional advantage would be economy in the number of subjects, since each subject would provide more than one observation. A design in which treatments are given in sequence to each subject is called a *cross-over* (or, in many non-medical applications, *change-over*) design.

In many, perhaps most, clinical trials, such a design would be infeasible, because the treatments are intended to produce irreversible changes in the patient's health, or because they must be administered for long periods of time. A cross-over design is most suitable for treatments intended for rapid relief of symptoms in chronic diseases, where the long-term condition of the patient remains fairly stable. The design is used extensively for Phase I and Phase II studies, and for equivalence trials (see below).

Extensive accounts of cross-over trials are given in the books by Jones and Kenward (1989), Ratkowsky *et al.* (1993) and Senn (1993), in several articles in a special issue of *Statistical Methods in Medical Research* (1994, Volume 3, No. 4), and in the article by Senn (1998).

The simple cross-over design

In the simplest case, with two treatments, A and B, one randomly chosen group of patients (group I) receives treatments in the order AB, while the other group (group II) receives them in the order BA. There may be different numbers of patients in the two groups. The design is variously called the *simple cross-over*, the *two-treatment, two-period design* or the *AB/BA design*.

The design has the following layout:

	Run-in	Period 1	Wash-out	Period 2
Reading	z_{ij}	y_{ij1}		y_{ij2}
Group I (n_1)	—	A	—	B
Group II (n_2)	—	B	—	A

Here, the 'readings' are observations of some appropriate measure of the patient's condition (e.g. respiratory test measurement, frequency of attacks of some sort, etc.). The two periods of administration are separated by a 'wash-out' period to enable the patient's condition to return to a level uninfluenced as far as possible by the treatment previously received. (In a drug trial, for instance, it should be long enough to allow for virtual elimination of a drug used in period 1.) The 'run-in' period is optional, but it may provide an opportunity for the patients to settle down and for the investigator to make a 'baseline' observation z_{ij}. The responses y_{ij1} and y_{ij2} will often be made towards the end of the treatment periods, to allow maximal effect of the treatments, but they may be averages or maxima of a series of observations taken throughout the periods. Observations may also be made at the end of the wash-out period, immediately before period 2, or after period 2.

The notation for the readings is as follows: the subscript i indicates the group, sometimes also called the 'sequence' ($i = 1$ for group I, $i = 2$ for group II); j identifies the subject within the group; the final subscript indicates the first or second response. The crucial measurements are the active responses y_{ij1} and y_{ij2}, but, as we shall see, the baseline readings z_{ij} may also be useful.

We first assume a simple additive model for the active responses:

$$y_{ijk} = \alpha_{ik} + \xi_{ij} + \varepsilon_{ijk}, \qquad (18.3)$$

where the α term is common to all subjects in a particular group and particular period, and depends on the treatment received, the ξ term is a characteristic of the individual subject, and the ε term is a random error, which we shall initially assume to be distributed as $N(0, \sigma^2)$. The question now is: how does the α term reflect the effects of group, period and treatment? Our model for α_{ik} is as follows:

	Period 1	Period 2	
Group I (AB)	$\mu + \tau_A + \pi_1$	$\mu + \tau_B + \pi_2 + \gamma_{AB}$	(18.4)
Group II (BA)	$\mu + \tau_B + \pi_1$	$\mu + \tau_A + \pi_2 + \gamma_{BA}$	

Here, μ is a general mean, the τ terms represent treatment effects, the π terms represent period effects, and the γ terms represent the treatment $\times$ period interaction. We shall discuss the interaction term later, but for the moment we shall use the model with merely main effects; that is, we assume that the two γ terms are both zero.

It is possible to analyse such data by an analysis of variance (Hills & Armitage, 1979), although when n_1 and n_2 are unequal the analysis becomes a little more complex. It is, in fact, easier to use t tests, as illustrated by Example 18.4.

Example 18.4

In a clinical trial for a new drug for the treatment of enuresis, each of 29 patients was given the drug for a period of 14 days and a placebo for a separate period of 14 days, the order of administration being chosen randomly for each patient. Table 18.5 shows the number of dry nights experienced during each treatment period.

A test for the relative efficacy of drug and placebo could be obtained from the complete series of 29 paired observations. We should need the 29 differences for (drug − placebo). For group I these are the (period 1− period 2) differences d_{1j} shown in Table 18.5. For group II we should need to change the sign of the differences d_{2j}. Writing $d_{1j}{}^* = d_{1j}$ and $d_{2j}{}^* = -d_{2j}$, we can do a t test on the 29 values of $d_{ij}{}^*$. This gives

Table 18.5 Number of dry nights out of 14 nights experienced by patients with enuresis treated by drug and placebo.

Group I

Period:	1	2		
Treatment:	A (drug)	B (placebo)	Difference	Sum
Patient			(1 − 2)	(1 + 2)
number, j	y_{1j1}	y_{1j2}	d_{1j}	s_{1j}
1	8	5	3	13
2	14	10	4	24
3	8	0	8	8
4	9	7	2	16
5	11	6	5	17
6	3	5	−2	8
7	6	0	6	6
8	0	0	0	0
9	13	12	1	25
10	10	2	8	12
11	7	5	2	12
12	13	13	0	26
13	8	10	−2	18
14	7	7	0	14
15	9	0	9	9
16	10	6	4	16
17	2	2	0	4

Group II

Period:	1	2		
Treatment:	B (placebo)	A (drug)	Difference	Sum
Patient			(1 − 2)	(1 + 2)
number, j	y_{2j1}	y_{2j2}	d_{2j}	s_{2j}
1	12	11	1	23
2	6	8	−2	14
3	13	9	4	22
4	8	8	0	16
5	8	9	−1	17
6	4	8	−4	12
7	8	14	−6	22
8	2	4	−2	6
9	8	13	−5	21
10	9	7	2	16
11	7	10	−3	17
12	7	6	1	13

$$\bar{d}* = 2{\cdot}172$$

$$s^2 = 11{\cdot}005$$

$$\mathrm{SE}(\bar{d}*) = \sqrt{(11{\cdot}005/29)} = 0{\cdot}616$$

$$t = \bar{d}*/\mathrm{SE}(\bar{d}*) = 3{\cdot}53 \text{ on 28 DF} \quad (P = 0{\cdot}001).$$

This analysis suggests strongly that the drug increases the number of dry nights as compared with the placebo. However, it is unsatisfactory as it takes no account of the order in which each patient received the two treatments. This might be particularly important if there were a systematic period effect—for example, if patients tended to obtain better relief in period 1 than in period 2.

The mean responses in the two periods for the two groups are as follows:

Period	1	2	Difference (1 − 2)
Group I: Treatment	A $\bar{y}_{11} = 8{\cdot}118$	B $\bar{y}_{12} = 5{\cdot}294$	$\bar{d}_1 = 2{\cdot}824$
Group II: Treatment	B $\bar{y}_{21} = 7{\cdot}667$	A $\bar{y}_{22} = 8{\cdot}917$	$\bar{d}_2 = -1{\cdot}250$

To test for the presence of a treatment effect, we can test the difference between $\bar{d}_1$ and $\bar{d}_2$, since, from (18.4), ignoring interaction terms, $\mathrm{E}(\bar{d}_1 - \bar{d}_2) = 2(\tau_\mathrm{A} - \tau_\mathrm{B})$. This comparison involves a two-sample t test, giving

$$t = (\bar{d}_1 - \bar{d}_2)/\mathrm{SE}(\bar{d}_1 - \bar{d}_2) \text{ on } n_1 + n_2 - 2 \text{ DF},$$

where

$$\mathrm{SE}(\bar{d}_1 - \bar{d}_2) = \sqrt{\left[s_d^2\left(\frac{1}{n_1} + \frac{1}{n_2}\right)\right]},$$

and s_d^2 is the pooled within-groups estimate of variance of the d_{ij}. In this example, $\bar{d}_1 - \bar{d}_2 = 4{\cdot}074$, $s_d^2 = 10{\cdot}767$ and $\mathrm{SE}(\bar{d}_1 - \bar{d}_2) = 1{\cdot}237$, giving $t = 4{\cdot}074/1{\cdot}237 = 3{\cdot}29$ on 27 DF $(P = 0{\cdot}003)$. The result is close to that given by the earlier, crude, analysis.

If there is a treatment effect, the expectation of the difference $\bar{d}_1 - \bar{d}_2$ will, from (18.4), be $2(\tau_\mathrm{A} - \tau_\mathrm{B})$. The treatment effect $\tau_\mathrm{A} - \tau_\mathrm{B}$ is therefore estimated as $\frac{1}{2}(\bar{d}_1 - \bar{d}_2) = 2{\cdot}037$ dry nights out of 14, and its standard error as $\frac{1}{2}\mathrm{SE}(\bar{d}_1 - \bar{d}_2) = 0{\cdot}618$. The 95% confidence interval for the treatment effect is thus $2{\cdot}037 \pm (2{\cdot}052)(0{\cdot}618) = 0{\cdot}77$ to $3{\cdot}31$ days. The multiplier here is $t_{27,\,0{\cdot}05} = 2{\cdot}052$.

To test for a period effect, we use $\bar{d}_1 + \bar{d}_2$, since, from (18.4), ignoring interaction terms, $\mathrm{E}(\bar{d}_1 + \bar{d}_2) = 2(\pi_1 - \pi_2)$. The same standard error is used as for $\bar{d}_1 - \bar{d}_2$. In the example, this gives $t = 1{\cdot}574/1{\cdot}237 = 1{\cdot}27$ on 27 DF $(P = 0{\cdot}21)$, providing no evidence of a period effect.

Treatment × period interaction, and carry-over

The analysis illustrated in Example 18.4 assumes that the response is affected additively by treatment and period effects, i.e. that there is no treatment × period (TP) interaction. The terms γ_{AB} and γ_{BA} in (18.4) represent such an interaction. Note that it is only their difference that matters: if these two terms were equal they could be absorbed into the period parameter π_2 and we should be back with the no-interaction model. There are various possible reasons for an interaction:

1 If the wash-out period is too short, the response in period 2 may be affected by the treatment received in period 1 as well as that in period 2.

2 Even if the wash-out period is sufficiently long for a period 1 drug to be eliminated, its psychological or physiological effect might persist into period 2.

3 If there is a strong period effect, changing the general level of response from period 1 to period 2, the treatment effect might be changed merely because it varies with different portions of the scale of measurement.

A test for the existence of a TP interaction may be obtained as follows. Denote the sum of the two responses for subject j in group i by

$$s_{ij} = y_{ij1} + y_{ij2}.$$

If there is no TP interaction, the expectation of s_{ij} for this subject is, from (18.3) and (18.4), $2\mu + \xi_{ij} + (\tau_A + \tau_B) + (\pi_1 + \pi_2)$. Since the subjects were assigned randomly, the ξ_{ij} can be taken to be randomly distributed with the same mean (which can be taken as zero, since the overall mean is accounted for by the term μ in (18.4)), and a variance σ_0^2, say. The expectations of s_{1j} and s_{2j} are thus equal. If, on the other hand, there is a TP interaction, the expectations will differ: if $\gamma_{AB} > \gamma_{BA}$, for instance, as might happen if the two treatments had different carry-over effects, the expectation of s_{1j} will exceed that of s_{2j}. We can therefore test the difference between the two mean values of s_{ij}, $\bar{s}_1$ and $\bar{s}_2$, again using a two-sample t test. Here, however, the within-group variance estimate s_s^2 is that of the s_{ij}, not (as before) the d_{ij}. Since the s_{ij} vary in part because of the variability between subjects, we should expect $s_s^2 > s_d^2$.

Example 18.4, continued

The values of s_{ij} are given in Table 18.5. The two means are $\bar{s}_1 = 13\cdot412, \bar{s}_2 = 16\cdot583$. The pooled variance estimate is $s_s^2 = 41\cdot890$ (substantially larger than s_d^2, as expected) and

$$\text{SE}(\bar{s}_1 - \bar{s}_2) = \sqrt{\left[(41\cdot890)\left(\frac{1}{17} + \frac{1}{12}\right)\right]} = 2\cdot440.$$

Thus, $t = (13\cdot412 - 16\cdot583)/2\cdot440 = -1\cdot30$ on 27 DF ($P = 0\cdot20$). There is no clear evidence of a TP interaction, and the earlier analysis therefore seems reasonable.

If there is a TP interaction, there will usually be little point in testing and estimating the treatment effect from the whole set of data, as in Example 18.4. Period 1 alone provides a perfectly valid test of A versus B, since subjects were assigned randomly to the two treatments. Period 2 is of doubtful value, since the subjects (although originally randomized) have undergone different experiences before entering period 2. A reasonable procedure might therefore seem to be to estimate the treatment effect from the difference between the two means, $\bar{y}_{11} - \bar{y}_{21}$. Unfortunately, there are a number of difficulties about this approach.

1   The comparison of the two period 1 means is subject to between-subject variation, and is therefore less precise than the full crossover approach.

2   The test for the TP interaction, based on $\bar{s}_1 - \bar{s}_2$, is also affected by between-subject variation. A substantial, and important, TP interaction may therefore exist but fail to be detected as significant. The loss in precision, both here and in the treatment comparison in **1**, may be mitigated by use of the baseline (run-in) readings, z_{ij}, which can either be subtracted from the observations made during the treatment periods or used as covariates.

3   The implication has been that a two-stage procedure would be applied: the TP interaction is tested, and if it is significant the treatment effect is tested and estimated from period 1; if TP is not significant the usual crossover analysis is used. Freeman (1989) pointed out that this would have an important consequence. If the null hypothesis is true, so that the treatment and TP effects are zero, and all tests are done at, say, the 5% level, the overall Type I error probability can be as high as 9·5%. If TP effects are non-zero, the inflation of Type I error can be much greater. The reason for this inflation is that the null hypothesis can be rejected at either of the two stages. Moreover, when TP is significant purely by chance (implying an unbalanced outcome of the randomization) it is quite likely that the period 1 difference will also be significant, since the two test statistics are positively correlated.

4   For much the same reason, if there is a non-zero TP effect, the estimate of treatment effect will be biased in the subset of cases when the period 1 estimate is used, and therefore biased overall. If there is no TP effect, the bias disappears.

These considerations have cast serious doubt on the two-stage approach to the simple crossover. The inflation of Type I error probability is not too serious if the user is made aware: it is a consequence of many other situations in which different tests are used in sequential order. On the other hand, the interpretation of the results may clearly be difficult, and much of the advantage of the crossover, in economizing in the number of subjects required, may have been lost. The best advice is to avoid this simple design unless the user is confident that the TP interaction is negligible. Such confidence may be provided by the results of similar studies conducted in the past, or from pharmacokinetic considerations in cases where the two preparations are chemically very similar. Grieve (1994) has described a Bayesian approach to this problem.

Extended designs

The two-treatment, two-period design can be extended by the use of more than two sequence groups, treatments or periods, or by combinations of these. These larger designs provide the opportunity to compare several treatments or to cover longer sequences of treatment changes. They may also help to remove some of the ambiguities of the simple design by permitting the assumptions underlying the model to be more rigorously tested.

The four combinations of groups, periods and treatments in a simple cross-over can be thought of as forming a 2×2 Latin square, with replication provided by the individual subjects. An obvious extension is to use a larger Latin square when there are more than two treatments. Some Latin squares are balanced for residual effects of earlier treatments, and have been used in agricultural research. They are due mainly to E.J. Williams and are described by Cochran and Cox (1957, §4.6a).

Examples of the use of cross-over designs with more than two periods are given by Ebbutt (1984) (for a trial with two treatments, but four periods and sequences), McCrory and Matthews (1990) and Woffindin *et al.* (1992).

For full accounts of extended designs, the reader should consult the books listed at the start of this section and the article by Matthews (1994). A few general points may be made here.

1 The extension to more than two periods and/or treatments provides more degrees of freedom for the TP interaction. It is usual to assume that this can be explained mainly by the effect of carry-over, and most of the literature concentrates on these carry-over effects.

2 The usual assumption is that each treatment has a unique carry-over effect on the next treatment period. This has been criticized—for example, by Fleiss (1989) and Senn (1993)—as being unduly simplistic. For example, the carry-over might extend to more than one subsequent period; its effect might depend on the current, as well as the previous, treatment; and it might be reasonable to assume that the carry-over effect of a particular treatment was related to its direct effect.

3 If the model with direct treatment and period effects and one-period carry-over effects is valid, extended designs permit the estimation and testing of the carry-over effects to be made within subjects. Also, the direct treatment effects can be estimated within subjects, even in the presence of carry-over. The main problem of the simple cross-over is thus overcome.

4 In the simple cross-over, the within-subject random error was assumed to be independently distributed for different observations. In a design with more

than two periods, the possibility must be allowed that the error terms are serially correlated, as in other longitudinal studies (§12.6). Unfortunately, a single cross-over trial is likely to be too small a data set to enable the nature of the serial correlation to be established at all precisely.

5   For any particular specification of the numbers of treatments, periods and sequence groups, there will be many alternative designs to choose from. Much research has been devoted to the establishment of optimal designs, providing maximum precision in the estimation of treatment comparisons. Since optimality depends on many of the unknown features discussed here, such as the nature of carry-over and serial correlation, it is difficult to arrive at clear recommendations. One such recommendation might be to do one's best to avoid carry-over by providing long wash-out periods, and making use of external information about the duration needed to achieve this aim.

Other response variables

The discussion so far has assumed that the response variable is continuous and can be regarded as normally distributed. Most research on extended designs makes this assumption. Most of the points about design strategy, made above, apply also for non-normal response data, although special methods have been devised for some standard situations. Tudor and Koch (1994) describe non-parametric methods, and Kenward and Jones (1994) describe models for binary and ordinal categorical data, based mainly on the logistic transform.

n-of-1 trials

In any clinical trial, patients may have different treatment effects; that is, there may be a subject $\times$ treatment interaction. In a parallel-groups trial, this cannot be isolated from the random error, although it may be possible to detect interactions between treatments and specific subgroups of subjects.

In an extended cross-over design, it may be possible in principle to see whether the treatment effects differ between subjects, although this is not commonly done. In the simple cross-over, this is not possible, as the patient $\times$ treatment interaction is absorbed into the within-subject error term.

The n-of-1 trial (Guyatt et al., 1990) is an attempt to obtain a reliable estimate of a treatment effect separately for each subject. In most clinical situations this is unlikely to be possible without considerable replication, which implies a rather long series of treatment changes. This, in turn, introduces the possibility that the treatment effect changes with time and increases the risk of withdrawal from the trial.

The simplest, and perhaps most satisfactory, design is to assign treatments in an entirely random order. The successive readings can then be regarded as independent, and can be analysed by standard methods, such as a two-sample t test. If the serial observations are subject to trend or to serial correlation, the effects of these disturbances will be reflected by inflation of the random error. If necessary, the effect of trend could be reduced by a systematic design such as permuted blocks, each containing a random permutation of the treatments. However, such designs make it more difficult to impose masking of treatment identity, and this may be particularly important in a single-patient trial requiring a high level of patient cooperation. The use of permutation tests (§10.6) in such circumstances is discussed by Senn (1993, §7.4.2).

In general, it seems unlikely that n-of-1 trials can be conducted on a sufficiently wide scale to provide personal guidance on treatment choice for all patients, and it is therefore likely that this choice will usually be made on the basis of evidence provided by orthodox trials on groups of patients.

Equivalence trials

The aim in an *equivalence trial* is not to detect possible differences in efficacy, but rather to show that treatments are, within certain narrow limits, equally effective. This need arises in two different contexts. A *bioequivalence trial* is a Phase I study, conducted within the pharmaceutical industry, to compare two different formulations or methods of administration of a drug. The intention is that the formulations should be regarded as interchangeable. The response variable will be based on pharmacokinetic studies, where, for each subject, the plasma concentration of the drug is measured during a short period after administration and some key feature of the concentration–time curve, such as the area under the curve, is recorded. Such variables are often skewly distributed, and a log transformation may simplify the analysis. Requirements are often based on the ratio of the pharmacokinetic responses for different formulations, and these can conveniently be expressed in terms of the difference between the means of the logarithmic transforms, which are required to lie within certain limits. Bioequivalence trials usually involve very small numbers of subjects and often follow a simple cross-over design, with suitable precautions to avoid carry-over.

The other scenario is a trial to compare the efficacies of two therapeutic regimes, where a new treatment, T, is compared against a standard, S. Interest centres on whether the response for S differs from that for T by less than some small margin. The comparison may be one-sided, in that a small disadvantage to T may be tolerated because it produces less severe side-effects than S, or is otherwise more acceptable, whereas no limit need be placed on a possible advantage of T over S; the term *non-inferiority trial* is often used for this situation.

An important point is that a test of the null hypothesis of zero difference is completely irrelevant, partly because a small non-zero true difference may be quite acceptable as being within the tolerated range of equivalence, but also because a non-significant result gives no indication as to whether or not the true difference lies within the tolerated interval.

Suppose the parameter θ measures the difference in efficacy between T and S, with high values favouring T. In a two-sided equivalence trial, the limits of equivalence may be denoted by $\theta_L < 0$ and $\theta_U > 0$. The investigator will be in a position to claim equivalence if it can be asserted that θ lies within the range (θ_L, θ_U). A simple approach is to assert equivalence if an appropriate confidence interval for θ lies wholly within this range.

Suppose that, for this purpose, we use $100(1 - 2\alpha)\%$ confidence limits; e.g. 95% limits would have $\alpha = 0.025$. An equivalent approach would be to carry out significance tests using each of the equivalence limits for the null hypothesis:

1   Test the null hypothesis H_L that $\theta = \theta_L$ against the one-sided alternative that $\theta > \theta_L$, with one-sided significance level α.
2   Test the null hypothesis H_U that $\theta = \theta_U$ against the one-sided alternative that $\theta < \theta_U$, with one-sided significance level α.

Equivalence is asserted if and only if *both* these null hypotheses are rejected. For a non-inferiority trial, only test **1** is necessary, and this corresponds to the requirement that a one-sided $100(1 - \alpha)\%$ confidence interval, extending to plus infinity, falls wholly to the right of θ_L.

A Bayesian interpretation

A Bayesian formulation for equivalence might require that the posterior probabilities that $\theta < \theta_L$ and that $\theta > \theta_U$ are *both* less than some small value α. With the usual assumptions of a non-informative prior and a normally distributed estimator, this is equivalent to the frequentist approach given above. For a non-inferiority trial, only the first of these two requirements is needed.

A slightly less rigorous Bayesian requirement would be that the posterior probability that θ lies within the equivalence range (θ_L, θ_U) is $1 - 2\alpha$. This is slightly more lenient towards equivalence than the previous approach, since an estimate near the upper limit of θ_U might give a posterior probability for exceeding that bound which was rather greater than α, and yet equivalence would be conceded because the probability that $\theta < \theta_L$ was very small and the total probability outside the range was still less than 2α. The frequentist analogue of this approach is a proposal by Westlake (1979) that a $100(1 - 2\alpha)\%$ confidence interval should be centred around the mid-point of the range, rather than about the parameter estimate. This would be equivalent to doing separate tests of H_L and H_U at the one-sided α level when the estimate is near the centre of the range, but a test of the nearest limit at the one-sided 2α level when the estimate is near that limit.

Sample size

The determination of sample size for an equivalence trial follows similar principles to those used in §4.6, with the subtle difference that the role of the null hypothesis is assumed by the hypotheses H_L and H_U, representing the borders of non-equivalence, while the alternative hypothesis is that θ lies within the range of equivalence (θ_L, θ_U).

We assume that the trial involves two groups, with n subjects in each, that the individual observations are normally distributed with variance σ^2, and that the estimate of treatment effect, d, is the difference between the two sample means, distributed as $N(\theta, 2\sigma^2/n)$. Assume for simplicity that the limits of equivalence are equally spaced around zero, so that $\theta_L = -\delta$, say, and $\theta_U = \delta$.

The determination of sample size requires specifications for Type I and Type II error probabilities. The Type I error is that of asserting equivalence when the treatments are not equivalent. This will be at a maximum when $\theta = \pm\delta$, when it becomes the Type I error probability, α, of the one-sided significance tests **1** and **2** above. The Type II error is that of failing to assert equivalence when the treatments are in fact equivalent. This will depend on the value of θ: when θ is just inside the range, the Type II error probability will be almost $1 - \alpha$, and it decreases to a minimum of, say, 2β, when $\theta = 0$. (Here, $1 - \beta$ is the power of either significance test against the alternative hypothesis that $\theta = 0$, but the Type II error can apply to either test, so its probability is doubled and the power becomes $1 - 2\beta$. This step is not required for a non-inferiority trial, since only one hypothesis is tested.) We shall, therefore, specify the values α and β and seek the value of n required.

As in (4.41),

$$n = 2\left[\frac{(z_{2\alpha} + z_{2\beta})\sigma}{\delta}\right]^2. \tag{18.5}$$

This can be used for either equivalence or non-inferiority trials, provided that the probabilities 2α and 2β are correctly interpreted, as indicated in the last paragraph.

The use of (18.5) provides an approximate framework for non-normal response variables and other designs. For a simple cross-over design, for instance, the variance $2\sigma^2/n$ for the estimated treatment effect, d, is replaced by the appropriate formula from the theory given earlier in this section. For binary responses, σ^2 is replaced by $\pi(1 - \pi)$, where π is a rough estimate of the overall probability of a positive response.

Example 18.5

A trial of laparoscopic hernia repair (LHR) in comparison with conventional hernia repair (CHR) is being planned. With conventional repair about 5% of patients will have a recurrence of their hernia within 5 years, due to breakdown of the repair. How many patients are required to demonstrate that the breakdown rate with LHR is at most 5% higher than with CHR (i.e. increased to at most 10%)?

This is a non-inferiority trial, and accords with the account above if we work with the non-breakdown rate (0·95 for LHR) and set $\delta = 0·05$. We might require that a one-sided 95% confidence interval should exclude a difference of 0·05, giving $2\alpha = 0·10$; and seek a power of 80% if there is no efficacy difference, giving $2\beta = 0·40$. The number of patients in each group is, from (18.5),

$$2(0·95)(0·05)\left(\frac{1·645 + 0·842}{0·05}\right)^2 = 235.$$

Thus a total of 470 patients would be required. As in other sample-size calculations, the result depends on rather arbitrary choices of probability levels and other parameters, and should be regarded as a guideline rather than a precise prescription.

Machin *et al.* (1997) give tables for sample-size determination in equivalence trials.

Cluster randomization

We have assumed so far that subjects are individually randomized to different treatment groups. In some situations it may be more convenient to consider clusters into which individuals fall naturally, and to assign treatments at random to the clusters rather than to the individuals. Some examples are as follows.

1 In a comparison of immunization schedules for application in rural communities, it may be convenient to apply the same schedule to all the inhabitants of a particular village. A similar plan was adopted for a trial of vitamin A supplementation for preschool children in Indonesia (Sommer *et al.*, 1986).

2 In a comparison of particular health strategies for urban schoolchildren, it may be more convenient to apply the same strategy to all the children in a particular school, or perhaps use the class as the relevant cluster.

3 An approach to the treatment of sexually transmitted diseases in rural communities involved a programme of enhanced training of staff, improved laboratory facilities and more reliable supply of drugs (Grosskurth *et al.*, 1995). In a comparison of this programme with a control scheme, the natural cluster is the health centre.

4 The Community Intervention Trial for Smoking Cessation (COMMIT) randomized 22 North American communities in a community-based trial (Gail *et al.*, 1992).

This approach is variously called *cluster randomization, group randomization*, or *community-based intervention*. Variants in the design of these studies include the use of matched pairs of clusters, based on the similarity of baseline variables;

and the restriction of response measurements to a random sample of individuals in each cluster, rather than the whole cluster population.

The most important point about cluster randomization is that, although response measurements may be made on individual subjects, the treatment comparisons are less precise than they would be if subjects were individually randomized. The reason is that responses of subjects within the same cluster are likely to be positively correlated. In the extreme case of perfect correlation, the advantage of replication within clusters is completely lost, so that the effective sample size is the number of clusters rather than the number of subjects. Essentially the same point arises with two-stage sampling (§19.2).

Suppose that there are $2K$ clusters, to be assigned randomly to two treatments, with K clusters in each, and that the ith cluster contains n_i individuals, with a total sample size $N = \Sigma n_i$ for each treatment. It can be shown that the variance of the overall mean response in either group is inflated by a factor $1 + \rho[(\Sigma n_i^2/N) - 1]$, called the *design effect*, where ρ is the correlation between responses for individuals in the same cluster (the *intraclass correlation*; see §19.11). If the clusters are all the same size n, this factor becomes $1 + \rho(n - 1)$. If $\rho = 1$, the design effect becomes n, and the variance of the overall mean is proportional to $1/K$ rather than $1/N$, as noted in the previous paragraph. At the design stage, sample sizes determined by the methods described earlier should be multiplied by the design effect (Donner, 1992).

One simple approach to the analysis of a cluster-randomized trial is to summarize the responses in each cluster by their mean and use these cluster means in a standard two-sample analysis—for example, by a two-sample t test or a Mann–Whitney non-parametric test. A theoretical disadvantage in this approach is that the cluster means will have different variances if the n_i differ. This is unlikely to be a serious problem unless the n_i differ grossly.

A more formal approach is to represent the data by a random-effects model (§§8.3, 12.5), with variance components σ_B^2 for the variation between clusters, and σ_W^2 within clusters. These variance components can be estimated from the data (§8.3). If the n_i vary, the modification given by (8.22) may be used. The variance components are related to the intraclass correlation by the equation $\rho = \sigma_B^2/(\sigma_B^2 + \sigma_W^2)$ (see §19.11), which may be used to estimate the design effect given above.

The more elaborate analysis of §12.5 may be used if the effects of covariates (defined either for the cluster or for the individual subject) are to be taken into account.

A comprehensive account of cluster-randomized trials is given by Murray (1998).

18.10 **Meta-analysis**

Glass (1976) defined *meta-analysis* as 'the statistical analysis of a large collection of analysis results from individual studies for the purpose of integrating the findings'. The etymology of the term can be criticized, but it is used more widely than competitors, such as *overviews*. To most scientists it would seem self-evident that all the available evidence on a particular question should be combined; any failure to do so runs the risk of imprecision and selection bias. Meta-analyses of clinical trial results were rare before about 1980, and there are various reasons for their late appearance. There has often been a paucity of precisely replicated trials, in contrast to the general scientific dictum that results are to be treated with scepticism unless they can be repeated. Repetition of trials with positive outcomes has often been regarded as involving unethical randomization, whilst repetition of negative studies has been rejected as not worthwhile. These objections gradually became less persuasive. Replication of trials with positive results was often regarded as ethically permissible, on the grounds that minor differences in protocol or in patient characteristics might affect the outcome; and replication of negative trials (for which there was no objection on medical ethical grounds) became more feasible as resources increased, making it possible to build a more precise picture of treatment efficacy.

We are concerned here primarily with meta-analysis of clinical trials, but it may be noted that the integration of study results is an active feature of other branches of medical research, such as epidemiological surveys (§19.4), diagnostic tests (§19.9) and bioassay (§20.1), none of which present the ethical features of clinical trials. Non-medical areas of scientific research in which methods of meta-analysis are used include agricultural field trials and educational research.

The present account is necessarily brief. More extensive accounts are given in the special journal issues edited by Yusuf *et al.* (1987) and Spitzer (1995), that of *Statistical Methods in Medical Research* (1993, Volume 2, No. 2), the booklet edited by Chalmers and Altman (1995) (who use the term *systematic review* in a rather more general sense), and many review articles, such as Jones (1995) and Thompson (1998).

Planning

The planning of a meta-analysis needs almost as much thought as that of a single trial, and the rules of procedure should be formalized in a protocol. There are differences in practice between different practitioners, but there would be fairly wide agreement on the following general principles.

1   The data from different trials should be kept separate, so that treatment contrasts derived from individual trials are pooled, rather than the

original data. Pooling the data at the outset would unnecessarily reduce precision if there were systematic differences in response between trials, and bias might be caused if some trials departed from equal assignment proportions.

2 Although trials will never be exactly identical in treatments used, patient characteristics, outcome variables, etc., they should be broadly similar in all these respects. This is a vague recommendation, and differences of view as to the choice of trials for inclusion are inevitable.

3 The trials should all involve random assignment and adequately masked assessment. Protocol departures should be treated in the same way, preferably by ITT.

4 All relevant and available data should be used.

Precept **4** is clearly open to different interpretations and practices. A widely held view is that efforts should be made to retrieve unpublished data, partly to avoid delays in publication, but more importantly to avoid publication bias (§18.8), discussed further below. Completeness of coverage may be relatively easy in some major areas of research, such as the acute treatment of myocardial infarction, where all current research is known to senior practitioners, but will be more difficult in less highly publicized areas. As noted in §18.8, a general system for registration of trials, at their outset, would be beneficial (Simes, 1986b; Dickersin *et al.*, 1995).

Publication bias may sometimes be detected by a *funnel plot*, in which an estimate of a parameter representing an efficacy difference for each trial is plotted against the trial size (or some similar measure, such as the reciprocal of the variance or standard error of the estimate). The estimates should cluster round a constant value, with variability decreasing with trial size (and hence producing the 'funnel' shape). For small trial sizes, however, where non-significant results are more likely, publication bias may cause the absence of points near zero effect, and hence a skewness in the shape of the funnel. Examples, mainly from epidemiology, are provided by Givens *et al.* (1997), who discuss methods of adjusting for the bias. Other relevant work is by Dear and Begg (1992) and Hedges (1992).

Many early meta-analyses worked merely with the summary statistics provided in the published reports of each trial. Current practice favours the use of individual patient data, enabling data checking and standardization (Stewart & Parmar, 1993; Stewart & Clarke, 1995).

Different meta-analysis investigators are likely to differ in their approach to some of the choices indicated in **1–4** above. It is, therefore, not too surprising if different meta-analysis on ostensibly the same question occasionally reach different conclusions (Chalmers *et al.*, 1987). An example is provided by two meta-analyses of trials comparing the anti-caries efficacy of sodium fluoride and sodium monofluorophosphate dentifrices (Johnson,

1993; Proskin, 1993). There is thus scope for overviews of related meta-analyses (M^2-*analyses?*), with the looming possibility of M^3-*analyses*, and so on!

Analysis

A useful starting-point is the method of weighting described in §8.2. The difference in efficacy between two treatments will be measured by a suitable parameter, typically chosen as the difference in mean responses or (for binary responses) the difference in proportions or the log odds ratio. Suppose there are k trials, and that for the ith trial the true value of the difference parameter is θ_i, estimated by the statistic y_i, with estimated sampling variance v_i. Define the weight $w_i = 1/v_i$. Then, if all the θ_i are equal to some common value θ, a suitable estimate of θ is the weighted mean

$$\bar{y} = \frac{\sum w_i y_i}{\sum w_i}, \tag{18.6}$$

as in (8.13), and, approximately, $\text{var}(\bar{y}) = 1/\sum w_i$. The assumption that the θ_i are constant may be tested, as in (8.14) and (8.15), by the heterogeneity statistic

$$G = \sum w_i(y_i - \bar{y})^2 = \sum w_i y_i^2 - \left(\sum w_i y_i\right)^2 / \sum w_i, \tag{18.7}$$

distributed approximately as $\chi^2_{(k-1)}$.

For trials with a binary outcome, these formulae may be applied to provide combined estimates of log relative risk (using (4.24) for $\sqrt{v_i}$) or log odds ratio (using (4.26). In the latter case, an alternative approach is to use the method of Yusuf *et al.* (1985) given in (4.33). If O_i and E_i are the observed and expected numbers of critical events for one of the treatments, the log odds ratio is estimated by $y_i = (O_i - E_i)/V_i$, with $\text{var}(y_i) = 1/V_i$, where V_i is calculated, as in (4.32), from the 2×2 table for the trial. Then the weighted mean (18.6) becomes

$$\bar{y} = \frac{\sum(O_i - E_i)}{\sum V_i},$$

with $\text{var}(\bar{y}) = 1/\sum V_i$. The heterogeneity statistic (18.7), distributed approximately as $\chi^2_{(k-1)}$, becomes

$$G' = \sum \frac{(O_i - E_i)^2}{V_i} - \frac{\left[\sum(O_i - E_i)\right]^2}{\sum V_i}.$$

As noted in §4.5, this method is biased when the treatment effect is large (i.e. when the odds ratio departs greatly from unity). The report by the Early Breast Cancer Trialists' Collaborative Group (1990) suggests that the bias is not serious if the odds ratio is within twofold in either direction and there are at least several dozen critical events in total. In more doubtful situations, it is preferable to apply the method of weighting to the direct estimates of the log odds ratio given by the log of (4.25).

Figure 18.2 illustrates a common method of visual display, sometimes called a *forest plot*, showing the results for separate trials and for their combinations. In this particular meta-analysis, the methods of Yusuf *et al.* (1985) were used for estimates and confidence limits for the log odds ratio, which were then transformed back to the odds ratio scale. Here, none of the individual trials shows a clear treatment effect, but the results for the various trials are consistent and the combined values for each of the two subgroups and for the whole data set have narrow confidence ranges, showing clear evidence of an effect.

An alternative method, the *Galbraith plot* (Galbraith, 1988; Thompson, 1993), plots the standardized estimate, $y_i/\text{SE}(y_i)$, against $1/\text{SE}(y_i)$. This is illustrated in Fig. 18.3. If the results of different trials are homogeneous, the points should be scattered about a line through the origin with a slope estimating the parameter θ, the scatter being homoscedastic. Outliers indicate heterogeneity.

The methods described so far follow a *fixed-effects* model, in that the difference parameter, θ, is assumed to take the same value for all trials. This, of course, is very unlikely to be true, although the variation in θ may be small and undetectable by the heterogeneity test. If there is clear evidence of heterogeneity, either from the test or from a visual presentation, the first step should be to explore its nature by identifying any outlying trials, and seeking to define subgroups of trials with similar characteristics which might reveal homogeneity within and heterogeneity between subgroups. Alternatively, the variability might be explained by regression of the parameter estimate on covariates characterizing the trial (Thompson & Sharp, 1999).

If no such rational explanations can be found for the heterogeneity, it is sometimes argued that the fixed-effects model is still valid (Early Breast Cancer Trialists' Collaborative Group, 1990; Peto *et al.*, 1995). These authors prefer the term 'assumption-free' to 'fixed-effects'. Their argument is that the analysis described here provides correct inferences for the particular mix of patients included in the specific trials under consideration. The inferences would not necessarily apply for patients in other trials, but this apparent defect is analogous to the fact that any single trial contains patients with different characteristics and prognoses, and its results will not necessarily apply to other groups of patients.

A more widely accepted view is that heterogeneity which cannot be explained by known differences in trial characteristics should be represented by a further source of random variation, leading to a *random-effects* model, as in §§8.3 and 12.5. The inferences to be made from the meta-analysis then relate to a

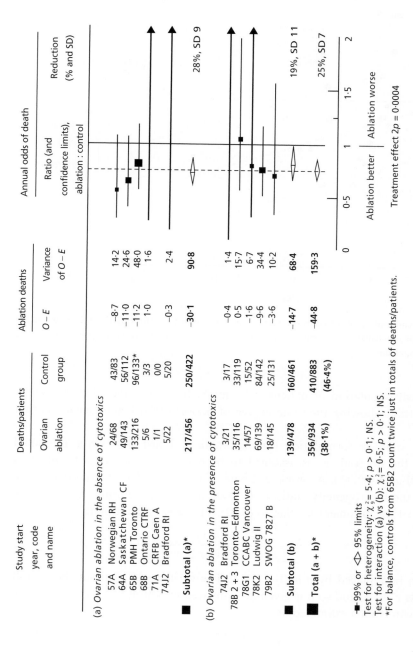

Study start year, code and name	Deaths/patients		Ablation deaths		Annual odds of death	Reduction (% and SD)
	Ovarian ablation	Control group	O − E	Variance of O − E	Ratio (and confidence limits), ablation : control	
(a) Ovarian ablation in the absence of cytotoxics						
57A Norwegian RH	24/68	43/83	−8·7	14·2		
64A Saskatchewan CF	49/143	56/112	−11·0	24·6		
65B PMH Toronto	133/216	96/133*	−11·2	48·0		
68B Ontario CTRF	5/6	3/3	1·0	1·6		
71A CRFB Caen A	1/1	0/0				
74J2 Bradford RI	5/22	5/20	−0·3	2·4		
Subtotal (a)*	217/456	250/422	−30·1	90·8		28%, SD 9
(b) Ovarian ablation in the presence of cytotoxics						
74J2 Bradford RI	3/21	3/17	−0·4	1·4		
78B 2 + 3 Toronto–Edmonton	35/116	33/119	0·5	15·7		
78G1 CCABC Vancouver	14/57	15/52	−1·6	6·7		
78K2 Ludwig II	69/139	84/142	−9·6	34·4		
79B2 SWOG 7827 B	18/145	25/131	−3·6	10·2		
Subtotal (b)	139/478	160/461	−14·7	68·4		19%, SD 11
Total (a + b)*	356/934 (38·1%)	410/883 (46·4%)	−44·8	159·3		25%, SD 7

Ablation better | Ablation worse

Treatment effect $2p$ = 0·0004

⊢■⊣ 99% or ◇ 95% limits

Test for heterogeneity: χ_9^2 = 5·4; p > 0·1; NS.
Test for interaction (a) vs (b): χ_1^2 = 0·5; p > 0·1; NS.
*For balance, controls from 65B2 count twice just in totals of deaths/patients.

Fig. 18.2 A meta-analysis of mortality results from trials of ovarian ablation in women with early breast cancer below age 50, subdivided by the presence or absence of cytotoxic chemotherapy (Early Breast Cancer Trialists' Collaborative Group, 1992, Fig. 9). In this presentation the area of a black square is proportional to V_i, and thus represents the precision of the estimate from that trial or group of trials. The significance level for a two-sided test is shown as '$2p$'. Reproduced by permission of the authors and publishers.

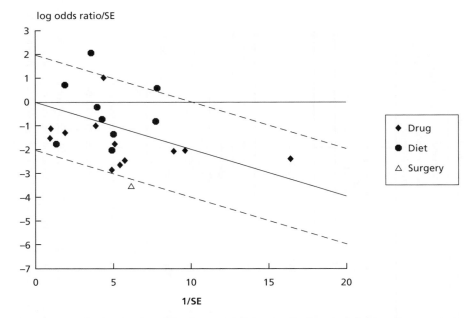

Fig. 18.3 A Galbraith plot for trials of serum cholesterol reduction, showing the effects on the log odds ratio for ischaemic heart disease events (Thompson, 1993). Reproduced by permission of the author and publishers.

hypothetical population of patients who might have been included in a wider group of trials showing the same degree of between-trial heterogeneity as that observed.

In the simplest formulation (DerSimonian & Laird, 1986), the estimated effect for the ith trial, y_i, is assumed to be distributed as $N(\theta_i, v_i)$, and θ_i is distributed as $N(\theta^*, v^*)$. A simple estimate of v^* is provided by considering the excess of the heterogeneity statistic, G, over its null expectation, $k - 1$, by an extension of the argument leading to (8.22). This gives the estimate

$$\hat{v}^* = \frac{G - (k - 1)}{\sum w_i - (\sum w_i^2)/\sum w_i},$$

which can be replaced by 0 if $G < k - 1$. The variance of y_i about the overall mean θ^* is $v^* + v_i$, and so it is given an estimated weight $w_i^* = 1/(\hat{v}^* + v_i)$. The overall mean is then estimated as

$$\hat{\theta}^* = \frac{\sum w_i^* y_i}{\sum w_i^*},$$

with estimated variance $1/\sum w_i^*$. This procedure is called *semi-weighting*. Note that since heterogeneity between the y_i will lead to $\hat{v}^* > 0$, and hence $w_i^* < w_i$, the combined estimate of efficacy, $\hat{\theta}*$, will have greater variance than the estimate $\bar{y}$ obtained from the fixed-effects model.

A slightly more efficient procedure is to estimate by maximum likelihood, which involves an iterative calculation (see, for instance, Normand, 1999, equation (8)).

Both these procedures are in the spirit of empirical Bayesian methods (§6.5), whereby the between-trial variation can be estimated from the available data. In contrast to this approach is the fully Bayesian analysis, in which (with the model described above) prior distributions are specified for the parameters v_i, $\theta*$ and $v*$, either based on specific prior judgements or using non-informative distributions to represent ignorance (Smith *et al.*, 1995; Normand, 1999).

19 Statistical methods in epidemiology

19.1 Introduction

The branch of medical science called *epidemiology* has been defined as 'the study of the distribution and determinants of health-related states or events in specified populations, and the application of this study to control of health problems' (Last, 1995, p. 55). In broad terms epidemiology is concerned with the distribution of disease, or of a physiological condition, and of the factors that influence the distribution. It includes within its orbit the study of chronic diseases, as well as the communicable diseases which give rise to epidemics of the classical sort. The subject overlaps to some extent with *social medicine, community medicine* or *public health*, which would usually be understood to include social and administrative topics, such as the provision and use of health services.

Epidemiology is concerned with certain characteristics of groups of individuals rather than single subjects, and inevitably gives rise to statistical problems. Many of these are conceptually similar to statistical problems arising in other branches of medical science, and, indeed, in the non-medical sciences, and can be approached by the methods of analysis described earlier in this book; several examples in earlier chapters have been drawn from epidemiological studies. Other methodological problems in epidemiology, although of statistical interest, are bound up with considerations of a non-statistical nature and cannot be discussed here. Examples are the interpretation of vital and health statistical data, which requires a close knowledge of administrative procedures for the recording of such data and of the classification of diseases and causes of death (Benjamin, 1968; World Health Organization, 1992); and the proper use and potential development of medical records of various sorts (Acheson, 1967). There is also a considerable body of literature concerned with the mathematical theory of epidemic disease; the monographs by Bailey (1975) and Becker (1989) provide useful summaries of this work. For general accounts of epidemiological methods, the reader may consult Kleinbaum *et al.* (1982), Miettinen (1985), Hennekens *et al.* (1987), Elwood (1988), Kelsey *et al.* (1996) and Rothman and Greenland (1998).

In this chapter we consider briefly certain problems arising in epidemiological research for which special statistical methods have been developed.

19.2 **The planning of surveys**

It is useful to distinguish between *descriptive surveys*, designed to provide estimates of some simple characteristics of populations, and *analytical surveys*,
designed to investigate associations between certain variables. Examples of the
first type are surveys to estimate the prevalence of some illness in a population or
the frequency distribution of medical consultations during a certain period. An
example of the second type would be a study of the association between the use
of a certain drug and the occurrence of a particular adverse effect. The distinction is by no means clear-cut. In a population survey we may be interested also in
associations—for example, that between the prevalence of an illness and a
person's age. Conversely, in an association survey it would be quite reasonable
to regard the association in question as a population parameter and to enquire
how it varies from one population to another. Nevertheless, in population
surveys the main emphasis is on the provision of reliable estimates of the features
of a well-defined population; in analytical surveys (to be considered further in
§19.4), the definition of the population is less important than the relationship
between the variables.

Statistical interest in population surveys arises primarily when these are
carried out by sampling methods. Some surveys are, of course, performed by
complete enumeration; population censuses are familiar examples. The advantages of sampling lie in the economy of cost, manpower and time. Any of these
factors may make complete enumeration out of the question. Furthermore, the
smaller scale of a sampling enquiry may permit more reliable observations to be
made.

The first step is usually to define the *sampling frame*, which is essentially a list
or form of identification of the individuals in the population to be sampled. For
example, if the aim is to sample adults resident in England, one useful way is to
define the sampling frame as the individuals listed in the current electoral
registers (lists of people entitled to vote at elections). If the intention is to sample
small areas of a country, the sampling frame may be defined by marking a map
into appropriate subdivisions by a grid. Once the individuals to be sampled have
been defined they can be numbered, and the problem will now be to decide which
numbers to select for the sample.

How is the sample to be chosen? If some characteristics of the population are
known, perhaps as a result of previous surveys, it is sometimes suggested that the
sample should be chosen by *purposive selection*, whereby certain features of the
sample are made to agree exactly or almost exactly with those of the population.
For example, in sampling for market research or opinion polls, some organizations use *quota sampling*, a method by which each interviewer is given instructions about certain characteristics (such as age, sex and social status of the
individuals to be selected), the proportions in various subgroups being chosen

to agree with the corresponding proportions in the population. The difficulty with this method is that serious discrepancies between the sample and the population may arise in respect of characteristics which have not been taken into account. There is nothing in the sampling procedure to give any general confidence about the representativeness of the sample.

In general, it is preferable to use some form of random sampling. In *simple random sampling*, which was introduced in §4.1, every possible sample of a given size from the population has an equal probability of being chosen.

To draw a simple random sample from a population we could imagine some physical method of randomization. For instance, if 10 people were to be selected at random from a population of 100, a card could be produced for each member of the population, the cards thoroughly shuffled, and 10 cards selected. Such a method would be tedious, particularly with large population sizes, and it is convenient to use a computer to make a random selection using appropriate software with computer-generated random numbers.

We now discuss some alternative forms of random sampling.

Systematic sampling

When the units or individuals in the population are listed or otherwise ordered in a systematic fashion, it may be convenient to arrange that the units chosen in any one sample occupy related positions in the sampling frame, the first unit being selected at random. For example, in drawing a sample of 1 in 50 of the entries in a card index, the first card may be selected by choosing a number at random from 1 to 50, after which every 50th card would be included. If the initial selection was 39 the selected cards would be those occupying positions 39, 89, 139, 189, . . . , etc. This is called a *systematic sample*. Another example might arise in two-dimensional sampling. Suppose a health survey is to be conducted in geographical units determined by a rectangular grid. If, say, 1 in 25 units are to be selected, the initial 'vertical' and 'horizontal' coordinates could be chosen at random, each from the numbers 1 to 5. If the initial random numbers were 5 and 3, the selected units would be

$$. \quad . \quad . \quad (5,3) \, . \quad . \quad . \, (5,8) \, . \quad . \quad . \, (5,13) \, . \quad .$$
$$. \qquad\qquad . \qquad\qquad .$$
$$. \qquad\qquad . \qquad\qquad .$$
$$. \quad . \quad . \, (10,3) \, . \quad . \quad . \, (10,8) \, . \quad . \quad . \, (10,13) \, . \quad .$$
$$. \qquad\qquad . \qquad\qquad .$$
$$. \qquad\qquad . \qquad\qquad .$$
$$. \quad . \quad . \, (15,3) \, . \quad . \quad . \, (15,8) \, . \quad . \quad . \, (15,13) \, . \quad .$$
$$. \qquad\qquad . \qquad\qquad .$$
$$. \qquad\qquad . \qquad\qquad .$$

where the first number specifies the 'vertical' position and the second the 'horizontal' position.

Systematic sampling is often at least as precise as random sampling. It is particularly dangerous, though, if the ordering of the units in the sampling frame imposes a positive correlation between units whose distance apart is equal to the sampling interval. In the geographical example above, if there were a series of populated valleys running east to west about five sampling units apart, the chosen units might almost all be rather heavily populated or almost all lightly populated. The sampling error of the method would therefore be unusually high. In general, it will be difficult to estimate the sampling error from a single systematic sample unless it is assumed that such correlations do not exist and that the sample can therefore be regarded as effectively random. One useful device is to choose simultaneously several systematic samples by different choices of the starting-point. A mean value or other relevant statistic could then be worked out separately for each systematic sample, and the sampling variance of the overall mean obtained by the usual formula in terms of the variance of the separate means.

Stratified sampling

In this method the population is divided into subgroups, or *strata*, each of which is sampled randomly with a known sample size. Suppose that we wish to estimate the mean value of a certain variable in the population and that strata are defined so that the mean varies considerably from one stratum to another. In simple random sampling, the distribution of observations over the strata will vary from sample to sample, and this lack of control will contribute to the variability of the sample mean. In contrast, in repeated sampling with the *same* distribution over the strata, this component of variability is irrelevant.

Strata may be defined qualitatively; for example, in a national health survey different regions of the country may be taken as strata. Or they may be defined in terms of one or more quantitative variables—for example, as age groups. The fraction of the stratum to be sampled may be constant or it may vary from stratum to stratum. The important points are: (i) that the distribution of both the population and the sample over the strata should be known; and (ii) that the between-strata variability should be as high as possible, or equivalently that each stratum should be as homogeneous as possible.

Suppose there are k strata and that in the ith stratum the population size is N_i, and the mean and variance of variable x are μ_i and σ_i^2. A random sample of size n_i is taken from the ith stratum; the sampling fraction n_i/N_i will be denoted by f_i. The sample mean and estimate of variance in the ith stratum are $\bar{x}_i$ and s_i^2. The total population size is

$$N = \sum_{i=1}^{k} N_i,$$

and the total sample size is

$$n = \sum_{i=1}^{k} n_i.$$

The mean value of x in the whole population is clearly

$$\mu = \frac{\sum N_i \mu_i}{N}.$$

The appropriate estimate of μ is

$$\hat{\mu} = \frac{\sum N_i \bar{x}_i}{N}, \tag{19.1}$$

which is easily seen to be unbiased. Its variance is

$$\mathrm{var}(\hat{\mu}) = \frac{1}{N^2} \sum N_i^2 \, \mathrm{var}(\bar{x}_i)$$

$$= \frac{1}{N^2} \sum \frac{N_i^2 \sigma_i^2}{n_i} (1 - f_i) \tag{19.2}$$

by (4.2), and this is estimated from the sample as

$$\mathrm{var}(\hat{\mu}) = \frac{1}{N^2} \sum \frac{N_i^2 s_i^2}{n_i} (1 - f_i). \tag{19.3}$$

If all the f_i are small, the terms $1 - f_i$ may be replaced by unity. In general, (19.2) will be smaller than the variance of the mean of a random sample because the terms σ_i^2 measure only the variability within strata. Variability between the μ_i is irrelevant.

If n is fixed and the f_i are small, $\mathrm{var}(\hat{\mu})$ becomes a minimum if the n_i are chosen to be as nearly as possible proportional to $N_i \sigma_i$. Thus, if σ_i is constant from one stratum to another, the n_i should be chosen in proportion to N_i, i.e. the sampling fraction should be constant. Strata with relatively large σ_i have correspondingly increased sampling fractions. Usually, little will be known about the σ_i before the survey is carried out and the choice of a constant sampling fraction will be the most reasonable strategy.

If the survey is designed to estimate a proportion π, the above formulae hold with $\bar{x}_i$ and μ_i replaced by p_i and π_i, the observed and true proportions in the ith stratum, σ_i^2 by $\pi_i(1 - \pi_i)$ and s_i^2 by $n_i p_i (1 - p_i)/(n_i - 1)$ (this being the estimate of variance in a sample of size n_i in which $n_i p_i$ observations are 1 and $n_i(1 - p_i)$ are 0).

Apart from the increased precision in the estimation of the population mean, stratification may be adopted to provide reasonably precise estimates of the means for each of the strata. This may lead to departures from the optimal allocation described above, so that none of the sample sizes in the separate strata become too small.

Example 19.1

It is desired to estimate the prevalence of a certain condition (i.e. the proportion of affected individuals) in a population of 5000 people by taking a sample of size 100. Suppose that the prevalence is known to be associated with age and that the population can be divided into three strata defined by age, with the following numbers of individuals:

Stratum, i	Age (years)	N_i
1	0–14	1200
2	15–44	2200
3	45–	1600
		5000

Suppose that the true prevalences, π_i, in the different strata are as follows:

Stratum, i	π_i
1	0·02
2	0·08
3	0·15

It is easily verified that the overall prevalence, $\pi \; (= \sum N_i \pi_i / \sum N_i)$, is 0·088. A simple random sample of size $n = 100$ would therefore give an estimate p with variance $(0·088)(0·912)/100 = 0·000803$.

For stratified sampling with optimal allocation the sample sizes in the strata should be chosen in proportion to $N_i \sqrt{[\pi_i(1 - \pi_i)]}$. The values of this quantity in the three strata are 168, 597 and 571, which are in the proportions 0·126, 0·447 and 0·427, respectively. The optimal sample sizes are, therefore, $n_1 = 12, n_2 = 45$ and $n_3 = 43$, or numbers very close to these (there being a little doubt about the effect of rounding to the nearest integer). Let us call this allocation A. This depends on the unknown π_i, and therefore could hardly be used in practice. If we knew very little about the likely variation in the π_i, we might choose the $n_i \propto N_i$, ignoring the effect of the changing standard deviation. This would give, for allocation B, $n_1 = 24, n_2 = 44$ and $n_3 = 32$. Thirdly, we might have some idea that the prevalence (and therefore the standard deviation) increased with age, and therefore adjust the allocation rather arbitrarily to give, say, $n_1 = 20, n_2 = 40$ and $n_3 = 40$ (allocation C). The estimate of $\hat{\pi}$ is, in each case, given by the formula equivalent to (19.1),

$$\hat{\pi} = \frac{\sum N_i p_i}{N},$$

where p_i is the estimated prevalence in the ith stratum. The variance of $\hat{\pi}$ is given by the equivalent of (19.2), in which we shall drop the terms f_i as being small:

$$\text{var}(\pi) = \frac{1}{N^2} \sum \frac{N_i^2 \pi_i (1 - \pi_i)}{n_i}.$$

The values of var($\hat{\pi}$) for the three allocations are as follows:

Allocation	var($\hat{\pi}$)
A	0·000714
B	0·000779
C	0·000739

As would be expected, the lowest variance is for A and the highest for B, the latter being only a little lower than the variance for a random sample.

Multistage sampling

In this method the sampling frame is divided into a population of 'first-stage sampling units', of which a 'first-stage' sample is taken. This will usually be a simple random sample, but may be a systematic or stratified sample; it may also, as we shall see, be a random sample in which some first-stage units are allowed to have a higher probability of selection than others. Each sampled first-stage unit is subdivided into 'second-stage sampling units', which are sampled. The process can continue through as many stages as are appropriate.

There are two main advantages of multistage sampling. First, it enables the resources to be concentrated in a limited number of portions of the whole sampling frame with a consequent reduction in cost. Secondly, it is convenient for situations in which a complete sampling frame is not available before the investigation starts. A list of first-stage units is required, but the second-stage units need be listed only within the first-stage units selected in the sample.

Consider as an example a health survey of men working in a certain industry. There would probably not exist a complete index of all men in the industry, but it might be easy to obtain a list of factories, which could be first-stage units. From each factory selected in the first-stage sample, a list of men could be obtained and a second-stage sample selected from this list. Apart from the advantage of having to make lists of men only within the factories selected at the first stage, this procedure would result in an appreciable saving in cost by enabling the investigation to be concentrated at selected factories instead of necessitating the examination of a sample of men all in different parts of the country.

The economy in cost and resources is unfortunately accompanied by a loss of precision as compared with simple random sampling. Suppose that in the example discussed above we take a sample of 20 factories and second-stage samples of 50 men in each of the 20 factories. If there is systematic variation between the factories, due perhaps to variation in health conditions in different parts of the country or to differing occupational hazards, this variation will be represented by a sample of only 20 first-stage units. A random sample of 1000 men, on the other hand, would represent 1000 random choices of first-stage units (some of which may, of course, be chosen more than once) and would consequently provide a better estimate of the national mean.

A useful device in two-stage sampling is called *self-weighting*. Each first-stage unit is given a probability of selection which is proportional to the number of second-stage units it contains. Second-stage samples are then chosen to have equal size. It follows that each second-stage unit in the whole population has an equal chance of being selected and the formulae needed for estimation are somewhat simplified.

Cluster sampling

Sometimes, in the final stage of multistage sampling, complete enumeration of the available units is undertaken. In the industrial example, once a survey team has installed itself in a factory, it may cost little extra to examine all the men in the factory; it may indeed be useful to avoid the embarrassment that might be caused by inviting some men but not others to participate. When there is no sampling at the final stage, the method is referred to as *cluster sampling*. The investigator has no control over the number of sampling units in the clusters and this means that the loss of precision, compared with simple random sampling, is even greater than that in multistage sampling.

Design effect

The ratio of the variance of an estimator from a sampling scheme to the variance of the estimator from simple random sampling with the same total number of sampling units is known as the *design effect*, often abbreviated to *Deff*. In Example 19.1 the *Deff* for allocation C is $0.000739/0.000803 = 0.92$. Another way of looking at the *Deff* is in terms of sample size. The same precision could have been achieved with a stratified sample of 92 people with allocation C as for a simple random sample of 100 people. The stratified sample is more efficient (*Deff* < 1) than simple random sampling and this will occur generally provided that there is a component of variation between strata. The efficiency of stratified sampling increases with the increasing heterogeneity between strata and the consequent greater homogeneity within strata.

In contrast, multistage and cluster sampling will usually have a *Deff* > 1. That is, a larger sample size will be required than with simple random sampling.

For cluster sampling with m members per cluster and a correlation within clusters of ρ for the variable under study, the *Deff* is given by

$$Deff = 1 + (m - 1)\rho,$$

which will always exceed 1 (except in the unlikely scenario of negative correlations within clusters). A similar expression was given in §18.9 for sample size calculations in a cluster randomized trial. If m differs between clusters, then, in the above formula, m is replaced by $\sum m^2 / \sum m$, which is approximately $\bar{m}$, provided that the coefficient of variation of cluster size is small.

The above discussion of the efficiency of different sampling schemes relative to simple random sampling is in terms of sample size. As we noted when discussing multistage sampling, one of the advantages of this method is a reduction in cost and the overall efficiency of a sampling scheme should be assessed in terms of the cost of carrying out the sampling, not just in terms of total sample size. If the cost of a sampling scheme is c per sample member, relative to the cost per member of a simple random sample, then the overall efficiency of the sampling scheme is

$$\frac{100\%}{c \times Deff}.$$

Thus, a sampling scheme is more, or less, efficient than simple random sampling according as $c \times Deff$ is less, or greater, than unity, respectively. Thus, a cluster sampling scheme with six members per cluster and a correlation within clusters of $0\cdot2$ ($Deff = 2\cdot0$) will be more efficient than simple random sampling, provided that the average cost of conducting the survey per sample member is less than a half of the cost per member of a simple random sample. In this case the increase in sample size required to achieve a specified precision has been more than offset by a reduction in costs.

Mark–recapture sampling

The name of this technique is derived from its application to the estimation of the number of animals or birds in an area. Traps are set and the captured animals form a sample of the population. They are marked and released. A second set of trappings yields a second sample consisting of unmarked animals and some that were marked on the first trapping occasion. Again, animals are marked and released and the process is continued for several sets of trappings.

The numbers of animals captured on each occasion, together with the numbers of recaptures of previously marked animals, can be used to estimate the total population. Assumptions must be made on whether the population is closed (no gains or losses over the total sampling period) or not, on whether the probability of capture depends on the previous capture history, and on heterogeneity between animals in probability of capture. The more information that is available—for example, more trapping occasions and a marking system that allows identification of the occasions on which each animal was captured—the more readily can assumptions be checked and modified.

This technique may be applied for the purpose of estimating the size of a population of individuals with some health-related characteristic. It is particularly useful for rare characteristics, which would require a very large sample using more traditional methods; for habits which people may be reluctant to disclose on a questionnaire, such as intravenous drug use; or for groups which may be differentially omitted from a sampling frame, such as homeless people in a city. Lists containing members of such a group may be available in agencies that provide services for the group, and if several lists are available then each may be considered to correspond to a 'trapping' occasion. If there is sufficient information on identity, then it can be established whether a person is on more than one list ('recaptures'). A difference from the animal trapping situation is that there may be no time sequence involved and the lists may be treated symmetrically in respect of each other.

If there are k lists, then the observations can be set out as a 2^k table, denoting presence or absence on each list. The number in the cell corresponding to absence on all k lists is, of course, unobserved and the aim of the method is to estimate this number and hence the total number. It will usually be reasonable to anticipate that the probability of being on a list is dependent on whether or not a person is on some of the other lists. That is, there will be list dependency (corresponding to capture being dependent on previous capture history). A method of proceeding is to fit a log-linear model to the $2^k - 1$ observed cells of the 2^k table and use this model to estimate the number in the unobserved cell. Dependencies between the lists can be included as interaction terms but the highest-order interaction between all k lists is set to zero, since it cannot be estimated from the incomplete table.

A text on the methodology is given by Seber (1982), and Cormack (1989) describes the use of the log-linear model. A brief review is given by Chao (1998). The method gives an estimate of the total population size and its standard error. A problem is that the estimate may be dependent on non-verifiable assumptions, so that the standard error does not adequately describe the uncertainty. Nevertheless, in situations where more robust methods, based on random sampling, are infeasible, the method does allow some estimation.

Imputation

Sample surveys usually have missing data through some people failing to answer some of the questions, either inadvertently or by refusing to answer particular questions. The analysis of the whole data set is facilitated if the missing data are replaced by imputed values. Imputed values may be obtained using a model based on the observed values. For example, a multiple regression of x_1 on $x_2, x_3, \ldots, x_p$ might be fitted on the complete data and used to estimate values of x_1 for those individuals with this variable missing but with observed values of $x_2, x_3, \ldots, x_p$. This gives the best predicted values but it is unsatisfactory to substitute these values because to do so excludes variability, and any analysis of the augmented data would appear more accurate than is justified. Instead, the random variability has to be built into the imputed values, not only the variability about the fitted regression line but also the variability due to uncertainty in estimating the regression coefficients. Thus imputed values contain random components and there is no unique best set of imputed values. Even for an imputed set of data with random variation incorporated, a single analysis will give standard errors of estimated parameters that are too small. This can be avoided by *multiple imputation*; that is, the missing data are imputed several times independently, and each imputed set is analysed in the same way. Variances of estimated parameters can then be produced by combining the within-imputation variance with the between-imputation variance. For further discussion of missing data and the importance of considering whether the fact that data are missing is informative in some way see §12.6.

Multiple imputation has generally been used with large sample surveys but may be more widely applied as suitable software becomes available. Readers wishing to learn more about this technique are referred to Rubin (1987) and Barnard *et al.* (1998).

Barnard *et al.* (1998) also describe applications of multiple imputation to a wider range of problems than non-response. These include imputation of the true ages of children when the collected data on ages were insufficiently precise, and the imputation of dates of acquired immune deficiency syndrome (AIDS) diagnosis in people with human immunodeficiency virus (HIV) infection who had not yet contracted AIDS, using a model based on a set of covariates (Taylor *et al.*, 1990).

Other considerations

The planning, conduct and analysis of sample surveys give rise to many problems that cannot be discussed here. The books by Moser and Kalton (1979) and Yates (1981) contain excellent discussions of the practical aspects of sampling. The books by Cochran (1977) and Yates (1981) may be consulted for the main theoretical results.

The statistical theory of sample surveys is concerned largely with the measurement of sampling error. This emphasis may lead the investigator to overlook the importance of non-sampling errors. In a large survey the sampling errors may be so small that systematic non-sampling errors may be much the more important. Indeed, in a complete enumeration, such as a complete population census, sampling errors disappear altogether, but there may be very serious non-sampling errors.

Some non-sampling errors are non-systematic, causing no bias in the average. An example would be random inaccuracy in the reading of a test instrument. These errors merely contribute to the variability of the observation in question and therefore diminish the precision of the survey. Other errors are systematic, causing a bias in a mean value which does not decrease with increasing sample size; for example, in a health survey certain types of illness may be systematically under-reported.

One of the most important types of systematic error is that due to inadequate coverage of the sampling frame, either because of non-cooperation by the individual or because the investigator finds it difficult to make the correct observations. For example, in an interview survey some people may refuse to be interviewed and others may be hard to find, may have moved away from the supposed address or even have died. Individuals who are missed for any of these reasons are likely to be atypical of the population in various relevant respects. Every effort must therefore be made to include as many as possible of the chosen individuals in the enquiry, by persistent attempts to make the relevant observations on all the non-responders or by concentrating on a subsample of them so that the characteristics of the non-responders can at least be estimated. This allows the possibility of weighting the subsample of initial non-responders to represent all non-responders (Levy & Lemeshow, 1991, p. 308), or, when background data are available on all subjects, to use multiple imputation to estimate other missing variables (Glynn *et al.*, 1993).

Reference must finally be made to another important type of study, the *longitudinal survey*. Many investigations are concerned with the changes in certain measurements over a period of time: for example, the growth and development of children over a 10-year period, or the changes in blood pressure during pregnancy. It is desirable where possible to study each individual over the relevant period of time rather than to take different samples of individuals at different points of time. The statistical problems arising in this type of study are discussed in §12.6.

19.3 **Rates and standardization**

Since epidemiology is concerned with the distribution of disease in populations, summary measures are required to describe the amount of disease in a population. There are two basic measures, incidence and prevalence.

Incidence is a measure of the rate at which new cases of disease occur in a population previously without disease. Thus, the incidence, denoted by I, is defined as

$$I = \frac{\text{number of new cases in period of time}}{\text{population at risk}}.$$

The period of time is specified in the units in which the rate is expressed. Often the rate is multiplied by a base such as 1000 or 1 000 000 to avoid small decimal fractions. For example, there were 280 new cases of cancer of the pancreas in men in New South Wales in 1997 out of a population of 3·115 million males. The incidence was $280/3 \cdot 115 = 90$ per million per year.

Prevalence, denoted by P, is a measure of the frequency of existing disease at a given time, and is defined as

$$P = \frac{\text{total number of cases at given time}}{\text{total population at that time}}.$$

Both incidence and prevalence usually depend on age, and possibly sex, and sex- and age-specific figures would be calculated.

The prevalence and incidence rates are related, since an incident case is, immediately on occurrence, a prevalent case and remains as such until recovery or death (disregarding emigration and immigration). Provided the situation is stable, the link between the two measures is given by

$$P = It, \tag{19.4}$$

where t is the average duration of disease. For a chronic disease from which there is no recovery, t would be the average survival after occurrence of the disease.

Standardization

Problems due to confounding (Example 15.6) arise frequently in vital statistics and have given rise to a group of methods called standardization. We shall describe briefly one or two of the most well-known methods, and discuss their relationship to the methods described in §15.6.

Mortality in a population is usually measured by an annual death rate—for example, the number of individuals dying during a certain calendar year divided by the estimated population size midway through the year. Frequently this ratio is multiplied by a convenient base, such as 1000, to avoid small decimal fractions; it is then called the annual death rate per 1000 population. If the death rate is calculated for a population covering a wide age range, it is called a *crude death rate*.

In a comparison of the mortality of two populations, say, those of two different countries, the crude rates may be misleading. Mortality depends strongly on age. If the two countries have different age structures, this contrast alone may explain a difference in crude rates (just as, in Table 15.6, the contrast between the 'crude' proportions with factor A was strongly affected by the different sex distributions in the disease and control groups). An example is given in Table 19.1 (on p. 664), which shows the numbers of individuals and numbers of deaths separately in different age groups, for two countries: A, typical of highly industrialized countries, with a rather high proportion of individuals at the older ages; and B, a developing country with a small proportion of old people. The death rates at each age (which are called *age-specific death rates*) are substantially higher for B than for A, and yet the crude death rate is higher for A than for B.

The situation here is precisely the same as that discussed at the beginning of §15.6, in connection with Example 15.6. Sometimes, however, mortality has to be compared for a large number of different populations, and some form of adjustment for age differences is required. For example, the mortality in one country may have to be compared over several different years; different regions of the same country may be under study; or one may wish to compare the mortality for a large number of different occupations. Two obvious generalizations are: (i) in standardizing for factors other than, or in addition to, age—for example, sex, as in Table 15.6; and (ii) in morbidity studies where the criterion studied is the occurrence of a certain illness rather than of death. We shall discuss the usual situation—the standardization of mortality rates for age.

The basic idea in standardization is that we introduce a *standard population* with a fixed age structure. The mortality for any *special population* is then adjusted to allow for discrepancies in age structure between the standard and special populations. There are two main approaches: *direct* and *indirect* methods of standardization. The following brief account may be supplemented by reference to Liddell (1960), Kalton (1968) or Hill and Hill (1991).

The following notation will be used.

Age group	Standard			Special		
	(1)	(2)	(3)	(4)	(5)	(6)
	Population	Deaths	Death rate (2)/(1)	Population	Deaths	Death rate (5)/(4)
1	N_1	R_1	P_1	n_1	r_1	p_1
$\vdots$						
i	N_i	R_i	P_i	n_i	r_i	p_i
$\vdots$						
k	N_k	R_k	P_k	n_k	r_k	p_k

Direct method

In the direct method the death rate is standardized to the age structure of the standard population. The directly standardized death rate for the special population is, therefore,

$$p' = \frac{\sum N_i p_i}{\sum N_i}. \tag{19.5}$$

It is obtained by applying the special death rates, p_i, to the standard population sizes, N_i. Alternatively, p' can be regarded as a weighted mean of the p_i, using the N_i as weights. The variance of p' may be estimated as

$$\text{var}(p') = \frac{\sum (N_i^2 p_i q_i / n_i)}{(\sum N_i)^2}, \tag{19.6}$$

where $q_i = 1 - p_i$; if, as is often the case, the p_i are all small, the binomial variance of p_i, $p_i q_i / n_i$, may be replaced by the Poisson term p_i / n_i $(= r_i / n_i^2)$, giving

$$\text{var}(p') \simeq \frac{\sum (N_i^2 p_i / n_i)}{(\sum N_i)^2}. \tag{19.7}$$

To compare two special populations, A and B, we could calculate a standardized rate for each (p'_A and p'_B), and consider

$$\bar{d} = p'_A - p'_B.$$

From (19.5),

$$\bar{d} = \frac{\sum N_i (p_{Ai} - p_{Bi})}{\sum N_i},$$

which has exactly the same form as (15.15), with $w_i = N_i$, and $d_i = p_{Ai} - p_{Bi}$ as in (15.14). The method differs from that of Cochran's test only in using a different system of weights. The variance is given by

$$\text{var}(\bar{d}) = \frac{\sum N_i^2 \text{var}(d_i)}{(\sum N_i)^2}, \tag{19.8}$$

with $\text{var}(d_i)$ given by (15.17). Again, when the p_{0i} are small, q_{0i} can be put approximately equal to 1 in (15.17).

If it is required to compare two special populations using the ratio of the standardized rates, p'_A / p'_B, then the variance of the ratio may be obtained using (19.6) and (5.12).

The variance given by (19.7) may be unsatisfactory for the construction of confidence limits if the numbers of deaths in the separate age groups are small, since the normal approximation is then unsatisfactory and the Poisson limits are asymmetric (§5.2). The standardized rate (19.5) is a weighted sum of the Poisson counts, r_i. Dobson *et al.* (1991) gave a method of calculating an approximate confidence interval based on the confidence interval of the total number of deaths.

Example 19.2

In Table 19.1 a standardized rate p' could be calculated for each population. What should be taken as the standard population? There is no unique answer to this question. The choice may not greatly affect the comparison of two populations, although it will certainly affect the absolute values of the standardized rates. If the contrast between the age-specific rates is very different at different age groups, we may have to consider whether we wish the standardized rates to reflect particularly the position at certain parts of the age scale; for example, it might be desirable to give less weight to the higher age groups because the purpose of the study is mainly to compare mortality at younger ages, because the information at higher ages is less reliable, or because the death rates at high ages are more affected by sampling error.

At the foot of Table 19.1 we give standardized rates with three choices of standard population: (a) population A, (b) population B, and (c) a hypothetical population, C, whose *proportionate* distribution is midway between A and B, i.e.

$$N_{Ci} \propto \frac{1}{2} \left(\frac{n_{Ai}}{\sum n_{Ai}} + \frac{n_{Bi}}{\sum n_{Bi}} \right).$$

Note that for method (a) the standardized rate for A is the same as the crude rate; similarly for (b) the standardized rate for B is the same as the crude rate. Although the absolute values of the standardized rates are different for the three choices of standard population, the contrast is broadly the same in each case.

Indirect method

This method is more conveniently thought of as a comparison of observed and expected deaths than in terms of standardized rates. In the special population the total number of deaths observed is $\sum r_i$. The number of deaths expected if the age-specific death rates were the same as in the standard population is $\sum n_i P_i$. The overall mortality experience of the special population may be expressed in terms of that of the standard population by the ratio of observed to expected deaths:

$$M = \frac{\sum r_i}{\sum n_i P_i}. \tag{19.9}$$

When multiplied by 100 and expressed as a percentage, (19.9) is known as the *standardized mortality ratio* (SMR).

To obtain the variance of M we can use the result $\text{var}(r_i) = n_i p_i q_i$, and regard the P_i as constants without any sampling fluctuation (since we shall often

Table 19.1 Death rate for two populations, A and B, with direct standardization using A, B and a midway population C.

Age (years)	A				B				C	
	Population		Deaths	Age-specific DR per 1000	Population		Deaths	Age-specific DR per 1000	Population	
	1000s	%			1000s	%			1000s	%
0–	2100	8·97	10000	4·76	185	14·51	4100	22·16	1174	11·74
5–	1900	8·12	800	0·42	170	13·33	100	0·59	1072	10·72
10–	1700	7·26	700	0·41	160	12·55	100	0·62	990	9·90
15–	1900	8·12	2000	1·05	120	9·41	180	1·50	876	8·76
20–	1700	7·26	1700	1·00	100	7·84	190	1·90	755	7·55
25–	1500	6·41	1400	0·93	80	6·27	160	2·00	634	6·34
30–	1500	6·41	1700	1·13	70	5·49	170	2·43	595	5·95
35–	1500	6·41	2700	1·80	65	5·10	200	3·08	576	5·76
40–	1600	6·84	4800	3·00	65	5·10	270	4·15	597	5·97
45–	1500	6·41	7800	5·20	60	4·71	370	6·17	556	5·56
50–	1500	6·41	14200	9·47	55	4·31	530	9·64	536	5·36
55–	1500	6·41	23800	15·87	40	3·14	690	17·25	478	4·78
60–	1300	5·56	34900	26·85	30	2·35	880	29·33	396	3·96
65–	900	3·85	40700	45·22	30	2·35	1500	50·00	310	3·10
70–	600	2·56	42000	70·00	20	1·57	1520	76·00	207	2·07
75–	700	2·99	98100	140·14	25	1·96	4100	164·00	248	2·48
Total	23400	99·99	287300		1275	99·99	15060		10000	100·00
Crude rate				**12·28**				**11·81**		
(a) *Standardization by population A*										
Expected deaths			287300				365815			
Standardized rate				**12·28**				**15·63**		
(b) *Standardization by population B*										
Expected deaths			10242				15060			
Standardized rate				**8·03**				**11·81**		
(c) *Standardization by population C*										
Expected deaths			101657				137338			
Standardized rate				**10·17**				**13·73**		

want to compare one SMR with another using the same standard population; in any case the standard population will often be much larger than the special population, and var(P_i) will be much smaller than var(p_i)). This gives

$$\text{var}(M) = \frac{\sum n_i p_i q_i}{\left(\sum n_i P_i\right)^2}. \tag{19.10}$$

As usual, if the p_i are small, $q_i \simeq 1$ and

$$\text{var}(M) \simeq \frac{\sum r_i}{\left(\sum n_i P_i\right)^2}. \tag{19.11}$$

Confidence limits for M constructed using (19.11) are equivalent to method **3** of §5.2 (p. 154). Where the total number of deaths, $\sum r_i$, is small, this is unsatisfactory and either the better approximations of methods **1** or **2** or exact limits should be used (see Example 5.3).

If the purpose of calculating var(M) is to see whether M differs significantly from unity, var(r_i) could be taken as $n_i P_i Q_i$, on the assumption that p_i differs from a population value P_i by sampling fluctuations. If again the P_i are small, $Q_i \simeq 1$, we have

$$\text{var}(M) \simeq \frac{\sum n_i P_i}{\left(\sum n_i P_i\right)^2} = \frac{1}{\sum n_i P_i}, \tag{19.12}$$

the reciprocal of the total expected deaths. Denoting the numerator and denominator of (19.9) by O and E (for 'observed' and 'expected'), an approximate significance test would be to regard O as following a Poisson distribution with mean E. If E is not too small, the normal approximation to the Poisson leads to the use of $(O - E)/\sqrt{E}$ as a standardized normal deviate, or, equivalently, $(O - E)^2/E$ as a $\chi^2_{(1)}$ variate. This is, of course, the familiar formula for a $\chi^2_{(1)}$ variate.

Example 19.3

Table 19.2 shows some occupational mortality data, a field in which the SMR is traditionally used. The special population is that of farmers in 1951, aged 20 to 65 years. The standard population is that of all males in these age groups, whether occupied or retired. Deaths of farmers over a 5-year period are used to help reduce the sampling errors, and the observed and expected numbers are expressed on a 5-year basis.

The SMR is

$$100 \, M = \frac{(100)(7678)}{11\,005} = 69 \cdot 8\%$$

and

Table 19.2 Mortality of farmers in England and Wales, 1949–53, in comparison with that of the male population. Source: Registrar General of England and Wales (1958).

Age i	(1) Annual death rate per 100 000, all males (1949–53) $\frac{1}{5}P_i \times 10^5$	(2) Farmers, 1951 census population n_i	(3) Deaths of farmers 1949–53 r_i	(4) Deaths expected in 5 years $5 \times (1) \times (2) \times 10^{-5}$ n_iP_i
20–	129·8	8 481	87	55
25–	152·5	39 729	289	303
35–	280·4	65 700	733	921
45–	816·2	73 376	1998	2 994
55–64	2312·4	58 226	4571	6 732
			7678	11 005

$$\text{var(SMR)} = 10^4\text{var}(M)$$
$$= \frac{(10^4)(7678)}{(11\,005)^2} \text{ from (19.11),}$$
$$= 0\cdot634,$$

and

$$\text{SE(SMR)} = 0\cdot80\%.$$

The smallness of the standard error (SE) of the SMR in Example 19.3 is typical of much vital statistical data, and is the reason why sampling errors are often ignored in this type of work. Indeed, there are problems in the interpretation of occupational mortality statistics which often overshadow sampling errors. For example, occupations may be less reliably stated in censuses than in the registration of deaths, and this may lead to biases in the estimated death rates for certain occupations. Even if the data are wholly reliable, it is not clear whether a particularly high or low SMR for a certain occupation reflects a health risk in that occupation or a tendency for selective groups of people to enter it. In Example 19.3, for example, the SMR for farmers may be low because farming is healthy, or because unhealthy people are unlikely to enter farming or are more likely to leave it. Note also that in the lowest age group there is an *excess* of deaths among farmers (87 observed, 55 expected). Any method of standardization carries the risk of oversimplification, and the investigator should always compare age-specific rates to see whether the contrasts between populations vary greatly with age.

The method of indirect standardization is very similar to that described as the comparison of observed and expected frequencies on p. 520. Indeed if, in the comparison of two groups, A and B, the standard population were defined as the pooled population A + B, the method would be precisely the same as that used in the Cochran–Mantel–Haenszel method (p. 520). We have seen (p. 662) that Cochran's test is equivalent to a comparison of two direct standardized rates. There is thus a very close relationship between the direct and indirect methods when the standard population is chosen to be the sum of the two special populations.

The SMR is a weighted mean, over the separate age groups, of the ratios of the observed death rates in the special population to those in the standard population, with weights (n_iP_i) that depend on the age distribution of the special population. This means that SMRs calculated for several special populations are not strictly comparable (Yule, 1934), since they have been calculated with different weights. The SMRs will be comparable under the hypothesis that the ratio of the death rates in the special and standard populations is independent of age—that is, in a proportional-hazards situation (§17.8).

The relationship between standardization and generalized linear models is discussed by Breslow and Day (1975), Little and Pullum (1979) and Freeman and Holford (1980).

19.4 **Surveys to investigate associations**

A question commonly asked in epidemiological investigations into the aetiology of disease is whether some manifestation of ill health is associated with certain personal characteristics or habits, with particular aspects of the environment in which a person has lived or worked, or with certain experiences which a person has undergone. Examples of such questions are the following.

1   Is the risk of death from lung cancer related to the degree of cigarette smoking, whether current or in previous years?
2   Is the risk that a child dies from acute leukaemia related to whether or not the mother experienced irradiation during pregnancy?
3   Is the risk of incurring a certain illness increased for individuals who were treated with a particular drug during a previous illness?

Sometimes questions like these can be answered by controlled experimentation in which the presumptive personal factor can be administered or withheld at the investigator's discretion; in example **3**, for instance, it might be possible for the investigator to give the drug in question to some patients and not to others and to compare the outcomes. In such cases the questions are concerned with causative effects: 'Is this drug a partial *cause* of this illness?' Most often, however, the experimental approach is out of the question. The investigator must then be satisfied to observe whether there is an *association* between factor and disease, and to take the risk which was emphasized in §7.1 if he or she wishes to infer a causative link.

These questions, then, will usually be studied by surveys rather than by experiments. The precise population to be surveyed is not usually of primary interest here. One reason is that in epidemiological surveys it is usually administratively impossible to study a national or regional population, even on a sample basis. The investigator may, however, have facilities to study a particular occupational group or a population geographically related to a particular medical centre. Secondly, although the mean values or relative frequencies of the different variables may vary somewhat from one population to another, the magnitude and direction of the associations between variables are unlikely to vary greatly between, say, different occupational groups or different geographical populations.

There are two main designs for aetiological surveys—the *case–control study*, sometimes known as a *case–referent* study, and the *cohort* study. In a case–control study a group of individuals affected by the disease in question is compared with a control group of unaffected individuals. Information is obtained, usually in a retrospective way, about the frequency in each group of the various environmental or personal factors which might be associated with the disease. This type of survey is convenient in the study of rare conditions which would appear too seldom in a random population sample. By starting with a group of affected individuals one is effectively taking a much higher sampling fraction of the cases than of the controls. The method is appropriate also when the classification by disease is simple (particularly for a dichotomous classification into the presence or absence of a specific condition), but in which many possible aetiological factors have to be studied. A further advantage of the method is that, by means of the retrospective enquiry, the relevant information can be obtained comparatively quickly.

In a cohort study a population of individuals, selected usually by geographical or occupational criteria rather than on medical grounds, is studied either by complete enumeration or by a representative sample. The population is classified by the factor or factors of interest and followed prospectively in time so that the rates of occurrence of various manifestations of disease can be observed and related to the classifications by aetiological factors. The prospective nature of the cohort study means that it will normally extend longer in time than the case–control study and is likely to be administratively more complex. The corresponding advantages are that many medical conditions can be studied simultaneously and that direct information is obtained about the health of each subject through an interval of time.

Case–control and cohort studies are often called, respectively, *retrospective* and *prospective* studies. These latter terms are usually appropriate, but the nomenclature may occasionally be misleading since a cohort study may be based entirely on retrospective records. For example, if medical records are available of workers in a certain factory for the past 30 years, a cohort study may relate to workers employed 30 years ago and be based on records of their health in the succeeding 30 years. Such a study is sometimes called a *historical prospective study*.

A central problem in a case–control study is the method by which the controls are chosen. Ideally, they should be on average similar to the cases in all respects except in the medical condition under study and in associated aetiological factors. Cases will often be selected from one or more hospitals and will then share the characteristics of the population using those hospitals, such as social and environmental conditions or ethnic features. It will usually be desirable to select the control group from the same area or areas, perhaps even from the same hospitals, but suffering from quite different illnesses unlikely to share the same aetiological factors. Further, the frequencies with which various factors are found will usually vary with age and sex. Comparisons between the case and control groups must, therefore, take account of any differences there may be in the age and sex distributions of the two groups. Such adjustments are commonly avoided by arranging that each affected individual is paired with a control individual who is deliberately chosen to be of the same age and sex and to share any other demographic features which may be thought to be similarly relevant.

The remarks made in §19.2 about non-sampling errors, particularly those about non-response, are also relevant in aetiological surveys. Non-responses are always a potential danger and every attempt should be made to reduce them to as low a proportion as possible.

Example 19.4

Doll and Hill (1950) reported the results of a retrospective study of the aetiology of lung cancer. A group of 709 patients with carcinoma of the lung in 20 hospitals was compared with a control group of 709 patients without carcinoma of the lung and a third group of 637 patients with carcinoma of the stomach, colon or rectum. For each patient with lung cancer a control patient was selected from the same hospital, of the same sex and within the same 5-year age group. Each patient in each group was interviewed by a social worker, all interviewers using the same questionnaire.

The only substantial differences between the case and control groups were in their reported smoking habits. Some of the findings are summarized in Table 19.3. The difference in the proportion of non-smokers in the two groups is clearly significant, at any rate for males. (If a significance test for data of this form were required, an appropriate method would be the test for the difference of two paired proportions, described in §4.5.) The group of patients with other forms of cancer had similar smoking histories to those of the control group and differed markedly from the lung cancer group. The comparisons involving this third group are more complicated because the individual patients were not paired with members of the lung cancer or control groups and had a somewhat different age distribution. The possible effect of age had to be allowed for by methods of age standardization (see §19.3).

Table 19.3 Recent tobacco consumption of patients with carcinoma of the lung and control patients without carcinoma of the lung (Doll and Hill, 1950).

		Daily consumption of cigarettes					
	Non-smoker	1–	5–	15–	25–	50–	Total
Male							
Lung carcinoma	2	33	250	196	136	32	649
Control	27	55	293	190	71	13	649
Female							
Lung carcinoma	19	7	19	9	6	0	60
Control	32	12	10	6	0	0	60

This paper by Doll and Hill is an excellent illustration of the care which should be taken to avoid bias due to unsuspected differences between case and control groups or to different standards of data recording. This study, and many others like it, strongly suggest an association between smoking and the risk of incurring lung cancer. In such retro-spective studies, however, there is room for argument about the propriety of a particular choice of control group, little information is obtained about the time relationships involved, and nothing is known about the association between smoking and diseases other than those selected for study. Doll and Hill (1954, 1956, 1964) carried out a cohort study prospectively by sending questionnaires to all the 59 600 doctors in the UK in October 1951. Adequate replies were received from 68·2% of the population (34 439 men and 6194 women). The male doctors were followed for 40 years and notifications of deaths from various causes were obtained, only 148 being untraced (Doll *et al.*, 1994). Some results are shown in Table 19.4. The groups defined by different smoking categories have different age distributions, and the death rates shown in the table have again been standardized for age (§19.3). Cigarette smoking is again shown to be associated with a sharp increase in the death rate from lung cancer, there is almost as strong an association for chronic obstructive lung disease, and a relatively weak association with the death rates from ischaemic heart disease.

This prospective study provides strong evidence that the association between smoking and lung cancer is causative. In addition to the data in Table 19.4, many doctors who smoked at the outset of the study stopped smoking during the follow-up period, and by 1971 doctors were smoking less than half as much as people of the same ages in the general population (Doll & Peto, 1976). This reduction in smoking was matched by a steady decline in the death rate from lung cancer for the whole group of male doctors (age-standardized, and expressed as a fraction of the national mortality rate) over the first 20 years of follow-up.

In a cohort study in which the incidence of a specific disease is of particular interest, the case–control approach may be adopted by analysing the data of all the cases and a control group of randomly selected non-cases. This approach was termed a *synthetic retrospective study* by Mantel (1973). Often the controls are

Table 19.4 Standardized annual death rates among male doctors for three causes of death, 1951–91, related to smoking habits (Doll *et al.*, 1994).

		Standardized death rate per 100 000 men					
					Cigarette smokers (cigarettes per day)		
	Number of deaths	Non-smokers	Ex-smokers	Current smokers	1–14	15–24	25–
Lung cancer	893	14	58	209	105	208	355
Chronic obstructive lung disease	542	10	57	127	86	112	225
Ischaemic heart disease	6438	572	678	892	802	892	1025

chosen matched for each case by random sampling from the members of the cohort who are non-cases at the time that the case developed the disease (Liddell *et al.*, 1977), and this is usually referred to as a *nested case–control study*. Care may be needed to avoid the repeated selection of the same individuals as controls for more than one case (Robins *et al.*, 1989). A related design is the *case–cohort study*, which consists of a random sample of the whole cohort; some members of this sample will become cases and they are supplemented by the cases that occur in the remainder of the cohort, with the non-cases in the random subcohort serving as controls for the total set of cases (Kupper *et al.*, 1975; Prentice, 1986). These designs are useful in situations where it is expensive to extract the whole data, or when expensive tests are required; if material, such as blood samples, can be stored and then analysed for only a fraction of the cohort, then there may be a large saving in resources with very little loss of efficiency.

The measurement of the degree of association between the risk of disease and the presence of an aetiological factor is discussed in detail in the next section.

19.5 **Relative risk**

Cohort and case–control methods for studying the aetiology of disease were discussed in the previous section. In such studies it is usual to make comparisons between groups with different characteristics, in particular between a group of individuals exposed to some factor and a group not exposed. A measure of the increased risk (if any) of contracting a particular disease in the exposed compared with the non-exposed is required. The measure usually used is the ratio of the incidences in the groups being compared and is referred to as *relative risk* (ϕ). Thus,

$$\phi = I_E/I_{NE}, \tag{19.13}$$

where I_E and I_{NE} are the incidence rates in the exposed and non-exposed, respectively. This measure may also be referred to as the *risk ratio*.

In a cohort study the relative risk can be estimated directly, since estimates are available of both I_E and I_{NE}. In a case–control study the relative risk cannot be estimated directly since neither I_E nor I_{NE} can be estimated, and we now consider how to obtain a useful solution.

Suppose that each subject in a large population has been classified as positive or negative according to some potential aetiological factor, and positive or negative according to some disease state. The factor might be based on a current classification or (more usually in a retrospective study) on the subject's past history. The disease state may refer to the presence or absence of a certain category of disease at a particular instant, or to a certain occurrence (such as diagnosis or death) during a stated period—that is, to *prevalence* and *incidence*, respectively.

For any such categorization the population may be enumerated in a 2×2 table, as follows. The entries in the table are *proportions* of the total population.

$$
\begin{array}{ccccc}
 & & \multicolumn{3}{c}{\text{Disease}} \\
 & & + & - & \\
 & + & P_1 & P_3 & P_1 + P_3 \\
\text{Factor} & & & & \\
 & - & P_2 & P_4 & P_2 + P_4 \\
\hline
 & & P_1 + P_2 & P_3 + P_4 & 1
\end{array}
\tag{19.14}
$$

If these proportions were known, the association between the factor and the disease could be measured by the ratio of the risks of being disease-positive for those with and those without the factor.

$$
\begin{aligned}
\text{Risk ratio} &= \frac{P_1}{(P_1 + P_3)} \div \frac{P_2}{(P_2 + P_4)} \\
&= \frac{P_1(P_2 + P_4)}{P_2(P_1 + P_3)}.
\end{aligned}
\tag{19.15}
$$

Where the cases are incident cases the risk ratio is the relative risk.

Now, in many (although not all) situations in which aetiological studies are done, the proportion of subjects classified as disease-positive will be small. That is, P_1 will be small in comparison with P_3, and P_2 will be small in comparison with P_4. In such a case, (19.15) will be very nearly equal to

$$\frac{P_1}{P_3} \div \frac{P_2}{P_4} = \frac{P_1 P_4}{P_2 P_3} (= \psi, \text{say}). \tag{19.16}$$

The ratio (19.16) is properly called the *odds ratio* (because it is the ratio of P_1/P_3 to P_2/P_4, and these two quantities can be thought of as odds in favour of having the disease), but it is often referred to as *approximate relative risk* (because of the approximation referred to above) or simply as *relative risk*. Another term is *cross-ratio* (because the two products $P_1 P_4$ and $P_2 P_3$ which appear in (19.16) are obtained by multiplying diagonally across the table).

The odds ratio (19.16) could be estimated from a random sample of the population, or from a sample stratified by the two levels of the factor (such as a prospective cohort study started some time before the disease assessments are made). It could also be estimated from a sample stratified by the two disease states (i.e. from a case–control study), and it is this fact which makes it such a useful measure of relative risk. Suppose a case–control study is carried out by selecting separate random samples of diseased and non-diseased individuals, and that the *frequencies* (not proportions) are as follows, using the notation of §4.5:

		Disease		
		+ (cases)	− (controls)	
Factor	+	a	c	$a + c$
	−	b	d	$b + d$
		$a + b$	$c + d$	n

$$\tag{19.17}$$

Frequently, of course, the sampling plan will lead to equal numbers of cases and controls; then $a + b = c + d = \frac{1}{2}n$. Now, a/b can be regarded as a reasonable estimate of P_1/P_2, and c/d similarly estimates P_3/P_4. The observed odds ratio,

$$\hat{\psi} = \frac{ad}{bc}, \tag{19.18}$$

is the ratio of a/b to c/d, and therefore can be taken as an estimate of

$$\frac{P_1}{P_2} \div \frac{P_3}{P_4} = \frac{P_1 P_4}{P_2 P_3} (= \psi), \tag{19.19}$$

the population odds ratio or approximate relative risk defined by (19.16).

The assumption that the case and control groups are random samples from the same relevant population group is difficult to satisfy in case–control studies. Nevertheless, the estimates of relative risk derived from case–control studies often agree quite well with those obtained from corroborative cohort studies, and the theory seems likely to be useful as a rough guide. In retrospective studies, cases are often matched with control individuals for various factors; the effect of this matching is discussed below.

Equation (19.18) is identical to (4.25), and the sampling variation of an odds ratio is best considered on the logarithmic scale, as in (4.26), so that approximate limits, known as the *logit limits*, can be obtained, as in Example 4.11. If any of the cell frequencies are small, more complex methods, as discussed in §4.5, must be used. Apart from exact limits (Baptista & Pike, 1977), the limits due to Cornfield (1956) are the most satisfactory (see (4.27) to (4.29)).

Example 19.5

In a case–control study of women with breast cancer (Ellery *et al.*, 1986), the data on whether oral contraceptives were used before first full-term pregnancy were:

		Cases	Controls	
	Yes	4	11	15
OC before FFTP				
	No	63	107	170
		67	118	185

Proceeding as in Example 4.11, the estimated odds ratio is 0·62 with 95% logit limits of 0·19 and 2·02. Using the notation of (4.27) to (4.29), the upper Cornfield limit is for $A = 7·62$. Substituting this value in (4.28) gives $\psi_U = 1·92$, from (4.29) var(a; $\psi = 1·92$) = 3·417, and evaluating (4.27) gives $-1·96$. The lower limit was found for $A = 1·66$, giving $\psi_L = 0·20$. Therefore the Cornfield limits are 0·20 and 1·92.

Frequently an estimate of relative risk is made from each of a number of subsets of the data, and there is some interest in the comparison and combination of these different estimates. There may, for example, be several studies of the same aetiological problem done at different times and places, or, in any one study, the data may have been subdivided into one or more categories, such as age groups, which affect the relative proportions in the rows of the 2×2 table or in the columns or in both rows and columns. One approach, illustrated in Example 19.6 below, is to take the separate estimates of ln $\hat{\psi}$ and weight them by the reciprocal of the sampling variance (4.26). The estimates can then be combined by taking a weighted mean, and they can be tested for heterogeneity by a χ^2 index like (8.15) (Woolf, 1955). This method breaks down when the subsets contain few subjects and therefore becomes unsuitable with increasing stratification of a data set. Although in these circumstances the method may be improved by adding $\frac{1}{2}$ to each observed frequency, it is preferable to use an alternative method of combination due to Mantel and Haenszel (1959). For many situations this method gives similar results to the method of Woolf, but the

Mantel–Haenszel method is more robust when some of the strata contain small frequencies; in particular, it may still be used without modification when some of the frequencies are zero. The method was introduced in §15.6 as a significance test. We now give further details from the viewpoint of estimation. Denote the frequencies in the 2×2 table for the ith subdivision by the notation of (19.17) with subscript i. The Mantel–Haenszel pooled estimate of ψ is then

$$R_{MH} = \frac{\sum (a_i d_i / n_i)}{\sum (b_i c_i / n_i)}. \tag{19.20}$$

Mantel and Haenszel gave a significance test of the hypothesis that $\psi = 1$. If there were no association between the factor and the disease, the expected value and the variance of a_i would, as in (15.18) and (17.12), be given by

$$\left.\begin{aligned} \mathrm{E}(a_i) &= \frac{(a_i + b_i)(a_i + c_i)}{n_i}, \\ \mathrm{var}(a_i) &= \frac{(a_i + b_i)(c_i + d_i)(a_i + c_i)(b_i + d_i)}{n_i^2 (n_i - 1)} \end{aligned}\right\}. \tag{19.21}$$

The test is calculated by adding the differences between the observed and expected values of a_i over the subsets. Since these subsets are independent, the variance of the sum of differences is equal to the sum of the separate variances. This gives as a test statistic

$$X_{MH}^2 = \frac{[\sum a_i - \sum \mathrm{E}(a_i)]^2}{\sum \mathrm{var}(a_i)}, \tag{19.22}$$

which is approximately a $\chi_{(1)}^2$ (see (15.20)). If desired, a continuity correction may be included.

A number of options are now available for estimating the variance of R_{MH}, and hence constructing confidence limits. First, using the method proposed by Miettinen (1976), *test-based* confidence limits may be constructed. If the standard error of $\ln R_{MH}$ were known, then, under normal theory, a test statistic of the hypothesis $\psi = 1$ ($\ln \psi = 0$) would be

$$z = \ln R_{MH} / \mathrm{SE}(\ln R_{MH}),$$

taken as an approximate standardized normal deviate. The test statistic X_{MH}^2 is approximately a $\chi_{(1)}^2$, and taking the square root gives an approximate standardized normal deviate (§5.1). The test-based method consists of equating these two test statistics to give an estimate of $\mathrm{SE}(\ln R_{MH})$. That is,

$$\mathrm{SE}(\ln R_{MH}) = (\ln R_{MH}) / X_{MH}. \tag{19.23}$$

This method is strictly only valid if $\psi = 1$, but in practice gives reasonable results provided R_{MH} is not extreme (see Breslow & Day (1980, §4.3), who recommend using X_{MH} calculated without the continuity correction for this purpose). Unfortunately, the method breaks down if $R_{MH} = 1$. The calculations are illustrated in Example 19.6.

The most satisfactory method was proposed by Robins *et al.* (1986). This method is suitable when a large data set is subdivided into many strata, some containing small frequencies, as well as when there are only a few strata, none containing small frequencies. Using their notation,

$$P_i = (a_i + d_i)/n_i, \quad Q_i = (b_i + c_i)/n_i,$$
$$R_i = a_i d_i/n_i, \quad S_i = b_i c_i/n_i, \quad R_+ = \sum R_i$$

and

$$S_+ = \sum S_i \text{ (so that } R_{MH} = R_+/S_+);$$

then

$$\text{var}(\ln R_{MH}) = \frac{\sum P_i R_i}{2R_+^2} + \frac{\sum (P_i S_i + Q_i R_i)}{2R_+ S_+} + \frac{\sum Q_i S_i}{2S_+^2}. \tag{19.24}$$

Breslow and Day (1980, §4.4) set out a method for testing the homogeneity of the odds ratio over the strata. However, like the method of Woolf discussed above, the method breaks down with increasing stratification.

A special case of subdivision occurs in case–control studies, in which each case is matched with a control subject for certain important factors, such as age, sex, residence, etc. Strictly, each pair of matched subjects should form a subdivision for the calculation of relative risk, although, of course, the individual estimates from such pairs would be valueless. The Mantel–Haenszel pooled estimate (19.20) can, however, be calculated, and takes a particularly simple form. Suppose there are altogether $\frac{1}{2}n$ matched pairs. These can be entered into a 2×2 table according to whether the two individuals are factor-positive or factor-negative, with frequencies as follows:

		Control		
		Factor +	Factor −	
Case	Factor +	t	r	a
	Factor −	s	u	b
		c	d	$\frac{1}{2}n$

(19.25)

The marginal totals in (19.25) are the cell frequencies in the earlier table (19.17). The Mantel–Haenszel estimate is then

$$R = \frac{r}{s}. \tag{19.26}$$

This can be shown to be a particularly satisfactory estimate if the true relative risk, as measured by the cross-ratio of the probabilities (19.16), is the same for every pair. The Mantel–Haenszel test statistic is identical to that of McNemar's test (4.17).

Inferences are made by treating r as a binomial variable with sample size $r + s$. The methods of §4.4 may then be applied and the confidence limits of the relative risk, ψ_L and ψ_U, obtained from those of the binomial parameter π, using the relation

$$\psi = \frac{\pi}{1 - \pi}.$$

Liddell (1983) showed that the limits given by (4.16) simplify after the above transformation to give

$$\left. \begin{aligned} \psi_L &= \frac{r}{(s + 1)F_{0.025,\, 2(s+1),\, 2r}} \\ \psi_U &= \frac{(r + 1)F_{0.025,\, 2(r+1),\, 2s}}{s} \end{aligned} \right\}, \tag{19.27}$$

and that an exact test of $\psi = 1$ is given by

$$F = \frac{r}{s + 1}, \tag{19.28}$$

tested against the F distribution with $2(s + 1)$ and $2r$ degrees of freedom (in this formulation, if $r < s$, r and s should be interchanged). This exact test may be used instead of the approximate McNemar test (§4.5).

A general point is that the logarithm of ψ is, from (19.16),

$$\ln(P_1/P_3) - \ln(P_2/P_4) = \text{logit (probability of disease when factor +)}$$
$$- \text{logit (probability of disease when factor −)}.$$

The methods of analysis suggested in this section can thus be seen to be particularly appropriate if the effect of changing from factor + to factor − is to change the probability of being in the diseased state by a constant amount *on the logit scale*. It has been indicated in §14.2 that this is a reasonable general approach to a wide range of problems, but in any particular instance it may be far from true. The investigator should therefore guard against too ready an assumption that a relative risk calculated in one study is necessarily applicable under somewhat different circumstances.

Example 19.6 uses the above methods to combine a number of studies into a summary analysis. It may be regarded as a simple example of meta-analysis (§18.10).

Example 19.6

Table 19.5 summarizes results from 10 retrospective surveys in which patients with lung cancer and control subjects were classified as smokers or non-smokers. In most or all of these surveys, cases and controls would have been matched, but the original data are usually not presented in sufficient detail to enable relative risks to be estimated from (19.26) and matching is ignored in the present analysis. (The effect of ignoring matching when it is present is, if anything, to underestimate the departure of the relative risk from unity.) The data were compiled by Cornfield (1956) and have been referred to also by Gart (1962).

Defining w_i as the reciprocal of $\text{var}(\ln \hat{\psi}_i)$ from (4.26), the weighted mean is

$$\frac{\sum w_i \ln \hat{\psi}_i}{\sum w_i} = \frac{161\cdot36}{105\cdot4} = 1\cdot531,$$

and the pooled estimate of ψ is $\exp(1\cdot531) = 4\cdot62$.

For the heterogeneity test (8.15), the $\chi^2_{(9)}$ statistic is

$$\sum w_i (\ln \hat{\psi}_i)^2 - \frac{(\sum w_i \ln \hat{\psi}_i)^2}{\sum w_i} = 253\cdot678 - 247\cdot061 = 6\cdot62 \quad (P = 0\cdot68).$$

There is no strong evidence of heterogeneity between separate estimates. It is, of course, likely that the relative risk varies to some extent from study to study, particularly as the factor 'smoking' covers such a wide range of activity. However, the sampling variation of the separate estimates is evidently too large to enable such real variation to emerge. If we assume that all the variation is due to sampling error, the variance of the weighted mean of $\ln \hat{\psi}_i$ can be obtained as

$$\frac{1}{\sum w_i} = 0\cdot00949.$$

Approximate 95% confidence limits for $\ln \psi$ are

$$1\cdot531 \pm (1\cdot96)\sqrt{0\cdot00949} = 1\cdot340 \text{ and } 1\cdot722.$$

The corresponding limits for ψ are obtained by exponentials as $3\cdot82$ and $5\cdot60$.

The Mantel–Haenszel estimator of ψ is

$$R_{MH} = \frac{302\cdot840}{64\cdot687} = 4\cdot68.$$

The statistic for testing that this estimate differs from unity is

$$X^2_{MH} = (3793 - 3554\cdot85)^2 / 193\cdot17$$
$$= 293\cdot60 \quad (P < 0\cdot001).$$

The test-based method of calculating confidence limits from (19.23) gives

$$SE(\ln R_{MH}) = \ln(4\cdot68)/\sqrt{293\cdot60}$$
$$= 1\cdot543/17\cdot13$$
$$= 0\cdot0901,$$

and approximate 95% confidence limits for $\ln \psi$ are

Table 19.5 Combination of relative risks from 10 retrospective surveys on smoking and lung cancer (Cornfield, 1956; Gart 1962).

Study number	Lung cancer patients Smokers a_i	Non-smokers b_i	Control patients Smokers c_i	Non-smokers d_i	Woolf's method $\hat\psi_i$	$\ln\hat\psi_i$	(1) $1/a_i +$ $1/b_i +$ $1/c_i +$ $1/d_i$	$w_i = \frac{1}{(1)}$	$w_i \ln\hat\psi_i$	Mantel–Haenszel n_i	$a_i d_i/n_i$	$b_i c_i/n_i$	$E(a_i)$	$var(a_i)$
1	83	3	72	14	5·38	1·683	0·4307	2·3	3·87	172	6·756	1·256	77·50	3·85
2	90	3	227	43	5·68	1·737	0·3721	2·7	4·69	363	10·661	1·876	81·21	7·68
3	129	7	81	19	4·32	1·463	0·2156	4·6	6·73	236	10·386	2·403	121·02	5·67
4	412	32	299	131	5·64	1·730	0·0447	22·4	38·75	874	61·753	10·947	361·19	33·18
5	1350	7	1296	61	9·08	2·206	0·1608	6·2	13·68	2714	30·343	3·343	1323·00	16·58
6	60	3	106	27	5·09	1·627	0·3965	2·5	4·07	196	8·265	1·622	53·36	5·57
7	459	18	534	81	3·87	1·353	0·0720	13·9	18·81	1092	34·047	8·802	433·76	22·17
8	499	19	462	56	3·18	1·157	0·0747	13·4	15·50	1036	26·973	8·473	480·50	17·41
9	451	39	1729	636	4·25	1·447	0·0300	33·3	48·19	2855	100·468	23·619	374·15	73·30
10	260	5	259	28	5·62	1·726	0·2434	4·1	7·08	522	13·188	2·346	249·16	7·76
Total	3793	136	5065	1096				105·4	161·37		302·840	64·687	3554·85	193·17

$$1 \cdot 543 \pm 1 \cdot 96 \times 0 \cdot 0901 = 1 \cdot 366 \text{ and } 1 \cdot 720.$$

The corresponding limits for ψ are the exponentials, $3 \cdot 92$ and $5 \cdot 58$. The point estimate and the confidence limits are very similar indeed to those derived using Woolf's method. Details of the calculation are not given here but (19.24) gives SE (ln R_{MH}) $= 0 \cdot 0977$ to give 95% confidence limits of $3 \cdot 86$ and $5 \cdot 67$, similar to both sets of limits derived earlier.

Another frequently occurring situation is when the factor, instead of having just two levels, presence or absence, has three or more levels that have a definite order. For example, instead of classifying people as non-smokers or smokers, the smokers could be divided further according to the amount smoked. Such a situation was discussed in §15.7. Mantel (1963) extended the Mantel–Haenszel procedure to provide a test for trend and to combine a number of subsets of the data (15.21). An example of the method is given in Example 15.8.

The methods discussed above are powerful in the commonly occurring situation where it is required to analyse the association between a disease and a single exposure factor, making allowance for one other factor, or at most a few, and where the effect of the other factors may be adequately represented by subdivision of the data into strata. The methods are inconvenient where several exposure factors are of interest and for each factor allowance must be made for the others, as was the case in Example 14.1. Also, where several factors are to be adjusted for, stratification would involve a large number of strata; in the limit each stratum would contain only one subject, so that comparisons within strata would be impossible. In these cases more general methods must be used and logistic regression (§14.2) is appropriate. This is because of the combination of two features. First, as observed above, the odds ratio can be estimated from a case–control study and, secondly, the logarithm of the odds ratio is a difference of logits. For a case-control study all the coefficients of (14.6) may be estimated except for the constant term β_0, which is distorted by the investigator's choice of the size of the case and control groups. The estimate of a regression coefficient measures the logarithm of the odds ratio for a change of unity in the corresponding variable, and so the exponentials of the regression coefficients give estimated odds ratios or approximate relative risks.

It was observed above that, for a case–control study where a matched control is chosen for each case, the Mantel–Haenszel method may be applied, and leads to McNemar's test. When the number of cases available is limited, the precision of a study may be increased, to some extent, by choosing more than one matched control per case. The Mantel–Haenszel method can be applied, treating each set of a case and its controls as a subset. The analysis may be simplified by grouping together sets providing identical information; for example, with three controls per case those sets where the case and just two of the three controls are positive for the exposure factor all provide identical information. This is an extension of

(19.25). For further details of the analysis, see Miettinen (1969, 1970) and Pike and Morrow (1970).

In a matched case–control study there may be covariates recorded on each individual and it may be necessary to take account of the possible influence of the covariates on the probability of disease. The covariates may be included in a logistic regression model but account also has to be taken of the matching. This is done by working conditionally within each set. Suppose that x represents the set of covariates, including the exposure factor of principal interest, and use a subscript of zero for the case and 1 to c for the c controls. Then, using the logistic regression model (14.6) and assuming that the probability of disease is small, so that the logit is approximately equal to the logarithm of the probability of disease, the probability of disease of each member of the set is $\exp(\beta_{0s} + \boldsymbol{\beta}^{\mathrm{T}} x_i)$, $i = 0, 1, \ldots, c$. The parameter β_0 has a subscript s to indicate that it depends on the particular set. Now each set has been chosen to include exactly one case of disease. Arguing conditionally that there is just one individual with disease in the set, the probability that it is the observed case is

$$\exp(\beta_{0s} + \boldsymbol{\beta}^{\mathrm{T}} x_0) / \sum \exp(\beta_{0s} + \boldsymbol{\beta}^{\mathrm{T}} x_i),$$

where summation is over all members of the set, $i = 0, 1, \ldots, c$. The numerator and denominator contain the common factor $\exp(\beta_{0s})$ and so the probability may be expressed as

$$\exp(\boldsymbol{\beta}^{\mathrm{T}} \mathbf{x_0}) / \sum \exp(\boldsymbol{\beta}^{\mathrm{T}} x_i), \tag{19.29}$$

a result first given by Thomas in Liddell *et al.* (1977). An expression of the form of (19.29) is obtained for each case and combined to form a likelihood; then $\boldsymbol{\beta}$ is estimated by the method of maximum likelihood (§14.2). By working conditionally within sets the large number of parameters β_{0s} (one per case) have been eliminated. This exposition has been relatively brief and readers interested in further details of the analysis of case–control studies are referred to the monographs by Breslow and Day (1980) and Schlesselman (1982).

In §17.6 it was observed that the logrank test for analysing survival data was similar to the Mantel–Haenszel test. Comparing (19.29) with (17.27) shows that the method of logistic regression in a matched case–control study is similar to the proportional-hazards model for survival analysis. A case–control study may be considered as a sample from a hypothetical cohort study; indeed, for validity it should be just that. It is, therefore, no coincidence that methods originally derived for the analysis of cohort studies should also be applicable to case–control studies. An analysis based on (19.29) can be carried out using PROC PHREG in the SAS program, with each case–control set defining a stratum.

19.6 **Attributable risk**

The full implications of an excess risk depend not only on the size of the relative risk but also on the proportion of the population positive for the aetiological factor. A moderate relative risk applicable to a high proportion of the population would produce more cases of disease than a high relative risk applicable to just a small proportion of the population. A measure of association, due to Levin (1953), that takes account of the proportion of the population at risk is the *attributable risk*. Terminology is not completely standard and other names for this measure are *aetiological fraction* and *attributable fraction*. Also these measures may be used to refer either to the whole population or just to the exposed subgroup and, to avoid ambiguity, it is preferable to be specific and to use the terms *population attributable risk* and *attributable risk among the exposed*.

The population attributable risk is defined as the proportion of cases in the total population that are attributable to the risk factor. It is usually calculated in circumstances in which it is considered justifiable to infer causation from an observed association. Then it may be interpreted as the proportion of cases in the population that are due to the factor, and hence as a measure of the importance of eliminating the factor as part of a disease-prevention strategy. The circumstances in which this interpretation is justified are probably few and there are particular difficulties when more than one cause is operating.

Suppose I_P is the incidence of the disease in the population and, as in §19.5, I_E and I_{NE} are the incidences in the exposed and non-exposed, respectively. Then the excess incidence attributable to the factor is $I_P - I_{NE}$ and dividing by the population incidence gives the population attributable risk,

$$\lambda_P = \frac{I_P - I_{NE}}{I_P}. \tag{19.30}$$

Now suppose a proportion θ_E of the population are exposed to the factor, then

$$\begin{aligned} I_P &= \theta_E I_E + (1 - \theta_E) I_{NE} \\ &= \theta_E \phi I_{NE} + (1 - \theta_E) I_{NE} \\ &= I_{NE}[1 + \theta_E(\phi - 1)], \end{aligned} \tag{19.31}$$

where ϕ is the relative risk and the second line is obtained using (19.13). Substituting in (19.30) gives

$$\lambda_P = \frac{\theta_E(\phi - 1)}{1 + \theta_E(\phi - 1)}, \tag{19.32}$$

and the attributable risk can be estimated from the relative risk and the proportion of the population exposed. Often the attributable proportion is multiplied by 100 to give a result in percentage terms and this may be referred to as the *population attributable risk per cent*.

An alternative expression may be derived using the notation of (19.14). If the probability of disease in those positive for the factor were the same as for those negative, then the proportion of the population positive for both factor and disease would be

$$(P_1 + P_3) \times \frac{P_2}{P_2 + P_4}.$$

Subtracting this from the actual proportion, P_1, gives the excess proportion related to the factor, and, dividing by the proportion with disease, the population attributable risk is given by

$$
\begin{aligned}
\lambda_P &= \left[P_1 - \frac{P_2(P_1 + P_3)}{P_2 + P_4} \right] \div (P_1 + P_2) \\
&= \frac{P_1}{P_1 + P_2} \left[1 - \frac{P_2(P_1 + P_3)}{P_1(P_2 + P_4)} \right] \\
&= \frac{P_1}{P_1 + P_2} \left(1 - \frac{I_{NE}}{I_E} \right) \\
&= \theta_1 \frac{\phi - 1}{\phi},
\end{aligned}
\tag{19.33}
$$

where θ_1 is the proportion of cases exposed to the factor.

It follows from (19.32) that the population attributable risk can be estimated from any study that provides estimates both of relative risk and the proportion of the population exposed to the factor. Thus, it may be estimated from a case–control study, since the relative risk can be estimated approximately and the proportion of the population exposed can be estimated from the controls (again assuming that the disease is rare). Alternatively, (19.33) could be used, since θ_1 can be estimated in a case–control study. Clearly, population attributable risk may be estimated from a cohort study of a random sample of the total population, but only from a sample stratified by the two levels of exposure if the proportion of the population exposed is known.

The attributable risk among the exposed may be defined as the proportion of exposed cases attributable to the factor. This measure is

$$\lambda_E = \frac{I_E - I_{NE}}{I_E} = \frac{\phi - 1}{\phi}. \tag{19.34}$$

The above formulation has been in terms of a factor which increases risk, i.e. relative risk greater than unity. For a factor which is protective, i.e. relative risk less than unity, a slightly different formulation is necessary; this is discussed by Kleinbaum *et al.* (1982, Chapter 9), although often the simplest approach is to reverse the direction of the relative risk, e.g. 'exercise is protective against heart disease' is equivalent to 'lack of exercise is a risk factor'.

We now consider the sampling variation of an estimate of population attributable risk from a case–control study, and give an example.

Consider data of the form (19.17) from a case–control study. Since $a/(a + b)$ estimates $P_1/(P_1 + P_2)$ or θ_1, and ad/bc estimates ψ, which is approximately ϕ, substitution in (19.33) gives as an estimate of λ_P

$$\hat{\lambda}_P = \frac{a}{a + b} \left(1 - \frac{bc}{ad} \right)$$
$$= \frac{ad - bc}{d(a + b)}. \tag{19.35}$$

Exactly the same expression may be obtained substituting $c/(c + d)$ for θ_E in (19.32). It is convenient to work with $\ln(1 - \hat{\lambda}_P)$ since, as shown by Walter (1975), this variable is approximately normally distributed.

$$1 - \hat{\lambda}_P = \frac{bd + bc}{d(a + b)}$$
$$= \frac{b}{a + b} \div \frac{d}{c + d}$$
$$= \frac{1 - \hat{\theta}_1}{1 - \hat{\theta}_2}$$

and

$$\ln(1 - \hat{\lambda}_P) = \ln(1 - \hat{\theta}_1) - \ln(1 - \hat{\theta}_2),$$

where $\hat{\theta}_1$ is an estimator of $P_1/(P_1 + P_2)$ and $\hat{\theta}_2$ of $P_3/(P_3 + P_4)$. $\hat{\theta}_1$ and $\hat{\theta}_2$ are independent estimators of proportions, so, using (4.13) and (5.19), we obtain

$$\text{var}[(1 - \hat{\lambda}_P)] = \frac{a}{b(a + b)} + \frac{c}{d(c + d)}. \tag{19.36}$$

Example 19.7

Consider the data from study 1 of Table 19.5, in which 83 out of 86 lung cancer patients were smokers compared with 72 out of 86 controls. Then, using (19.35) and (19.36),

$$\hat{\lambda}_P = \frac{83 \times 14 - 3 \times 72}{14 \times 86}$$
$$= 0 \cdot 7857,$$
$$\ln(1 - \hat{\lambda}_P) = -1 \cdot 540,$$
$$\text{var}[\ln(1 - \hat{\lambda}_P)] = \frac{83}{3 \times 86} + \frac{72}{14 \times 86}$$
$$= 0 \cdot 3815.$$

Therefore approximate 95% confidence limits for $\ln(1 - \hat{\lambda}_P)$ are

$$-1 \cdot 540 \pm (1 \cdot 96)\sqrt{0 \cdot 3815} = -2 \cdot 751 \text{ and } -0 \cdot 329,$$

and the corresponding limits for $\hat{\lambda}_P$ are 0·281 and 0·936.

Whittemore (1983) extended Levin's measure to account for a qualitative confounding variable by forming a weighted average of the attributable risks in each stratum of the confounder with weights equal to the proportion of cases estimated to be within each stratum in the whole population. This does not require any assumption of a uniform relative risk across strata, and so also adjusts for interaction effects. Where the confounders are accounted for by a stratified analysis, then a pooled relative risk is often estimated using the Mantel–Haenszel approach, and this estimate can be used to estimate the attributable risk, using (19.33). Kuritz and Landis (1988) used this approach for a matched case–control study and proposed a method of calculating the confidence interval. Greenland (1987) gave variance estimators for the attributable risk based on the sampling variability of R_{MH} (19.24); these estimators are satisfactory for both large strata and sparse data—that is, data divided into a large number of strata with small numbers within each stratum. The interpretation of these adjusted measures of population attributable risk as the proportion of cases that could be eliminated by removing exposure to the factor depends on all other factors remaining unchanged. In most situations it would be impossible to modify one factor without influencing other factors and so this interpretation would be invalid.

Further details of the estimation of attributable risk and the problems of interpretation are given in a review article by Benichou (1998).

19.7 **Subject-years method**

As noted in §19.4, a commonly used research method is the *cohort study*, in which a group is classified by exposure to some substance, followed over time and the vital status of each member determined up to the time at which the analysis is being conducted. A review of methods of cohort study design and application was given by Liddell (1988). It may be possible to use existing records to determine exposure in the past, and this gives the *historical prospective cohort* study, used particularly in occupational health research. Such studies often cover periods of over 20 years. The aim is to compare the mortality experience of subgroups, such as high exposure with low exposure, in order to establish whether exposure to the agent might be contributing to mortality. As such studies cover a long period of time, individuals will be ageing and their mortality risk will be changing. In addition, there may be period effects on mortality rate. Both the age and period effects will need to be taken account of. One approach is the *subject-years* or *person-years method*, sometimes referred to as the *modified life-table approach*; an early use of this method was by Doll (1952). In this approach the number of deaths in the group, or in the subgroups, is expressed in terms of the number of deaths expected if the individuals had experienced the same death rates as the population of which the group is a part.

The expected mortality is calculated using published national or regional death rates. The age of each subject, both at entry to the study and as it changes through the period of follow-up, has to be taken into account. Also, since age-specific death rates depend on the period of time at which the risk occurs, the cohort of each subject must be considered. Official death rates are usually published in 5-year intervals of age and period and may be arranged as a rectangular array consisting of cells, such as the age group 45–49 during the period 1976–80. Each subject passes through several of these cells during the period of follow-up and experiences a risk of dying according to the years of risk in each cell and the death rate. This risk is accumulated so long as a subject is at risk of dying in the study—that is, until the date of death or until the end of the follow-up period for the survivors. This accumulated risk is the same as the cumulative hazard (17.29). The expected number of deaths is obtained by adding over all subjects in the group, and it is computationally convenient to add the years at risk in each cell over subjects before multiplying by the death rates. This is the origin of the name of the method, since subject-years at risk are calculated.

The method can be applied for total deaths and also for deaths from specific causes. The same table of subject-years at risk is used for each cause with different tables of death rates and, when a particular cause of death is being considered, deaths from any other cause are effectively treated as censored survivals. For any cause of death, the observed number is treated as a Poisson variable with expectation equal to the expected number (Example 5.2). The method is similar to indirect standardization of death rates (§19.3) and the ratio of observed to expected deaths is often referred to as the standardized mortality ratio (SMR).

Example 19.8

A group of 512 men working in an asbestos factory was followed up (Newhouse *et al.*, 1985). All men who started work in particular jobs at any time after 1933 were included and mortality was assessed over the period from 10 years after start of employment in the factory for each man up to the end of 1980. Mortality from lung cancer was of particular relevance. The subject-years at risk and the death rates for lung cancer in England and Wales are shown in Table 19.6 in 5-year age groups and 10-year periods (in the original application 5-year periods were used).

Table 19.6 Subject-years at risk (y) of asbestos workers and death rates (d) per 100 000 for lung cancer in men in England and Wales.

Age group	Period							
	1941–50		1951–60		1961–70		1971–80	
	y	d	y	d	y	d	y	d
25–29	82	2	62	1	13	1	3	1
30–34	148	3	273	4	156	3	43	2
35–39	74	9	446	10	435	8	141	6
40–44	41	21	395	25	677	22	290	16
45–49	33	46	229	58	749	54	485	46
50–54	23	78	172	124	590	119	642	106
55–59	14	112	158	216	399	226	621	201
60–64	11	137	109	294	288	370	479	346
65–69	4	137	78	343	185	508	273	530
70–74	0	107	47	325	124	562	151	651
75+	0	86	16	270	58	518	72	756

The expected number of deaths due to lung cancer is

$$(82 \times 2 + 62 \times 1 + 13 \times 1 + \ldots + 72 \times 756) \times 10^{-5} = 13 \cdot 8.$$

The observed number was 67, so the SMR is $67/13 \cdot 8 = 4 \cdot 9$. Using the methods given in §5.2, a test of the null hypothesis that the asbestos workers experienced national death rates is

$$z = (67 - 13 \cdot 8)/\sqrt{13 \cdot 8} = 14 \cdot 3 \ (P < 0 \cdot 001),$$

and approximate 95% confidence limits for the SMR are $3 \cdot 8$ and $6 \cdot 2$.

The method has usually been applied to compare observed and expected mortality within single groups but may be extended to compare the SMR between different subgroups or, more generally, to take account of covariates recorded for each individual, by expressing the SMR as a proportional-hazards regression model (Berry, 1983)—that is, by the use of a generalized linear model (§14.4). For subgroup i, if m_i is the cumulative hazard from the reference population and γ_i the proportional-hazards multiplier, then μ_i, the expected number of deaths, is given by

$$\ln \mu_i = \ln m_i + \ln \gamma_i.$$

If γ_i is modelled in terms of a set of covariates by

$$\ln \gamma_i = \beta_0 + \beta_1 x_{i1} + \beta_2 x_{i2} + \ldots + \beta_p x_{ip}$$

then

$$\ln \mu_i = \ln m_i + \beta_0 + \beta_1 x_{i1} + \beta_2 x_{i2} + \ldots + \beta_p x_{ip}. \tag{19.37}$$

This model is similar to the generalized linear model of a Poisson variable (14.12) but contains the additional term $\ln m_i$, sometimes referred to as the *offset*, which ensures that age and period are both adjusted for. An example, in which the covariates are represented by a three-factor structure, is given in Berry (1983).

A disadvantage of the above approach is that it involves the assumption of proportional hazards between the study population and the external reference population across all the age–period strata, that is, that the reference death rates apply to the study population at least to a constant of proportionality. The simplest alternative approach that does not depend on this assumption is to work entirely within the data set without any reference to an external population. The death rates are calculated for each age–period cell from the data for the whole cohort. These internal rates are then used to calculate the expected numbers of deaths for subgroups defined in terms of the covariates, and so SMRs are produced for each of the subgroups based on the observed death rates of the whole population in each cell, instead of on external death rates (Breslow & Day, 1987, §3.5). If there are more than two subgroups, comparison of these internal SMRs still depends on proportional hazards of the subgroups across the age–period strata, but a proportional-hazards assumption between the study population and a reference population is no longer necessary. This approach is known to be conservative and may be improved by a Mantel–Haenszel approach (Breslow, 1984b; Breslow & Day, 1987, §3.6). This method is referred to as *internal standardization*.

A second approach is to use direct standardization with an internal subgroup as standard. An appropriate choice for this internal reference may be an unexposed group or the least exposed group in the study. This method produces *standardized rate ratios* (SRRs), which are ratios of the directly standardized rate for each subgroup to the rate in the standard reference subgroup. The method avoids the possible problems associated with comparing SMRs from more than two groups (§19.3), but the SRRs may be less precisely estimated than SMRs if the subgroups contain cells with few deaths. For a fuller discussion and an example analysed both by the external SMR method and the internal SRR method, see Checkoway *et al.* (1989, Chapter 5).

The most comprehensive approach is that of Poisson modelling. For subgroup i and age–period stratum j, if n_{ij} is the number of subject-years and γ_{ij} the death rate then, μ_{ij}, the expected number of deaths is given by

$$\ln \mu_{ij} = \ln n_{ij} + \ln \gamma_{ij}.$$

If γ_{ij} is modelled in terms of the age–period stratum and a set of covariates by

$$\ln \gamma_{ij} = \beta_{0j} + \beta_1 x_{ij1} + \beta_2 x_{ij2} + \ldots + \beta_p x_{ijp},$$

then

$$\ln \mu_{ij} = \ln n_{ij} + \beta_{0j} + \beta_1 x_{ij1} + \beta_2 x_{ij2} + \ldots + \beta_p x_{ijp}. \qquad (19.38)$$

This is a generalized linear model of a Poisson variable (14.12), with the additional term $\ln n_{ij}$ (see (14.13)). An application is given as Example 14.4 (p. 501). Breslow and Day (1987, Chapter 4) give fuller details and worked examples.

In many cases the external method (19.37) and the internal method (19.38) will give similar inferences on the effect of the covariates. The latter has the advantage that there is no assumption that the death rates in all the age–period strata follow a proportional-hazards model with respect to the reference population, but the precision of the comparisons is slightly inferior to the external method. A combination of the two approaches, using (19.37) for the overall group and main subgroups and (19.38) for regression modelling, has the advantage of estimating the effects of the covariates and also estimating how the mortality in the overall group compares with that in the population of which it is a part. An example where this was done is given by Checkoway *et al.* (1993).

19.8 **Age–period–cohort analysis**

In §17.2 we discussed the life-table and noted two forms, the current life-table and the cohort life-table (Table 17.1). The former is based on the death rates in a particular period of time (1930 to 1932 in Table 17.1) for people of different ages, whilst the latter is based on the death rates of people born in particular years (1929–33 in Table 17.1) as they age. There are three time-related variables that may influence death rates:
1 *Age*—death rates are clearly related to age.
2 Calendar *period*—age-specific death rates may change over time.
3 *Cohort*—a group born at a particular time, referred to as a cohort, may have
    different age-specific death rates from those born at different times.
The effects, of the three variables are referred to as the age, period and cohort effects, respectively. Although the above refers to death rates, the outcome could be any health-related variable, such as disease rates, blood pressure or respiratory function.

Period effects would occur if a change took place at a particular time and applied to all age groups. For example, if a new treatment were introduced that improved the prognosis for those who contracted a particular disease with a high fatality rate, then this would show as a period effect for death rates due to that disease. Cohort effects are sometimes referred to as *generational* effects. These effects are associated with events that influence people born at a particular time. For example, adult height is influenced by nutrition in the first few years of life and so would be low for those born at times when nutrition was poor—for example, during a war when supplies were short. Again, the adoption of smoking has tended to be a generational effect and this gives rise to cohort effects on lung cancer and other diseases associated with smoking.

The analysis of an outcome in relation to all three of these time-related variables is termed an *age–period–cohort analysis*. Such analyses are useful in determining trends which might be used for prediction, and for assessing the effects of measures introduced to improve health or of changing habits. For example, is there a reduction in lung cancer incidence that might be associated with health promotional activities aimed at persuading smokers to stop smoking, and with the extent of a corresponding reduction in smoking? There is, however, a fundamental problem in conducting such analyses, which is easily illustrated.

Suppose there are data on an outcome, for people in different cohorts, at different periods of time and for a range of ages. For an individual denote the date of birth by a cohort variable, c, the time of observation by the period variable p, and age by a. Then these three variables are clearly related by

$$a = p - c. \tag{19.39}$$

Now suppose, for an outcome y, a linear regression model was applied of the form

$$E(y) = \beta_0 + \beta_a a + \beta_p p + \beta_c c. \tag{19.40}$$

Then when this model is fitted to the data there will be a problem due to collinearity (§11.9). In fact, as (19.39) represents exact collinearity there will be no unique fitted regression. If one solution is

$$Y_1 = b_0 + b_a a + b_p p + b_c c, \tag{19.41}$$

then

$$Y_2 = b_0 + b_a' a + b_p' p + b_c' c \tag{19.42}$$

will be an equivalent fit, for any value of a constant u, provided that

$$\left. \begin{array}{l} b_a' = b_a + u \\ b_p' = b_p - u \\ b_c' = b_c + u \end{array} \right\}, \tag{19.43}$$

since for any data point the difference between the two fitted values,

$$Y_2 - Y_1 = u(a - p + c),$$

will be zero because of the identity (19.39), i.e. the fitted values for any legitimate age–period–cohort combination will be the same. There is, therefore, no unique best-fitted regression line. This is known as the *identifiability* problem.

In practice, (19.40) may not apply exactly, because of the accuracy to which the variables are recorded. If each variable is recorded as an integer, then someone born in 1937 and recorded in 2000 will be age 62 or 63 years, according to whether the study was done before or after the date of birth. Sometimes, particularly in studies of death rates, the variables are recorded in 5-year groups and the 1935–39 cohort will overlap the 55–59 and 60–64 age groups during the period 1995–99. The identifiability problem nevertheless remains, as the lack of exact collinearity is an artefact due to the coarseness of the variable grouping.

At first sight, it might appear that, if there is no unique regression, there can be no unique solutions for any quantities that the regression can be used to estimate. Fortunately, this is not the case and there is a wide range of situations where the fitted regression, in spite of its lack of uniqueness, gives a unique solution. The simplest of these is prediction using fitted trends. Suppose data are available up to a year defined by $p = p_0$ and it is required to make predictions for the following year $p = p_0 + 1$. Those aged a in that year will be from the cohort defined by $c = p_0 + 1 - a$. Then, using (19.42),

$$Y = b_0 + b'_a a + b'_p(p_0 + 1) + b'_c(p_0 + 1 - a)$$
$$= b_0 + (b'_a - b'_c)a + (b'_p + b'_c)p_0 + (b'_p + b'_c).$$

Now in the second line of this expression all the terms in parentheses are, from (19.43), independent of u. Hence the predicted value does not depend on the arbitrary constant u and is, therefore, uniquely estimable.

The identifiability problem has arisen because of the linear relationship (19.39). If the fitted regression includes non-linear terms in age, period or cohort, then these terms will not be exactly collinear. It would still be necessary to check, using regression diagnostics (§11.9), that there was not collinearity due to the ranges over which the data are available, but this is a separate matter from the identifiability problem. Therefore, non-linear trends in the age, period and cohort effects can be separately estimated.

Suppose some change has been introduced or has occurred in year p_0, and it is postulated that this may have produced an immediate effect at all ages and for all later years. That is,

$$E(y) = \beta_0 + \beta_a a + \beta_p p + \beta_c c \text{ for } p \le p_0$$

and

$$E(y) = \beta_0 + \beta_a a + \beta_p p + \beta_c c + \beta_e \text{ for } p > p_0,$$

where β_e is the effect due to the change. Then these two equations can be combined by defining the dummy variable (§11.7), e, taking the value 0 for $p \le p_0$ and 1 for $p > p_0$, into

$$E(y) = \beta_0 + \beta_a a + \beta_p p + \beta_c c + \beta_e e.$$

The variable e is not collinear with any combination of a, p and c so that β_e is estimable.

The above discussion has been deliberately simplistic in order to illustrate the problem of identifiability and some of the circumstances in which this does not matter as far as using data to make inferences is concerned. In practice, it would be rare to fit a simple linear model of the form (19.40). If the outcome were a death rate, then the relationship with age would be far from linear and the analysis might be of ln y, or the age groups might be represented by a set of dummy variables (§11.7). It would also be unexpected that the effect of any change would be as simple as that just considered.

The quantities that are estimable are the non-linear components of trends in age, period and cohort. The linear components of trend are not separately estimable, but linear functions of them that take account of the identity (19.39) are (Holford, 1983).

The most general model would be that all of the age, period and cohort effects were represented by a full set of indicator variables. This again gives rise to the problem of identifiability and, to obtain a unique solution, a constraint has to be introduced. Possible approaches to providing a constraint are discussed by Holford (1998) but, unless there is some reason, from sources outside the data, to regard a particular constraint as the most plausible, any constraint contains an arbitrary element, and it is then preferable to accept the problem of identifiability and only to consider quantities that are estimable.

Another problem is that, as an age–period–cohort analysis covers several decades of data, any changes in definition of the outcome variable will enter the model. For example, if there were changes in diagnostic criteria over time, then these would appear as period effects even if there had been no real period changes.

Examples of the use of age–period–cohort analyses were given by Armstrong and Doll (1974), Holford *et al.* (1994) and Zheng *et al.* (1996).

19.9 Diagnostic tests

In epidemiological studies much use is made of diagnostic tests, based either on clinical observations or on laboratory techniques, by means of which individuals are classified as healthy or as falling into one of a number of disease categories. Such tests are, of course, important throughout the whole of medicine, and in particular form the basis of screening programmes for the early diagnosis of disease. Most such tests are imperfect instruments, in the sense that healthy individuals will occasionally be classified wrongly as being ill, while some individuals who are really ill may fail to be detected. How should we measure the ability of a particular diagnostic test to give the correct diagnosis both for healthy and for ill subjects?

The reliability of diagnostic tests

Suppose that each individual in a large population can be classified as truly positive or negative for a particular diagnosis. This true diagnosis may be based on more refined methods than are used in the test; or it may be based on evidence which emerges after the passage of time—for instance, at autopsy. For each class of individual, true positive and true negative, we can consider the probabilities that the test gives a positive or negative verdict, as in the table below.

$$
\begin{array}{ccccc}
 & & \text{Test} & & \\
 & & + & - & \\
\text{True} & + & 1-\beta & \beta & 1 \\
 & - & \alpha & 1-\alpha & 1
\end{array}
\qquad (19.44)
$$

An individual in the top right corner of this 2×2 table is called a *false negative*; β is the probability of a false negative, and $1 - \beta$ is called the *sensitivity* of the test. Those in the lower left corner are called *false positives*; α is the probability of a false positive, and $1 - \alpha$ is the *specificity* of the test. There is an analogy here with significance tests. If the null hypothesis is that an individual is a true negative, and a positive test result is regarded as 'significant', then α is analogous to the significance level and $1 - \beta$ is analogous to the power of detecting the alternative hypothesis that the individual is a true positive (p. 139).

Clearly it is desirable that a test should have small values of α and β, although other considerations, such as cost and ease of application, are highly relevant. Other things being equal, if test A has smaller values of both α and β than test B, it can be regarded as a better test. Suppose, though, that A has a smaller value of α but a larger value of β. Unless some relative weight can be attached to the two forms of error—false positives and false negatives—no clear judgement is possible. If the two errors are judged to be of approximately equal importance, a natural method of combination is by the sum of two error probabilities, $\alpha + \beta$. Youden (1950) proposed an essentially equivalent index,

$$J = 1 - (\alpha + \beta). \qquad (19.45)$$

If the test has no diagnostic value, $\alpha = 1 - \beta$ and $J = 0$. If the test is invariably correct, $\alpha = \beta = 0$ and $J = 1$. Values of J between -1 and 0 could arise if the test result were negatively associated with the true diagnosis, but this situation is unlikely to arise in practice.

The use of Youden's index implicitly assumes that the sensitivity and specificity have equal importance, since α and β are given equal weight in (19.45).

There may be good reasons against this view. First, the two types of error will have very different consequences, and it will often be reasonable to attach much more weight to a false negative than to a false positive; this consideration would suggest giving more weight to β than to α, and would lead to the choice of a procedure with a relatively small value of β/α. On the other hand, if the disease is rare, the false negatives will be numerically few, and the number of individuals wrongly diagnosed would be minimized by choosing $\beta > \alpha$. These two considerations clearly conflict, and a resolution must be achieved in the light of the consequences of diagnostic errors for the disease in question.

The discussion so far has been in terms of probabilities. In practice these could be estimated from surveys. Suppose a special survey of a random sample of a population gave the following frequencies:

$$
\begin{array}{c c c c}
 & & \multicolumn{2}{c}{\text{Test}} \\
 & & + & - \\
\text{True} & + & a & b \\
 & - & c & d
\end{array}
\qquad (19.46)
$$

The probability of a false negative would be estimated by $\hat{\beta} = b/(a+b)$; the probability of a false positive by $\hat{\alpha} = c/(c+d)$. Youden's index J would be estimated by $\hat{J} = 1 - (\hat{\alpha} + \hat{\beta})$. The sampling errors of these estimates follow from standard binomial expressions.

An important point to note is that the expected proportions of misdiagnoses among the *apparent* positives and negatives, i.e. the test positives and negatives, depend not only on α and β but on the true prevalence of the disease. This may be seen from the following two sets of frequencies. In each case the sensitivity and specificity are both 0·9.

Case (a)

		\multicolumn{2}{c}{Test}		
		+	−	
True	+	450	50	500
	−	50	450	500
		500	500	1000

Case (b)

		\multicolumn{2}{c}{Test}		
		+	−	
True	+	90	10	100
	−	90	810	900
		180	820	1000

$$(19.47)$$

| Proportion of true +ves | 0·90 | 0·10 | | 0·50 | 0·01 |

The proportion of true positives among the apparent positives is sometimes called the *predictive value of a positive test*; the proportion of true negatives among the apparent negatives is the *predictive value of a negative test*. In case (a), the true prevalence is 500/1000 = 0·5 and the predictive value of a positive test is high (0·9). In case (b), however, where the true prevalence is 100/1000 = 0·1, the same predictive value is only 0·5. The predictive values are conditional probabilities of the test results and may be calculated using Bayes' theorem (§3.3), with the prevalences of disease and non-disease as the prior probabilities and the likelihoods of the test results obtained from the sensitivity and specificity.

Case (b) illustrates the position in many presymptomatic screening procedures where the true prevalence is low. Of the subjects found positive by the screening test, a rather high proportion may be false positives. To avoid this situation the test may sometimes be modified to reduce α, but such a step often results in an increased value of β and hence a reduced value of $1 - \beta$; the number of false positives among the apparent positives will have been reduced, but so will the number of true positives detected.

The sort of modification referred to in the last sentence is particularly relevant when the test, although dichotomous, is based on a continuous measurement. Examples are the diagnosis of diabetes by blood-sugar level or of glaucoma by intraocular pressure. Any change in the critical level of the measurement will affect α and β. One very simple model for this situation would be to assume that the variable, x, on which the test is based is normally distributed with the same variance σ^2 for the normal and diseased populations, but with different means, μ_N and μ_D (Fig. 19.1). For any given α, the value of β depends solely on the standardized distance between the means,

$$\Delta = \frac{\mu_D - \mu_N}{\sigma}.$$

If the critical value for the test is the mid-point between the means, $\frac{1}{2}(\mu_N + \mu_D)$, α and β will both be equal to the single-tail area of the normal distribution beyond a standardized deviate of $\frac{1}{2}\Delta$. To compare the merits of different tests one could, therefore, compare their values of Δ; tests with high values of Δ will differentiate between normal and diseased groups better than those with low values. There is a clear analogy here with the generalized distance as a measure of the effectiveness of a discriminant function (p. 467); the discrimination is performed here by the single variable x.

Instead of an all-or-none classification as healthy or diseased, it may sometimes be useful to express the strength of the evidence for any individual falling into each of the two groups. For the model described above, the logarithm of the likelihood ratio is linearly related to x, as shown in the lower part of Fig. 19.1. (This is a particular case of the more general result for discriminant functions

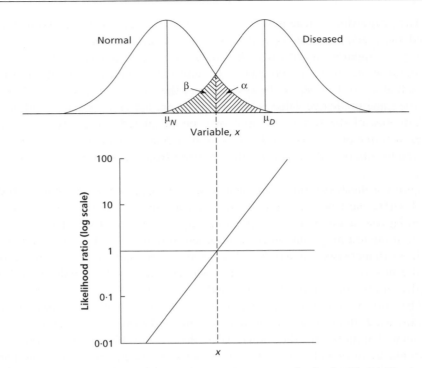

Fig. 19.1 The performance of a diagnostic test based on a normally distributed variable when the normal and diseased groups differ in the mean but have the same variance. The lower diagram shows on a log scale the ratio of the likelihood that an observation comes from the diseased group to that of its coming from the normal group.

referred to on p. 467.) The likelihood ratio may, from Bayes' theorem (§3.3), be combined with the ratio of prior probabilities to give the ratio of posterior probabilities. Suppose, for example, that a particular value of x corresponds to a likelihood ratio of 10, and that the prior probability of a diseased individual (i.e. the population prevalence) is 0·01. The posterior odds that the individual is diseased are then

$$\frac{10}{1} \times \frac{0\cdot01}{0\cdot99} = \frac{0\cdot10}{0\cdot99},$$

corresponding to a posterior probability of being diseased of 0·09. It is thus much more likely that the individual is healthy than that he or she is diseased; as in case (b) of (19.47), where the prevalence was low, a high proportion of apparent positives are in fact false positives.

The assumptions underlying the above discussion are unlikely to be closely fulfilled in practice. Distributions may be non-normal and have different variances; there may be various categories of disease, each with a different distribution of x. Nevertheless, the concepts introduced here usually provide a good basis for discussing the performance of a diagnostic test.

The above discussion on predictive values assessed using Bayes' theorem was based on the assumption that the sensitivity and specificity of a test are fixed quantities and, in particular, independent of the prevalence of disease. This is not always a reasonable assumption (Walter & Irwig, 1988), and it has increasingly been questioned (e.g. Lachs *et al.*, 1992; Moons *et al.*, 1997) in settings where there is variability in patients' presenting features, because the spectrum of disease is different in groups defined by severity of symptoms or by whether they are seen in primary or tertiary care. It is perhaps a more reasonable assumption for a screening test, for which people being tested are asymptomatic.

Another way of expressing the situation shown in Fig. 19.1 is the *receiver operating characteristic* (ROC) *curve*. This is a line diagram with the sensitivity, $1 - \beta$, plotted vertically and the false positive rate, α, on the horizontal axis. The horizontal axis may also be shown by a reversed scale of the specificity, $1 - \alpha$. The ROC curve is constructed by finding the sensitivity and specificity for a range of values of x. Figure 19.2 shows the ROC curve corresponding to Fig. 19.1. The possible combinations of sensitivity and specificity that may be chosen by varying the critical values of the test may be read off the curve. Tests with the ROC curves furthest into the top left corner are the better tests.

Misclassification errors are not restricted to the classification of disease. In a retrospective–case-control study, for example, the disease classification is likely to be based on highly accurate diagnostic methods, but the factor classification often depends on personal recollection and will not, therefore, be completely accurate. False positives and false negatives can be defined in terms of the factor classification in an obvious way. If the specificity and sensitivity are the same for

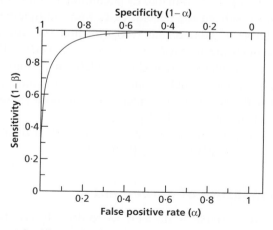

Fig. 19.2 Receiver operating characteristic curve corresponding to Fig. 19.1.

the disease group as for the control group, i.e. non-differential misclassification, the effect is to reduce any measures of association between factor and disease; for instance, the relative risk is brought nearer to unity than it would be if the errors were not present, and the difference between the two proportions of positives is reduced numerically.

If either the specificity or the sensitivity (or both) differs between groups, the bias in risk estimate may be in either direction (Diamond & Lilienfeld, 1962a, b; Newell, 1962). A particular danger in a case–control study where classification of the exposure factor depends on recollection and the disease is traumatic is that the cases may be likely to recall events that the controls either might not recall or might dismiss as unimportant; this would lead to an exaggeration of the estimate of risk. The situation is further complicated if a confounder is misclassified. There is a large literature on the effects of misclassification errors and methods of assessing the consequent size of the bias on the association between disease and an exposure variable. If sufficient information is available, it may be possible to produce corrected estimates. For further discussion, see Kleinbaum *et al.* (1982, Chapter 12), Kelsey *et al.* (1996, Chapter 13) and Rothman and Greenland (1998, pp. 347–55).

Our discussion of diagnostic tests has been restricted to a comparison of the result of a single test with the true diagnosis. In many situations, the true diagnosis cannot conveniently be established in a large survey population but there may be an opportunity to compare a new test against a reference test. Buck and Gart (1966) (also Gart & Buck, 1966) discuss the rather complicated analysis of data of this type; if the reference test were assumed to have no error, then this would lead to estimates of the error rates of the new test being biased upwards. Hui and Walter (1980) showed that, if the two tests were applied to two populations with different prevalences of disease, then the error rates of both tests and the two prevalences might be estimated by maximum likelihood methods. Walter and Irwig (1988) considered the general case, with multiple tests and multiple populations, in terms of models that recognize that the true disease status is unknown; such models are referred to as *latent class models*. Torrance-Rynard and Walter (1997) considered latent class models for a single population and evaluated the bias arising through assuming conditional independence between tests—that is, that the two tests are independent in both those with and those without disease, when there is truly dependence.

Special considerations arise for meta-analyses (§18.10) of diagnostic tests (Glasziou & Irwig, 1998; Walter *et al.*, 1999).

19.10 Kappa measure of agreement

When a categorical variable is difficult to record objectively, it is common practice to use more than one rater to assess the variable, and to use the mean, or median, values in the main data analysis. It is, however, prudent to confirm before the calculation of any sort of average value that the raters are using the categories similarly, since otherwise it would be unclear what the average values represented. Examples are the classification of a condition on a scale with two or more categories based on an assessment of presenting signs and symptoms, and the reading of chest radiographs.

Consider first the case where there are just two categories, presence or absence of some condition, and suppose that two raters assess n subjects independently. Then the results can be set out in a 2×2 table as follows:

	Rater 2		
Rater 1	Present	Absent	
Present	a	b	$a+b$
Absent	c	d	$c+d$
	$a+c$	$b+d$	n

A natural way of assessing agreement between the raters would be to note that the raters agree on $a+d$ of the subjects and to express this in terms of the number of patients as the ratio $(a+d)/n$. Two examples illustrate the disadvantage of this simple approach:

A	Rater 2				B	Rater 2		
Rater 1	Present	Absent			Rater 1	Present	Absent	
Present	5	5	10		Present	35	5	40
Absent	5	85	90		Absent	5	55	60
	10	90	100			40	60	100

In both of these examples the raters agree on 90% of the subjects, but the disagreement appears greater in example A than in example B since, in the former, there is agreement that the condition is present for only five subjects out of the 15 assessed by at least one of the raters as having the condition, whilst in the latter it is agreed that the condition is present in 35 out of 45 subjects assessed as having the condition by at least one of the raters.

The difficulty has arisen because no account has been taken of agreements that could occur due to chance. If there were no real agreement between the raters, then the expected frequencies in the cells of the 2×2 table would be determined by chance. For example A, it would be expected that there would be 81 subjects rated negative by both raters and one subject rated positive by both raters, where these expected numbers have been calculated by exactly the same methods as used to calculate expected frequencies in a χ^2 test (§4.5). The observed agreement for 90 subjects does not appear so impressive when contrasted with an expected agreement for 82 patients. In example B, the expected number of agreements is only 52 and the observed number is much greater than this.

The above rationale is the basis for the *kappa* (κ) measure of agreement, introduced by Cohen (1960). The method is as follows. First define I_o as the observed measure of agreement, and I_e as the corresponding expected measure. Then

$$I_o = \frac{a+d}{n}$$
$$I_e = \frac{(a+c)(a+b) + (b+d)(c+d)}{n^2}.$$

Secondly, κ is defined as the difference between observed and expected agreement, expressed as a fraction of the maximum difference. Since the maximum value of I_o is 1, this gives

$$\kappa = \frac{I_o - I_e}{1 - I_e}. \tag{19.48}$$

For examples A and B the values of κ are 0·44 and 0·79, respectively. The maximum value of κ is 1, which represents perfect agreement, and κ will take the value zero if there is only chance agreement. Although negative values are mathematically possible, representing an agreement to disagree, these are unlikely to occur in practice.

Example 19.9

In a study by Bergen *et al.* (1992), tardive dyskinesia was assessed by two raters by scoring seven items on a 5-point scale, coded 0 to 4. One definition of tardive dyskinesia is that there should be either two scores of at least 2 or one of at least 3. For one series of assessments there were 168 subjects and the agreement was as follows:

	Rater a		
Rater b	Present	Absent	
Present	123	10	133
Absent	6	29	35
	129	39	168

Then

$$I_o = \frac{152}{168} = 0 \cdot 905$$

$$I_e = \frac{129 \times 133 + 39 \times 35}{168^2} = 0 \cdot 656$$

$$\kappa = \frac{0 \cdot 905 - 0 \cdot 656}{1 - 0 \cdot 656} = 0 \cdot 72.$$

The agreement between the two raters was good, and so the two assessments were combined and tardive dyskinesia recorded for those patients who were diagnosed by both raters.

Weighted kappa

Where there are more than two categories and the categories are ordered, a difference between raters of just one category is less disagreement than a difference of two categories, and a difference of three categories would indicate even more disagreement, etc. It is clearly desirable to incorporate this in a measure of agreement and this is done using the *weighted kappa* (Cohen, 1968). This measure is calculated by assigning a weight, w_i, to subjects for whom the raters differ by i categories. When the raters agree, the weight is unity—that is, $w_0 = 1$. If there are k categories, then the maximum disagreement is of $k - 1$ categories and this is given weight zero. The most common set of weights for the intermediate values is that they are equally spaced and this gives

$$w_i = 1 - \frac{i}{k - 1}. \tag{19.49}$$

Then the observed index of agreement is defined as

$$I_o = \frac{\sum w_i r_i}{n},$$

where r_i is the number of subjects for whom the raters differ by i categories. The expected value is calculated similarly, using expected frequencies, and the weighted κ is evaluated using (19.48).

Example 19.10

In a study by Cookson *et al.* (1986), chest radiographs were classified by two readers according to the 1980 International Labour Organization (ILO) Classification of Radiographs of Pneumoconiosis. The readings are given in Table 19.7.

Table 19.7 Readings of chest radiographs by two readers (Cookson *et al.*, 1986). The frequencies with agreement between raters are shown in bold type, and disagreements by one category in italics. (Reproduced with permission from the authors and publishers).

Reader 1	Reader 2 0/0	0/1	1/0	1/1	1/2	2/1	2/2	2/3	Total
0/0	**626**	*32*	26	3					687
0/1	*53*	**20**	*17*	3					93
1/0	22	*3*	**21**	8		1	1		56
1/1	2	2	*6*	**1**	2	1			14
1/2	3		1	*3*		4			11
2/1									0
2/2									0
2/3								**1**	1
Total	706	57	71	18	2	6	1	1	862

The observed number of exact agreements is obtained by summing the frequencies, shown in bold type, in the diagonal extending from the top left cell to the bottom right cell of the table. Observed numbers of disagreements are obtained similarly by summing the frequencies in parallel lines displaced either side of the main diagonal. For example, the disagreements by one category are shown in italics. The expected numbers are obtained from the marginal totals, and summed in the same way. This gives:

Number of categories of disagreement	Obs	Exp	w	$w \times$ Obs	$w \times$ Exp
0 (agreement)	669	573·8	1	669·0	573·8
1	128	135·6	0·86	109·7	116·2
2	55	106·5	0·71	39·3	76·1
3	6	27·2	0·57	3·4	15·5
4	4	11·4	0·43	1·7	4·9
5	0	5·0	0·29	0	1·4
6	0	1·0	0·14	0	0·1
7	0	1·6	0	0	0
	862	862·0		823·1	788·0

Summarizing we have

$$I_o = 823 \cdot 1/862 = 0 \cdot 955 \quad I_e = 788 \cdot 0/862 = 0 \cdot 914$$

$$\kappa = \frac{0 \cdot 955 - 0 \cdot 914}{1 - 0 \cdot 914} = 0 \cdot 48.$$

There is fair agreement.

An alternative set of weights, which penalizes disagreements by the square of the number of categories of disagreement, is

$$w_i = 1 - \frac{i^2}{(k-1)^2}. \tag{19.50}$$

Although κ provides a measure of agreement within a particular set of data its use as a more general measure is limited. This is because its value is dependent not only on the intrinsic agreement of the two raters but also on the prevalence of the condition being assessed or, for multicategorical conditions, the distribution across the categories (Kraemer, 1979). Thus κ is not a general measure of agreement between raters but only of their agreement in a particular situation.

The problems discussed in the previous paragraph are analysed in detail by Cicchetti and Feinstein (1990) and Feinstein and Cicchetti (1990). They proposed that, just as agreement between a diagnostic test and disease status would not normally be summarized in terms of a single index, but in terms of sensitivity for the disease positives and specificity for the disease negatives, so also agreement between raters should be expressed by two measures. The situations are not identical, since in the former disease status represents the true situation against which the diagnostic test is assessed, whereas in the latter the two raters have to be treated on an equal basis. The measures proposed are p_pos, the number of agreed positives divided by the average number of positives for the two raters, and p_neg defined similarly for the negatives. That is,

$$p_\text{pos} = \frac{a}{\frac{1}{2}[(a+b)+(a+c)]} = \frac{2a}{2a+b+c}$$

$$p_\text{neg} = \frac{d}{\frac{1}{2}[(c+d)+(b+d)]} = \frac{2d}{2d+b+c}.$$

For the three situations considered earlier

	A	B	Example 19.9
p_pos	0·50	0·88	0·94
p_neg	0·94	0·92	0·78
κ	0·44	0·79	0·72

In A and B the two raters have similar agreement when the condition is absent, but in B the raters have much better agreement when the condition is present. The two measures provide information about the areas of agreement and disagreement which is not identifiable from a single measure.

The standard error of κ may be evaluated (Fleiss, 1981, Chapter 13) and used to test that agreement is better than chance and to set confidence limits. However, the estimation of agreement is not usually an end to itself, and usually agreement is known to be better than chance, so that a significance test of the null hypothesis that there is no agreement is unnecessary.

Landis and Koch (1977) suggest arbitrary subdivisions of κ into ranges: 0 to 0·2 representing slight agreement, $>0·2$–$0·4$ fair agreement, $>0·4$–$0·6$ moderate, $>0·6$–$0·8$ substantial and $>0·8$ almost perfect agreement. Fleiss (1981, p. 218) modified this and recommends that values of κ exceeding 0·75 represent excellent agreement, values between 0·4 and 0·75 fair to good agreement and values less than 0·4 poor agreement. There would be little purpose in using a measure with such poor agreement, since it would be unclear what the measure represented.

In some studies a large number of items may be assessed by different members of a panel of raters; for example, a set of chest radiographs might be divided into batches and each batch read by three members of a larger team of readers. An overall measure of agreement can be constructed, although separate measures for each pair of readers would usually be calculated in order to identify the components of the overall measure. Overall measures of agreement may be more conveniently evaluated using intraclass correlation (§19.11) techniques (see Shoukri, 1998), which give measures that are closely related to κ.

19.11 Intraclass correlation

Another situation in which components of variance are used is that in which there are a number of correlated members within classes. This can arise in a number of ways; for example, a class might be a pair of twins, or a class might be a sample or individual with an item measured using a number of different methods. One measure sometimes used in this situation is termed the *intraclass correlation coefficient*.

For a pair of identical twins, there is ambiguity in calculating the correlation coefficient using (7.8), since the two values have no particular order that could be used to label them as x and y. This could be done at random but then the result would depend on the randomization used. To avoid this, all possibilities are considered and this means that each pair is looked at both ways round—that is, as (x, y) and as (y, x). The correlation coefficient is calculated from the $2n$ pairs thus formed and this provides an estimate of the required correlation, although the precision of this estimate would be much closer to that based on a sample of n pairs, not $2n$. The correlation calculated in this way achieves its maximum value of 1 only if all the pairs of values fall on a straight line through the origin with slope unity.

Suppose a new method is available for measuring some variable and it is required to assess the agreement between values obtained using the new method and those obtained with an existing method. Data could be collected in which a number of individuals were measured using each method to give a pair of values for each individual. A high correlation about a line not passing through the origin or with a slope different from 1 would not represent useful agreement between the methods as far as the user was concerned, although if this occurred it might be possible to calibrate the new method to give better agreement. Thus although, unlike the twins, there is no ambiguity on the identification within pairs, we require a measure of correlation with the property that it will only equal unity if the two measurements are identical within each individual.

The intraclass correlation coefficient is a measure of the correlation between the values obtained with any two randomly chosen methods within the same individual (class) and has the above property. The correlation calculated from $2n$ pairs as above is approximately equal to the intraclass correlation coefficient except when n is small. The method is closely related to components of variance (§§8.3 and 9.6), and using this methodology is more convenient and more accurate than forming multiple pairs. In general, there may be more than two methods under test, and we suppose that there are m methods, each assessed on n subjects. Then the design is equivalent to randomized blocks (§9.2), in which the methods are tested within the subjects, i.e. the blocks. There are three sources of variation, each with its component of variance:

1 Variation between subjects, with a variance component σ_s^2.
2 Systematic variation between methods, with a variance component σ_m^2. This variability represents differences between methods.
3 Random variation from one measurement to another, with a variance component σ^2, additional to the sources of variation **1** and **2**.

Then the two-way analysis of variance has the form:

	DF	MSq	Expected MSq
Between subjects (classes)	$n - 1$	M_s	$\sigma^2 + m\sigma_s^2$
Between methods	$m - 1$	M_m	$\sigma^2 + n\sigma_m^2$
Residual	$(n - 1)(m - 1)$	M_r	σ^2

The intraclass correlation coefficient is defined as the correlation between any two measurements in the same subject using randomly chosen methods. All three components of variation contribute to the variance of each measurement and, since the two measurements are for the same subject, the variance component representing variation between subjects is common to the two measurements. Therefore the intraclass correlation coefficient is

$$\rho_I = \frac{\sigma_s^2}{\sigma_s^2 + \sigma_m^2 + \sigma^2}.$$

Equating the mean squares (MSq) in the analysis of variance with their expectations gives the following estimate of ρ_I (Bartko, 1966):

$$r_I = \frac{M_s - M_r}{M_s + (m-1)M_r + \frac{m}{n}(M_m - M_r)}. \tag{19.51}$$

For $m = 2$ the intraclass correlation coefficient can be obtained as follows. Let x_{i1} and x_{i2} be the values for methods 1 and 2, respectively, for subject i. Define $t_i = x_{i1} + x_{i2}$ and $d_i = x_{i1} - x_{i2}$ as the sum and difference of the pair of values. Calculate the mean difference, $\bar{d}$, and the standard deviations of t_i and d_i, s_t and s_d, respectively. Then

$$r_I = \frac{s_t^2 - s_d^2}{s_t^2 + s_d^2 + \frac{2}{n}(n\bar{d}^2 - s_d^2)}. \tag{19.52}$$

It is easy to see from this form that the systematic difference between the methods reduces the intraclass correlation coefficient, due to the inclusion of $\bar{d}^2$ in the denominator. A closely related index, the concordance correlation coefficient, was given by Lin (1992).

An alternative formulation is appropriate when there is no reason to suppose there are any systematic differences between the values within a class—for example, pairs of twins. There is then no entry in the analysis of variance for Between methods; M_r is estimated from a one-way analysis of variance (§8.1) with $n(m-1)$ degrees of freedom (DF) and the last term in the denominator of (19.51) is omitted (Snedecor & Cochran, 1989, §13.5).

Another situation where the method may be useful is where a characteristic that cannot be measured objectively is assessed by two or more raters and the level of agreement between the raters, which may be referred to as the reliability of the ratings, is critical to the way the data are used.

Example 19.11

In a study by Bergen *et al.* (1992), tardive dyskinesia was assessed by two assessors on a scale taking integer values from 0 to 28. For one series of assessments there were 168 subjects with the following summary statistics:

$$\bar{t} = 16 \cdot 39, s_t = 7 \cdot 71, \bar{d} = 0 \cdot 28, s_d = 1 \cdot 89.$$

Applying (19.52) gives

$$r_I = \frac{7 \cdot 71^2 - 1 \cdot 89^2}{7 \cdot 71^2 + 1 \cdot 89^2 + \frac{2}{168}(168 \times 0 \cdot 28^2 - 1 \cdot 89^2)}$$

$$= 0 \cdot 885.$$

The agreement between the two raters was very good, and the mean difference of 0·28 and variation in the difference (standard deviation (SD) 1·89) were small compared with the mean total of 16·4 with SD of 7·7. Therefore it was considered acceptable to combine the assessments of the two raters and use the mean value in the main analysis.

The intraclass correlation coefficient is closely related to the weighted κ measure of agreement (§19.10) used when the ratings are recorded on a categorical scale (Fleiss, 1975); if the weights (19.50) were used, then the weighted κ and the intraclass correlation coefficient would be equal except for terms in $1/n$. In Example 19.10 the weighted κ using these weights was 0·620 and the intraclass correlation coefficient, giving the categories values, $0, 1, \ldots, 7$, was 0·621.

The intraclass correlation coefficient has the same feature as the product–moment correlation coefficient—namely, that its value is influenced by the selection of subjects over which it is defined. If the subjects are highly variable, then the intraclass correlation coefficient will tend to be high, whereas for a more homogeneous group of subjects it will be lower. Another problem is that the intraclass correlation coefficient also combines information from the systematic difference between methods with the random measurement variation. Thus, the intraclass correlation coefficient is a measure which combines three features of the data from which it is calculated. This may not matter if the only purpose of calculating the coefficient is to assess agreement between methods within a particular study, but comparisons of intraclass correlation coefficients between studies are difficult to interpret.

A fuller evaluation of the agreement between methods is provided by an analysis of the differences, d_i (Altman, 1991, pp. 397–401). A plot of d_i against the mean, $\frac{1}{2}t_i$, allows the determination of whether the systematic difference between the methods or the random variation differs according to the mean value, and if they do not, the difference between the methods can be summarized by $\bar{d}$ and s_d. If the random variation increases with the mean value, an analysis of the differences after a logarithmic transformation may be appropriate (§11.3).

19.12 **Disease screening**

The effectiveness of a programme for the early screening of disease depends not only on the reliability of the tests used, but even more on the availability of treatment capable of improving the prognosis for an individual in whom the early stages of disease have been detected.

If the disease is commonly fatal, the primary aim of screening will be to reduce the risk of death or at least to increase survival time. The effectiveness of a screening programme may therefore sometimes be assessed by observing any trend in the cause-specific mortality rate for the community in which the programme is introduced. However, trends in mortality rates occur for various reasons, and cannot unambiguously be attributed to the screening programme. In a few instances it has been possible to carry out randomized trials, in which volunteers are assigned to receive or not to receive screening. After an appropriate follow-up period, the mortality experiences of the two groups can be compared.

It is often useful to study the time periods between certain stages in the development of a disease. The following comments indicate briefly some of the basic concepts. Figure 19.3 shows the principal events.

The sojourn time, y, is the period during which the disease is asymptomatic but detectable by screening, and will vary between individuals, with a mean value m. The lead time, x, is of interest because: (i) it measures the time gained for potentially effective treatment; and (ii) in comparing duration of survival between screened and unscreened groups, it would be misleading to measure survival from T_3 for the unscreened group but from t for the screened group. The lead time provides a correction for this bias.

The estimation of sojourn and lead time is somewhat complex (Walter & Day, 1983; Day & Walter, 1984; Brookmeyer *et al.*, 1986). The following points should be noted, for the situation where there is a single screening.

1 Lead time is a random variable, partly because y varies between individuals, but also because t can occur at any point between T_2 and T_3 (or, indeed, outside that range, in which case the disease will be undetected by the screen). If y were constant, the mean lead time, L, for those individuals whose disease was detected by the screen, would be $\frac{1}{2}m$. However, since y varies, the longer sojourn times will be more likely to contain a screening point, and are correspondingly more highly represented in the 'detected' group than in the whole group of cases. (This is an example of '*length-biased sampling*'). A consequence is that $L = \frac{1}{2}[m + (\sigma^2/m)]$, where σ^2 is the variance of y.

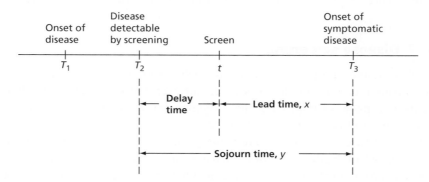

Fig. 19.3 Schematic representation of events in the development of a chronic disease, with a screening procedure during the asymptomatic phase.

2 We shall be interested in the mean lead time for the whole group of cases, including those in whom the disease is not detected. This is called the programme lead time, and is equal to $(1 - \beta)\,L$, where β is the proportion of false negatives (i.e. cases missed).

3 To estimate m, use may be made of the relation (19.4),

$$P = Im,$$

where P is the prevalence of presymptomatic disease (which can be estimated from the results of the screen, allowing for the false negatives), and I is the incidence of symptomatic disease (which might be estimated from a control series).

4 The estimation of σ^2, which is needed for the calculation of L, is more troublesome than that of m, and may require a further assumption about the functional form of the distribution of y.

The discussion so far has been in terms of a single screening occasion. In practice, it will be preferable to consider a series of screening occasions, so that each individual who develops the disease at some time has a reasonable chance of being screened whilst the disease is presymptomatic (see Walter & Day, 1983; Day & Walter, 1984).

It has been assumed above that all cases detectable by screening would, if undetected and therefore untreated, progress to symptomatic disease. This is not always the case and the sojourn time may be subdivided into two stages. Presymptomatic disease in the first stage may not progress to the second stage, and may even regress, whilst those who progress to the second stage would progress to symptomatic disease. This situation is considered by Brookmeyer and Day (1987).

A comprehensive review of modelling the disease-screening process is given by Stevenson (1998).

The effectiveness of a screening programme may be assessed by a randomized controlled trial in which individuals are randomized to either a screening group or a control group. The considerations discussed in Chapter 18 would apply and there are also special considerations. The primary analysis would be of the end-point that it is the aim of screening to modify, often mortality. The analysis would follow the intent-to-treat—that is, intent-to-screen—approach, for the reasons discussed in §18.6. The data from such a trial offer the opportunity for secondary analyses concerned with modelling the natural history of the disease. The timing of the outcome is also important, as follow-up continues for several years; in the *stop-screen* design, follow-up continues for several years after the screening regimen has been completed and any effect of screening would be expected to decline towards the end of the follow-up period.

Randomized controlled trials of screening are usually large studies continuing over several years and are infrequently conducted. If screening is available and being utilized by part of a population, then an epidemiological study, comparing those who participate in screening with those that do not, might be considered. If it were possible to identify a population offered screening, assess for each member of the population whether they accepted the offer or not and follow this population over several years, then this would be a cohort study (§19.4). In the comparison of the screened with the non-screened, there is the possibility of selection bias if those who accept the offer of screening have a different risk profile from those who do not. If information is available, it may be possible to make some adjustments for the confounding effect of known risk factors. Such a study would be very difficult to carry out, requiring the same large numbers and length of follow-up as a randomized controlled trial.

Since any benefit of screening is through earlier diagnosis followed by effective treatment, a study comparing survival time in cases diagnosed in those participating in screening with those who do not participate in screening might seem attractive. There are a number of difficulties in evaluating such studies. Most of the cases in the screening group will have been diagnosed at screening and all of those in the non-screened group clinically. It is invalid to compare survival times from the time of diagnosis, since this involves lead-time bias—that is, cases diagnosed at screening would survive longer, even if the screening were ineffective, because of lead time. There is also length–time bias, as a consequence of length-biased sampling, if those with the longer sojourn times would also be the more slowly progressing when they reached the clinical stage. If some cases detected at screening are in a preclinical stage for which progression is not inevitable, this constitutes a further bias. All these biases are in the direction of seeming to improve prognosis in the cases detected at screening compared with those diagnosed on clinical grounds. The difficulties of estimating the sizes of these biases are so great that an epidemiological study of this type is unlikely to produce any useful information on the efficacy of screening.

A more promising option is a case–control study (§19.4), which, as the outcome is rare, avoids the large numbers and long follow-up necessary in a cohort study. Cases would be deaths due to the disease or incident cases of invasive disease. A comparison of whether or not the cases and controls had been screened could be carried out to produce data of the form of (19.17), and a more detailed analysis involving the number of screening examinations and their timing could be undertaken. Selection bias may still be a problem, and it may not always be clear if a 'screening' examination was a true screening examination or had been initiated by symptoms. There are also difficulties in classifying the timing of screening in terms of what is known about the duration of the sojourn time. A great deal has been published on the use of case–control methods to assess the efficacy of screening; readers interested in more details are referred to Sasco *et al.* (1986), Weiss *et al.* (1992), Etzioni and Weiss (1998) and the review by Cronin *et al.* (1998).

If a screening programme is available to a complete population and a large proportion participate, then the effectiveness of the programme may be assessed by comparing trends over time both before and after the screening was first in operation. An effect would be expected to provide an estimable period effect in an age–period–cohort analysis (§19.8). Such an analysis would be stronger if contemporaneous data could be obtained from a similar area where screening was not available.

19.13 **Disease clustering**

Many epidemiological investigations are concerned with the detection of some form of clustering of cases of a certain disease—clustering in time, in space or in both time and space. For example, one might enquire whether cases of a certain congenital malformation (which might normally occur at a fairly constant rate in a community) appear with unduly high frequency in certain years. Such a tendency towards clustering in time might indicate aetiological factors, such as maternal virus infections, which were particularly severe in certain years. Again, one might suspect that certain forms of illness are more common among people who work or live in certain areas, perhaps because of environmental factors peculiar to these places. The groups in which cases tend to be clustered may be families or households; such familial aggregation might again be caused by environmental factors, but it might be due also to intrafamilial infection or to genetic predisposition to disease. In the study of the possible infectious aetiology of rare diseases such as leukaemia or certain congenital malformations, clustering in either space or time will be less interesting than a space–time association. By the latter we mean a tendency for those cases which are relatively close together in space also to be relatively close together in time.

Many such problems give rise to quite complicated considerations; it is not possible to explore the subject fully here. This section contains a brief account of some of these considerations. Further details may be obtained from the references in this section and from the review of Cuzick (1998).

Epidemiological studies are often carried out after some unusual coincidences have been noticed. For example, Westley-Wise et al. (1999) describe an investigation of a cluster of leukaemia cases in people living in suburbs adjacent to a coke by-products plant. The investigation was triggered by local concern following four cases in former students of the secondary school in the area. Further investigation found a total of 12 cases in people younger than 50 years over an 8-year period when the expected number was 3·5. Clearly this was a highly significant excess, since the probability of observing 12 or more cases when the expectation is 3·5 is about 3 in 10 000 (§3.7). After a careful investigation the cause of the cluster remained uncertain. It is rare that such studies throw much light on the cause of the cluster.

A general warning should be issued against the overinterpretation of striking instances of clustering when there is no further supportive evidence. In the example above the degree of clustering exhibited by the first four cases may well have been 'significant' when taken in isolation, and yet may nevertheless have been a purely random phenomenon. Many other possible opportunities for clustering, in other places or at other times, might have been put under scrutiny; if they had been studied, perhaps nothing remarkable would have been found except in the original instance which caused the enquiry. Our attention may, therefore, have been focused on merely the most extreme of a large number of random fluctuations. Similarly, in any one study there are often many ways of examining the data for possible clusters. To report only that method of analysis that gives the most significant finding is to provide a misleading interpretation of the true situation. The problem is similar to that of multiple comparisons (§8.4), but in the present context the number of possible comparisons is likely to be so large, and so difficult to define, that no satisfactory method of adjustment is available. In the example, the existence of a cluster was confirmed by the discovery of more excess cases, and a more stringent, but conservative, test of the excess is to discount the original four cases.

Clustering in time

A rather simple approach to many problems of this sort is to divide the time period into equal intervals, to express the incidence rate in each interval as a proportion and to test the significance of differences between these proportions by standard $2 \times k$ contingency table methods. If the population at risk is almost constant and the incidence rate is low, the number of cases appearing in the different intervals will, on the null hypothesis of constant risk, follow a Poisson distribution and the usual heterogeneity test (§8.8) may be used. A test, due to Edwards (1961), that is particularly sensitive to seasonal clustering of cases is described in §12.4 (p. 418).

It may be sensible to concentrate attention on the maximum of the various numbers of cases, on the grounds that occasional clustering may affect only one or two of the time intervals. Ederer *et al.* (1964) describe some methods for doing this, and Grimson (1993) has provided an exact version of the test.

Clustering in space

Rather similar methods can be applied to detect clustering in space, which may result in differences in incidence between different groups of people. It will usually be convenient to subdivide the total population into administrative areas containing quite different numbers of individuals; the Poisson distribution is not then applicable, but contingency table methods can be used.

If the geographical distribution of the population is unknown, it is sometimes useful to carry out a case–control study to show whether the cases are in some sense closer together than a comparable group of controls. Lloyd and Roberts (1973), for example, applied this method to the study of spatial clustering of congenital limb defects in Cardiff. The distribution of differences between all pairs of cases can be compared with that of distances between pairs of controls, to see whether small distances occur more frequently for cases than for controls. Suppose there are n cases and m controls. A Monte Carlo test (§10.6) may be carried out, by making repeated random selections of n individuals from the total of $m + n$, and counting the number of close pairs, Z, within each set of n. The significance of the *observed* value of Z for the n cases can then be adjudged by seeing whether it falls in the tails of the distribution of Z formed by the random permutations. Alternatively, the values of E(Z) and var(Z) in the permutation distribution can be calculated by an adaptation of exact formulae derived for Knox's test for space–time clustering described on p. 714 (David & Barton, 1966; Mantel, 1967; Smith & Pike, 1974). Cuzick and Edwards (1990) proposed a test based on the distribution of cases and controls in space. For each case the nearest k neighbours are found and the number of these that are cases forms the basis of a test. The test is carried out for different values of k and the results are combined into an overall test.

The question sometimes arises whether cases of a particular disease occurring within a certain time period tend to cluster near a well-defined location, such as an industrial plant suspected of emitting toxic material. Here, the population could be divided into subgroups according to distance from the focus, and a test performed to show whether the incidence of the disease was particularly high in the subgroup nearest to the focus, or perhaps whether it declined with distance from the focus. If the spatial distribution of the population is unknown, a case–control study may provide evidence as to whether cases within a certain region are more likely to be close to the focus than are a comparable group of controls. Gardner (1989) considered the problems associated with establishing whether there was an association between childhood cancers and proximity to nuclear installations.

Clustering in time and space

Knox (1964) pointed out that, if a relatively rare condition were in part caused by an infectious agent, one would expect to find a space–time interaction in the sense that cases which occurred close together in space would tend also to be close in time. In a study of childhood leukaemia in north-east England, he obtained information about 96 cases occurring in a certain area during a particular period of time, and tabulated each pair of cases in a 2×2 table according to certain 'closeness' criteria. A pair of cases was called 'adjacent' in time if the

Table 19.8 Pairs of cases of childhood leukaemia tabulated according to adjacency in time and space (Knox, 1964).

Time	Space Adjacent	Not adjacent	Total
Adjacent	5	147	152
Not adjacent	20	4388	4408
	25	4535	4560

interval between times of onset was less than 60 days, and 'adjacent' in space if the distance was less than 1 km. The results are shown in Table 19.8. The total frequency, 4560, is the number of pairs formed from 96 cases, $96 \times 95/2$.

If there were no relationship between the time at which a case occurred and the spatial position, the cell frequencies in Table 19.8 would have been expected to be proportional to the marginal totals. In particular, the expected value for the smallest frequency is $(152)(25)/4560 = 0.83$. The deviations of observed from expected frequencies cannot be tested by the usual methods for 2×2 tables since the entries are not independent (if cases A and B form an adjacent pair, and so do B and C, it is rather likely that A and C will also do so). However, it can be shown that, when the proportions of both types of adjacency are small, a good approximation to the correct significance test is to test the observed frequency as a possible observation from a Poisson distribution with mean equal to the expected frequency. In a Poisson distribution with mean 0.83, the probability of observing five or more events is 0.0017, so the excess must be judged highly significant.

A number of developments have been made since Knox's paper was published. In particular, account can be taken of the actual distances in time and space, rather than the dichotomies used in Knox's test (Mantel, 1967); and allowance can be made for known periods of time, or spatial distances, within which infection could have taken place (Pike & Smith, 1968). For a general review, see Smith (1982). Raubertas (1988) proposed a method of analysis which separates the effects of clustering in space, clustering in time and space–time clustering. The method involves estimating main effects associated with regions, main effects of the time intervals and their interaction. Then for each region a weighted average is formed consisting of the effects of nearby regions, with each region weighted by a measure of closeness in space. These weighted averages are combined into a test statistic that is sensitive to space clustering. A test for time clustering is produced in a similar manner, and the test for space–time clustering is based on weighted averages of the interaction terms, with weights taken as the product of the weights used for space and time. The method was applied to the

329 cases of Creutzfeld–Jakob disease identified in France over the period 1968–82, with space defined in terms of 94 departments.

Clustering in families

Clustering of disease in families may be due to an infective agent or to a genetic cause. These are the main reasons for studying familial aggregation, but other possible causes often complicate the issue. Members of the same family or household share the same natural environment and social conditions, all of which may affect the incidence of a particular disease. Age is a further complication, particularly in sibling studies, since siblings tend to be more similar in age than are members of different sibships.

These considerations imply that an analysis must take into account both the effects of a shared environment and the genetic effects. The former are related to living in the same household, irrespective of the genetic relationship, whilst the latter involve the degree of genetic relationship, irrespective of the extent of living in the same household. The situation is further complicated by the possibility of interactions between genetic factors and the environment. Twin studies have proved popular since they automatically match for age, and often for a shared environment, so that a comparison of the correlations within twin pairs, between monozygotic and dizygotic twins, tests for a genetic effect.

The aim of an analysis is to subdivide the covariance between family members into components representing the component due to shared environment and that due to shared genes. The genetic correlation is dependent on degree of relationship and a method of dealing with this is through pedigree analysis (Elston & Stewart, 1971). An example is given by Hopper and Mathews (1983) in which the blood lead level of 617 subjects in 80 families was analysed with respect to a shared environment and a number of covariates.

A principal aim of family studies will be to see whether the distribution of the number of affected individuals per family is overdispersed. For example, for traits governed by recessive Mendelian inheritance, the distribution of the number of affected offspring in sibships of a given size, would be expected to be binomial, with a probability of $\frac{1}{4}$, but there would in addition be a large number of families with no genetic risk and therefore no affected offspring. In other situations, the risk might vary more continuously from family to family. In studies of this sort there is a special problem of *ascertainment*. The form of distribution that might be expected in a complete enumeration of families may be distorted by the process of selection. For example, if families are selected through the notification of cases, those families with many cases are more likely to be selected than those with few, and families with no cases will not be selected at all. Methods have been proposed for the analysis of family distributions in a number of clearly defined situations. However, the method of ascertainment, and the nature of the consequent biases, may be complex and difficult to define clearly. Adjustment for ascertainment bias may therefore be difficult. For a review, see Hodge (1998).

The whole area of assessment of association between a health effect and genetic factors is under rapid development due to a number of advances. These include genetic mapping, linkage analysis (Ott, 1999), linkage disequilibrium analysis, and the human genome project, which has opened up the possibility of finding a simple or complex genetic effect through DNA analysis. It is beyond our scope to pursue this, but readers are referred to the book by Khoury *et al.* (1993).

20 Laboratory assays

20.1 **Biological assay**

In this chapter the term 'assay' is used rather loosely to cover a variety of laboratory studies in which specified properties of preparations are measured and calibrated. *Biological assays*, or *bioassays*, form an important subset, defined below. The general principles were established mainly during the 1930s and 1940s, and the methods of analysis developed then and later are comprehensively described by Finney (1978).

A biological assay is an experiment to determine the concentration of a key substance S in a preparation P by measuring the activity of P in a biological system B. The latter is usually a response in experimental animals which should as far as possible be specific to S. For example, vitamin D can be assayed by its anti-rachitic activity in rats. The biological material may, however, be humans, plants or microorganisms. The important point is that the system is purely a measuring device: the effect of S on B is of interest only in so far as it permits one to measure the concentration of S in P.

The strength of S in P cannot usually be measured directly as a function of the response, since this is likely to vary according to experimental conditions and the nature of the biological material B. This difficulty may be overcome by the use of a standard preparation containing S at constant concentration in an inert diluent and maintained under conditions that preserve its activity. The adoption of a standard preparation usually leads to the definition of a *standard unit* as the activity of a certain amount of the standard. Any test preparation, T, can then be assayed against the standard, S, by simultaneous experimentation. If, say, S is defined to contain 1000 units per g and T happens to contain 100 units per g, a dose $10X$ g of T should give the same response as X g of S. The *relative potency* or *potency ratio* of T in terms of S is then said to be 1/10, or equivalently T may be said to have a *potency* of 100 units per g.

In the ideal situation described above, we have assumed that S and T both contain different concentrations of the same substance S in inert diluents, and any assay with a response specific to S will measure the unique potency ratio. Such an assay is called an *analytical dilution assay*; it perhaps rarely exists in the real world. In practice, most biological responses are specific to a range of substances, perhaps closely related chemically, like the various penicillins. In such cases, the potency may depend to some extent on the assay system, because different varieties of the active substances may have differential effects in different biological systems. An assay which for a particular biological system behaves *as though* the ideal situation were true is called a *comparative dilution assay*.

The term 'bioassay' is often used in a more general sense, to denote any experiment in which specific responses to externally applied agents are observed in animals or some other biological system. This usage is, for example, common in the extensive programmes for the testing of new drugs, pesticides, food additives, etc., for potential carcinogenic effects. Some of these broader types of assays are considered in §20.6. At present, we are concerned solely with bioassays in the more specific sense described earlier, in which the central purpose is the estimation of relative potency.

Direct assays

The simplest form of assay is the *direct assay*, in which increasing doses of S and T can be administered to an experimental unit until a certain critical event takes place. This situation is rare; an example is the assay of prepared digitalis in the guinea-pig, in which the critical event is arrest of heart beat. The critical dose given to any one animal is a measure of the individual tolerance of that animal, which can be expected to vary between animals through biological and environmental causes. On any one occasion for a particular animal, suppose that the tolerance dose of S is X_S and that of T is X_T; in practice, of course, only one of these can be observed. Then the potency, ρ, of T in terms of S is given by X_S/X_T. (Note the crucial assumption here that the occurrence of the critical event depends merely on the amount of the key substance administered, and not on its concentration in the diluent.)

If S and T were each administered to large random samples from a population of animals, the tolerance doses X_S and X_T would form two distributions related to each other, as in Fig. 20.1(a); the distribution of X_S would differ from that of X_T by a multiplying factor ρ, exactly as if the scale were extended or contracted by this factor. From random samples on T and S, ρ could be estimated from the distributions of X_T and X_S.

The estimation problem is simplified if the doses are recorded logarithmically, as in Fig. 20.1(b). If $x_S = \log X_S$ and $x_T = \log X_T$, we can estimate $\log \rho$ from the two sample means $\bar{x}_S$ and $\bar{x}_T$, by $M = \bar{x}_S - \bar{x}_T$. The distributions of x_S and x_T are automatically guaranteed to be the same shape, and in practice they are likely to be reasonably normal, since tolerance doses tend to be positively skewly distributed and the logarithmic transformation will reduce the skewness. The standard theory of the t distribution in the two-sample case thus provides confidence limits for $\log \rho$, and (by taking antilogs) the corresponding limits for ρ. Unfortunately, the continuous administration of doses and the

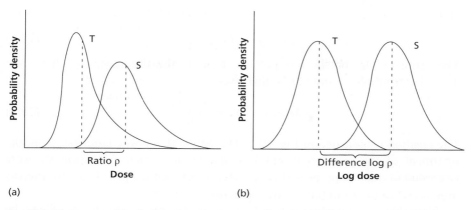

Fig. 20.1 Direct assay. Distributions of tolerance doses and their logarithms for standard and test preparations.

immediate response needed for direct assays are rarely feasible. Instead, the assayer has to rely on *indirect assays*, in which predetermined doses of T and S are given to groups of experimental units and the resulting responses are observed. Two different models for this situation are considered in the next two sections.

20.2 **Parallel-line assays**

Suppose that, for a particular assay system, the mean response, y, is linearly related to the log dose, x. That is, for a log dose x_S of S, the expected response is

$$E(y) = \alpha + \beta x_S. \tag{20.1}$$

Now, the same expected response would be obtained by a log dose x_T of T, where $x_S - x_T = \log \rho$, the log potency ratio of T in terms of S. Consequently the equation of the regression line for T is

$$\left. \begin{aligned} E(y) &= \alpha + \beta(x_T + \log \rho) \\ &= (\alpha + \beta \log \rho) + \beta x_T \end{aligned} \right\}. \tag{20.2}$$

The regression lines (20.1) and (20.2) for S and T, respectively, are parallel, but differ in position if $\log \rho$ is different from zero (i.e. if ρ is different from 1). The horizontal distance between the two lines is $\log \rho$.

In any one assay, values of y will be observed at various values of x_S for S and at values of x_T for T. The regression relationships (20.1) and (20.2) are estimated by fitting two parallel lines exactly as in §11.4 (equation (11.24)), giving equations

$$Y_S = \bar{y}_S + b(x_S - \bar{x}_S) \tag{20.3}$$

and

$$Y_T = \bar{y}_T + b(x_T - \bar{x}_T). \tag{20.4}$$

The estimate, M, of the log potency ratio is the difference $x_S - x_T$ when $Y_S = Y_T$; from (20.3) and (20.4), this gives

$$M = \bar{x}_S - \bar{x}_T - \frac{\bar{y}_S - \bar{y}_T}{b}. \tag{20.5}$$

The position is indicated in Fig. 20.2. The only difference in emphasis from the treatment of the problem in §11.4 is that in the earlier discussion we were interested in estimating the vertical difference between the parallel lines, whereas now we estimate, from (20.5), the horizontal distance.

Note that, if the regression is not linear, the two regression curves will still be 'parallel' in the sense that their *horizontal* distance on the log-dose scale will be constant. In general, though, the *vertical* distance will not be constant unless the regression is linear. An approach using polynomial or other non-linear regression (§§12.1 and 12.4) might be considered, but it is more usual, and more convenient, to seek a transformation of the response variable which more nearly achieves linearity (§10.8). For the methods of analysis described below, we assume linearity and also that the residual variation about the regression is normal, with constant variance.

Suppose that there are n_S and n_T observations on S and T, respectively, and that the residual mean square (MSq) about parallel lines (the s_c^2 of (11.34)) is s^2. An approximate formula for var(M) is, from (5.12),

$$\text{var}(M) \simeq \frac{s^2}{b^2} \left[\frac{1}{n_S} + \frac{1}{n_T} + \frac{(\bar{y}_S - \bar{y}_T)^2}{b^2 \sum (S_{xx})} \right], \tag{20.6}$$

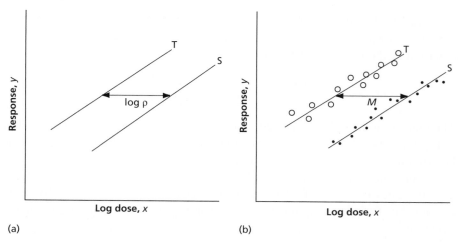

(a)   (b)

Fig. 20.2 Parallel-line assay. True (a) and fitted (b) regression lines for standard and test preparations.

where $\sum(S_{xx})$ is the pooled Within-Preparations sum of squares (SSq) of x. The last term in the square brackets can also be written, from (20.5), as

$$\frac{(M - \bar{x}_S + \bar{x}_T)^2}{\sum(S_{xx})}.$$

It will be relatively small if the doses of S and T are chosen so that the mean responses $\bar{y}_S$ and $\bar{y}_T$ are nearly equal. (To achieve this, one needs either luck or some preliminary estimate of the potency.) To a further degree of approximation, then,

$$\text{var}(M) \simeq \frac{s^2}{b^2}\left(\frac{1}{n_S} + \frac{1}{n_T}\right). \tag{20.7}$$

This formula shows that the precision of the estimate of potency depends mainly on: (i) the numbers n_S and n_T which are at the experimenter's disposal; and (ii) the value of $\lambda = s/b$. The latter quantity is sometimes called the *index of precision* (although 'imprecision' would be a better description); it represents the inherent imprecision of the assay method. To improve the precision of the assay per unit observation, it would be useful to modify the experimental method so that s decreases, b increases, or both. Unfortunately, s and b often tend to increase or decrease together and improvement may be difficult. Furthermore, reductions in λ may be attainable only by increased cost and the question then arises whether it is more economical to improve precision by increasing the number of observations made rather than by modifying the technique.

Approximate confidence limits for log ρ may be obtained by setting limits around M, using (20.6) and the t distribution on the degrees of freedom (DF) appropriate for $s^2, n_S + n_T - 3 \ (= v, \text{ say})$. Corresponding limits for ρ are then obtained by taking antilogs. A more exact expression is available by applying Fieller's theorem ((5.15) and (5.16)) to the ratio forming the final term in (20.5). The $100(1 - \alpha)\%$ limits for log ρ are then

$$\bar{x}_S - \bar{x}_T + \frac{M - \bar{x}_S + \bar{x}_T \pm \frac{t_{v,\alpha}s}{b}\left[(1 - g)\left(\frac{1}{n_S} + \frac{1}{n_T}\right) + \frac{(M - \bar{x}_S + \bar{x}_T)^2}{\sum(S_{xx})}\right]^{\frac{1}{2}}}{1 - g}, \tag{20.8}$$

where

$$g = \frac{t_{v,\alpha}^2 s^2}{b^2 \sum(S_{xx})}. \tag{20.9}$$

As noted in §5.3, the quantity g depends on the significance level of the departure of b from zero. When g is very small, the limits (20.8) will be close to those given by the approximate method using (20.6). If $g > 1$, the slope is not significant at the α level, and the limits from (20.8) will either be infinite or will exclude the estimate M.

The validity of a parallel-line assay depends crucially on the assumptions of linearity and parallelism. Non-linearity can often be corrected by a transformation of the response scale. Non-parallelism when the regressions are apparently linear is more troublesome, and may indicate a basically invalid assay system. With a suitable choice of design, these assumptions can be tested by an analysis of variance, essentially following the steps illustrated in Tables 11.2 and 11.5.

Suppose there are k_S dose groups of S, and k_T of T (a so-called $k_S + k_T$ design). An analysis of variance of y for the whole data set could have the following subdivision of DF:

Between doses	$k_S + k_T - 1$	
Between preparations		1
Common slope		1
Between slopes		1
Non-linearity		$k_S + k_T - 4$
Within doses	$n_S + n_T - (k_S + k_T)$	
Total	$n_S + n_T - 1$	

The 'Between preparations' term is of no particular interest, since the difference in mean response between preparations depends on the choice of dose levels. Parallelism and linearity are tested by the MSqs from the 'Between slopes' and 'Non-linearity' lines, with F tests against the MSq from the 'Within doses' line. Non-significance in these validity tests does not guarantee complete validity, since the departures from the model may be too small to be detected from the data being analysed. Confidence in the assay system can best be provided by knowledge of previous assays on similar substances, using the same assay system.

Note that a $2 + 2$ design is too small to test linearity, the DF being zero. If the regressions are in fact non-linear, the effect may be to inflate the 'Between slopes' SSq, and the two types of departure cannot be clearly distinguished. A $2 + 3$ or larger design avoids this problem. Finney (1978) provides a very detailed account of experimental design in biological assays.

Radioligand assays

In a *radioligand assay* (RLA) the system $\mathcal{B}$ is an antigen–antibody reaction. In one form of RLA, the *radioimmunoassay* (RIA), the substance to be assayed is an antigen. A quantity of antigen is initially labelled with a radioisotope, a known dose of the test or standard preparation is added and the response is measured by a radiation count of antibody-bound labelled antigen. The bound count is affected by the dose of the substance under assay, a large dose diluting the labelled antigen so that the count is low. The dose–response curve is typically sigmoid in shape, with an upper asymptote, D, to the mean response, at zero dose, and a lower asymptote, C, at very high doses. If the mean bound count at log dose x is U, the quantity

$$Y = \ln\left(\frac{U - C}{D - U}\right) \tag{20.10}$$

is analogous to the logit transformation for proportions (14.5) and it is often (though not always) found that Y is approximately linearly related to x.

In an *immunoradiometric assay* (IRMA) the roles of antigen and antibody are interchanged, but the principles are otherwise the same as for RIAs.

RIAs are used routinely in clinical chemistry, and specimens from many different patients may be assayed against the same standard. The precision of RIAs is relatively high, and it is common for responses to be made at a single dose of each test preparation, for comparison with a standard curve determined from readings at several doses. This design may achieve potency estimates of adequate precision, but it permits no test of parallelism, and should only be used if the assay validity has already been established by a larger design.

Although potencies are often estimated by eye, a formal approach, providing estimates of error and validity tests, is preferable. Finney (1978) gives details of such an approach, and the author also (Finney, 1979) describes the desiderata for computer programs intended for the routine analysis of RIAs. See also Govindarajulu (2000). The statistical methodology is a direct extension of that described earlier in this section, with some additional features. In particular: (i) the lower and upper asymptotes, C and D, need to be estimated from the data (counts will usually have been observed at each of the extremes of dose level); and (ii) the variance of the observed count u is likely to increase with the mean U. Ideally, u might be expected to follow a Poisson distribution, but there is often some additional source of variation, causing the variance to be greater than the mean. A full analysis may assume a normal approximation, but the need to estimate the asymptotes and to take account of the logit transformation (20.10) leads to an iterative least squares or maximum likelihood solution, as in §12.4. The relationship of $\mathrm{var}(u)$ to U may be estimated as part of the solution, or it may be possible to assume some functional relationship on the basis of past experience.

Combination of assays

Assays to determine the relative potency of a particular (S, T) pair may be replicated, as in other scientific experiments, to improve precision and extend the validity of the results. More specifically, T may be intended as a future standard preparation, and collaborative studies to compare T with the previous standard S may involve many different laboratories.

The general principles established in §8.2 and (in the meta-analysis of clinical trials) §18.10 also apply here. In particular, combined estimates of log potency ratio and corresponding heterogeneity tests can be obtained approximately by the methods of §8.2. The weights for the individual estimates M_i are the reciprocals of the approximate variances ((20.6) in the case of parallel-line assays).

There is one important difference between the combination of results from assays and those from clinical trials. In the meta-analysis of trials (§18.10), the efficacy parameter may vary between trials because of different patient characteristics or variations in treatment. In replicate assays of an (S, T) pair, the relative potency *ought* to be constant, since it depends on physical properties of the two preparations. However, variation may occur, partly through imperfect control of laboratory procedures but, more importantly, because the preparations may not contain a single active constituent but may instead include mixtures of closely related variants, which may be more active in some assay systems than in others. Heterogeneity, therefore, is often a possibility in replicate assays, although it will usually be relatively unimportant.

The approximate nature of the methods of §8.2 arises mainly through the random error associated with the weights. In (20.6), for example, the slope b will have a random error which may be proportionately large. For parallel-line assays a maximum likelihood solution is available for a formulation that assumes constant error variance across the assays but allows variation in slope (Armitage, 1970; Williams, 1978). This approach, with associated heterogeneity tests, is described by Finney (1978, §14.3).

20.3 **Slope-ratio assays**

In some assay systems the response, y, can conveniently be related to the dose, rather than the log dose, the residual variation being approximately normal and having approximately constant variance. This situation arises particularly in microbiological assays where the response is a turbidometric measure of growth of microorganisms. If the potency of T in terms of S is ρ, the same expected response will be given by doses X_T of T and X_S of S, where $X_S = \rho X_T$. If, therefore, the regression equation for S is

$$\mathrm{E}(y) = \alpha + \beta_S X_S, \tag{20.11}$$

that for T will be

$$\begin{aligned} \mathrm{E}(y) &= \alpha + \beta_S(\rho X_T) \\ &= \alpha + \beta_T X_T, \end{aligned} \tag{20.12}$$

where $\beta_T = \rho\beta_S$. Equations (20.11) and (20.12) represent two straight lines with the same intercept, α, on the vertical axis and with slopes in the ratio $1 : \rho$. Hence the term *slope ratio*. The intercept α is the expected response at zero dose, whether of T or of S. The position is shown in Fig. 20.3.

In the analysis of results from a slope-ratio assay the observed responses at various doses X_S of S and X_T of T must be fitted by two lines of the form

$$Y = a + b_S X_S \tag{20.13}$$

and

$$Y = a + b_T X_T, \tag{20.14}$$

which are, like the true regression lines, constrained to pass through the same intercept on the vertical axis (Fig. 20.3). This is a form of regression analysis not previously considered in this book. The problem can conveniently be regarded as one of multiple regression. For each observation we define three variables, y, X_S and X_T, of which y is the dependent variable and X_S and X_T are predictor variables. For any observation on S, X_S is non-zero and $X_T = 0$; for an observation on T, $X_S = 0$ and X_T is non-zero. The assay may include control observations (so-called *blanks*) without either S or T; for these, $X_S = X_T = 0$. The true regression equations (20.11) and (20.12) can now be combined into one multiple regression equation:

$$E(y) = \alpha + \beta_S X_S + \beta_T X_T, \tag{20.15}$$

and the estimated regressions (20.13) and (20.14) are combined in the estimated multiple regression

$$Y = a + b_S X_S + b_T X_T. \tag{20.16}$$

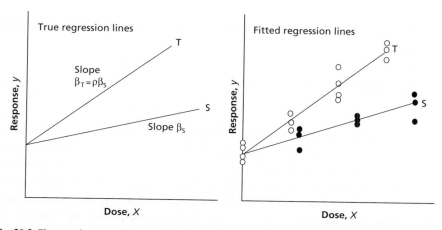

Fig. 20.3 Slope-ratio assay. True and fitted regression lines for standard and test preparations.

This relationship can be fitted by standard multiple regression methods (§11.6), and the potency $\rho \, (= \beta_T/\beta_S)$ estimated by

$$R = b_T/b_S. \tag{20.17}$$

The residual variance of y is estimated by the usual residual MSq, s^2, and the variances and covariance of b_S and b_T are obtained from (11.43) and (11.44):

$$\mathrm{var}(b_S) = c_{11}s^2, \mathrm{var}(b_T) = c_{22}s^2, \mathrm{cov}(b_S, b_T) = c_{12}s^2. \tag{20.18}$$

Approximate confidence limits for ρ are obtained by the following formula derived from (5.17):

$$\mathrm{var}(R) = \frac{s^2}{b_S^2}(c_{22} - 2Rc_{12} + R^2c_{11}). \tag{20.19}$$

A more exact solution, using Fieller's theorem, is available, as in (5.15), but is not normally required with assays of this type.

For numerical examples of the calculations, see Finney (1978, Chapter 7).

The adequacy of the model in a slope-ratio assay can be tested by a rather elegant analysis of variance procedure. Suppose the design is of a $1 + k_S + k_T$ type; that is, there is one group of 'blanks' and there are k_S dose groups of S and k_T dose groups of T. Suppose also that there is replication at some or all of the dose levels, giving n observations in all. A standard analysis (as described on p. 360) leads to the following subdivision of DF:

Between doses	$k_S + k_T$	
Regression		2
Deviations from model		$k_S + k_T - 2$
Within doses	$n - k_S - k_T - 1$	
	$n - 1$	

The SSq for deviations from the model can be subdivided into the following parts:

Blanks	1
Intersection	1
Non-linearity for non-zero doses	$k_S + k_T - 4$
	$k_S + k_T - 2$

The SSq for 'blanks' indicates whether the 'blanks' observations are sufficiently consistent with the remainder. It can be obtained by refitting the multiple regression with an extra dummy variable (1 for 'blanks', 0 otherwise), and noting the reduction in the deviations SSq. A significant variance-ratio test for 'blanks' might indicate non-linearity for very low doses; if the remaining tests were satisfactory, the assay could still be analysed adequately by omitting the 'blanks'.

The SSq for 'intersection' shows whether the data can justifiably be fitted by two lines intersecting on the vertical axis. Significance here is more serious and usually indicates invalidity of the assay system. It can be obtained by fitting two separate lines to the observations at non-zero doses of S and T. The difference in residual between this analysis and that referred to above (for the 'blanks' test) gives the required SSq.

The third component, due to non-linearity at non-zero doses, can be obtained either by subtraction or directly from the two separate regressions ($k_S - 2$ DF for S and $k_T - 2$ for T adding to the required $k_S + k_T - 4$).

Further details, with examples, are given by Finney (1978, Chapter 7), who also discusses the use of symmetric designs which permit simplification of the analysis by the use of linear contrasts.

20.4 **Quantal-response assays**

Frequently the response is quantal (i.e. binary), as in direct assays, and yet the assay has to be done indirectly by selection of doses and observation of the responses elicited. For instance, in an assay of viral preparations, the response may be the presence or absence of viral growth in each of a group of egg membranes inoculated with a fixed quantity of a particular dilution of a preparation. In general, if a particular dose of one preparation is applied to n_i experimental units, the investigator observes that a certain number of responses, say, r_i, are positive and $n_i - r_i$ are negative. For any one preparation, the response curve relating the expected response (expressed as the probability of a positive response) to the dose or to the log dose is likely to be sigmoid in shape, as in the continuous curve in Fig. 20.4. The fitting of such a response curve presents precisely the sort of problem considered in §14.2 and, as we shall see, the methods described there are immediately applicable.

A further point is worth noting. The response curve, rising from 0 to 1 on the vertical scale, may be regarded as the cumulative distribution function of a random variable, which can be called the *tolerance* of experimental units to the agent under test. The tolerances are precisely the critical doses that would be observed in a direct assay. If, for example, a dose X corresponds to a response P, we can interpret this as showing that a proportion P of the units have a tolerance less than X (and therefore succumb to X), and $1 - P$ have a tolerance greater than X. The response function P is thus the distribution function of tolerance; the corresponding density function is called the *tolerance distribution* (see Fig. 20.4). A very similar situation holds in psychological tests of the stimulus–response type. An individual given a stimulus X will respond if the threshold (corresponding to the tolerance in biological assay) is less than X. Neither in the psychological example nor in biological assay is there any need to suppose that X is a constant quantity for any individual; it may vary from occasion to occasion in the same individual.

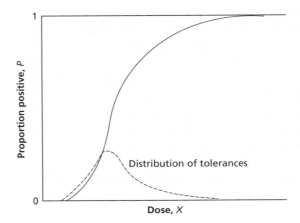

Fig. 20.4 Quantal-response curve with the corresponding tolerance distribution.

In an assay of T and S, the response curves, plotted against $x = \log X$, will be parallel in the sense that they differ by a constant horizontal distance, $\log \rho$, and a full analysis requires that the data be fitted by two parallel curves of this sort. A natural approach is to linearize the response curves by applying to the response one of the standard transformations for binary data (§§10.8 and 14.1). One can then suppose that the expectations of the transformed values are linearly related to the log dose, x, by the equations

$$\left.\begin{array}{l} Y = \alpha_S + \beta x \text{ for S} \\ Y = \alpha_T + \beta x \text{ for T} \end{array}\right\}.$$ (20.20)

and

The slope parameter β is inversely proportional to the standard deviation of the log-tolerance distribution. For the logistic transformation (14.5) with $Y = \ln[P/(1 - P)]$, for instance, the proportionality factor is $\pi/\sqrt{3} = 1 \cdot 814$.

Although (20.20) has essentially the same form as (20.3) and (20.4), the methods described in §20.1 for parallel-line assays cannot be used, since the random variation about the lines is not normally distributed with constant variance. The model may be fitted iteratively by the maximum likelihood procedure for logistic regression described in §14.2, using a dummy variable to distinguish between S and T, as in (11.55). Writing $\alpha_T = \alpha_S + \delta$, the log potency ratio is given by $\log \rho = \delta/\beta$. A computer program for logistic regression may be used to obtain the estimates a_S, d and b of α_S, δ and β, respectively, and hence $\log \rho$ is estimated by $M = d/b$. From (5.17), an approximate formula for var(M) is

$$\text{var}(M) \simeq \frac{V_d}{b^2} - \frac{2dC_{db}}{b^3} + \frac{d^2 V_b}{b^4},$$

where $V_d = \text{var}(d)$, $C_{db} = \text{cov}(d, b)$ and $V_b = \text{var}(b)$. These variances and the covariance should be obtainable from the computer output. Approximate $100(1 - \alpha)\%$ confidence limits for log ρ are then

$$M \pm z_\alpha \sqrt{\text{var}(M)},$$

where z_α is the usual standardized normal deviate. Limits for ρ are obtained by taking antilogs.

By analogy with (20.8), Fieller's theorem can be used to give more reliable approximations. From (5.13) the limits for log ρ then become

$$\frac{M - \dfrac{gC_{db}}{V_b} \pm \dfrac{z_\alpha}{b}\left[V_d - 2MC_{db} + M^2 V_b - g\left(V_d - \dfrac{C_{db}^2}{V_b}\right)\right]^{\frac{1}{2}}}{1 - g},$$

where $g = z_\alpha^2 V_b / b^2$.

Approximate χ^2 tests for (i) parallelism and (ii) linearity may be obtained by the analysis of deviance, by taking: (i) the difference between the deviances of the fitted model and a model with separate slopes for S and T; and (ii) the deviance of the latter model.

An alternative approach to the analysis of quantal-response data, *probit analysis*, is widely used. This method, which is fully described by Finney (1971), provides the maximum likelihood solution for the *probit* or *normal equivalent deviate* (NED) transformation (§14.1) rather than for the logit. Here P is the distribution function for a standard normal deviate Y (a constant 5 being added to the NED to give the probit). This transformation thus implies that the tolerance distribution for the log dose is normal, and the slope parameter β in (20.20) is the reciprocal of the standard deviation. There is no evidence to suggest that either model is more consistent with real data than the other, and curves fitted by the two methods are invariably very similar.

Before the advent of computer programs for the efficient analysis of quantal-response data, a number of simple methods were in common use. These mainly aimed to estimate the location of the tolerance distribution as summarized by its median. This is the dose at which $P = 0.5$, and is called the *median effective dose* (ED$_{50}$). In the comparison of two response curves, the ED$_{50}$ for T and S are in the ratio $1 : \rho$. If they are estimated by X_{0T} and X_{0S}, the ratio X_{0S}/X_{0T} will provide an estimate of ρ. The ED$_{50}$ is sometimes given slightly different names according to the type of response: e.g. LD$_{50}$ or median lethal dose if the response is lethal. A full account of these short-cut methods is given by Finney (1978, §§18.6–18.8).

The up-and-down (or staircase) method

In experiments or assays in which the main purpose is to estimate the ED$_{50}$, the choice of dose levels is important. Doses yielding very low or very high values of

P contribute little to the precision of the ED_{50} estimate, and the aim should be to use doses giving values of P closer to 0·5. Since the dose–response curve is initially unknown, an adaptive design may be needed.

In the *up-and-down* (or *staircase*) *method*, the doses are changed after each observation, being increased by one step after a negative response and decreased after a positive. The dose levels should be predetermined as equally spaced log doses, with a spacing guessed to be about one standard deviation of the log-dose tolerance distribution. The effect of the adaptive choice of dose levels is to cluster the doses around the ED_{50}. When the experiment has stopped, the results can be analysed in the usual way, e.g. by using the maximum likelihood solution for logistic regression.

Note that although the design tends to use doses giving high precision to the ED_{50} estimate, it performs badly in estimating the slope β of the linear relationship (for which purpose a wider spread of dose levels would have been desirable), and hence may provide a poor estimate of the precision of the ED_{50} estimate, since this depends importantly on β. It may, therefore, be wise to allow some divergence from the strict rule by the occasional use of more extreme doses.

The adaptive design clearly requires that the positive or negative result of each observation should become known quickly, before the next dose is chosen. It is particularly suitable for the determination of auditory, visual or pain thresholds for individual subjects, where immediate responses to stimuli are available.

For further details, see Dixon (1988).

20.5 **Some special assays**

This section discusses three special forms of assay: Michaelis–Menten assays, which arise in the study of enzyme kinetics; limiting dilution assays, which occur in various applications, most recently in immunology; and mutagenicity assays, which are often used in testing compounds for the potential genetic damage they may cause.

It must be conceded that this is a rather arbitrary selection from the numerous specialist assays that could have been included. However, these three forms of assay have given rise to substantial discussion of their statistical analysis, both in the biometrical literature and in the relevant specialist literature. It should also be conceded that the purist may object to their description as assays at all, as there is frequently no standard against which an unknown is assayed. For example, the first two methods seek to determine a parameter such as a concentration or rate constant on the basis of an equation derived from theory. Nevertheless, the term 'assay' is often applied to these procedures and this is a convenient place to discuss them.

Michaelis–Menten assays

In the presence of an enzyme, certain biochemical reactions convert substrate into product at a rate y which depends on substrate concentration x. For many reactions these quantities are related by the Michaelis–Menten equation,

$$y = \frac{V_{\max} x}{K_M + x}, \tag{20.21}$$

where $V_{\max}$ (the asymptotic rate) and K_M (the *Michaelis constant*) are quantities which it is important to know in the study of the enzyme.

The experimenter will observe reaction velocities $y_i (i = 1, \ldots, n)$ at a variety of substrate concentrations, $x_i, (i = 1, \ldots, n)$ and will use these data to estimate $V_{\max}$ and K_M or, occasionally, the *specificity constant* $V_{\max}/K_M$, which is the limit of the slope of (20.21) when the substrate concentration tends to zero.

As was noted in §12.4, (20.21) is not linear in its parameters and over the last 60 years this has given rise to several methods for solving this problem. Three methods rely on simple transformations of (20.21) that give equations that are linear in some set of parameters. The first is the double-reciprocal or *Lineweaver–Burk* transformation already encountered in Example 12.5:

$$\frac{1}{y} = \frac{1}{V_{\max}} + \frac{K_M}{V_{\max}} \frac{1}{x}. \tag{20.22}$$

An alternative comes from multiplying (20.22) by x, namely,

$$\frac{x}{y} = \frac{K_M}{V_{\max}} + \frac{1}{V_{\max}} x, \tag{20.23}$$

which is sometimes known as the *Woolf* transformation. The final alternative, associated with the name of *Scatchard* or *Eadie–Hofstee*, notes that (20.21) can be written as

$$y = V_{\max} - K_M \frac{y}{x}. \tag{20.24}$$

Some background on each of these transformations can be found in §2.5 of Cornish-Bowden (1995a). These equations are used by transforming each observed point (x_i, y_i) in the prescribed way and estimating the parameters from the least squares estimates of slope and intercept.

Ruppert *et al.* (1989) discuss various papers that have compared these methods, together with the method which fits (20.21) directly, using non-linear methods (see §12.4). Of course, while (20.22)–(20.24) are legitimate transformations of the Michaelis–Menten equation (20.21), they are insufficently specified to permit discussion of statistical properties. If the observed reaction velocity is related to the substrate concentration by (20.21), plus an additive residual with constant variance, then a fuller investigation of the properties of the transformations is possible (see, for example, Currie, 1982). Clearly, if the error has constant variance on the scale of (20.21), then the residual will not have constant variance on the scale implicit in (20.22) or (20.23), so ordinary least squares, which has good properties only if the variance of the residuals is constant, will inevitably produce estimates with poor properties when used after one of these transformations has been applied.

Indeed, contrasts between the linearizing transformations have often focused more on practical aspects than on the statistical properties of the estimators. The double-reciprocal plot when applied to a point with a small substrate concentration often leads to a point whose position is highly variable and often very influential (see §11.9). Consequently, various methods have been devised which are intended to be less susceptible to such problems. One of the most unusual is the *direct linear plot* (Cornish-Bowden & Eisenthal, 1974). This is quite widely used in the area of application and will be described below. Another approach is to accept that some points will be highly variable and try to allow for this using some form of weighted least squares (see Cornish-Bowden, 1995b).

The direct linear plot proceeds as follows. Suppose (x_i, y_i) obeys (20.21); then the equivalent formulation (20.24) can be viewed as constraining the values of K_M and V_{max} to lie on the line

$$V_{max} = y_i + K_M \frac{y_i}{x_i}. \tag{20.25}$$

A similar equation can be formed for each of the n points in the data set. If the n points all obey (20.21), i.e. there is no error, then the n lines corresponding to equations of the form (20.25) will intersect at the true values of K_M and V_{max}. In practice, the points will depart from (20.21) by an error term and so the pairs of lines corresponding to (20.25) will intersect in $\frac{1}{2}n(n-1)$ points, each of which provides a separate value for K_M and V_{max}. Cornish-Bowden and Eisenthal (1974) propose that the estimate of each parameter is the median of these separate values. These authors point out that this method is particularly well suited for use at the laboratory bench, as well as being less susceptible than other methods to outlying values. Valid estimates of error for the parameter estimates are harder to obtain but have been provided by Cressie and Keightley (1979). It should be noted that the version of the direct linear plot described is driven by (20.24) and an alternative, based on (20.23), will provide estimates in terms of V_{max} and V_{max}/K_M.

While the performance of ordinary least squares when applied following transformations such as (20.22) and (20.23) is questionable if the errors have constant variance on the scale of (20.21), this would not, of course, be the case if the errors were constant on the transformed scale. In practice, satisfactory statistical modelling of data from a Michaelis–Menten equation requires knowledge of the form of the error term, and this is usually unavailable. Ruppert *et al.*

(1989) propose an approach which tries to identify appropriate error structures from the data themselves. These authors assume that the data obey the model

$$y_i^{(\lambda)} = \left(\frac{V_{\max} x_i}{K_M + x_i} \right)^{(\lambda)} + x_i^\theta \varepsilon_i,$$

where ε_i are independent normal random variables with mean 0 and variance σ^2 and $z^{(\lambda)}$ denotes the Box–Cox transformation (see §10.8). The parameters λ and θ, as well as K_M, $V_{\max}$ and σ, are estimated by maximum likelihood. The form of error model induced by certain pairs of values for λ and θ are described in Table 1 of Ruppert *et al.* (1989).

An alternative approach to estimating the form of the error from the data was discussed by Nelder (1991) in a rejoinder to Ruppert *et al.* Nelder advocated using a generalized linear model, with mean given by (20.21) and variance function $V(\mu) = \mu^\theta$; a reciprocal link applied to (20.21) gives a form that is linear in $K_M / V_{\max}$ and $1 / V_{\max}$. Parameters are estimated by extended quasi-likelihood (see McCullagh & Nelder, 1989, p. 349): values of θ close to zero will correspond to the model that has constant variance on the scale of (20.21) and values close to 2 correspond to errors with a constant coefficient of variation. The relative merits of the approaches advocated by Nelder and by Ruppert *et al.* are discussed by the authors at the end of Nelder's article.

Example 20.1

The data from Forsyth *et al.* (1993) considered in Example 12.5 are now reconsidered. The Michaelis–Menten equation is fitted in six ways. Figure 20.5(a) shows (20.21) fitted directly using non-linear methods and assuming a constant error variance on the scale of the reaction velocities: Fig. 20.5 (b, c and d) shows, respectively, the data transformed by (20.22), (20.23) and (20.24), together with the ordinary least squares regression line.

From Fig. 20.5(a) it appears that the data conform closely to the Michaelis–Menten equation but this impression is not fully sustained in the other plots. In each of the other plots there is a discrepant point which, in each case, corresponds to the observation with the smallest substrate concentration. In Fig. 20.5(b) the discrepancy is perhaps less obvious because the discrepant point is so influential that it forces the fitted line to depart from the obvious line of the remaining points.

Figure 20.6 is the direct linear plot for these data: three of the 10 intersections between the five lines result in intersections with negative values for both K_M and $V_{\max}$. These points all involve intersection with the line corresponding to the point which appeared discrepant in Fig. 20.5. The one intersection with this line that is in the first quadrant is clearly distant from the other intersections, which are relatively closely clustered.

The estimates of K_M and $V_{\max}$ from these methods are shown in Table 20.1.

The estimated values are clearly highly dependent on the method of fitting. Admittedly this is what might be expected when only five points are analysed, but this number is not atypical in applications. The negative values from the Lineweaver–Burk transformation emphasize the sensitivity of this method to even slightly unusual observations. As

Table 20.1 Estimates of K_M and V_{max} derived by various methods for data plotted in Fig. 20.5

| Method | Intercept | | Slope | | K_M | V_{max} |
	Meaning	Value	Meaning	Value		
Non-linear fit	—		—		11·3	1114
Lineweaver–Burk	$1/V_{max}$	−0·00066	K_M/V_{max}	0·0290	−43·9	−1515
Woolf	K_M/V_{max}	0·0152	$1/V_{max}$	0·00082	18·6	1225
Scatchard	V_{max}	802	$-K_M$	−6·2	6·2	802
Direct linear plot	—		—		7·7	979
GLM: gamma errors	$1/V_{max}$	0·000717	K_M/V_{max}	0·01444	20·2	1395

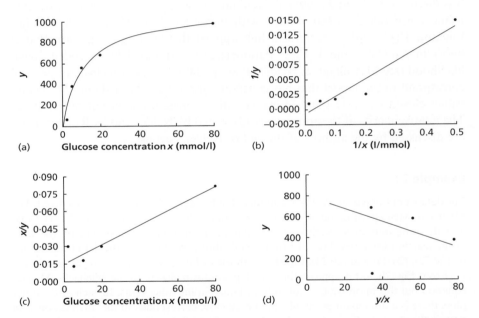

Fig. 20.5 Data from Forsyth *et al.* (1993): raw data and data plotted according to various linearizing transformations.

explained in Example 12.5, the non-linear fit is equivalent to a generalized linear model (GLM) with reciprocal link and normal errors, and the substantial difference between this and the GLM with gamma errors highlights the effect that the form of error can have in these calculations.

Limiting dilution assays

Limiting dilution assays allow a concentration of an agent, which could be a chemical, a particular cell type or a pathogen, to be measured when the analyst only has the means to detect the presence or absence of the agent. The idea is that if the assay starts with a solution containing the agent, then the presence or absence of an agent can be discerned in each of a succession of dilutions. The degree of dilution needed essentially to eliminate the agent can, on the basis of certain assumptions, be used to calculate the concentration of the agent in the original sample. This type of assay has been used to assess concentrations of pollutants or pathogens in water and, more recently, has found widespread application in immunology, where the aim is to determine the proportion of cells in a sample that are of a particular type, such as T cells (see, for example, Fazekas de St Groth, 1982).

A more specific description requires some notation. Suppose that the concentration of the agent in the original sample is θ, and a succession of dilutions in which the concentrations will be $\theta d_1, \theta d_2, \ldots, \theta d_m$, are prepared. A typical selection for the dilutions might be $d_i = 2^{-i}$: the number of dilutions m would be chosen by the experimenter. It is usual to assay several specimens at each dilution; if n_i specimens are assayed at dilution d_i, then r_i will be found to contain the agent. The probability that a specimen at dilution d_i contains the agent is, in general, some function of the dilution and θ, say, $\pi(\theta, d_i) = \pi_i$. The number of assays which were found to contain the agent, r_i, will follow a binomial distribution with parameters n_i and π_i, so a maximum likelihood analysis would maximize

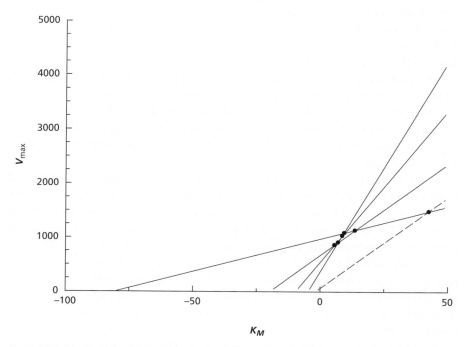

Fig. 20.6 Direct linear plot (based on (20.24)): seven of the 10 intersections are shown: the line corresponding to the point with smallest substrate concentration is dashed.

$$\sum_{i=1}^{m} r_i \log[\pi(\theta, d_i)] + (n_i - r_i) \log[1 - \pi(\theta, d_i)]$$

as a function of θ. In order to do this, it is necessary to specify how the probability that the agent is present varies with the dilution.

Most limiting dilution assays use a formula for $\pi(\theta, d_i)$ based on the Poisson distribution (see §3.7); Ridout (1995) discusses an alternative. Suppose the application is to measure the concentration of a certain type of bacteria in a water-supply. Suppose also that the experimenter has the means to detect the presence of one or more bacteria in a sample. It is natural to suppose that the number of bacteria per unit volume of the water-supply is Poisson, with mean θ. If the original sample is diluted with an equal volume of uncontaminated water, then the number of bacteria in the diluted sample will have a Poisson distribution with mean $\frac{1}{2}\theta$. Similarly a more general dilution would give a Poisson distribution with mean θd. It follows that the probability that a sample at this dilution will contain no bacteria is $\exp(-\theta d)$ and consequently

$$\pi(\theta, d) = 1 - \exp(-\theta d). \tag{20.26}$$

In immunological applications this is known as the single-hit Poisson model, because it corresponds to assuming that the number of T cells in a sample is Poisson and a positive result will be obtained in the presence of only one T cell. Lefkovits and Waldmann (1999) discuss other forms for $\pi(\theta, d_i)$, such as multihit models and models representing different types of interaction between cell sub-types, such as B cells and T cells.

The analysis of a limiting dilution assay by maximum likelihood is generally satisfactory. It can be implemented as a generalized linear model, using a complementary log-log link and binomial errors (see Healy, 1988, p. 93). Problems arise if almost all results are positive or almost all are negative, but it is clear that such data sets are intrinsically unsatisfactory and no method of analysis should be expected to redeem them.

Several alternative methods of analysis have been suggested. Lefkovits and Waldmann (1999) proposed ordinary linear regression through the origin with $\log_e[(n_i - r_i)/n_i]$ as the response variable and dilution d_i as the independent variable. This is plausible because $\log_e[(n_i - r_i)/n_i]$ estimates the log of the proportion of assays that contain no agent which, from (20.26), is expected to be $-\theta d_i$. Lefkovits and Waldmann indicate that the form of the plot of $\log_e[(n_i - r_i)/n_i]$ against d_i not only allows θ to be estimated but allows systematic deviations from (20.26) to be discerned. Nevertheless, the method has serious drawbacks; it takes no account of the different variances of each point, and dilutions with $r_i = n_i$ are illegitimately excluded from the analysis.

Taswell (1981) compares several methods of estimation and advocates minimum-χ^2 estimation. This method appears to do well but this is largely because it generally provides a close approximation to maximum likelihood. In Does *et al.* (1988) the jackknife (see §10.7) is applied to reduce the bias in the maximum likelihood estimate: this issue is also addressed by other authors (see Mehrabi & Matthews, 1995, and references therein).

How the dilutions used in the experiment are chosen is another topic that has received substantial attention. Fisher (1966, §68, although the remark is in much earlier editions) noted that the estimate of log θ would be at its most precise when all observations are made at a dilution $d = 1 \cdot 59/\theta$. Of course, this has limited value in itself because the purpose of the assay is to determine the value of θ, which a priori is unknown. Nevertheless, several methods have been suggested that attempt to combine Fisher's observation with whatever prior knowledge the experimenter has about θ. Fisher himself discussed geometric designs, i.e. those with $d_j = c^{j-1} d_1$, particularly those with c equal to 10 or a power of 2. Geometric designs have been the basis of many of the subsequent suggestions: see, for example, Abdelbasit and Plackett (1983) or Strijbosch *et al.* (1987). Mehrabi and Matthews (1998) use a Bayesian approach to the problem; they found optimal designs that did not use a geometric design but they also noted that there were some highly efficient geometric designs. Most of the literature on the design of limiting dilution assays has focused on obtaining designs that provide precise estimates of θ or log θ. Two aspects of this ought to be noted. First, the designs assume that the single-hit Poisson model is correct and some of the designs offer little opportunity to verify this from the collected data. Secondly, the experimenters are often more interested in mechanism than precision, i.e. they want to know that, for example, the single-hit Poisson model applies, with precise knowledge about the value of associated parameter being a secondary matter. Although the design literature contains some general contribution in this direction, there appears to be little specific to limiting dilution assays.

Mutagenicity assays

There is widespread interest in the potential that various chemicals have to cause harm to people and the environment. Indeed, the ability of a chemical or other agent to cause genetic mutations—for example, by damaging an organism's DNA—is often seen as important evidence of possible carcinogenicity. Consequently, many chemicals are subjected to *mutagenicity assays* to assess their propensity to cause this kind of damage. There are many assays in this field and most of these require careful statistical analysis. Here we give a brief description of the statistical issues surrounding the commonest assay, the Ames *Salmonella* microsome assay; more detailed discussion can be found in Kirkland (1989) and in Piegorsch (1998) and references therein.

The Ames *Salmonella* microsome assay exposes the bacterium *Salmonella typhimurium* to varying doses of the chemical under test. This organism cannot

synthesize histidine, an amino acid that is needed for growth. However, mutations at certain locations of the bacterial genome reverse this inability, so, if the
bacteria are grown on a Petri dish or plate containing only minimal histidine,
then colonies will only grow from mutated cells. If there are more colonies on
plates subjected to greater concentrations of the chemical, then this provides
evidence that the mutation rate is dose-dependent. It is usual to have plates with
zero dose of the test chemical—negative controls—and five concentrations of the
chemical. There may also be a positive control—a substance known to result in a
high rate of mutations—although this is often ignored in the analysis. It is also
usual to have two, three or even more replicates at each dose.

The data that arise in these assays comprise the number of mutants in the jth
replicate at the ith dose, Y_{ij}, $j = 1, \ldots, r_i, i = 1, \ldots, D$. A natural assumption is
that these counts will follow a Poisson distribution. This is because: (i) there are
large numbers of microbes placed on each plate and only a very small proportion
will mutate; and (ii) the microbes mutate independently of one another. However, it is also necessary for the environment to be similar between plates that are
replicates of the same dose of test chemical and also between these plates the
number of microbes should not vary.

If the Poisson assumption is tenable, then the analysis usually proceeds by
applying a test for trend across the increasing doses. In order to perform a test of
the null hypothesis of no change of mutation rate with dose against an alternative of the rate increasing with dose, it is necessary to associate an increasing
score, x_i, with each dose group (often x_i will be the dose or log dose given to that
group). The test statistic is

$$Z_P = \frac{\sum_{i=1}^{D} x_i r_i (\overline{Y}_i - \overline{Y})}{\sqrt{(\overline{Y} S_x^2)}}, \tag{20.27}$$

where $\overline{Y}_i = \sum_j Y_{ij}/r_i, \overline{Y} = \sum_i r_i \overline{Y}_i / \sum_i r_i$ and $S_x^2 = \sum_i r_i (x_i - \bar{x})^2$, with $\bar{x}$
$= \sum_i r_i \bar{x}_i / \sum_i r_i$. Under the null hypothesis, (20.27) has approximately a stand-
ard normal distribution.

This straightforward analysis is usually satisfactory, provided the conditions
outlined above to justify the assumption of a Poisson distribution hold and that
the mutation rate does increase monotonically with dose. It is quite common for
one of these not to hold, and in such cases alternative or amended analyses must
be sought.

The mutation rate is often found to drop at the highest doses. This can be due
to various mechanisms—e.g. at the highest doses toxic effects of the chemical
under test may kill some microbes before they can mutate. Consequently a test
based on Z_P may be substantially less powerful than it would be in the presence
of monotone dose response. A sophisticated approach to this problem is to

attempt to model the processes that lead to this downturn; see, for example, Margolin *et al.* (1981) and Breslow (1984a). A simpler, but perhaps less satisfying approach is to identify the dose at which the downturn occurs and to test for a monotonic dose response across all lower doses; see, for example, Simpson and Margolin (1986).

It is also quite common for the conditions relating to the assumptions of a Poisson distribution not to be met. This usually seems to arise because the variation between plates within a replicate exceeds what you would expect if the counts on the plates all came from the same Poisson distribution. A test of the hypothesis that all counts in the *i*th dose group come from the same Poisson distribution can be made by referring

$$\frac{\sum_{j=1}^{r_i} (Y_{ij} - \overline{Y}_i)^2}{\overline{Y}_i}$$

to a χ^2 distribution with $r_i - 1$ degrees of freedom. A test across all dose groups can be made by adding these quantities from $i = 1$ to D and referring the sum to a χ^2 distribution with $\sum r_i - D$ degrees of freedom.

A plausible mechanism by which the assumptions for a Poisson distribution are violated is for the number of microbes put on each plate within a replicate to vary. Suppose that the mutation rate at the *i*th dose is λ_i and the number of microbes placed on the *j*th plate at this dose is N_{ij}. If experimental technique is sufficiently rigorous, then it may be possible to claim that the count N_{ij} is constant from plate to plate. If the environments of the plates are sufficiently similar for the same mutation rate to apply to all plates in the *i*th dose group, then it is likely that Y_{ij} is Poisson, with mean $\lambda_i N_{ij}$. However, it may be more realistic to assume that the N_{ij} vary about their target value, and variation in environments for the plates, perhaps small variations in incubation temperatures, leads to mutation rates that also vary slightly about their expected values. Conditional on these values, the counts from a plate will still be Poisson, but unconditionally the counts will exhibit extra-Poisson variation.

In this area of application, extra-Poisson variation is often encountered. It is then quite common to assume that the counts follow a *negative binomial distribution*. If the mean of this distribution is μ, then the variance is $\mu + \alpha\mu^2$, for some non-negative constant α ($\alpha = 0$ corresponds to Poisson variation). A crude justification for this, albeit based in part on mathematical tractability, is that the negative binomial distribution would be obtained if the $\lambda_i N_{ij}$ varied about their expected values according to a gamma distribution.

If extra-Poisson variation is present, the denominator of the test statistic (20.27) will tend to be too small and the test will be too sensitive. An amended version is obtained by changing the denominator to $\sqrt{[\overline{Y}(1 + \hat{\alpha}\overline{Y})S_x^2]}$, with $\hat{\alpha}$ an estimate of α obtained from the data using a method of moments or maximum likelihood.

20.6 **Tumour incidence studies**

In §20.5, reference was made to the use of mutagenicity assays as possible indicators of carcinogenicity. A more direct, although more time-consuming, approach to the detection and measurement of carcinogenicity is provided by tumour incidence experiments on animals. Here, doses of test substances are applied to animals (usually mice or rats), and the subsequent development of tumours is observed over an extended period, such as 2 years. In any one experiment, several doses of each test substance may be used, and the design may include an untreated control group and one or more groups treated with known carcinogens. The aim may be merely to screen for evidence of carcinogenicity (or, more properly, tumorigenicity), leading to further experimental work with the suspect substances; or, for substances already shown to be carcinogenic, the aim may be to estimate 'safe' doses at which the risk is negligible, by extrapolation downwards from the doses actually used.

Ideally, the experimenter should record, for each animal, whether a tumour occurs and, if so, the time of occurrence, measured from birth or some suitable point, such as time of weaning. Usually, a particular site is in question, and only the first tumour to occur is recorded. Different substances may be compared on the 'response' scale, by some type of measurement of the differences in the rate of tumour production; or, as in a standard biological assay, on the 'dose' scale, by comparing dose levels of different substances that produce the same level of tumour production.

The interpretation of tumour incidence experiments is complicated by a number of practical considerations. The most straightforward situation arises (i) when the tumour is detectable at a very early stage, either because it is easily visible, as with a skin tumour, or because it is highly lethal and can be detected at autopsy; and (ii) when the substance is not toxic for other reasons. In these circumstances, the tumorigenic response for any substance may be measured either by a simple 'lifetime' count of the number of tumour-bearing animals observed during the experiment, or by recording the time to tumour appearance and performing a survival analysis. With the latter approach, deaths of animals due to other causes can be regarded as censored observations, and the curve for tumour-free survival estimated by life-table or parametric methods, as in Chapter 17. Logrank methods may be used to test for differences in tumour-free survival between different substances.

The simple lifetime count may be misleading if substances differ in their non-tumour-related mortality. If, for instance, a carcinogenic substance is highly lethal, animals may die at an early stage before the tumours have had a chance to appear; the carcinogenicity will then be underestimated. One approach is to remove from the denominator animals dying at an early stage (say, before the first tumour has been detected in the whole experiment). Alternatively, in a life-table analysis these deaths can be regarded as withdrawals and the animals removed from the numbers at risk.

A more serious complication arises when the tumours are not highly lethal. If they are completely non-lethal, and are not visible, they may be detected after the non-specific deaths of some animals and subsequent autopsy, but a complete count will require the sacrifice of animals either at the end of the experiment or by *serial sacrifice* of random samples at intermediate times. The latter plan will provide information on the time distribution of tumour incidence. The relevant measures are now the *prevalences* of tumours at the various times of sacrifice, and these can be compared by standard methods for categorical data (Chapter 15).

In practice, tumours will usually have intermediate lethality, conforming neither to the life-table model suitable for tumours with rapid lethality nor to the prevalence model suitable for non-lethal tumours. If tumours are detected only after an animal's death and subsequent autopsy, and a life-table analysis is performed, bias may be caused by non-tumour-related mortality. Even if substances under test have the same tumorigenicity, a substance causing high non-specific mortality will provide the opportunity for detection of tumours at autopsy at early stages of the experiment, and will thus wrongly appear to have a higher tumour incidence rate.

To overcome this problem, Peto (1974) and Peto *et al.* (1980) have suggested that individual tumours could be classified as *incidental* (not affecting longevity and observed as a result of death from unrelated causes) or *fatal* (affecting mortality). Tumours discovered at intermediate sacrifice, for instance, are incidental. Separate analyses would then be based on prevalence of incidental tumours and incidence of fatal tumours, and the contrasts between treatment groups assessed by combining data from both analyses. This approach may be impracticable if pathologists are unable to make the dichotomous classification of tumours with confidence.

Animal tumour incidence experiments have been a major instrument in the assessment of carcinogenicity for more than half a century. Recent research on methods of analysis has shown that care must be taken to use a method appropriate to the circumstances of the particular experiment. In some instances it will not be possible to decide on the appropriate way of handling the difficulties outlined above, and a flexible approach needs to be adopted, perhaps with alternative analyses making different assumptions about the unknown factors.

For more detailed discussion, see Peto *et al.* (1980) and Dinse (1998).

Appendix tables

Table A1 Areas in tail of the normal distribution

Single-tail areas in terms of standardized deviates. The function tabulated is $\frac{1}{2}P$, the probability of obtaining a standardized normal deviate greater than z, *in one direction*. The two-tail probability, P, is twice the tabulated value.

z	0·00	0·01	0·02	0·03	0·04	0·05	0·06	0·07	0·08	0·09
0·0	0·5000	0·4960	0·4920	0·4880	0·4840	0·4801	0·4761	0·4721	0·4681	0·4641
0·1	0·4602	0·4562	0·4522	0·4483	0·4443	0·4404	0·4364	0·4325	0·4286	0·4247
0·2	0·4207	0·4168	0·4129	0·4090	0·4052	0·4013	0·3974	0·3936	0·3897	0·3859
0·3	0·3821	0·3783	0·3745	0·3707	0·3669	0·3632	0·3594	0·3557	0·3520	0·3483
0·4	0·3446	0·3409	0·3372	0·3336	0·3300	0·3264	0·3228	0·3192	0·3156	0·3121
0·5	0·3085	0·3050	0·3015	0·2981	0·2946	0·2912	0·2877	0·2843	0·2810	0·2776
0·6	0·2743	0·2709	0·2676	0·2643	0·2611	0·2578	0·2546	0·2514	0·2483	0·2451
0·7	0·2420	0·2389	0·2358	0·2327	0·2296	0·2266	0·2236	0·2206	0·2177	0·2148
0·8	0·2119	0·2090	0·2061	0·2033	0·2005	0·1977	0·1949	0·1922	0·1894	0·1867
0·9	0·1841	0·1814	0·1788	0·1762	0·1736	0·1711	0·1685	0·1660	0·1635	0·1611
1·0	0·1587	0·1562	0·1539	0·1515	0·1492	0·1469	0·1446	0·1423	0·1401	0·1379
1·1	0·1357	0·1335	0·1314	0·1292	0·1271	0·1251	0·1230	0·1210	0·1190	0·1170
1·2	0·1151	0·1131	0·1112	0·1093	0·1075	0·1056	0·1038	0·1020	0·1003	0·0985
1·3	0·0968	0·0951	0·0934	0·0918	0·0901	0·0885	0·0869	0·0853	0·0838	0·0823
1·4	0·0808	0·0793	0·0778	0·0764	0·0749	0·0735	0·0721	0·0708	0·0694	0·0681
1·5	0·0668	0·0655	0·0643	0·0630	0·0618	0·0606	0·0594	0·0582	0·0571	0·0559
1·6	0·0548	0·0537	0·0526	0·0516	0·0505	0·0495	0·0485	0·0475	0·0465	0·0455
1·7	0·0446	0·0436	0·0427	0·0418	0·0409	0·0401	0·0392	0·0384	0·0375	0·0367
1·8	0·0359	0·0351	0·0344	0·0336	0·0329	0·0322	0·0314	0·0307	0·0301	0·0294
1·9	0·0287	0·0281	0·0274	0·0268	0·0262	0·0256	0·0250	0·0244	0·0239	0·0233

	.00	.01	.02	.03	.04	.05	.06	.07	.08	.09
2·0	0·02275	0·02222	0·02169	0·02118	0·02068	0·02018	0·01970	0·01923	0·01876	0·01831
2·1	0·01786	0·01743	0·01700	0·01659	0·01618	0·01578	0·01539	0·01500	0·01463	0·01426
2·2	0·01390	0·01355	0·01321	0·01287	0·01255	0·01222	0·01191	0·01160	0·01130	0·01101
2·3	0·01072	0·01044	0·01017	0·00990	0·00964	0·00939	0·00914	0·00889	0·00866	0·00842
2·4	0·00820	0·00798	0·00776	0·00755	0·00734	0·00714	0·00695	0·00676	0·00657	0·00639
2·5	0·00621	0·00604	0·00587	0·00570	0·00554	0·00539	0·00523	0·00508	0·00494	0·00480
2·6	0·00466	0·00453	0·00440	0·00427	0·00415	0·00402	0·00391	0·00379	0·00368	0·00357
2·7	0·00347	0·00336	0·00326	0·00317	0·00307	0·00298	0·00289	0·00280	0·00272	0·00264
2·8	0·00256	0·00248	0·00240	0·00233	0·00226	0·00219	0·00212	0·00205	0·00199	0·00193
2·9	0·00187	0·00181	0·00175	0·00169	0·00164	0·00159	0·00154	0·00149	0·00144	0·00139
3·0	0·00135									
3·1	0·00097									
3·2	0·00069									
3·3	0·00048									
3·4	0·00034									
3·5	0·00023									
3·6	0·00016									
3·7	0·00011									
3·8	0·00007									
3·9	0·00005									
4·0	0·00003									

Standardized deviates in terms of two-tail areas

P	1·0	0·9	0·8	0·7	0·6	0·5	0·4
z	0	0·126	0·253	0·385	0·524	0·674	0·842

P	0·3	0·2	0·1	0·05	0·02	0·01	0·001
z	1·036	1·282	1·645	1·960	2·326	2·576	3·291

Reproduced in part from Table 3 of Murdoch and Barnes (1968) by permission of the authors and publishers.

Table A2 **Percentage points of the χ^2 distribution**

The function tabulated is $\chi^2_{\nu,P}$, the value exceeded with probability P in a χ^2 distribution with ν degrees of freedom (the $100P$ percentage point).

Degrees of freedom, ν	Probability of greater value, P									
	0·975	0·900	0·750	0·500	0·250	0·100	0·050	0·025	0·010	0·001
1	—	0·02	0·10	0·45	1·32	2·71	3·84	5·02	6·63	10·83
2	0·05	0·21	0·58	1·39	2·77	4·61	5·99	7·38	9·21	13·82
3	0·22	0·58	1·21	2·37	4·11	6·25	7·81	9·35	11·34	16·27
4	0·48	1·06	1·92	3·36	5·39	7·78	9·49	11·14	13·28	18·47
5	0·83	1·61	2·67	4·35	6·63	9·24	11·07	12·83	15·09	20·52
6	1·24	2·20	3·45	5·35	7·84	10·64	12·59	14·45	16·81	22·46
7	1·69	2·83	4·25	6·35	9·04	12·02	14·07	16·01	18·48	24·32
8	2·18	3·49	5·07	7·34	10·22	13·36	15·51	17·53	20·09	26·12
9	2·70	4·17	5·90	8·34	11·39	14·68	16·92	19·02	21·67	27·88
10	3·25	4·87	6·74	9·34	12·55	15·99	18·31	20·48	23·21	29·59
11	3·82	5·58	7·58	10·34	13·70	17·28	19·68	21·92	24·72	31·26
12	4·40	6·30	8·44	11·34	14·85	18·55	21·03	23·34	26·22	32·91
13	5·01	7·04	9·30	12·34	15·98	19·81	22·36	24·74	27·69	34·53
14	5·63	7·79	10·17	13·34	17·12	21·06	23·68	26·12	29·14	36·12
15	6·27	8·55	11·04	14·34	18·25	22·31	25·00	27·49	30·58	37·70

df										
16	6·91	9·31	11·91	15·34	19·37	23·54	26·30	28·85	32·00	39·25
17	7·56	10·09	12·79	16·34	20·49	24·77	27·59	30·19	33·41	40·79
18	8·23	10·86	13·68	17·34	21·60	25·99	28·87	31·53	34·81	42·31
19	8·91	11·65	14·56	18·34	22·72	27·20	30·14	32·85	36·19	43·82
20	9·59	12·44	15·45	19·34	23·83	28·41	31·41	34·17	37·57	45·32
21	10·28	13·24	16·34	20·34	24·93	29·62	32·67	35·48	38·93	46·80
22	10·98	14·04	17·24	21·34	26·04	30·81	33·92	36·78	40·29	48·27
23	11·69	14·85	18·14	22·34	27·14	32·01	35·17	38·08	41·64	49·73
24	12·40	15·66	19·04	23·34	28·24	33·20	36·42	39·36	42·98	51·18
25	13·12	16·47	19·94	24·34	29·34	34·38	37·65	40·65	44·31	52·62
26	13·84	17·29	20·84	25·34	30·43	35·56	38·89	41·92	45·64	54·05
27	14·57	18·11	21·75	26·34	31·53	36·74	40·11	43·19	46·96	55·48
28	15·31	18·94	22·66	27·34	32·62	37·92	41·34	44·46	48·28	56·89
29	16·05	19·77	23·57	28·34	33·71	39·09	42·56	45·72	49·59	58·30
30	16·79	20·60	24·48	29·34	34·80	40·26	43·77	46·98	50·89	59·70
40	24·43	29·05	33·66	39·34	45·62	51·80	55·76	59·34	63·69	73·40
50	32·36	37·69	42·94	49·33	56·33	63·17	67·50	71·42	76·15	86·66
60	40·48	46·46	52·29	59·33	66·98	74·40	79·08	83·30	88·38	99·61
70	48·76	55·33	61·70	69·33	77·58	85·53	90·53	95·02	100·42	112·32
80	57·15	64·28	71·14	79·33	88·13	96·58	101·88	106·63	112·33	124·84
90	65·65	73·29	80·62	89·33	98·64	107·56	113·14	118·14	124·12	137·21
100	74·22	82·36	90·13	99·33	109·14	118·50	124·34	129·56	135·81	149·45

Condensed from Table 8 of Pearson and Hartley (1966) by permission of the authors and publishers.

Table A3 **Percentage points of the t distribution**
The function tabulated is $t_{v, P}$, the value exceeded in both directions with probability P in a t distribution with v degrees of freedom (the $100P$ percentage point).

Degrees of freedom, v	Probability of greater value, P												
	0.9	0.8	0.7	0.6	0.5	0.4	0.3	0.2	0.1	0.05	0.02	0.01	0.001
1	0.158	0.325	0.510	0.727	1.000	1.376	1.963	3.078	6.314	12.706	31.821	63.657	636.619
2	0.142	0.289	0.445	0.617	0.816	1.061	1.386	1.886	2.920	4.303	6.965	9.925	31.598
3	0.137	0.277	0.424	0.584	0.765	0.978	1.250	1.638	2.353	3.182	4.541	5.841	12.924
4	0.134	0.271	0.414	0.569	0.741	0.941	1.190	1.533	2.132	2.776	3.747	4.604	8.610
5	0.132	0.267	0.408	0.559	0.727	0.920	1.156	1.476	2.015	2.571	3.365	4.032	6.869
6	0.131	0.265	0.404	0.553	0.718	0.906	1.134	1.440	1.943	2.447	3.143	3.707	5.959
7	0.130	0.263	0.402	0.549	0.711	0.896	1.119	1.415	1.895	2.365	2.998	3.499	5.408
8	0.130	0.262	0.399	0.546	0.706	0.889	1.108	1.397	1.860	2.306	2.896	3.355	5.041
9	0.129	0.261	0.398	0.543	0.703	0.883	1.100	1.383	1.833	2.262	2.821	3.250	4.781
10	0.129	0.260	0.397	0.542	0.700	0.879	1.093	1.372	1.812	2.228	2.764	3.169	4.587
11	0.129	0.260	0.396	0.540	0.697	0.876	1.088	1.363	1.796	2.201	2.718	3.106	4.437
12	0.128	0.259	0.395	0.539	0.695	0.873	1.083	1.356	1.782	2.179	2.681	3.055	4.318
13	0.128	0.259	0.394	0.538	0.694	0.870	1.079	1.350	1.771	2.160	2.650	3.012	4.221
14	0.128	0.258	0.393	0.537	0.692	0.868	1.076	1.345	1.761	2.145	2.624	2.977	4.140
15	0.128	0.258	0.393	0.536	0.691	0.866	1.074	1.341	1.753	2.131	2.602	2.947	4.073

Total for both tails, P

$-t_{v, P}$ $t_{v, P}$

16	0.128	0.258	0.392	0.535	0.690	0.865	1.071	1.337	1.746	2.120	2.583	2.921	4.015
17	0.128	0.257	0.392	0.534	0.689	0.863	1.069	1.333	1.740	2.110	2.567	2.898	3.965
18	0.127	0.257	0.392	0.534	0.688	0.862	1.067	1.330	1.734	2.101	2.552	2.878	3.922
19	0.127	0.257	0.391	0.533	0.688	0.861	1.066	1.328	1.729	2.093	2.539	2.861	3.883
20	0.127	0.257	0.391	0.533	0.687	0.860	1.064	1.325	1.725	2.086	2.528	2.845	3.850
21	0.127	0.257	0.391	0.532	0.686	0.859	1.063	1.323	1.721	2.080	2.518	2.831	3.819
22	0.127	0.256	0.390	0.532	0.686	0.858	1.061	1.321	1.717	2.074	2.508	2.819	3.792
23	0.127	0.256	0.390	0.532	0.685	0.858	1.060	1.319	1.714	2.069	2.500	2.807	3.767
24	0.127	0.256	0.390	0.531	0.685	0.857	1.059	1.318	1.711	2.064	2.492	2.797	3.745
25	0.127	0.256	0.390	0.531	0.684	0.856	1.058	1.316	1.708	2.060	2.485	2.787	3.725
26	0.127	0.256	0.390	0.531	0.684	0.856	1.058	1.315	1.706	2.056	2.479	2.779	3.707
27	0.127	0.256	0.389	0.531	0.684	0.855	1.057	1.314	1.703	2.052	2.473	2.771	3.690
28	0.127	0.256	0.389	0.530	0.683	0.855	1.056	1.313	1.701	2.048	2.467	2.763	3.674
29	0.127	0.256	0.389	0.530	0.683	0.854	1.055	1.311	1.699	2.045	2.462	2.756	3.659
30	0.127	0.256	0.389	0.530	0.683	0.854	1.055	1.310	1.697	2.042	2.457	2.750	3.646
40	0.126	0.255	0.388	0.529	0.681	0.851	1.050	1.303	1.684	2.021	2.423	2.704	3.551
60	0.126	0.254	0.387	0.527	0.679	0.848	1.046	1.296	1.671	2.000	2.390	2.660	3.460
120	0.126	0.254	0.386	0.526	0.677	0.845	1.041	1.289	1.658	1.980	2.358	2.617	3.373
∞	0.126	0.253	0.385	0.524	0.674	0.842	1.036	1.282	1.645	1.960	2.326	2.576	3.291

Table A4 Percentage points of the *F* distribution

The function tabulated is F_{P, ν_1, ν_2}, the value exceeded with probability P in the F distribution with ν_1 degrees of freedom for the numerator and ν_2 degrees of freedom for the denominator (the $100P$ percentage point). The values for $P = 0.05$ and 0.01 are shown in bold type.

DF for denominator, ν_2	P	DF for numerator, ν_1										
		1	2	3	4	5	6	7	8	12	24	∞
1	0.05	**161.4**	**199.5**	**215.7**	**224.6**	**230.2**	**234.0**	**236.8**	**238.9**	**243.9**	**249.1**	**254.3**
	0.025	647.8	799.5	864.2	899.6	921.8	937.1	948.2	956.7	976.7	997.2	1018
	0.01	**4057**	**5000**	**5403**	**5625**	**5764**	**5859**	**5928**	**5981**	**6106**	**6235**	**6366**
	0.005	16211	20000	21615	22500	23056	23437	23715	23925	24426	24940	25465
2	0.05	**18.51**	**19.00**	**19.16**	**19.25**	**19.30**	**19.33**	**19.35**	**19.37**	**19.41**	**19.45**	**19.50**
	0.025	38.51	39.00	39.17	39.25	39.30	39.33	39.36	39.37	39.41	39.46	39.50
	0.01	**98.50**	**99.00**	**99.17**	**99.25**	**99.30**	**99.33**	**99.36**	**99.37**	**99.42**	**99.46**	**99.50**
	0.005	198.5	199.0	199.2	199.2	199.3	199.3	199.4	199.4	199.4	199.5	199.5
3	0.05	**10.13**	**9.55**	**9.28**	**9.12**	**9.01**	**8.94**	**8.89**	**8.85**	**8.74**	**8.64**	**8.53**
	0.025	17.44	16.04	15.44	15.10	14.88	14.73	14.62	14.54	14.34	14.12	13.90
	0.01	**34.12**	**30.82**	**29.46**	**28.71**	**28.24**	**27.91**	**27.67**	**27.49**	**27.05**	**26.60**	**26.13**
	0.005	55.55	49.80	47.47	46.19	45.39	44.84	44.43	44.13	43.39	42.62	41.83
4	0.05	**7.71**	**6.94**	**6.59**	**6.39**	**6.26**	**6.16**	**6.09**	**6.04**	**5.91**	**5.77**	**5.63**
	0.025	12.22	10.65	9.98	9.60	9.36	9.20	9.07	8.98	8.75	8.51	8.26
	0.01	**21.20**	**18.00**	**16.69**	**15.98**	**15.52**	**15.21**	**14.98**	**14.80**	**14.37**	**13.93**	**13.46**
	0.005	31.33	26.28	24.26	23.15	22.46	21.97	21.62	21.35	20.70	20.03	19.32

5	0·05	**6·61**	**5·79**	**5·41**	**5·19**	**5·05**	**4·95**	**4·88**	**4·82**	**4·68**	**4·53**	**4·36**
	0·025	10·01	8·43	7·76	7·39	7·15	6·98	6·85	6·76	6·52	6·28	6·02
	0·01	**16·26**	**13·27**	**12·06**	**11·39**	**10·97**	**10·67**	**10·46**	**10·29**	**9·89**	**9·47**	**9·02**
	0·005	22·78	18·31	16·53	15·56	14·94	14·51	14·20	13·96	13·38	12·78	12·14
6	0·05	**5·99**	**5·14**	**4·76**	**4·53**	**4·39**	**4·28**	**4·21**	**4·15**	**4·00**	**3·84**	**3·67**
	0·025	8·81	7·26	6·60	6·23	5·99	5·82	5·70	5·60	5·37	5·12	4·85
	0·01	**13·75**	**10·92**	**9·78**	**9·15**	**8·75**	**8·47**	**8·26**	**8·10**	**7·72**	**7·31**	**6·88**
	0·005	18·63	14·54	12·92	12·03	11·46	11·07	10·79	10·57	10·03	9·47	8·88
7	0·05	**5·59**	**4·74**	**4·35**	**4·12**	**3·97**	**3·87**	**3·79**	**3·73**	**3·57**	**3·41**	**3·23**
	0·025	8·07	6·54	5·89	5·52	5·29	5·12	4·99	4·90	4·67	4·42	4·14
	0·01	**12·25**	**9·55**	**8·45**	**7·85**	**7·46**	**7·19**	**6·99**	**6·84**	**6·47**	**6·07**	**5·65**
	0·005	16·24	12·40	10·88	10·05	9·52	9·16	8·89	8·68	8·18	7·65	7·08
8	0·05	**5·32**	**4·46**	**4·07**	**3·84**	**3·69**	**3·58**	**3·50**	**3·44**	**3·28**	**3·12**	**2·93**
	0·025	7·57	6·06	5·42	5·05	4·82	4·65	4·53	4·43	4·20	3·95	3·67
	0·01	**11·26**	**8·65**	**7·59**	**7·01**	**6·63**	**6·37**	**6·18**	**6·03**	**5·67**	**5·28**	**4·86**
	0·005	14·69	11·04	9·60	8·81	8·30	7·95	7·69	7·50	7·01	6·50	5·95
9	0·05	**5·12**	**4·26**	**3·86**	**3·63**	**3·48**	**3·37**	**3·29**	**3·23**	**3·07**	**2·90**	**2·71**
	0·025	7·21	5·71	5·08	4·72	4·48	4·32	4·20	4·10	3·87	3·61	3·33
	0·01	**10·56**	**8·02**	**6·99**	**6·42**	**6·06**	**5·80**	**5·61**	**5·47**	**5·11**	**4·73**	**4·31**
	0·005	13·61	10·11	8·72	7·96	7·47	7·13	6·88	6·69	6·23	5·73	5·19
10	0·05	**4·96**	**4·10**	**3·71**	**3·48**	**3·33**	**3·22**	**3·14**	**3·07**	**2·91**	**2·74**	**2·54**
	0·025	6·94	5·46	4·83	4·47	4·24	4·07	3·95	3·85	3·62	3·37	3·08
	0·01	**10·04**	**7·56**	**6·55**	**5·99**	**5·64**	**5·39**	**5·20**	**5·06**	**4·71**	**4·33**	**3·91**
	0·005	12·83	9·43	8·08	7·34	6·87	6·54	6·30	6·12	5·66	5·17	4·64

Continued on p. 752

Table A4 (continued)

DF for denominator, v_2	P	DF for numerator, v_1										
		1	2	3	4	5	6	7	8	12	24	∞
12	0·05	4·75	3·89	3·49	3·26	3·11	3·00	2·91	2·85	2·69	2·51	2·30
	0·025	6·55	5·10	4·47	4·12	3·89	3·73	3·61	3·51	3·28	3·02	2·72
	0·01	9·33	6·93	5·95	5·41	5·06	4·82	4·64	4·50	4·16	3·78	3·36
	0·005	11·75	8·51	7·23	6·52	6·07	5·76	5·52	5·35	4·91	4·43	3·90
14	0·05	4·60	3·74	3·34	3·11	2·96	2·85	2·76	2·70	2·53	2·35	2·13
	0·025	6·30	4·86	4·24	3·89	3·66	3·50	3·38	3·29	3·05	2·79	2·49
	0·01	8·86	6·51	5·56	5·04	4·69	4·46	4·28	4·14	3·80	3·43	3·00
	0·005	11·06	7·92	6·68	6·00	5·56	5·26	5·03	4·86	4·43	3·96	3·44
16	0·05	4·49	3·63	3·24	3·01	2·85	2·74	2·66	2·59	2·42	2·24	2·01
	0·025	6·12	4·69	4·08	3·73	3·50	3·34	3·22	3·12	2·89	2·63	2·32
	0·01	8·53	6·23	5·29	4·77	4·44	4·20	4·03	3·89	3·55	3·18	2·75
	0·005	10·58	7·51	6·30	5·64	5·21	4·91	4·69	4·52	4·10	3·64	3·11
18	0·05	4·41	3·55	3·16	2·93	2·77	2·66	2·58	2·51	2·34	2·15	1·92
	0·025	5·98	4·56	3·95	3·61	3·38	3·22	3·10	3·01	2·77	2·50	2·19
	0·01	8·29	6·01	5·09	4·58	4·25	4·01	3·84	3·71	3·37	3·00	2·57
	0·005	10·22	7·21	6·03	5·37	4·96	4·66	4·44	4·28	3·86	3·40	2·87
20	0·05	4·35	3·49	3·10	2·87	2·71	2·60	2·51	2·45	2·28	2·08	1·84
	0·025	5·87	4·46	3·86	3·51	3·29	3·13	3·01	2·91	2·68	2·41	2·09
	0·01	8·10	5·85	4·94	4·43	4·10	3·87	3·70	3·56	3·23	2·86	2·42
	0·005	9·94	6·99	5·82	5·17	4·76	4·47	4·26	4·09	3·68	3·22	2·69

v_2	α											
30	0·05	**4·17**	**3·32**	**2·92**	**2·69**	**2·53**	**2·42**	**2·33**	**2·27**	**2·09**	**1·89**	**1·62**
	0·025	5·57	4·18	3·59	3·25	3·03	2·87	2·75	2·65	2·41	2·14	1·79
	0·01	**7·56**	**5·39**	**4·51**	**4·02**	**3·70**	**3·47**	**3·30**	**3·17**	**2·84**	**2·47**	**2·01**
	0·005	9·18	6·35	5·24	4·62	4·23	3·95	3·74	3·58	3·18	2·73	2·18
40	0·05	**4·08**	**3·23**	**2·84**	**2·61**	**2·45**	**2·34**	**2·25**	**2·18**	**2·00**	**1·79**	**1·51**
	0·025	5·42	4·05	3·46	3·13	2·90	2·74	2·62	2·53	2·29	2·01	1·64
	0·01	**7·31**	**5·18**	**4·31**	**3·83**	**3·51**	**3·29**	**3·12**	**2·99**	**2·66**	**2·29**	**1·80**
	0·005	8·83	6·07	4·98	4·37	3·99	3·71	3·51	3·35	2·95	2·50	1·93
60	0·05	**4·00**	**3·15**	**2·76**	**2·53**	**2·37**	**2·25**	**2·17**	**2·10**	**1·92**	**1·70**	**1·39**
	0·025	5·29	3·93	3·34	3·01	2·79	2·63	2·51	2·41	2·17	1·88	1·48
	0·01	**7·08**	**4·98**	**4·13**	**3·65**	**3·34**	**3·12**	**2·95**	**2·82**	**2·50**	**2·12**	**1·60**
	0·005	8·49	5·79	4·73	4·14	3·76	3·49	3·29	3·13	2·74	2·29	1·69
120	0·05	**3·92**	**3·07**	**2·68**	**2·45**	**2·29**	**2·17**	**2·09**	**2·02**	**1·83**	**1·61**	**1·25**
	0·025	5·15	3·80	3·23	2·89	2·67	2·52	2·39	2·30	2·05	1·76	1·31
	0·01	**6·85**	**4·79**	**3·95**	**3·48**	**3·17**	**2·96**	**2·79**	**2·66**	**2·34**	**1·95**	**1·38**
	0·005	8·18	5·54	4·50	3·92	3·55	3·28	3·09	2·93	2·54	2·09	1·43
∞	0·05	**3·84**	**3·00**	**2·60**	**2·37**	**2·21**	**2·10**	**2·01**	**1·94**	**1·75**	**1·52**	**1·00**
	0·025	5·02	3·69	3·12	2·79	2·57	2·41	2·29	2·19	1·94	1·64	1·00
	0·01	**6·63**	**4·61**	**3·78**	**3·32**	**3·02**	**2·80**	**2·64**	**2·51**	**2·18**	**1·79**	**1·00**
	0·005	7·88	5·30	4·28	3·72	3·35	3·09	2·90	2·74	2·36	1·90	1·00

Condensed from Table 18 of Pearson and Hartley (1966) by permission of the authors and publishers.

For values of v_1 and v_2 not given, interpolation is approximately linear in the reciprocals of v_1 and v_2.

Table A5 **Percentage points of the distribution of studentized range**

The function tabulated is $Q_{p,\alpha}$, the value exceeded with probability α in the distribution of studentized range, for p groups and f_2 DF within groups (the 100α percentage point). The values for $\alpha = 0.05$ are shown in bold type.

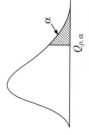

$Q_{p,\alpha}$

Number of groups, p

f_2	α	2	3	4	5	6	7	8	9	10
5	0.05	**3.64**	**4.60**	**5.22**	**5.67**	**6.03**	**6.33**	**6.58**	**6.80**	**6.99**
	0.01	5.70	6.98	7.80	8.42	8.91	9.32	9.67	9.97	10.24
6	0.05	**3.46**	**4.34**	**4.90**	**5.30**	**5.63**	**5.90**	**6.12**	**6.32**	**6.49**
	0.01	5.24	6.33	7.03	7.56	7.97	8.32	8.61	8.87	9.10
7	0.05	**3.34**	**4.16**	**4.68**	**5.06**	**5.36**	**5.61**	**5.82**	**6.00**	**6.16**
	0.01	4.95	5.92	6.54	7.01	7.37	7.68	7.94	8.17	8.37
8	0.05	**3.26**	**4.04**	**4.53**	**4.89**	**5.17**	**5.40**	**5.60**	**5.77**	**5.92**
	0.01	4.75	5.64	6.20	6.62	6.96	7.24	7.47	7.68	7.86
9	0.05	**3.20**	**3.95**	**4.41**	**4.76**	**5.02**	**5.24**	**5.43**	**5.59**	**5.74**
	0.01	4.60	5.43	5.96	6.35	6.66	6.91	7.13	7.33	7.49
10	0.05	**3.15**	**3.88**	**4.33**	**4.65**	**4.91**	**5.12**	**5.30**	**5.46**	**5.60**
	0.01	4.48	5.27	5.77	6.14	6.43	6.67	6.87	7.05	7.21
12	0.05	**3.08**	**3.77**	**4.20**	**4.51**	**4.75**	**4.95**	**5.12**	**5.27**	**5.39**
	0.01	4.32	5.05	5.50	5.84	6.10	6.32	6.51	6.67	6.81

14	0.05	**3.03**	**3.70**	**4.11**	**4.41**	**4.64**	**4.83**	**4.99**	**5.13**	**5.25**
	0.01	4.21	4.89	5.32	5.63	5.88	6.08	6.26	6.41	6.54
16	0.05	**3.00**	**3.65**	**4.05**	**4.33**	**4.56**	**4.74**	**4.90**	**5.03**	**5.15**
	0.01	4.13	4.79	5.19	5.49	5.72	5.92	6.08	6.22	6.35
18	0.05	**2.97**	**3.61**	**4.00**	**4.28**	**4.49**	**4.67**	**4.82**	**4.96**	**5.07**
	0.01	4.07	4.70	5.09	5.38	5.60	5.79	5.94	6.08	6.20
20	0.05	**2.95**	**3.58**	**3.96**	**4.23**	**4.45**	**4.62**	**4.77**	**4.90**	**5.01**
	0.01	4.02	4.64	5.02	5.29	5.51	5.69	5.84	5.97	6.09
30	0.05	**2.89**	**3.49**	**3.85**	**4.10**	**4.30**	**4.46**	**4.60**	**4.72**	**4.82**
	0.01	3.89	4.45	4.80	5.05	5.24	5.40	5.54	5.65	5.76
40	0.05	**2.86**	**3.44**	**3.79**	**4.04**	**4.23**	**4.39**	**4.52**	**4.63**	**4.73**
	0.01	3.82	4.37	4.70	4.93	5.11	5.26	5.39	5.50	5.60
60	0.05	**2.83**	**3.40**	**3.74**	**3.98**	**4.16**	**4.31**	**4.44**	**4.55**	**4.65**
	0.01	3.76	4.28	4.59	4.82	4.99	5.13	5.25	5.36	5.45
120	0.05	**2.80**	**3.36**	**3.68**	**3.92**	**4.10**	**4.24**	**4.36**	**4.47**	**4.56**
	0.01	3.70	4.20	4.50	4.71	4.87	5.01	5.12	5.21	5.30
∞	0.05	**2.77**	**3.31**	**3.63**	**3.86**	**4.03**	**4.17**	**4.29**	**4.39**	**4.47**
	0.01	3.64	4.12	4.40	4.60	4.76	4.88	4.99	5.08	5.16

Condensed from Table 29 of Pearson and Hartley (1966) by permission of the authors and publishers.

Table A6 **Percentage points for the Wilcoxon signed rank sum test**
The function tabulated is the critical value for the smaller of the signed rank sums, T_+ and T_-. An observed value equal to or less than the tabulated value is significant at the two-sided significance level shown (the actual tail-area probability being less than or equal to the nominal value shown). If ties are present, the result is somewhat more significant than is indicated here.

Sample size, n' (excluding zero differences)	Two-sided significance level	
	0·05	0·01
6	0	—
7	2	—
8	3	0
9	5	1
10	8	3
11	10	5
12	13	7
13	17	9
14	21	12
15	25	15
16	29	19
17	34	23
18	40	27
19	46	32
20	52	37
21	58	42
22	66	48
23	73	54
24	81	61
25	89	68

Condensed from the Geigy Scientific Tables (1982), by permission of the authors and publishers.

Table A7 **Percentage points for the Wilcoxon two-sample rank sum test**

Define n_1 as the smaller of the two sample sizes ($n_1 \leq n_2$). Calculate T_1 as the sum of the ranks in sample 1, and $E(T_1) = \frac{1}{2}n_1(n_1 + n_2 + 1)$. Calculate T' as T_1 if $T_1 \leq E(T_1)$ and as $n_1(n_1 + n_2 + 1) - T_1$ if $T_1 > E(T_1)$. The result is significant at the two-sided 5% (or 1%) level if T' is less than or equal to the upper (or lower) tabulated value (the actual tail-area probability being less than or equal to the nominal value). If ties are present, the result is somewhat more significant than is indicated here.

n_2	P	Smaller sample size, n_1 4	5	6	7	8	9	10	11	12	13	14	15
4	0·05	10											
	0·01	—											
5	0·05	11	17										
	0·01	—	15										
6	0·05	12	18	26									
	0·01	10	16	23									
7	0·05	13	20	27	36								
	0·01	10	16	24	32								
8	0·05	14	21	29	38	49							
	0·01	11	17	25	34	43							
9	0·05	14	22	31	40	51	62						
	0·01	11	18	26	35	45	56						
10	0·05	15	23	32	42	53	65	78					
	0·01	12	19	27	37	47	58	71					
11	0·05	16	24	34	44	55	68	81	96				
	0·01	12	20	28	38	49	61	73	87				
12	0·05	17	26	35	46	58	71	84	99	115			
	0·01	13	21	30	40	51	63	76	90	105			
13	0·05	18	27	37	48	60	73	88	103	119	136		
	0·01	13	22	31	41	53	65	79	93	109	125		
14	0·05	19	28	38	50	62	76	91	106	123	141	160	
	0·01	14	22	32	43	54	67	81	96	112	129	147	
15	0·05	20	29	40	52	65	79	94	110	127	145	164	184
	0·01	15	23	33	44	56	69	84	99	115	133	151	171

Condensed from the Geigy Scientific Tables (1982) by permission of the authors and publishers.

Table A8 **Sample size for comparing two proportions**
This table is used to determine the sample size necessary to find a significant difference (5% two-sided significance level) between two proportions estimated from independent samples where the true proportions are π_1 and π_2, and $\delta = \pi_1 - \pi_2$ is the specified difference ($\pi_1 > \pi_2$). Sample sizes are given for 90% power (upper value of pair) and 80% power (lower value). The sample size given in the table refers to *each* of the two independent samples. The table is derived using (4.42) with a continuity correction.

Note: If $\pi_2 > 0.5$, work with $\pi_1' = 1 - \pi_2$ and $\pi_2' = 1 - \pi_1$.

Smaller probability, π_2	$\delta = \pi_1 - \pi_2$									
	0.05	0.1	0.15	0.2	0.25	0.3	0.35	0.4	0.45	0.5
0.05	621	207	113	75	54	42	33	27	23	19
	475	160	88	59	43	33	27	22	19	16
0.1	958	286	146	92	65	48	38	30	25	21
	726	219	113	72	51	38	30	24	20	17
0.15	1252	354	174	106	73	54	41	33	27	22
	946	270	134	82	57	42	33	26	21	18
0.2	1504	412	198	118	80	58	44	34	28	23
	1134	313	151	91	62	45	35	27	22	18
0.25	1714	459	216	127	85	61	46	35	28	23
	1291	349	165	98	66	47	36	28	23	18
0.3	1883	496	230	134	88	62	46	36	28	23
	1417	376	176	103	68	49	36	28	23	18
0.35	2009	522	240	138	90	63	46	35	28	22
	1511	396	183	106	69	49	36	28	22	18
0.4	2093	538	244	139	90	62	46	34	27	21
	1574	407	186	107	69	49	36	27	21	17
0.45	2135	543	244	138	88	61	44	33	25	19
	1605	411	186	106	68	47	35	26	20	16
0.5	2135	538	240	134	85	58	41	30	23	18
	1605	407	183	103	66	45	33	24	19	15

Table A9 **Sample size for detecting relative risk in case–control study**

This table is used to determine the sample size necessary to find the odds ratio statistically significant (5% two-sided test) in a case–control study with an equal number of cases and controls. The specified odds ratio is denoted by OR, and p is the proportion of controls that are expected to be exposed. For each pair of values the upper figure is for a power of 90% and the lower for a power of 80%. The tabulated sample size refers to the number of *cases* required. The table is derived using (4.22) and (4.42) with a continuity correction.

Note: If $p > 0.5$, work with $p' = 1 - p$ and $OR' = 1/OR$.

Proportion of controls exposed, p	OR (odds ratio)							
	0·5	1·5	2·0	2·5	3·0	4·0	5·0	10·0
0·05	1369	2347	734	393	259	150	105	43
	1044	1775	560	301	200	117	82	34
0·1	701	1266	402	219	146	87	62	27
	534	958	307	168	113	68	48	22
0·15	479	913	295	163	110	67	48	23
	366	691	225	125	85	52	38	19
0·2	370	743	244	136	93	58	43	21
	282	562	187	105	72	45	34	17
0·25	306	647	216	122	85	53	40	21
	233	490	165	94	66	42	32	17
0·3	264	590	200	115	80	51	39	22
	202	447	153	88	62	40	31	18
0·35	236	556	192	111	79	51	39	23
	180	421	147	86	61	40	31	18
0·4	216	538	188	111	79	52	41	24
	165	407	144	85	61	41	32	20
0·45	203	533	189	112	81	54	43	26
	155	403	145	87	63	43	34	21
0·5	194	538	194	116	85	58	46	29
	148	407	148	90	66	45	36	23

References

Abdelbasit K.M. and Plackett, R.L. (1983) Experimental design for binary data. *J. Am. Stat. Ass.* **78**, 90–98.

Acheson E.D. (1967) *Medical Record Linkage.* Oxford University Press, London.

Adcock C.J. (1997) The choice of sample size and the method of maximum expected utility—comments on the paper by Lindley. *Statistician* **46**, 155–162.

Agresti A. (1989) A survey of models for repeated ordered categorical response data. *Stat. Med.* **8**, 1209–1224.

Agresti A. (1990) *Categorical Data Analysis.* Wiley, New York.

Agresti A. (1996) *An Introduction to Categorical Data Analysis.* Wiley, New York.

AIH National Perinatal Statistics Unit and Fertility Society of Australia (1991) *Assisted Conception—Australia and New Zealand 1989.* AIH NPSU, Sydney.

Aitkin M. (1987) Modelling variance heterogeneity in normal regression using GLIM. *Appl. Stat.* **36**, 332–339.

Aitkin M. and Clayton, D. (1980) The fitting of exponential, Weibull and extreme value distributions to complex censored survival data using GLIM. *Appl. Stat.* **29**, 156–163.

Altman D.G. (1991) *Practical Statistics for Medical Research.* Chapman and Hall, London.

Altman D.G., Whitehead J., Parmar, M.K.B. *et al.* (1995) Randomised consent designs in cancer clinical trials. *Eur. J. Cancer* **31**, 1934–1944.

Andersen P.K. and Keiding, N. (1998) Survival analysis, overview. In *Encyclopedia of Biostatistics*, eds P. Armitage and T. Colton, pp. 4452–4461. Wiley, Chichester.

Angrist J.D., Imbens, G.W. and Rubin D.B. (1996) Identification of causal effects using instrumental variables. *J. Am. Stat. Ass.* **91**, 444–472.

Appleton D.R. (1995) What do we mean by a statistical model? *Stat. Med.* **14**, 185–197.

Armitage P. (1955) Tests for linear trends in proportions and frequencies. *Biometrics* **11**, 375–386.

Armitage P. (1957) Studies in the variability of pock counts. *J. Hyg., Camb.* **55**, 564–581.

Armitage P. (1970) The combination of assay results. *Biometrika* **57**, 665–666.

Armitage P. (1975) *Sequential Medical Trials*, 2nd edn. Blackwell Scientific Publications, Oxford.

Armitage P. (1985) The search for optimality in clinical trials. *Int. Stat. Rev.* **53**, 15–24.

Armitage P. (1999) Data and safety monitoring in the Concorde and Alpha trials. *Cont. Clin. Trials* **20**, 207–228.

Armitage P., McPherson C.K. and Copas, J.C. (1969) Statistical studies of prognosis in advanced breast cancer. *J. Chron. Dis.* **22**, 343–360.

Armstrong B. and Doll R. (1974) Bladder cancer mortality in England and Wales in relation to cigarette smoking and saccharin consumption. *Br. J. Prev. Soc. Med.* **28**, 233–240.

Ashby D., Pocock S.J. and Shaper A.G. (1986) Ordered polytomous regression: an example relating serum biochemistry and haematology to alcohol consumption. *Appl. Stat.* **35**, 289–301.

Atkinson A.C. (1985) *Plots, Transformations, and Regression.* Clarendon Press, Oxford.

Australian Institute of Health and Welfare (1992) *Dapsone Exposure, Vietnam Service and Cancer Incidence.* Commonwealth of Australia, Canberra.

Babbie E.R. (1989) *The Practice of Social Research*, 5th edn. Wadsworth, Belmont, California.

Bacharach A.L., Chance M.R.A. and Middleton T.R. (1940) The biological assay of testicular diffusing factor. *Biochem. J.* **34**, 1464–1471.

Bailar J.C. III and Ederer F. (1964) Significance factors for the ratio of a Poisson variable to its expectation. *Biometrics* **20**, 639–643.

Bailey N.T.J. (1975) *The Mathematical Theory of Infectious Diseases and its Applications*, 2nd edn. Griffin, London.

Bailey N.T.J. (1977) *Mathematics, Statistics and Systems for Health*. Wiley, New York.

Baptista J. and Pike M.C. (1977) Exact two-sided confidence limits for the odds ratio in a 2×2 table. *Appl. Stat.* **26**, 214–220.

Barnard G.A. (1989) On alleged gains in power from lower P-values. *Stat. Med.* **8**, 1469–1477.

Barnard J., Rubin D.B. and Schenker, N. (1998) Multiple imputation methods. In *Encyclopedia of Biostatistics*, eds P. Armitage and T. Colton, pp. 2772–2780. Wiley, Chichester.

Barndorff-Nielsen O.E. and Cox D.R. (1989) *Asymptotic Techniques for Use in Statistics*. Chapman and Hall, London.

Barnett V. and Lewis T. (1994) *Outliers in Statistical Data*, 3rd edn. Wiley, Chichester.

Bartko J.J. (1966) The intraclass correlation coefficient as a measure of reliability. *Psychol. Rep.* **19**, 3–11.

Bartlett M.S. (1937) Properties of sufficiency and statistical tests. *Proc. R. Soc. A* **160**, 268–282.

Bartlett M.S. (1949) Fitting a straight line when both variables are subject to error. *Biometrics* **5**, 207–212.

Bartlett R.H., Roloff D.W., Cornell R.G. *et al.* (1985) Extracorporeal circulation in neonatal respiratory failure: a prospective randomized study. *Pediatrics* **76**, 479–487.

Bates D.M. and Watts D.G. (1980) Relative curvature measures of nonlinearity (with discussion). *J. R. Stat. Soc. B* **42**, 1–25.

Bather J.A. (1985) On the allocation of treatments in sequential medical trials. *Int. Stat. Rev.* **53**, 1–13.

Beach M.L. and Baron J. (1998) Regression to the mean. In *Encyclopedia of Biostatistics*, eds P. Armitage and T. Colton, pp. 3753–3755. Wiley, Chichester.

Beale E.M.L. (1960) Confidence regions in non-linear estimation (with discussion). *J. R. Stat. Soc. B* **22**, 41–88.

Becker N.G. (1989) *The Analysis of Infectious Disease Data*. Chapman and Hall, London.

Begg C.B. (1990) On inferences from Wei's biased coin design for clinical trials (with discussion). *Biometrika* **77**, 467–484.

Begg C.B. and Berlin J.A. (1988) Publication bias: a problem in interpreting medical data (with discussion). *J. R. Stat. Soc. A* **151**, 419–453.

Begg C.B. and Iglewicz B. (1980) A treatment allocation procedure for clinical trials. *Biometrics* **36**, 81–90.

Belsley D.A. (1991) *Conditioning Diagnostics, Collinearity and Weak Data in Regression*. Wiley, New York.

Benichou J. (1998) Attributable risk. In *Encyclopedia of Biostatistics*, eds P. Armitage and T. Colton, pp. 216–229. Wiley, Chichester.

Benjamin B. (1968) *Health and Vital Statistics*. Allen and Unwin, London.

Bergen J., Kitchin R. and Berry G. (1992) Predictors of the course of tardive dyskinesia in patients receiving neuroleptics. *Biol. Psychiatry* **32**, 580–594.

Berkson J. (1950) Are there two regressions? *J. Am. Stat. Ass.* **45**, 164–180.

Berkson J. and Gage R.P. (1950) Calculation of survival rates for cancer. *Proc. Staff Meet. Mayo Clin.* **25**, 270–286.

Bernardo J.M. and Ramón J.M. (1998) An introduction to Bayesian reference analysis: inference on the ratio of multinomial parameters. *Statistician* **47**, 101–135.

Bernardo J.M. and Smith A.F.M. (1994) *Bayesian Theory*. Wiley, Chichester.

Berry D.A. (1987) Interim analysis in clinical research. *Cancer Invest.* **5**, 469–477.

Berry D.A. and Fristedt B. (1985) *Bandit Problems: Sequential Allocation of Experiments*. Chapman and Hall, London.

Berry G. (1983) The analysis of mortality by the subject-years method. *Biometrics* **39**, 173–184.

Berry G. (1986, 1988) Statistical significance and confidence intervals. *Med. J. Aust.* **144**, 618–619; reprinted in *Br. J. Clin. Pract.* **42**, 465–468.

Berry G. and Armitage P. (1995) Mid-P confidence intervals: a brief review. *Statistician* **44**, 417–423.

Berry G. and Simpson J. (1998) Modeling strategy. In *Handbook of Public Health Methods*, eds C. Kerr, R. Taylor and G. Heard, pp. 321–330. McGraw-Hill, Sydney.

Berry G., Kitchin R.M. and Mock P.A. (1991) A comparison of two simple hazard ratio estimators based on the logrank test. *Stat. Med.* **10**, 749–755.

Berry G., Newhouse M.L. and Wagner J.C. (2000) Mortality from all cancers of asbestos factory workers in east London 1933–80. *Occ. Env. Med.* **57**, 782–785.

Besag J. (1974) Spatial interaction and the statistical analysis of lattice systems (with discussion). *J. R. Stat. Soc. B* **36**, 192–236.

Besag J. and Clifford P. (1991) Sequential Monte Carlo *p*-values. *Biometrika* **78**, 301–304.

Besag J., Green P., Higdon D. and Mengersen K. (1995) Bayesian computation and stochastic systems (with discussion). *Stat. Sci.* **10**, 3–66.

Bishop R.O. (2000) *Predictors of functional outcome after injury—a polytomous regression of Glasgow Outcome Score.* Treatise for the Degree of Master of Public Health, Department of Public Health and Community Medicine, University of Sydney, Sydney.

Bliss C.I. (1958) *Periodic Regression in Biology and Climatology.* Bulletin no. 615, Connecticut Agric. Exp. Station, New Haven.

BMDP (1993) *BMDP/Dynamic, Version 7* www.statsol.ie/bmdp.htm

Boardman T.J. (1974) Confidence intervals for variance components—a comparative Monte Carlo study. *Biometrics* **30**, 251–262.

Bowman A.W. and Azzalini A. (1997) *Applied Smoothing Techniques for Data Analysis.* Oxford University Press, Oxford.

Box G.E.P. (1954a) Some theorems on quadratic forms applied in the study of analysis of variance problems: I. Effect of inequality of variance in the one-way classification. *Ann. Math. Stat.* **25**, 290–302.

Box G.E.P. (1954b) Some theorems on quadratic forms applied in the study of analysis of variance problems: II. Effect of inequality of variance and of correlation between errors in the two-way classification. *Ann. Math. Stat.* **25**, 484–498.

Box G.E.P. and Cox D.R. (1964) An analysis of transformations (with discussion). *J. R. Stat. Soc. B* **26**, 211–252.

Box G.E.P. and Jenkins G.M. (1976) *Time Series Analysis: Forecasting and Control*, revised edn. Holden-Day, San Francisco.

Box G.E.P. and Tiao G.C. (1973) *Bayesian Inference in Statistical Analysis.* Addison-Wesley, Reading, Massachusetts.

Bradley R.A., Katti S.K. and Coons I.J. (1962) Optimal scaling for ordered categories. *Psychometrika* **27**, 355–374.

Breslow N. (1990) Biostatistics and Bayes (with discussion). *Stat. Sci.* **5**, 269–298.

Breslow N.E. (1974) Covariance analysis of censored survival data. *Biometrics* **30**, 89–99.

Breslow N.E. (1984a) Extra-Poisson variation in log-linear models. *Appl. Stat.* **33**, 38–44.

Breslow N.E. (1984b) Elementary methods of cohort analysis. *Int. J. Epidemiol.* **13**, 112–115.

Breslow N.E. and Day N.E. (1975) Indirect standardization and multiplicative models for rates, with reference to the age adjustment of cancer incidence and relative frequency data. *J. Chron. Dis.* **28**, 289–303.

Breslow N.E. and Day N.E. (1980) *Statistical Methods in Cancer Research*, Vol. 1—*The Analysis of Case–Control Studies.* International Agency for Research on Cancer Scientific Publications No. 32, Lyon.

Breslow N.E. and Day N.E. (1987) *Statistical Methods in Cancer Research*, Volume 2—*The Design and Analysis of Cohort Studies.* International Agency for Research on Cancer Scientific Publications No. 82, Lyon.

Brook D. (1964) On the distinction between the conditional probability and the joint probability approaches in the specification of nearest-neighbour systems. *Biometrika* **51**, 481–483.

Brookmeyer R. and Day N.E. (1987) Two-stage models for the analysis of cancer screening data. *Biometrics* **43**, 657–669.

Brookmeyer R., Day N.E. and Moss S. (1986) Case–control studies for estimation of the natural history of preclinical disease from screening data. *Stat. Med.* **5**, 127–138.

Brooks S.P. (1998) Markov chain Monte Carlo method and its application. *Statistician* **47**, 69–100.

Brown A., Mohamed S.D., Montgomery R.D., Armitage P. and Laurence D.R. (1960) Value of a large dose of antitoxin in clinical tetanus. *Lancet* **ii**, 227–230.

Brown C.C. (1982) On a goodness of fit test for the logistic model based on score statistics. *Commun. Stat.-Theor. Meth.* **11**, 1087–1105.

Brown M.B. (1992) A test for the difference between two treatments in a continuous measure of outcome when there are dropouts. *Cont. Clin. Trials* **13**, 213–225.

Buck A.A. and Gart J.J. (1966) Comparison of a screening test and a reference test in epidemiologic studies. I. Indices of agreement and their relation to prevalence. *Am J. Epidemiol.* **83**, 586–592.

Bull J.P. (1959) The historical development of clinical therapeutic trials. *J. Chron. Dis.* **10**, 218–248.

Bulmer M.G. (1980) *The Mathematical Theory of Quantitative Genetics.* Oxford University Press, Oxford.

Buyse M.E., Staquet M.J. and Sylvester R.J. (eds) (1984) *Cancer Clinical Trials: Methods and Practice*. Oxford University Press, Oxford.

Byar D.P. (1983) Analysis of survival data: Cox and Weibull models with covariates. In *Statistics in Medical Research: Methods and Issues with Applications in Cancer Research*, eds V. Miké and K. Stanley, pp. 365–401. Wiley, New York.

Carlin B.P. and Louis T.A. (2000) *Bayes and Empirical Bayes Methods for Data Analysis*, 2nd edn. Chapman and Hall/CRC, Boca Raton.

Carroll R.J. and Schneider H. (1985) A note on Levene's tests for equality of variances. *Stat. Prob. Letter* **3**, 191–194.

Casagrande J.T., Pike M.C. and Smith P.G. (1978) The power function of the 'exact' test for comparing two binomial distributions. *Appl. Stat.* **27**, 176–180.

Chalmers I. and Altman D.G. (eds) (1995) *Systematic Reviews*. British Medical Journal, London.

Chalmers T.C., Berrier J., Sacks H.S. *et al.* (1987) Meta-analysis of clinical trials as a scientific discipline. II: Replicate variability and comparison of studies that agree and disagree. *Stat. Med.* **6**, 733–744.

Chaloner K., Church T., Louis T.A. and Matts J.P. (1993) Graphical elicitation of a prior distribution for a clinical trial. *Statistician* **42**, 341–353.

Chao A. (1998) Capture–recapture. In *Encyclopedia of Biostatistics*, eds P. Armitage and T. Colton, pp. 482–486. Wiley, Chichester.

Chase P.J. (1970) Combinations of *M* out of *N* objects. *Comm. A. Comp. Mach.* **13**, 368.

Chatfield C. (1995) Model uncertainty, data mining and statistical inference (with discussion). *J. R. Stat. Soc. A* **158**, 419–466.

Chatfield C. (1996) *The Analysis of Time Series: an Introduction*, 5th edn. Chapman and Hall, London.

Chatfield C. and Collins A.J. (1980) *Introduction to Multivariate Analysis*. Chapman and Hall, London.

Checkoway H., Pearce N. and Crawford-Brown D.J. (1989) *Research Methods in Occupational Epidemiology*. Oxford University Press, New York.

Checkoway H., Heyer N.J., Demers P.A. and Breslow N.E. (1993) A cohort mortality study

of workers in the diatomaceous earth industry. *Br. J. Ind. Med.* **50**, 586–597.

Chen C.-H. and Wang P.C. (1991) Diagnostic plots in Cox's regression model. *Biometrics* **47**, 841–850.

Chernoff H. and Petkau A.J. (1981) Sequential medical trials involving paired data. *Biometrika* **68**, 119–132.

Chiang C.L. (1984) *The Life Table and its Applications*. Krieger, Malabar, Florida.

Cicchetti D.V. and Feinstein A.R. (1990) High agreement but low kappa: II. Resolving the paradoxes. *J. Clin. Epidemiol* **43**, 551–558.

Clayton D. and Cuzick J. (1985) Multivariate generalizations of the proportional hazards model (with discussion). *J. R. Stat. Soc. A* **148**, 82–117.

Clayton D. and Kaldor J. (1987) Empirical Bayes estimates of age-standardized relative risks for use in disease mapping. *Biometrics* **43**, 671–681.

Clayton D.G. (1991) A Monte Carlo method for Bayesian inference in frailty models. *Biometrics* **47**, 467–485.

Cleveland W.S. (1979) Robust locally weighted regression and smoothing scatterplots. *J. Am. Stat. Ass.* **74**, 829–836.

Cleveland W.S. (1985) *The Elements of Graphing Data*. Wadsworth, Monterey.

Cleveland W.S. (1993) *Visualizing Data*. Hobart Press, Summit.

Cochran W.G. (1954) Some methods for strengthening the common χ^2 tests. *Biometrics* **10**, 417–451.

Cochran W.G. (1977) *Sampling Techniques*, 3rd edn. Wiley, New York.

Cochran W.G. and Cox G.M. (1957) *Experimental Designs*, 2nd edn. Wiley, New York.

Cochrane A.L. (1972) *Effectiveness and Efficiency: Random Reflections on Health Services*. Nuffield Provincial Hospitals Trust, London.

Cockcroft A., Edwards J., Bevan C. *et al.* (1981) An investigation of operating theatre staff exposed to humidifier fever antigens. *Br. J. Ind. Med.* **38**, 144–151.

Cockcroft A., Berry G., Brown E.B. and Exall C. (1982) Psychological changes during a controlled trial of rehabilitation in chronic respiratory disability. *Thorax* **37**, 413–416.

Cohen J. (1960) A coefficient of agreement for nominal scales. *Educ. Psychol. Meas.* **20**, 37–46.

Cohen J. (1968) Weighted kappa: nominal scale agreement with provision for scale disagreement or partial credit. *Psychol. Bull.* **70**, 213–220.

Cole B.F., Gelber R.D. and Goldhirsch A. (1995) A quality-adjusted survival meta-analysis of adjuvant chemotherapy for premenstrual breast cancer. *Stat. Med.* **14**, 1771–1784.

Cole T.J. (1988) Fitting smoothed centile curves to reference data (with discussion). *J. R. Stat. Soc. A* **151**, 385–418.

Cole T.J. (1995) Conditional reference charts to assess weight gain in British infants. *Arch. Dis. Child.* **73**, 8–16.

Cole T.J. (1998) Presenting information on growth distance and conditional velocity in one chart: practical issues of chart design. *Stat. Med.* **17**, 2697–2707.

Cole T.J. and Green P.J. (1992) Smoothing reference centile curves: the LMS method and penalized likelihood. *Stat. Med.* **11**, 1305–1319.

Cole T.J., Morley C.J., Thornton A.J. and Fowler M.A. (1991) A scoring system to quantify illness in babies under 6 months of age. *J. R. Stat. Soc. A* **154**, 287–304.

Collett D. (1994) *Modelling Survival Data in Medical Research*. Chapman and Hall, London.

Collins R.L. and Meckler R.J. (1965) Histology and weight of the mouse adrenal: a diallel genetic study. *J. Endocrinol.* **31**, 95–105.

Concorde Coordinating Committee (1994) Concorde: MRC/ANRS randomised double-blind controlled trial of immediate and deferred zidovudine in symptom-free HIV infection. *Lancet* **343**, 871–881.

Connor R.J. (1987) Sample size for testing differences in proportions for the paired-sample design. *Biometrics* **43**, 207–211.

Conover W.J. (1999) *Practical Nonparametric Statistics*, 3rd edn. Wiley, New York.

Cook P., Doll R. and Fellingham S.A. (1969) A mathematical model for the age distribution of cancer in man. *Int. J. Cancer* **4**, 93–112.

Cook R.D. (1977) Detection of influential observations in linear regression. *Technometrics* **19**, 15–18.

Cook R.D. and Weisberg S. (1982) *Residuals and Influence in Regression*. Chapman and Hall, London.

Cookson W.O.C.M., de Klerk N.H., Musk A.W. *et al.* (1986) Prevalence of radiographic asbestosis in crocidolite miners and millers at Wittenoom, Western Australia. *Br. J. Ind. Med.* **43**, 450–457.

Cormack R.M. (1989) Log-linear models for capture–recapture. *Biometrics* **45**, 395–413.

Cornfield J. (1956) A statistical property arising from retrospective studies. *Proc. Third Berkeley Symp. Math. Stat. Prob.* **4**, 135–148.

Cornish E.A. and Fisher R.A. (1937) Moments and cumulants in the specification of distributions. *Rev. Inst. Int. Stat.* **5**, 307–322.

Cornish-Bowden A. (1995a) *Fundamentals of Enzyme Kinetics*, revised edn. Portland Press, London.

Cornish-Bowden A. (1995b) *Analysis of Enzyme Kinetic Data*. Oxford University Press, Oxford.

Cornish-Bowden A. and Eisenthal R. (1974) Statistical considerations in the estimation of enzyme kinetic parameters by the direct linear plot and other methods. *Biochem. J.* **139**, 721–730.

Cox D.R. (1958) *Planning of Experiments*. Wiley, New York.

Cox D.R. (1972) Regression models and life-tables (with discussion). *J. R. Stat. Soc. B* **34**, 187–220.

Cox D.R. (1990) Discussion of paper by C.B. Begg. *Biometrika* **77**, 483–484.

Cox D.R. and Hinkley D.V. (1974) *Theoretical Statistics*. Chapman and Hall, London.

Cox D.R. and Oakes D. (1984) *Analysis of Survival Data*. Chapman and Hall, London.

Cox D.R. and Snell E.J. (1968) A general definition of residuals (with discussion). *J. R. Stat. Soc. B* **30**, 248–275.

Cox D.R. and Snell E.J. (1989) *Analysis of Binary Data*, 2nd edn. Chapman and Hall, London.

Cox D.R. and Wermuth N. (1996) *Multivariate Dependencies: Models, Analysis and Interpretation*. Chapman and Hall, London.

Cox D.R., Fitzpatrick R., Fletcher A.E. *et al.* (1992) Quality of life assessment: can we keep it simple? (with discussion). *J. R. Stat. Soc. A* **155**, 353–393.

Cox T.F. and Cox M.A.A. (2001) *Multidimensional Scaling*, 2nd edn. Chapman and Hall/CRC, Boca Raton.

Cramér H. (1946) *Mathematical Methods of Statistics*. Princeton University Press, Princeton.

Cressie N.A.C. and Keightley D.D. (1979) The underlying structure of the direct linear plot with application to the analysis of hormone–

receptor interactions. *J. Ster. Biochem.* **11**, 1173–1180.

Cronin K.A., Weed D.L., Connor R.J. and Prorok P.C. (1998) Case–control studies of cancer screening: theory and practice. *J. Nat. Cancer Inst.* **90**, 498–504.

Crowder M.J. and Hand D.J. (1990) *Analysis of Repeated Measures*. Chapman and Hall, London.

Currie D.J. (1982) Estimating Michaelis–Menten parameters: bias, variance and experimental design. *Biometrics* **38**, 907–919.

Cutler S.J. and Ederer F. (1958) Maximum utilization of the life table method in analysing survival. *J. Chron. Dis.* **8**, 699–712.

Cuzick J. (1998) Clustering. In *Encyclopedia of Biostatistics*, eds P. Armitage and T. Colton, pp. 747–756. Wiley, Chichester.

Cuzick J. and Edwards R. (1990) Spatial clustering for inhomogeneous populations (with discussion). *J. R. Stat. Soc. B* **52**, 73–104.

Cytel (1995) *StatXact-3 for Windows. Software for Exact Nonparametric Inference*. Cytel Software Corporation, Cambridge, Massachusetts.

Daniel C. (1959) Use of half-normal plots in interpreting factorial two-level experiments. *Technometrics* **1**, 311–341.

Darby S.C. and Reissland J.A. (1981) Low levels of ionizing radiation and cancer—are we underestimating the risk? (with discussion). *J. R. Stat. Soc. A* **144**, 298–331.

David F.N. and Barton D.E. (1966) Two space–time interaction tests for epidemicity. *Br. J. Prev. Soc. Med.* **20**, 44–48.

Davidian M. and Giltinan D.M. (1995) *Nonlinear Models for Repeated Measurements Data*. Chapman and Hall, London.

Davison A.C. and Hinkley D.V. (1997) *Bootstrap Methods and their Application*. Cambridge University Press, Cambridge.

Day N.E. and Walter S.D. (1984) Simplified models of screening for chronic disease: estimation procedures from mass screening programmes. *Biometrics* **40**, 1–14.

Dear K.B.G. and Begg C.B. (1992) An approach for assessing publication bias prior to performing a meta-analysis. *Stat. Sci.* **7**, 237–245.

Dellaportas P. and Smith A.F.M. (1993) Bayesian inference for generalised linear and proportional hazards models via Gibbs sampling. *Appl. Stat.* **42**, 443–459.

DeMets D.L. and Lan K.K.G. (1994) Interim analysis: the alpha spending function approach. *Stat. Med.* **13**, 1341–1352.

DerSimonian R. and Laird N. (1986) Meta-analysis in clinical trials. *Cont. Clin. Trials*, **7**, 177–188.

Devroye L. (1986) *Non-Uniform Random Variate Generation*. Springer-Verlag, New York.

Diamond E.L. and Lilienfeld A.M. (1962a) Effects of errors in classification and diagnosis in various types of epidemiological studies. *Am. J. Public Health* **52**, 1137–1144.

Diamond E.L. and Lilienfeld A.M. (1962b) Misclassification errors in 2 × 2 tables with one margin fixed: some further comments. *Am. J. Public Health* **52**, 2106–2110.

Dickersin K. and Min Y.I. (1993) Publication bias: the problem that won't go away. *Ann. N.Y. Acad. Sci.* **703**, 135–148.

Dickersin K., Scherer R. and Lefebvre C. (1995) Identifying relevant studies for systematic reviews. In *Systematic Reviews*, eds D.G. Altman and I. Chalmers, pp. 17–36. British Medical Journal, London.

Diggle P.J. (1988) An approach to the analysis of repeated measures. *Biometrics* **44**, 959–971.

Diggle P.J. (1990) *Time Series—A Biostatistical Introduction*. Clarendon, Oxford.

Diggle P.J. (1998) Dealing with missing values in longitudinal studies. In *Statistical Analysis of Medical Data*, eds B.S. Everitt and G. Dunn, pp. 203–228. Edward Arnold, London.

Diggle P.J. and Kenward M.G. (1994) Informative drop-out in longitudinal data analysis (with discussion). *Appl. Stat.* **43**, 49–93.

Diggle P.J., Liang K.-Y. and Zeger S.L. (1994) *Analysis of Longitudinal Data*. Oxford University Press, Oxford.

Dinse G.E. (1998) Tumor incidence experiments. In *Encyclopedia of Biostatistics*, eds P. Armitage and T. Colton, pp. 4597–4609. Wiley, Chichester.

Dixon W.J. (1988) Staircase method (up-and-down). In *Encyclopedia of Statistical Sciences*, eds S. Kotz and N.L. Johnson, pp. 622–625. Wiley, New York.

Dobson A.J. (1990) *An Introduction to Generalized Linear Models*. Chapman and Hall, London.

Dobson A.J., Kuulasmaa K., Eberle E. and Scherer J. (1991) Confidence intervals for weighted sums of Poisson parameters. *Stat. Med.* **10**, 457–462.

Does R.J.M.M., Strijbosch L.W.G. and Albers W. (1988) Using jackknife methods for estimating the parameter in dilution series. *Biometrics* **44**, 1093–1102.

Doll R. (1952) The causes of death among gasworkers with special reference to cancer of the lung. *Br. J. Ind. Med.* **9**, 180–185.

Doll R. and Hill A.B. (1950) Smoking and carcinoma of the lung. Preliminary report. *Br. Med. J.* **ii**, 739–748.

Doll R. and Hill A.B. (1954) The mortality of doctors in relation to their smoking habits. A preliminary report. *Br. Med. J.* **i**, 1451–1455.

Doll R. and Hill A.B. (1956) Lung cancer and other causes of death in relation to smoking. A second report on the mortality of British doctors. *Br. Med. J.* **ii**, 1071–1081.

Doll R. and Hill A.B. (1964) Mortality in relation to smoking: ten years' observations of British doctors. *Br. Med. J.* **i**, 1399–1410, 1460–1467.

Doll R. and Peto R. (1976) Mortality in relation to smoking: 20 years' observations on male British doctors. *Br. Med. J.* **ii**, 1525–1536.

Doll R. and Pygott F. (1952) Factors influencing the rate of healing of gastric ulcers: admission to hospital, phenobarbitone, and ascorbic acid. *Lancet* **i**, 171–175.

Doll R., Peto R., Wheatley K., Gray R. and Sutherland I. (1994) Mortality in relation to smoking: 40 years' observations on male British doctors. *Br. Med. J.* **309**, 901–911.

Donner A. (1984) Approaches to sample size estimation in the design of clinical trials—a review. *Stat. Med.* **3**, 199–214.

Donner A. (1992) Sample size requirements for stratified cluster randomization designs. *Stat. Med.* **11**, 743–750.

Draper D. (1995) Assessment and propagation of model uncertainty (with discussion). *J. R. Stat. Soc. B* **57**, 45–97.

Draper N.R. and Smith H. (1998) *Applied Regression Analysis*, 3rd edn. Wiley, New York.

Dunn G. (1999) The problem of measurement error in modelling the effect of compliance in a randomized trial. *Stat. Med.* **18**, 2863–2877.

Dyke G.V. and Patterson H.D. (1952) Analysis of factorial arrangements when the data are proportions. *Biometrics* **8**, 1–12.

Early Breast Cancer Trialists' Collaborative Group (1990) *Treatment of Early Breast Cancer*, Vol. 1: *Worldwide Evidence 1985–1990*. Oxford University Press, Oxford.

Early Breast Cancer Trialists' Collaborative Group (1992) Systemic treatment of early breast cancer by hormonal, cytotoxic, or immune therapy. *Lancet* **339**, 1–15, 71–85.

Easterbrook P.J., Berlin J.A., Gopalan R. and Matthews D.R. (1991) Publication bias in clinical research. *Lancet* **337**, 867–872.

EaSt for Windows (1999) *Software for the Design and Interim Monitoring of Group Sequential Clinical Trials*. CYTEL Software Corporation, Cambridge, Massachusetts.

Ebbutt A.F. (1984) Three-period crossover designs for two treatments. *Biometrics* **40**, 219–224.

Ederer F., Myers M.H. and Mantel N. (1964) A statistical problem in space and time: do leukemia cases come in clusters? *Biometrics* **20**, 626–638.

Edgington E.S. (1987) *Randomization Tests*, 2nd edn. Marcel Dekker, New York.

Edwards J.H. (1961) The recognition and estimation of cyclical trends. *Ann. Hum. Genet.* **25**, 83–86.

Efron B. and Feldman D. (1991) Compliance as an explanatory variable (with discussion). *J. Am. Stat. Ass.* **86**, 9–26.

Efron B. and Morris C.N. (1975) Data analysis using Stein's estimator and its generalizations. *J. Am. Stat. Ass.* **70**, 311–319.

Efron B. and Tibshirani R.J. (1993) *An Introduction to the Bootstrap*. Chapman and Hall, London.

Ehrenberg A.S.C. (1968) The elements of lawlike relationships. *J. R. Stat. Soc. A* **131**, 280–302.

Ehrenberg A.S.C. (1975) *Data Reduction*. Wiley, London.

Ehrenberg A.S.C. (1977) Rudiments of numeracy. *J. R. Stat. Soc. A* **140**, 277–297.

Einot I. and Gabriel K.R. (1975) A study of the powers of several methods of multiple comparisons. *J. Am. Stat. Ass.* **70**, 574–583.

Ellery C., MacLennan R., Berry G. and Shearman R.P. (1986) A case–control study of breast cancer in relation to the use of steroid contraceptive agents. *Med. J. Aust.* **144**, 173–176.

Elston R.C. and Stewart J. (1971) A general model for the genetic analysis of pedigree data. *Hum. Hered.* **21**, 523–542.

Elwood J.M. (1988) *Causal Relationships in Medicine: A Practical System for Critical Appraisal*. Oxford University Press, Oxford.

Etzioni R.D. and Weiss N.S. (1998) Analysis of case–control studies of screening: impact of misspecifying the duration of detectable pre-clinical pathological changes. *Am. J. Epidemiol.* **148**, 292–297.

Everitt B. (1980) *Cluster Analysis*, 2nd edn. Heinemann, London.

Fazekas de St Groth S. (1982) The evaluation of limiting dilution assays. *J. Immun. Meth.* **49**, R11–R23.

Feinstein A.R. and Cicchetti D.V. (1990) High agreement but low kappa: I. The problems of two paradoxes. *J. Clin. Epidemiol.* **43**, 543–549.

Fieller E.C. (1940) The biological standardization of insulin. *J. R. Stat. Soc., Suppl.* **7**, 1–64.

Fienberg S.E. (1980) *The Analysis of Cross-Classified Categorical Data*, 2nd edn. MIT Press, Cambridge, Massachusetts.

Finkelstein D.M. (1986) A proportional hazards model for interval-censored failure time data. *Biometrics* **42**, 845–854.

Finney D.J. (1971) *Probit Analysis*, 3rd edn. Cambridge University Press, Cambridge.

Finney D.J. (1978) *Statistical Method in Biological Assay*, 3rd edn. Griffin, London.

Finney D.J. (1979) The computation of results from radioimmunoassays. *Meth. Inf. Med.* **18**, 164–171.

Finney D.J., Latscha R., Bennett B.M. and Hsu P. (1963) *Tables for Testing Significance in a 2 × 2 Contingency Table*. Cambridge University Press, Cambridge.

Fischer-Lapp K. and Goetghebeur E. (1999) Practical properties of some structural mean analyses of the effect of compliance in randomized trials. *Cont. Clin. Trials* **20**, 531–546.

Fisher R.A. (1950, 1964) The significance of deviations from expectation in a Poisson series. *Biometrics* **6**, 17–24; reprinted in **20**, 265–272.

Fisher R.A. (1966) *The Design of Experiments*, 8th edn. Oliver and Boyd, Edinburgh.

Fisher R.A. and Yates F. (1963) *Statistical Tables for Biological, Agricultural and Medical Research*, 6th edn. Oliver and Boyd, Edinburgh.

Fitzmaurice G.M., Molenberghs G. and Lipsitz S.R. (1995) Regression models for longitudinal binary responses with informative dropout. *J. R. Stat. Soc. B* **57**, 691–704.

Fleiss J.L. (1975) Measuring agreement between two judges on the presence or absence of a trait. *Biometrics* **31**, 651–659.

Fleiss J.L. (1981) *Statistical Methods for Rates and Proportions*, 2nd edn. Wiley, New York.

Fleiss J.L. (1989) A critique of recent research on the two-treatment crossover design. *Cont. Clin. Trials* **10**, 237–243.

Fleiss J.L., Tytun A. and Ury H.K. (1980) A simple approximation for calculating sample sizes for comparing independent proportions. *Biometrics* **36**, 343–346.

Fleming T.R., DeGruttola V. and DeMets D.L. (1998) Surrogate endpoints. In *Encyclopedia of Biostatistics*, eds P. Armitage and T. Colton, pp. 4425–4431. Wiley, Chichester.

Forsyth R.J., Bartlett K., Burchell A., Scott H.M. and Eyre J.A. (1993) Astrocytic glucose-6-phosphatase and the permeability of brain microsomes to glucose-6-phosphate. *Biochem. J.* **294**, 145–151.

Forsythe A.B. and Stitt F.W. (1977) *Randomization or Minimization in the Treatment Assignment of Patient Trials: Validity and Power of Tests*. Technical Report No. 28, BMDP Statistical Software, Health Sciences Computing Facility, University of California, Los Angeles.

Fraser P.M. and Franklin D.A. (1974) Mathematical models for the diagnosis of liver disease. Problems arising in the use of conditional probability theory. *Quart. J. Med.* **43**, 73–88.

Freedman L.S., Lowe D. and Macaskill P. (1984) Stopping rules for clinical trials incorporating clinical opinion. *Biometrics* **40**, 575–586.

Freeman D.H. and Holford T.R. (1980) Summary rates. *Biometrics* **36**, 195–205.

Freeman P.R. (1989) The performance of the two-stage analysis of two-treatment, two-period cross-over trials. *Stat. Med.* **8**, 1421–1432.

Freund R.J., Littell R.C. and Spector P.C. (1986) *SAS System for Linear Models*, 1986 edn. SAS Institute, Cary.

Friedman L.M., Furberg C.D. and DeMets D.L. (1998) *Fundamentals of Clinical Trials*, 3rd edn. Wright, Boston.

Friedman M. (1937) The use of ranks to avoid the assumption of normality implicit in the analysis of variance. *J. Am. Stat. Ass.* **32**, 675–701.

Gabriel K.R. (1962) Ante-dependence analysis of an ordered set of variables. *Ann. Math. Stat.* **33**, 201–212.

Gail M.H., Byar D.P., Pechacek T.F. and Corle D.K. (1992) Aspects of statistical design for the Community Intervention Trial for Smoking Cessation (COMMIT). *Cont. Clin. Trials* **13**, 6–21.

Galbraith R.F. (1988) A note on graphical presentation of estimated odds ratios from several clinical trials. *Stat. Med.* **7**, 889–894.

Gardner M.J. (1989) Review of reported increases of childhood cancer rates in the vicinity of nuclear installations in the UK. *J. R. Stat. Soc. A* **152**, 307–325.

Gardner M.J. and Altman D.G. (eds) (1989) *Statistics With Confidence: Confidence Intervals and Statistical Guidelines*. British Medical Journal, London.

Gardner M.J. and Heady J.A. (1973) Some effects of within-person variability in epidemiological studies. *J. Chron. Dis.* **26**, 781–795.

Gart J.J. (1962) On the combination of relative risks. *Biometrics* **18**, 601–610.

Gart J.J. and Buck A.A. (1966) Comparison of a screening test and a reference test in epidemiologic studies. II. A probabilistic model for the comparison of diagnostic tests. *Am. J. Epidemiol.* **83**, 593–602.

Gart J.J. and Nam J. (1988) Approximate interval estimation of the ratio of binomial parameters: a review and corrections for skewness. *Biometrics* **44**, 323–338.

Geary D.N., Huntington E. and Gilbert R.J. (1992) Analysis of multivariate data from four dental clinical trials. *J. R. Stat. Soc. A* **155**, 77–89.

Gehan E. (1965) A generalized Wilcoxon test for comparing arbitrarily singly censored samples. *Biometrika* **52**, 203–223.

Geigy Scientific Tables (1982) Vol. 2: *Introduction to Statistics, Statistical Tables, Mathematical Formulae*, 8th edn. Ciba-Geigy, Basle.

Gelber R.D., Gelman R.S. and Goldhirsch A. (1989) A quality-of-life oriented endpoint for comparing therapies. *Biometrics* **45**, 781–795.

Gelfand A.E. and Smith A.F.M. (1990) Sampling-based approaches to calculating marginal densities. *J. Am. Stat. Ass.* **85**, 398–409.

Geller N.L. and Pocock S.J. (1987) Interim analyses in randomized clinical trials: ramifications and guidelines for practitioners. *Biometrics* **43**, 213–223.

Gelman A. (1996) Inference and monitoring convergence. In *Markov Chain Monte Carlo in Practice*, eds W.R. Gilks, S. Richardson and D.J. Spiegelhalter, pp. 131–143. Chapman and Hall, London.

Gelman A. and Rubin D.B. (1992) Inference from iterative simulation using multiple sequences (with discussion). *Stat. Sci.* **7**, 457–511.

Gelman A., Carlin J.B., Stern H.S. and Rubin D.B. (1995) *Bayesian Data Analysis*. Chapman and Hall, London.

Geman S. and Geman D. (1984) Stochastic relaxation, Gibbs distributions and the Bayesian restoration of images. *IEEE Trans. Patt. Anal. Mach. Intell.* **6**, 721–741.

Gevins A.S. (1980) Pattern recognition of human brain electrical potentials. *IEEE Trans. Patt. Anal. Mach. Intell.* **PAMI-2**, 383–404.

Geyer C.J. (1992) Practical Markov chain Monte Carlo. *Stat. Sci.* **7**, 473–511.

Gilks W.R. (1996) Full conditional distributions. In *Markov Chain Monte Carlo in Practice*, eds W.R. Gilks, S. Richardson and D.J. Spiegelhalter, pp. 75–88. Chapman and Hall, London.

Gilks W.R. and Roberts G.O. (1996) Strategies for improving MCMC. In *Markov Chain Monte Carlo in Practice*, eds W.R. Gilks, S. Richardson and D.J. Spiegelhalter, pp. 89–114. Chapman and Hall, London.

Gilks W.R. and Wild P. (1992) Adaptive rejection sampling for Gibbs sampling. *Appl. Stat.* **41**, 337–348.

Gilks W.R., Richardson S. and Spiegelhalter D.J. (1996) *Markov Chain Monte Carlo in Practice*. Chapman and Hall, London.

Givens G.H., Smith D.D. and Tweedie R.L. (1997) Publication bias in meta-analysis: a Bayesian data-augmentation approach to account for issues exemplified in the passive smoking debate (with discussion). *Stat. Sci.* **12**, 221–250.

Glass G.V. (1976) Primary, secondary, and meta-analysis of research. *Educ. Res.* **5**, 3–8.

Glasser M. (1967) Exponential survival with covariance. *J. Am. Stat. Ass.* **62**, 561–568.

Glasziou P. and Irwig L. (1998) Meta-analysis of diagnostic tests. In *Encyclopedia of Biostatistics*, eds P. Armitage and T. Colton, pp. 2579–2585. Wiley, Chichester.

Glasziou P.P. and Schwartz S. (1991) Clinical decision analysis. *Med. J. Aust.* **154**, 105–110.

Glynn R., Laird N. and Rubin D.B. (1993) The performance of mixture models for nonignorable nonresponse with follow ups. *J. Am. Stat. Ass.* **88**, 984–993.

Godambe V.P. (1991) *Estimating Functions*. Oxford University Press, Oxford.

Goetghebeur E. and Lapp K. (1997) The effect of treatment compliance in a placebo-controlled trial: regression with unpaired data. *Appl. Stat.* **46**, 351–364.

Goetghebeur E. and van Houwelingen H. (eds) (1998) Issue no. 3: analysing non-compliance in clinical trials. *Stat. Med.* **17**, 247–389.

Goldstein H. (1995) *Multilevel Statistical Models*, 2nd edn. Arnold, London.

Goldstein H. and Healy M.J.R. (1995) The graphical representation of a collection of means. *J. R. Stat. Soc. A* **158**, 175–177.

Goldstein H. and Pan H. (1992) Percentile smoothing using piecewise polynomials, with covariates. *Biometrics* **48**, 1057–1068.

Goldstein H. and Spiegelhalter D.J. (1996) League tables and their limitations: statistical issues in comparisons of institutional performance (with discussion). *J. R. Stat. Soc. A* **159**, 385–443.

Goldstein H., Healy M.J.R. and Rasbash J. (1994) Multilevel time series models with applications to repeated measures data. *Stat. Med.* **13**, 1643–1655.

Goldstein H., Rasbash J., Plewis I. *et al.* (1998) *A User's Guide to MLwiN*. Institute of Education, University of London, London.

Goldstein R. (1998) Software, biostatistical. In *Encyclopedia of Biostatistics*, eds P. Armitage and T. Colton, pp. 4180–4187. Wiley, Chichester.

Goldstein R. and Harrell F. (1998) Survival analysis, software. In *Encyclopedia of Biostatistics*, eds P. Armitage and T. Colton, pp. 4461–4466. Wiley, Chichester.

Good I.J. (1950) *Probability and the Weighing of Evidence*. Griffin, London.

Gore S.M., Pocock S.J. and Kerr G.R. (1984) Regression models and non-proportional hazards in the analysis of breast cancer survival. *Appl. Stat.* **33**, 176–195.

Govindarajulu Z. (2000) *Statistical Techniques in Bioassay*, 2nd edn. Karger, New York.

Gratton R.J., Appleton D.R. and Alwiswasy M.R. (1978) The measurement of tumour growth rates. In *Developments in Cell Biology 2*, eds A.-J. Valleron and P.D.M. Macdonald, pp. 325–332. Elsevier, Amsterdam.

Gray J.B. and Woodall W.H. (1994) The maximum size of standardized and internally studentized residuals in regression analysis. *Am. Stat.* **48**, 111–113.

Green P.J. and Silverman B.W. (1994) *Nonparametric Regression and Generalized Linear Models*. Chapman and Hall, London.

Greenacre M.J. (1984) *Theory and Applications of Correspondence Analysis*. Academic Press, London.

Greenhouse S.W. and Geisser S. (1959) On methods in the analysis of profile data. *Psychometrika* **24**, 95–112.

Greenland S. (1987) Variance estimators for attributable fraction estimates consistent in both large strata and sparse data. *Stat. Med.* **6**, 701–708.

Greenland S. and Salvan A. (1990) Bias in the one-step method for pooling study results. *Stat. Med.* **9**, 247–252.

Greenwood M. (1926) *The Natural Duration of Cancer*. HM Stationery Office, London.

Grieve A.P. (1994) Bayesian analysis of two-treatment crossover studies. *Stat. Meth. Med. Res.* **3**, 407–429.

Griffiths D. and Sandland R. (1984) Fitting generalized allometric models to multivariate growth data. *Biometrics* **40**, 139–150.

Grimmett G.R. and Stirzacker D.R. (1992) *Probability and Random Processes*, 2nd edn. Oxford University Press, Oxford.

Grimson R.C. (1993) Disease clusters, exact distributions of maxima, and *P*-values. *Stat. Med.* **12**, 1773–1794.

Grosskurth H., Mosha F., Todd J. *et al.* (1995) Impact of improved treatment of sexually transmitted diseases on HIV infection in rural Tanzania: randomized controlled trial. *Lancet* **346**, 530–536.

Grossman J., Parmar M.K.B., Spiegelhalter D.J. and Freedman L.S. (1994) A unified method for monitoring and analysing controlled trials. *Stat. Med.* **13**, 1815–1826.

Guyatt G.H., Heyting A.H., Jaeschke R. *et al.* (1990) *N* of 1 trials for investigating new drugs. *Cont. Clin. Trials* **11**, 88–100.

Hammersley J.M. and Handscomb D.C. (1964) *Monte Carlo Methods*. Methuen, London.

Harrington D., Crowley J., George S.L. *et al.* (1994) The case against independent monitoring committees. *Stat. Med.* **13**, 1411–1414.

Hastie T.J. and Tibshirani R.J. (1990) *Generalized Additive Models*. Chapman and Hall, London.

Hastings W.K. (1970) Monte Carlo sampling methods using Markov chains and their applications. *Biometrika* **57**, 97–109.

Hauck W.W. and Donner A. (1977) Wald's test as applied to hypotheses in logit analysis. *J. Am. Stat. Ass.* **72**, 851–853.

Haybittle J.L. (1971) Repeated assessment of results in clinical trials of cancer treatment. *Br. J. Radiol.* **44**, 793–797.

Hayhoe F.G.J., Quaglino D. and Doll R. (1964) *The Cytology and Cytochemistry of Acute Leukaemias.* Med. Res. Coun. Spec. Rep. Ser., No. 304, HM Stationery Office, London.

Healy M.J.R. (1952) Some statistical aspects of anthropometry (with discussion). *J. R. Stat. Soc. B* **14**, 164–177.

Healy M.J.R. (1963) Fitting a quadratic. *Biometrics* **19**, 362–363.

Healy M.J.R. (1974) Notes on the statistics of growth standards. *Ann. Hum. Biol.* **1**, 41–46.

Healy M.J.R. (1979) Some statistical paradoxes of the normal range. In *Evaluation of Efficacy of Medical Action*, eds A. Alperovitch, F.T. de Dombal and F. Grémy, pp. 509–514. North-Holland, Amsterdam.

Healy M.J.R. (1981) Some problems of repeated measurements (with discussion). In *Perspectives in Medical Statistics*, eds J.F. Bithell and R. Coppi, pp. 155–171. Academic Press, London.

Healy M.J.R. (1984) The use of R^2 as a measure of goodness of fit. *J. R. Stat. Soc. A* **147**, 608–609.

Healy M.J.R. (1988) *GLIM: an Introduction.* Clarendon Press, Oxford.

Healy M.J.R. (1989) Growth curves and growth standards—the state of the art. In *Auxology 88: Perspectives in the Science of Growth and Development*, ed. J.M. Tanner, pp. 13–21. Smith-Gordon, London.

Healy M.J.R. (2000) *Matrices for Statistics*, 2nd edn. Oxford University Press, Oxford.

Healy M.J.R., Rasbash, J. and Yang, M. (1988) Distribution-free estimation of age-related centiles. *Ann. Hum. Biol.* **15**, 17–22.

Hedges L.V. (1992) Modeling publication selection effects in meta-analysis. *Stat. Sci.* **7**, 246–255.

Heitjan D.F. (1999) Ignorability and bias in clinical trials. *Stat. Med.* **18**, 2421–2434.

Hennekens C.H., Buring J.E. and Mayrent S.L. (eds) (1987) *Epidemiology in Medicine*. Little, Brown, Boston.

Hill A.B. (1962) *Statistical Methods in Clinical and Preventive Medicine*. Livingstone, Edinburgh.

Hill A.B. and Hill I.D. (1991) *Bradford Hill's Principles of Medical Statistics*, 12th edn. Arnold, London.

Hill D.J., White V.M. and Scollo M.M. (1998) Smoking behaviours of Australian adults in 1995: trends and concerns. *Med. J. Aust.* **168**, 209–213.

Hills M. (1966) Allocation rules and their error rates. *J. R. Stat. Soc. B.* **28**, 1–20.

Hills M. and Armitage, P. (1979) The two-period cross-over clinical trial. *Br. J. Clin. Pharmacol.* **8**, 7–20.

Hirji K.F. (1991) A comparison of exact, mid-P, and score tests for matched case–control studies. *Biometrics* **47**, 487–496.

Hirji K.F., Mehta C.R. and Patel N.R. (1988) Exact inference for matched case–control studies. *Biometrics* **44**, 803–814.

Hodge S.E. (1998) Ascertainment. In *Encyclopedia of Biostatistics*, eds P. Armitage and T. Colton, pp. 197–201. Wiley, Chichester.

Hogan J.W. and Laird N.M. (1997) Mixture models for joint distribution of repeated measures and event times. *Stat. Med.* **16**, 239–257.

Holford T.R. (1976) Life tables with concomitant information. *Biometrics* **32**, 587–597.

Holford T.R. (1983) The estimation of age, period and cohort effects for vital rates. *Biometrics* **39**, 311–324.

Holford T.R. (1998) Age–period–cohort analysis. In *Encyclopedia of Biostatistics*, eds P. Armitage and T. Colton, pp. 82–99. Wiley, Chichester.

Holford T.R., Zhang Z. and McKay L.A. (1994) Estimating age, period and cohort effects using the multistage model for cancer. *Stat. Med.* **13**, 23–41.

Hopper J.L. and Mathews J.D. (1983) Extensions to multivariate normal models for pedigree analysis. II. Modeling the effect of shared environment in the analysis of variation in blood levels. *Am. J. Epidemiol.* **117**, 344–355.

Horton N.J. and Laird N.M. (1999) Maximum likelihood analysis of generalized linear models with missing covariates. *Stat. Meth. Med. Res.* **8**, 37–50.

Hosmer D.W. and Lemeshow, S. (1980) A goodness-of-fit test for the multiple logistic regression model. *Commun. Stat.* **A10**, 1043–1069.

Hosmer D.W. and Lemeshow S. (1989) *Applied Logistic Regression*. Wiley, New York.

Hsu J.C. (1996) *Multiple Comparisons: Theory and Methods*. Chapman and Hall, London.

Hui S.L. and Walter S.D. (1980) Estimating the error rates of diagnostic tests. *Biometrics* **36**, 167–171.

Huynh H. and Feldt L.S. (1976) Estimation of the Box correction for degrees of freedom for sample data in randomized block and split-plot designs. *J. Educ. Stat.* **1**, 69–82.

Ipsen J. (1955) Appropriate scores in bio-assays using death-times and survivor symptoms. *Biometrics* **11**, 465–480.

Irwig L., Turnbull D. and McMurchie M. (1990) A randomised trial of general practitioner-written invitations to encourage attendance at screening mammography. *Community Health Stud.* **14**, 357–364.

Irwig L., Glasziou P., Wilson A. and Macaskill P. (1991) Estimating an individual's true cholesterol level and response to intervention. *J. Am. Med. Ass.* **266**, 1678–1685.

ISIS-4 (Fourth International Study of Infarct Survival) Collaborative Group (1995) ISIS-4: a randomised factorial trial assessing early oral captopril, oral mononitrate, and intravenous magnesium sulphate in 58 050 patients with suspected acute myocardial infarction. *Lancet* **345**, 669–685.

James G.S. (1951) The comparison of several groups of observations when the ratios of the population variances are unknown. *Biometrika* **38**, 324–329.

Jeffreys H. (1961) *Theory of Probability*, 3rd edn. Clarendon Press, Oxford.

Jennison C. and Turnbull B.W. (2000) *Group Sequential Methods with Applications to Clinical Trials*. Chapman and Hall/CRC, Boca Raton.

Johnson M.F. (1993) Comparative efficacy of NaF and SMFP dentifrices in caries prevention: a meta-analytic overview. *Caries Res.* **27**, 328–336.

Johnson, W.D. and George V.T. (1991) Effect of regression to the mean in the presence of within-subject variability. *Stat. Med.* **10**, 1295–1302.

Jones B. and Kenward M.G. (1989) *Design and Analysis of Cross-Over Trials*. Chapman and Hall, London.

Jones D.R. (1995) Meta-analysis: weighing the evidence. *Stat. Med.* **14**, 137–149.

Jones M.C. and Rice J.A. (1992) Displaying the important features of large collections of similar curves. *Am. Stat.* **46**, 140–145.

Kadane J.B. and Wolfson L.J. (1998) Experiences in elicitation. *Statistician* **47**, 3–19.

Kalbfleisch J.D. and Prentice R.L. (1980) *The Statistical Analysis of Failure Time Data*. Wiley, New York.

Kalton G. (1968) Standardization: a technique to control for extraneous variables. *Appl. Stat.* **17**, 118–136.

Kaplan E.L. and Meier P. (1958) Nonparametric estimation from incomplete observations. *J. Am. Stat. Ass.* **53**, 457–481.

Kay R. (1977) Proportional hazard regression models and the analysis of censored survival data. *Appl. Stat.* **26**, 227–237.

Kelsey J.L., Whittemore A.S., Evans A.S. and Thompson W.D. (1996) *Methods in Observational Epidemiology*. Oxford University Press, New York.

Kendall M.G. (1951) Regression, structure and functional relationship. Part I. *Biometrika* **38**, 11–25.

Kendall M.G. (1952) Regression, structure and functional relationship. Part II. *Biometrika* **39**, 96–108.

Kendall, M.G. and Gibbons J.D. (1990) *Rank Correlation Methods*, 5th edn. Arnold, London.

Kenward M.G. (1987) A method for comparing profiles of repeated measurements. *Appl. Stat.* **36**, 296–308. Correction, **40**, 379.

Kenward M.G. (1998) Selection models for repeated measurements with non-random dropout: an illustration of sensitivity. *Stat. Med.* **17**, 2723–2732.

Kenward M.G. and Jones B. (1994) The analysis of binary and categorical data from crossover trials. *Stat. Meth. Med. Res.* **3**, 325–344.

Kenward M.G. and Molenberghs G. (1998) Likelihood based frequentist inference when data are missing at random. *Stat. Sci.* **13**, 236–247.

Kenward M.G. and Molenberghs G. (1999) Parametric models for incomplete continuous and categorical longitudinal data. *Stat. Meth. Med. Res.* **8**, 51–83.

Keuls M. (1952) The use of 'Studentized range' in connection with an analysis of variance. *Euphytica* **1**, 112–122.

Khoury M.J., Beaty T.H. and Cohen B.H. (1993) *Fundamentals of Genetic Epidemiology*. Oxford University Press, New York.

Kim K. and DeMets D.L. (1987) Design and analysis of group sequential tests based on the type I error spending rate function. *Biometrika* **74**, 149–154.

Kinmonth A.L., Woodcock A., Griffin S., Spiegal N. and Campbell M.J. (1998) Randomised controlled trial of patient centred care of diabetes in general practice: impact on current wellbeing and future risk. *Br. Med. J.* **317**, 1202–1208.

Kirkland D.J. (1989) *Statistical Evaluation of Mutagenicity Test Data*. Cambridge University Press, Cambridge.

Kittleson J.M. and Emerson S.S. (1999) A unifying family of group sequential test designs. *Biometrics* **55**, 874–882.

Klein I.P. and Moeschberger M.L. (1997) *Survival Analysis: Techniques for Censored and Truncated Data*. Springer-Verlag, New York.

Kleinbaum D.G. (1994) *Logistic Regression—A Self-Learning Text*. Springer-Verlag, New York.

Kleinbaum D.G. (1996) *Survival Analysis: A Self-Learning Text*. Springer-Verlag, New York.

Kleinbaum D.G., Kupper L.L. and Morgenstern H. (1982) *Epidemiologic Research—Principles and Quantitative Methods*. Lifetime Learning Publications, Belmont, California.

Kleinbaum D.G., Kupper L.L., Muller K.E. and Nizam A. (1998) *Applied Regression Analysis and Other Multivariable Methods*. Duxbury Press, Pacific Grove.

Klotz J.H. (1964) On the normal scores two-sample rank test. *J. Am. Stat. Ass.* **59**, 652–664.

Knox E.G. (1964) Epidemiology of childhood leukaemia in Northumberland and Durham. *Br. J. Prev. Soc. Med.* **18**, 17–24.

Koenker R. and Bassett G.S. (1978) Regression quantiles. *Econometrica* **46**, 33–50.

Koopman P.A.R. (1984) Confidence intervals for the ratio of two binomial proportions. *Biometrics* **40**, 513–517.

Kraemer H.C. (1979) Ramifications of a population model for κ as a coefficient of reliability. *Psychometrika* **44**, 461–472.

Kruskal, W.H. and Wallis W.A. (1952) Use of ranks in one-criterion variance analysis. *J. Am. Stat. Ass.* **47**, 583–621.

Krzanowski W.J. and Marriott F.H.C. (1994) *Multivariate Analysis*: Part I. *Distributions, Ordination and Inference*. Arnold, London.

Krzanowski W.J. and Marriott F.H.C. (1995) *Multivariate Analysis*: Part 2. *Classification, Covariance Structures and Repeated Measurements*. Arnold, London.

Kupper L.L., McMichael A.J. and Spirtas R. (1975) A hybrid epidemiologic study design useful in estimating relative risk. *J. Am. Stat. Ass.* **70**, 524–528.

Kuritz S.J. and Landis J.R. (1988) Attributable risk estimation from matched case–control data. *Biometrics* **44**, 355–367.

Kuritz S.J., Landis J.R. and Koch G.G. (1988) A general overview of Mantel–Haenszel methods: applications and recent developments. *Ann. Rev. Public Health* **9**, 123–160.

Lachin J.M. (1998) Sample size determination. In *Encyclopedia of Biostatistics*, eds P. Armitage and T. Colton, pp. 3892–3902. Wiley, Chichester.

Lachs M.S., Nachamkin I., Edelstein P.H. *et al.* (1992) Spectrum bias in the evaluation of diagnostic tests: lessons from the rapid dipstick test for urinary tract infection. *Ann. Int. Med.* **117**, 135–140.

Laird N.M. and Ware J.H. (1982) Random-effects models for longitudinal data. *Biometrics* **38**, 963–974.

Lan K.K.G. and DeMets D.L. (1983) Discrete sequential boundaries for clinical trials. *Biometrika* **70**, 659–663.

Lan K.K.G., Simon R. and Halperin M. (1982) Stochastically curtailed tests in long-term clinical trials. *Commun. Stat.* **C1**, 207–219.

Lancaster H.O. (1950) Statistical control in haematology. *J. Hyg., Camb.* **48**, 402–417.

Lancaster H.O. (1952) Statistical control of counting experiments. *Biometrika* **39**, 419–422.

Lancaster H.O. (1961) Significance tests in discrete distributions. *J. Am. Stat. Ass.* **56**, 223–234.

Lancaster H.O. (1965) Symmetry in multivariate distributions. *Aust. J. Stat.* **7**, 115–126.

Landis J.R. and Koch G.G. (1977) The measurement of observer agreement for categorical data. *Biometrics* **33**, 159–174.

Last J.M. (1995) *A Dictionary of Epidemiology*. Oxford University Press, Oxford.

Lauritzen S.L. (1996) *Graphical Models*. Oxford University Press, Oxford.

Lawless J.F. (1982) *Statistical Models and Methods for Lifetime Data*. Wiley, New York.

Lawley, D.N. and Maxwell A.E. (1971) *Factor Analysis as a Statistical Method*, 2nd edn. Butterworths, London.

Lee P.M. (1997) *Bayesian Statistics: an Introduction*, 2nd edn. Arnold, London.

Lefkovits I. and Waldmann H. (1999) *Limiting Dilution Analysis of Cells in the Immune System*, 2nd edn. Oxford University Press, Oxford.

Lehmann E.L. (1975) *Nonparametrics: Statistical Methods Based on Ranks*. Holden-Day, San Francisco.

Lemeshow S. and Hosmer D.W. (1982) A review of goodness of fit statistics for use in the development of logistic regression models. *Am. J. Epidemiol.* **115**, 92–106.

Lemeshow S., Hosmer D.W., Klar, J. and Lwanga S.K. (1990) *Adequacy of Sample Size in Health Studies*. Wiley, Chichester.

Lesaffre E. and Pledger G. (1999) A note on the number needed to treat. *Cont. Clin. Trials* **20**, 439–447.

Levene H. (1960) Robust tests for equality of variances. In *Contributions to Probability and Statistics—Essays in Honor of Harold Hotelling*, eds I. Olkin, S.G. Ghurye, W. Hoeffding, W.G. Madow and H.B. Mann, pp. 278–292. Stanford University Press, Stanford, California.

Levin M.L. (1953) The occurrence of lung cancer in man. *Acta Un. Int. Cancer* **9**, 531–541.

Levy P.S. and Lemeshow S. (1991) *Sampling of Populations: Methods and Applications*. Wiley, New York.

Liang K.-Y. and Zeger S.L. (1986) Longitudinal data analysis using generalized linear models. *Biometrika* **73**, 13–22.

Liang K.-Y., Zeger S.L. and Qaqish B. (1992) Multivariate regression analyses for categorical data (with discussion). *J. R. Stat. Soc. B* **54**, 3–40.

Liddell F.D.K. (1960) The measurement of occupational mortality. *Br. J. Ind. Med.* **17**, 228–233.

Liddell F.D.K. (1983) Simplified exact analysis of case–reference studies: matched pairs; dichotomous exposure. *J. Epidemiol. Community Health* **37**, 82–84.

Liddell F.D.K. (1984) Simple exact analysis of the standardized mortality ratio. *J. Epidemiol. Community Health* **38**, 85–88.

Liddell F.D.K. (1988) The development of cohort studies in epidemiology: a review. *J. Clin. Epidemiol.* **41**, 1217–1237.

Liddell F.D.K., McDonald J.C. and Thomas D.C. (1977) Methods of cohort analysis: appraisal by application to asbestos mining (with discussion). *J. R. Stat. Soc. A* **140**, 469–491.

Liddell F.D.K., Thomas D.C., Gibbs G.W. and McDonald J.C. (1984) Fibre exposure and mortality from pneumoconiosis, respiratory and abdominal malignancies in chrysotile production in Quebec, 1926–75. *Ann. Acad. Med.* **13** (Suppl.), 340–342.

Lin L.I.-K. (1992) Assay validation using the concordance correlation coefficient. *Biometrics* **48**, 599–604.

Lindley D.V. (1957) A statistical paradox. *Biometrika* **44**, 187–192.

Lindley D.V. (1965) *Introduction to Probability and Statistics from a Bayesian Viewpoint*. Part 1, *Probability*. Part 2, *Inference*. Cambridge University Press, Cambridge.

Lindley D.V. (1997) The choice of sample size. *Statistician* **46**, 129–138.

Lindley D.V. (2000) The philosophy of statistics (with comments). *Statistician* **49**, 293–337.

Little R.J.A. (1976) Inference about means for incomplete multivariate data. *Biometrika* **63**, 593–604.

Little R.J.A. (1993) Pattern-mixture models for multivariate incomplete data. *J. Am. Stat. Ass.* **88**, 125–134.

Little R.J.A. and Pullum T.W. (1979) The general linear model and direct standardization—a comparison. *Sociol. Meth. Res.* **7**, 475–501.

Little R.J.A. and Rubin D.B. (1987) *Statistical Analysis with Missing Data*. Wiley, Chichester.

Lloyd S. and Roberts C.J. (1973) A test for space clustering and its application to congenital limb defects in Cardiff. *Br. J. Prev. Soc. Med.* **27**, 188–191.

Lombard H.L. and Doering C.R. (1947) Treatment of the four-fold table by partial correlation as it relates to public health problems. *Biometrics* **3**, 123–128.

McCrory J.W. and Matthews J.N.S. (1990) A comparison of four methods of pre-oxygenation. *Br. J. Anaes.* **64**, 571–576.

McCullagh P. and Nelder J.A. (1989) *Generalized Linear Models*, 2nd edn. Chapman and Hall, London.

McDonald C.J., Mazzuca S.A. and McCabe G.P. (1983) How much of the placebo 'effect' is really statistical regression? *Stat. Med.* **2**, 417–427.

McGilchrist C.A. and Aisbett C.W. (1991) Regression with frailty in survival analysis. *Biometrics* **47**, 461–466.

McKelvey M., Gottlieb J.A., Wilson H.E. *et al.* (1976) Hydroxyldaunomycin (Adriamycin) combination chemotherapy in malignant lymphoma. *Cancer* **38**, 1484–1493.

MacKenzie L.A. (1983) The analysis of the ultra-violet radiation doses required to produce erythemal responses in normal skin. *Br. J. Dermatol.* **108**, 1–9.

MacKie R., Hunter J.A.A., Aitchison T.C. *et al.* for the Scottish Melanoma Group (1992) Cutaneous malignant melanoma, Scotland, 1979–89. *Lancet* **339**, 971–975.

McPherson C.K. (1971) *Some problems in sequential experimentation.* PhD thesis, University of London.

Machin D. and Gardner M.J. (1989) Calculating confidence intervals for survival time analyses. In *Statistics with Confidence—Confidence Intervals and Statistical Guidelines*, eds M.J. Gardner and D.G. Altman, pp. 64–70. British Medical Journal, London.

Machin D., Campbell M.J., Fayers P.M. and Pinol A.P.Y. (1997) *Sample Size Tables for Clinical Studies*, 2nd edn. Blackwell, Oxford.

Macklin J. (1990) *Setting the Agenda for Change.* Background paper no. 1, National Health Strategy, Melbourne.

Manly B.F.J. (1994) *Multivariate Statistical Methods—A Primer.* Chapman and Hall, London.

Mantel N. (1963) Chi-square tests with one degree of freedom: extensions of the Mantel–Haenszel procedure. *J. Am. Stat. Ass.* **58**, 690–700.

Mantel N. (1966) Evaluation of survival data and two new rank order statistics arising in its consideration. *Cancer Chemother. Rep.* **50**, 163–170.

Mantel N. (1967) The detection of disease clustering and a generalized regression approach. *Cancer Res.* **27**, 209–220.

Mantel N. (1973) Synthetic retrospective studies and related topics. *Biometrics* **29**, 479–486.

Mantel N. and Haenszel W. (1959) Statistical aspects of the analysis of data from retrospective studies of disease. *J. Nat. Cancer Inst.* **22**, 719–748.

Mardia K.V., Kent J.T. and Bibby J.M. (1979) *Multivariate Analysis.* Academic Press, London.

Margolin B.H., Kaplan N. and Zeiger E. (1981) Statistical analysis of the Ames *Salmonella/* microsome test. *Proc. Nat. Acad. Sci.* **78**, 3779–3783.

Marks R.G. (1982) Measuring the correlation between time series of hormonal data. *Stat. Med.* **1**, 49–57.

Marriott F.H.C. (1974) *The Interpretation of Multiple Observations.* Academic Press, London.

Marshall R.J. (1991) Mapping disease and mortality rates using empirical Bayes estimators. *Appl. Stat.* **40**, 283–294.

Martin M.A. and Welsh A.H. (1998) Graphical displays. In *Encyclopedia of Biostatistics*, eds P. Armitage and T. Colton, pp. 1750–1771. Wiley, Chichester.

Martin W.J. (1949) *The Physique of Young Adult Males.* Med. Res. Coun. Mem., No. 20, HM Stationery Office, London.

Martuzzi M. and Elliott P. (1996) Empirical Bayes estimation of small area prevalence of non-rare conditions. *Stat. Med.* **15**, 1867–1873.

Marubini E. and Valsecchi M.G. (1995) *Analysing Survival Data from Clinical Trials and Observational Studies.* Wiley, Chichester.

Matthews J.N.S. (1994) Multi-period crossover trials. *Stat. Meth. Med. Res.* **3**, 383–405.

Matthews J.N.S. (1998) Time-by-time analysis of longitudinal data. In *Encyclopedia of Biostatistics*, eds P. Armitage and T. Colton, pp. 4522–4523. Wiley, Chichester.

Matthews J.N.S. (2000) *Randomized Controlled Clinical Trials: An Introduction for Statisticians.* Arnold, London.

Matthews J.N.S., Altman D.G., Campbell M.J. and Royston, P. (1990) Analysis of serial measurements in medical research. *Br. Med. J.* **300**, 230–255.

Matthews J.N.S., Matthews D.S.F. and Eyre J.A. (1999) A statistical method for the estimation of cerebral blood flow using the Kety–Schmidt technique. *Clin. Sci.* **97**, 485–492.

Medical Research Council (1948) Streptomycin treatment of pulmonary tuberculosis. *Br. Med. J.* **ii**, 769–782.

Medical Research Council (1950) Treatment of pulmonary tuberculosis with streptomycin and para-amino-salicylic acid. *Br. Med. J.* **ii**, 1073–1085.

Medical Research Council (1951) The prevention of whooping-cough by vaccination: a report of the Whooping-Cough Immunization Committee. *Br. Med. J.* **i**, 1463–1471.

Mehrabi Y. and Matthews J.N.S. (1995) Likelihood-based methods for bias reduction in limiting dilution assays. *Biometrics* **51**, 1543–1549.

Mehrabi Y. and Matthews J.N.S. (1998) Implementable Bayesian designs for limiting dilution assays. *Biometrics* **54**, 1398–1406.

Mehta C.R. (1994) The exact analysis of contingency tables in medical research. *Stat. Meth. Med. Res.* **3**, 135–156.

Mehta C.R. and Patel N.R. (1983) A network algorithm for performing Fisher's exact test in r × c contingency tables. *J. Am. Stat. Ass.* **78**, 427–434.

Mehta C.R. and Patel N.R. (1995) Exact logistic regression: theory and examples. *Stat. Med.* **14**, 2143–2160.

Mehta C.R. and Patel N.R. (1998) Exact inference for categorical data. In *Encyclopedia of Biostatistics*, eds P. Armitage and T. Colton, pp. 1411–1422. Wiley, Chichester.

Mehta C.R., Patel N.R. and Gray, R. (1985) Computing an exact confidence interval for the common odds ratio in several 2 by 2 contingency tables. *J. Am. Stat. Ass.* **80**, 969–973.

Mehta C.R., Patel N.R. and Senchaudhuri P. (1988) Importance sampling for estimating exact probabilities in permutational inference. *J. Am. Stat. Ass.* **83**, 999–1005.

Meier P. (1975) Statistics and medical experimentation. *Biometrics* **31**, 511–529.

Meinert C.L. (1986) *Clinical Trials: Design, Conduct, and Analysis.* Oxford University Press, Oxford.

Meinert C.L. (1998) Clinical trials and treatment effects monitoring. *Cont. Clin. Trials* **19**, 515–522.

Merrell M. and Shulman L.E. (1955) Determination of prognosis in chronic disease, illustrated by systemic lupus erythematosus. *J. Chron. Dis.* **1**, 12–32.

Metropolis N., Rosenbluth A.W., Rosenbluth M.N., Teller A.H. and Teller E. (1953) Equations of state calculations by fast computing machine. *J. Chem. Phys.* **21**, 1087–1091.

Miettinen O. and Nurminen M. (1985) Comparative analysis of two rates. *Stat. Med.* **4**, 213–226.

Miettinen O.S. (1969) Individual matching with multiple controls in the case of all-or-none responses. *Biometrics* **25**, 339–355.

Miettinen O.S. (1970) Estimation of relative risk from individually matched series. *Biometrics* **26**, 75–86.

Miettinen O.S. (1976) Estimability and estimation in case–referent studies. *Am. J. Epidemiol.* **103**, 226–235.

Miettinen O.S. (1985) *Theoretical Epidemiology: Principles of Occurrence Research in Medicine.* Wiley, New York.

Miller R.G. (1974) The jackknife—a review. *Biometrika* **61**, 1–15.

Miller R.G. Jr (1981) *Simultaneous Statistical Inference*, 2nd edn. Springer-Verlag, New York.

Minitab (2000) *MINITAB 13*. www.minitab.com

Mitchell J. and Mackerras D. (1995) The traditional humoral food habits of pregnant Vietnamese-Australian women and their effect on birth weight. *Aust. J. Public Health* **19**, 629–633.

Molenberghs G., Michiels B., Kenward M.G. and Diggle P.J. (1998) Monotone missing data and pattern-mixture models. *Stat. Neerland.* **52**, 153–161.

Moons K.G., van Es G.A., Deckers J.W., Habbema J.D. and Grobbee D.E. (1997) Limitations of sensitivity, specificity, likelihood ratio, and Bayes' theorem in assessing diagnostic probabilities: a clinical example. *Epidemiology* **8**, 12–17.

Morrison D.F. (1976) *Multivariate Statistical Methods*, 2nd edn. McGraw-Hill, New York.

Moser C. and Kalton G. (1979) *Survey Methods in Social Investigation*, 2nd edn. Gower, Aldershot.

MPS Research Unit (2000) *Pest 4: Operating Manual.* University of Reading, Reading.

MRC Vitamin Study Research Group (1991) Prevention of neural tube defects: results of the Medical Research Council Vitamin Study. *Lancet* **338**, 131–137.

Murdoch J. and Barnes J.A. (1968) *Statistical Tables for Science, Engineering and Management.* Macmillan, London.

Murray D.M. (1998) *Design and Analysis of Group-Randomized Trials.* Oxford University Press, Oxford.

Naylor A.F. (1964) Comparisons of regression constants fitted by maximum likelihood to four common transformations of binomial data. *Ann. Hum. Genet.* **27**, 241–246.

Naylor J.C. and Smith A.F.M. (1982) Applications of a method for the efficient computation of posterior distributions. *Appl. Stat.* **31**, 214–235.

Nelder J.A. (1991) Generalized linear models for enzyme-kinetic data. *Biometrics* **47**, 1605–1615.

Nelder J.A. and Wedderburn R.W.M. (1972) Generalized linear models. *J. R. Stat. Soc. A* **135**, 370–384.

Newcombe R.G. (1998a) Two-sided confidence intervals for the single proportion: comparison of seven methods. *Stat. Med.* **17**, 857–872.

Newcombe R.G. (1998b) Interval estimation for the difference between independent proportions: comparison of eleven methods. *Stat. Med.* **17**, 873–890.

Newcombe R.G. (1998c) Improved confidence intervals for the difference between binomial proportions based on paired data. *Stat. Med.* **17**, 2635–2650.

Newell D. and Simpson J. (1990) Regression to the mean. *Med. J. Aust.* **153**, 51–53.

Newell D.J. (1962) Errors in the interpretation of errors in epidemiology. *Am. J. Public Health* **52**, 1925–1928.

Newell D.J., Greenberg B.G., Williams T.F. and Veazey P.B. (1961) Use of cohort life tables in family studies of disease. *J. Chron. Dis.* **13**, 439–452.

Newey W.K. and Powell J.L. (1987) Asymmetric least square estimation and testing. *Econometrica* **55**, 819–847.

Newhouse M.L., Berry G. and Wagner J.C. (1985) Mortality of factory workers in east London 1933–80. *Br. J. Ind. Med.* **42**, 4–11.

Newman D. (1939) The distribution of range in samples from a normal population, expressed in terms of an independent estimate of standard deviation. *Biometrika* **31**, 20–30.

Normand S.T. (1999) Meta-analysis: formulating, evaluating, combining, and reporting. *Stat. Med.* **18**, 321–359.

O'Brien P.C. and Fleming T.R. (1979) A multiple testing procedure for clinical trials. *Biometrics* **35**, 549–556.

O'Hagan A. (1994) *Kendall's Advanced Theory of Statistics*: Vol. 2B, *Bayesian Inference*. Arnold, London.

Oldham P.D. (1968) *Measurement in Medicine: the Interpretation of Numerical Data*. English Universities Press, London.

Olschewski M. (1998) Quality of life and survival analysis. In *Encyclopedia of Biostatistics*, eds P. Armitage and T. Colton, pp. 3613–3618. Wiley, Chichester.

O'Quigley J., Pepe M. and Fisher L. (1990) Continual reassessment method: a practical design for phase I clinical trials in cancer. *Biometrics* **46**, 33–48.

O'Rourke P.P., Crone R.K., Vacanti J.P. *et al.* (1989) Extracorporeal membrane oxygenation and conventional medical therapy in neonates with persistent pulmonary hypertension of the newborn: a prospective randomized study. *Pediatrics* **84**, 957–963.

O'Sullivan M.C., Eyre J.A. and Miller S. (1991) Radiation of phasic stretch reflex in biceps brachii to muscles of the arm and its restriction during development. *J. Physiol.* **439**, 529–543.

Ott J. (1999) *Analysis of Human Genetic Linkage*. Johns Hopkins University Press, Baltimore.

Pan H.Q., Goldstein H. and Yang Q. (1990) Nonparametric estimation of age-related centiles over wide age ranges. *Ann. Hum. Biol.* **17**, 475–481.

Parker R.A. and Bregman D.J. (1986) Sample size for individually matched case–control studies. *Biometrics* **42**, 919–926.

Parmar M.K.B. and Machin D. (1995) *Survival Analysis: a Practical Approach*. Wiley, Chichester.

Parmar M.K.B., Spiegelhalter D.J. and Freedman L.S. (1994) The CHART trials: Bayesian design and monitoring in practice. *Stat. Med.* **13**, 1297–1312.

Patterson H.D. and Thompson R. (1971) Recovery of interblock information when blocks sizes are unequal. *Biometrika* **58**, 545–554.

Pauker S.G. and Kassirer J.P. (1992) Decision analysis. In *Medical Uses of Statistics*, 2nd edn., eds J.C. Bailar III and F. Mosteller, pp. 159–179. NEJM Books, Boston.

Pearce S.C. (1965) *Biological Statistics: an Introduction*. McGraw-Hill, New York.

Pearce S.C. (1983) *The Agricultural Field Experiment*. Wiley, Chichester.

Pearson E.S. and Hartley H.O. (1966) *Biometrika Tables for Statisticians*, Vol. 1, 3rd edn. Cambridge University Press, Cambridge.

Peirce C.S. and Jastrow J. (1885) On small differences of sensation. *Mem. Nat. Acad. Sci. for 1884* **3**, 75–83.

Peto R. (1974) Guidelines on the analysis of tumour rates and death rates in experimental animals. *Br. J. Cancer* **29**, 101–105.

Peto R. and Pike M.C. (1973) Conservatism of the approximation $\sum (O - E)^2/E$ in the logrank test for survival data or tumor incidence data. *Biometrics* **29**, 579–584.

Peto R., Pike M.C., Armitage P. *et al.* (1976, 1977) Design and analysis of randomized clinical trials requiring prolonged observation of each patient. I. Introduction and design. *Br. J. Cancer* **34**, 585–612. II. Analysis and examples. *Br. J. Cancer* **35**, 1–39.

Peto R., Pike M., Day N. *et al.* (1980) Guidelines for simple, sensitive significance test for carcinogenic effects in long-term animal experiments. In *Long-term and Short-term Screening Assays for Carcinogens: A Critical Appraisal,* IARC Monographs Supplement 2, Annex, International Agency for Research on Cancer, Lyon: pp. 311–426.

Peto R., Collins R. and Gray R. (1995) Large-scale randomized evidence: large, simple trials and overviews of trials. *J. Clin. Epidemiol.* **48**, 23–40.

Piantadosi S. (1997) *Clinical Trials: A Methodologic Perspective.* Wiley, New York.

Piegorsch, W.W. (1998) Mutagenicity study. In *Encyclopedia of Biostatistics,* eds. P. Armitage and T. Colton, pp. 2938–2943. Wiley, Chichester.

Pike M.C. (1966) A method of analysis of a certain class of experiments in carcinogenesis. *Biometrics* **22**, 142–161.

Pike M.C. and Morrow R.H. (1970) Statistical analysis of patient–control studies in epidemiology—factor under investigation an all-or-none variable. *Br. J. Prev. Soc. Med.* **24**, 42–44.

Pike M.C. and Smith P.G. (1968) Disease clustering: a generalization of Knox's approach to the detection of space–time interactions. *Biometrics* **24**, 541–556.

Pocock S.J. (1974) Harmonic analysis applied to seasonal variations in sickness absence. *Appl. Stat.* **23**, 103–120.

Pocock S.J. (1977) Group sequential methods in the design and analysis of clinical trials. *Biometrika* **64**, 191–199.

Pocock S.J. (1983) *Clinical Trials: A Practical Approach.* Wiley, Chichester.

Pocock S.J. and Abdalla M. (1998) The hope and hazards of using compliance data in randomized controlled trials. *Stat. Med.* **17**, 303–317.

Pocock S.J., Armitage P. and Galton D.A.G. (1978) The size of cancer clinical trials: an international survey. *UICC Tech. Rep. Ser.* **36**, 5–32.

Powell-Tuck J., MacRae K.D., Healy M.J.R., Lennard-Jones J.E. and Parkins R.A. (1986) A defence of the small clinical trial: evaluation of three gastroenterological studies. *Br. Med. J.* **292**, 599–602.

Pregibon D. (1980) Goodness of link tests for generalized linear models. *Appl. Stat.* **29**, 15–24.

Pregibon D. (1981) Logistic regression diagnostics. *Ann. Stat.* **9**, 705–724.

Prentice R.L. (1978) Linear rank tests with right censored data. *Biometrika* **65**, 167–179.

Prentice R.L. (1986) A case–cohort design for epidemiologic cohort studies and disease prevention trials. *Biometrika* **73**, 1–11.

Prentice R.L. (1989) Surrogate endpoints in clinical trials: definition and operational criteria. *Stat. Med.* **8**, 431–440.

Proskin H.M. (1993) Statistical considerations related to a meta-analytic evaluation of published caries clinical studies comparing the anticaries efficacy of dentifrices containing sodium fluoride and sodium monofluorophosphate. *Am. J. Dent.* **6** (Special issue), S44–S49.

Quenouille M.H. (1949) Approximate tests of correlation in time-series. *J. R. Stat. Soc. B* **11**, 68–84.

Radhakrishna S. (1965) Combination of results from several 2×2 contingency tables. *Biometrics* **21**, 86–98.

Raftery A.E. and Lewis S.M. (1992) How many iterations in the Gibbs sampler? In *Bayesian Statistics 4,* eds J.M. Bernardo J.O. Berger, A.P. Dawid and A.F.M. Smith, pp. 765–776. Oxford University Press, Oxford.

Raftery A.E. and Lewis S.M. (1996) Implementing MCMC. In *Markov Chain Monte Carlo in Practice,* eds W.R. Gilks, S. Richardson and D.J. Spiegelhalter, pp. 115–130. Chapman and Hall, London.

Räisänen M.J., Virkkunen M., Huttunen M.O., Furman B. and Kärkkäinen J. (1984) Letter to the Editor. *Lancet* **ii**, 700–701.

Ratkowsky D.A., Evans M.A. and Alldredge J.R. (1993) *Cross-over Experiments: Design, Analysis and Application.* Dekker, New York.

Raubertas R.F. (1988) Spatial and temporal analysis of disease occurrence for detection of clustering. *Biometrics* **44**, 1121–1129.

Registrar General of England and Wales (1958) *Decennial Supplement. Occupational Mortality,* Part II, Vol. 2. *Tables.* HM Stationery Office, London.

Reinsch C. (1967) Smoothing by spline functions. *Numer. Math.* **10**, 177–183.

Ridout M.S. (1995) Three-stage designs for seed testing experiments. *Appl. Stat.* **44**, 153–162.

Roberts E., Dawson W.M. and Madden M. (1939) Observed and theoretical ratios in Mendelian inheritance. *Biometrika* **31**, 56–66.

Roberts G.O. (1996) Markov chain concepts related to sampling algorithms. In *Markov Chain Monte Carlo in Practice*, eds W.R. Gilks, S. Richardson and D.J. Spiegelhalter, pp. 45–57. Chapman and Hall, London.

Roberts G.O. and Smith A.F.M. (1994) Simple conditions for the convergence of the Gibbs sampler and Hastings–Metropolis algorithms. *Stoch. Proc. Appl.* **49**, 207–216.

Robertson J.D. and Armitage P. (1959) Comparison of two hypotensive agents. *Anaesthesia* **14**, 53–64.

Robins J.M., Breslow N.E. and Greenland S. (1986) Estimators of the Mantel–Haenszel variance consistent in both sparse data and large-strata limiting models. *Biometrics* **42**, 311–323.

Robins J.M., Prentice R.L. and Blevins D. (1989) Designs for synthetic case–control studies in open cohorts. *Biometrics* **45**, 1103–1116.

Robinson G.K. (1991) That BLUP is a good thing: the estimation of random effects. *Stat. Sci.* **6**, 15–51.

Robinson G.K. (1998) Variance components. In *Encyclopedia of Biostatistics*, eds P. Armitage and T. Colton, pp. 4713–4719. Wiley, Chichester.

Rose G.A. (1962) A study of blood pressure among Negro schoolchildren. *J. Chron. Dis.* **15**, 373–380.

Rothman K. (1978) A show of confidence. *N. Engl. J. Med.* **299**, 1362–1363.

Rothman K.J. and Greenland S. (1998) *Modern Epidemiology*, 2nd edn. Lippincott-Raven, Philadelphia.

Rowlands R.J., Griffiths K., Kemp K.W. *et al.* (1983) Application of cusum techniques to the routine monitoring of analytical performance in clinical laboratories. *Stat. Med.* **2**, 141–145.

Royall R.M. (1986) Model robust confidence intervals using maximum likelihood estimators. *Int. Stat. Rev.* **54**, 221–226.

Royston P. (1992) Approximating the Shapiro–Wilk W-test for non-normality. *Stat. Comp.* **2**, 117–119.

Royston P. and Altman D.G. (1994) Regression using fractional polynomials of continuous covariates: parsimonious parametric modelling (with discussion). *Appl. Stat.* **43**, 429–467.

Royston P. and Thompson S.G. (1995) Comparing non-nested regression models. *Biometrics* **51**, 114–127.

Royston P. and Wright E.M. (1998) A method for estimating age-specific reference intervals ('normal ranges') based on fractional polynomials and exponential transformation. *J. R. Stat. Soc. A* **161**, 79–101.

Rubin D.B. (1976) Inference and missing data. *Biometrika* **63**, 581–592.

Rubin D.B. (1984) Bayesianly justifiable and relevant frequency calculations for the applied statistician. *Ann. Stat.* **12**, 1151–1172.

Rubin D.B. (1987) *Multiple Imputation for Non-response in Surveys*. Wiley, Chichester.

Ruppert D., Cressie N. and Carroll R.J. (1989) A transformation/weighting model for estimating Michaelis–Menten parameters. *Biometrics* **45**, 637–656.

Sackett D.L., Rosenberg W.M.C., Gray J.A.M. and Richardson, W.S. (1996) Evidence based medicine: what it is and what it isn't. *Br. Med. J.* **312**, 71–72.

Sarkar S.K. and Chang C.-K. (1997) The Simes method for multiple hypothesis testing with positively dependent test statistics. *J. Am. Stat. Ass.* **92**, 1601–1608.

SAS (2000) *SAS, Version 8*. www.sas.com

Sasco A.J., Day N.E. and Walter S.D. (1986) Case–control studies for the evaluation of screening. *J. Chron. Dis.* **39**, 399–405.

Satterthwaite F.E. (1946) An approximate distribution of estimates of variance components. *Biometrics Bull.* **2**, 110–114.

Savage L.J. (1954) *The Foundations of Statistics*. Wiley, New York.

Schafer J.L. (1997) *Analysis of Incomplete Multivariate Data*. Chapman and Hall, London.

Schafer J.L. (1999) Multiple imputation: a primer. *Stat. Meth. Med. Res.* **8**, 3–15.

Scheffé H. (1959) *The Analysis of Variance*. Wiley, New York.

Schlesselman J.J. (1982) *Case–Control Studies: Design, Conduct, Analysis*. Wiley, New York.

Schneiderman M.A. and Armitage, P. (1962) A family of closed sequential procedures. *Biometrika* **49**, 41–56.

Schwartz D. and Lellouch J. (1967) Explanatory and pragmatic attitudes in therapeutic trials. *J. Chron. Dis.* **20**, 637–648.

Schwartz D., Flamant R. and Lellouch, J. (1980) *Clinical Trials* (trans. M.J.R. Healy), Academic Press, London.

Schwarz G. (1978) Estimating the dimension of a model. *Ann. Stat.* **6**, 461–464.

Scott J.E.S., Hunter E.W., Lee R.E.J. and Matthews J.N.S. (1990) Ultrasound measurement of renal size in newborn infants. *Arch. Dis. Child.* **65**, 361–364.

Searle S.R. (1987) *Linear Models for Unbalanced Data.* Wiley, New York.

Seber G.A.F. (1982) *The Estimation of Animal Abundance and Related Parameters.* Griffin, London.

Seber G.A.F. and Wild, C.J. (1989) *Nonlinear Regression.* Wiley, Chichester.

Senn S. (1993) *Cross-over Trials in Clinical Research.* Wiley, Chichester.

Senn S. (1997) *Statistical Issues in Drug Development.* Wiley, Chichester.

Senn S. (1998) Crossover designs. In *Encyclopedia of Biostatistics*, eds P. Armitage and T. Colton, pp. 1033–1049. Wiley, Chichester.

Senn S.J. (1988) How much of the placebo 'effect' is really statistical regression? (letter). *Stat. Med.* **7**, 1203.

Shafer G. (1982) Lindley's paradox (with discussion). *J. Am. Stat. Ass.* **77**, 325–351.

Shapiro S.H. and Louis T.A. (eds) (1983) *Clinical Trials: Issues and Approaches.* Dekker, New York.

Shapiro S.S. and Wilk M.B. (1965) An analysis of variance test for normality (complete samples). *Biometrika* **52**, 591–611.

Shoukri M.M. (1998) Measurement of agreement. In *Encyclopedia of Biostatistics*, eds P. Armitage and T. Colton, pp. 103–117. Wiley, Chichester.

Siegel S. and Castellan N.J., Jr (1988) *Nonparametric Statistics for the Behavioral Sciences*, 2nd edn. McGraw-Hill, New York.

Silverman B.W. (1984) Spline smoothing: the equivalent variable kernel method. *Ann. Stat.* **12**, 898–916.

Silverman B.W. (1986) *Density Estimation for Statistics and Data Analysis.* Chapman and Hall, London.

Simes R.J. (1986a) An improved Bonferroni procedure for multiple tests of significance. *Biometrika* **73**, 751–754.

Simes R.J. (1986b) Publication bias: the case for an international registry of clinical trials. *J. Clin. Oncol.* **4**, 1529–1541.

Simon R. and Thall, P.F. (1998) Phase II trials. In *Encyclopedia of Biostatistics*, eds P. Armitage and T. Colton, pp. 3370–3376. Wiley, Chichester.

Simons L.A., Friedlander Y., McCallum J. *et al.* (1991) The Dubbo study of the health of elderly: correlates of coronary heart disease at study entry. *J. Am. Geriatr. Soc.* **39**, 584–590.

Simpson D.G. and Margolin B.H. (1986) Recursive nonparametric testing for dose–response relationships subject to downturns at high doses. *Biometrika* **73**, 589–596.

Smith A.F.M., West M., Gordon K., Knapp M.S. and Trimble I.M.G. (1983) Monitoring kidney transplant patients. *Statistician* **32**, 46–54.

Smith P.G. (1982) Spatial and temporal clustering. In *Cancer Epidemiology and Prevention*, eds D. Schottenfeld and J.F. Fraumeni, pp. 391–407. Saunders, Philadelphia.

Smith P.G. and Pike M.C. (1974) A note on a 'close pairs' test for space clustering. *Br. J. Prev. Soc. Med.* **28**, 63–64.

Smith T.C., Spiegelhalter D.J. and Thomas A. (1995) Bayesian approaches to random-effects meta-analysis: a comparative study. *Stat. Med.* **14**, 2685–2699.

Sneath P.H.A. and Sokal R.R. (1973) *Numerical Taxonomy.* Freeman, San Francisco.

Snedecor G.W. and Cochran W.G. (1989) *Statistical Methods*, 8th edn. Iowa State University Press, Ames.

Solomon P.J. (1984) Effect of misspecification of regression models in the analysis of survival data. *Biometrika* **71**, 291–298. Correction, **73**, 245.

Sommer A. and Zeger S.L. (1991) On estimating efficacy from clinical trials. *Stat. Med.* **10**, 45–52.

Sommer A., Tarwotjo I., Djunaedi E. *et al.* (1986) Impact of vitamin A supplementation on childhood mortality: a randomized controlled community trial. *Lancet* **i**, 1169–1173.

Spiegelhalter D.J. and Freedman L.S. (1986) A predictive approach to selecting the size of a clinical trial, based on subjective clinical opinion. *Stat. Med.* **5**, 1–13.

Spiegelhalter D.J. and Freedman L.S. (1988) Bayesian approaches to clinical trials (with discussion). In *Bayesian Statistics, 3*, eds J.M. Bernado, M.H. DeGroot, D.V. Lindley and A.F.M. Smith, pp. 453–477. Oxford University Press, Oxford.

Spiegelhalter D.J. and Knill-Jones R.P. (1984) Statistical and knowledge-based approaches to clinical decision-support systems, with an application to gastroenterology (with discussion). *J. R. Stat. Soc. A* **147**, 35–76.

Spiegelhalter D.J., Dawid A.P., Lauritzen S.L. and Cowell R.G. (1993) Bayesian analysis in expert systems. *Stat. Sci.* **8**, 219–283.

Spiegelhalter D.J., Freedman L.S. and Parmar M.K.B. (1994) Bayesian approaches to randomized trials (with discussion). *J. R. Stat. Soc. A* **157**, 357–416.

Spiegelhalter D.J., Best N.G., Gilks W.R. and Inskip H. (1996) Hepatitis B: a case study in MCMC methods. In *Markov Chain Monte Carlo in Practice*, eds W.R. Gilks, S. Richardson and D.J. Spiegelhalter, pp. 21–43. Chapman and Hall, London.

Spiegelhalter D.J., Myles J.P., Jones D.R. and Abrams K.R. (1999) An introduction to Bayesian methods in health technology assessment. *Br. Med. J.* **319**, 508–512.

Spiegelhalter D.J., Thomas A. and Best N. (2000) *WinBUGS Version 1.3 User Manual*. MRC Biostatistics Unit, Cambridge.

Spitzer W.O. (ed) (1995) The Potsdam International Consultation on Meta-analysis. *J. Clin. Epidemiol.* **48**, 1–171.

Sprent P. (1969) *Models in Regression and Related Topics*. Methuen, London.

Sprent P. and Dolby G.R. (1980) The geometric mean functional relationship. *Biometrics* **36**, 547–550.

Sprent P. and Smeeton N.C. (2001) *Applied Nonparametric Statistical Methods*, 3rd edn. Chapman and Hall / CRC Boca Raton.

S-PLUS (2000) *S-PLUS 6*. www.mathsoft.com

SPSS (1999) *SPSS10*. www.spss.com/spss10

Stata (2001) *Stata 7*. www.stata.com

StatsDirect (1999) *StatsDirect, Version 1*. www.statsdirect.com

Stevenson C. (1998) Models of screening. In *Encyclopedia of Biostatistics*, eds P. Armitage and T. Colton, pp. 3999–4022. Wiley, Chichester.

Stewart L.A. and Clarke M.J. (1995) Practical methodology of meta-analyses (overviews) using updated individual patient data. *Stat. Med.* **14**, 2057–2079.

Stewart L.A. and Parmar M.K.B. (1993) Meta-analysis of the literature or of individual patient data: is there a difference? *Lancet* **341**, 418–422.

Storer B. (1989) Design and analysis of Phase I clinical trials. *Biometrics* **45**, 925–937.

Storer B.E. (1998) Phase I trials. In *Encyclopedia of Biostatistics*, eds P. Armitage and T. Colton, pp. 3365–3370. Wiley, Chichester.

Strijbosch L.W.G., Buurman W.A., Does R.J.M.M., Zinken P.H. and Groenewegen G. (1987) Limiting dilution assays: experimental design and statistical analysis. *J. Immun. Meth.* **97**, 133–140.

'Student' (W.S. Gosset). (1907) On the error of counting with a haemocytometer. *Biometrika* **5**, 351–360.

Sutherland I. (1946) The stillbirth-rate in England and Wales in relation to social influences. *Lancet* **ii**, 953–956.

SYSTAT (2000) *SYSTAT 10*. www.spssscience.com/systat

Tarone R.E. and Ware J. (1977) On distribution-free tests for equality of survival distributions. *Biometrika* **64**, 156–160.

Tarwotjo I., Sommer A., West K.P. *et al.* (1987) Influence of participation on mortality in a randomized trial of vitamin A prophylaxis. *Am. J. Clin. Nut.* **45**, 1466–1471.

Taswell C. (1981) Limiting dilution assays for the determination of immunocompetent cell frequencies. *J. Immun.* **126**, 1613–1619.

Taves D.R. (1974) Minimization: a new method of assigning patients to treatment and control groups. *Clin. Pharmacol. Ther.* **15**, 443–453.

Taylor H.M. and Karlin S. (1984) *An Introduction to Stochastic Modeling*. Academic Press, Orlando.

Taylor J.M.G., Muñoz A., Bass S.M. *et al.* (1990) Estimating the distribution of times from HIV seroconversion to AIDS using multiple imputation. *Stat. Med.* **9**, 505–514.

Theobald G.W. (1937) Effect of calcium and vitamins A and D on incidence of pregnancy toxaemia. *Lancet* **ii**, 1397–1399.

Therneau T.M., Grambsch P.M. and Fleming T.R. (1990) Martingale-based residuals for survival models. *Biometrika* **77**, 147–160.

Thomas A., Spiegelhalter D.J. and Gilks W.R. (1992) BUGS: a program to perform Bayesian inference using Gibbs sampling. In *Bayesian Statistics, 4*, eds J.M. Bernardo, J.O. Berger, A.P. Dawid and A.F.M. Smith, Oxford University Press, Oxford.

Thomas D.G. (1971) AS36: exact confidence limits for the odds ratio in a 2×2 table. *Appl. Stat.* **20**, 105–110.

Thompson S.G. (1993) Controversies in meta-analysis: the case of the trials of serum cholesterol reduction. *Stat. Meth. Med. Res.* **2**, 173–192.

Thompson S.G. (1998) Meta-analysis of clinical trials. In *Encyclopedia of Biostatistics*, eds P. Armitage and T. Colton, pp. 2570–2579. Chichester: Wiley.

Thompson S.G. and Barber J.A. (2000) How should cost data in pragmatic randomised trials be analysed? *Br. Med. J.* **320**, 1197–1200.

Thompson S.G. and Sharp S.J. (1999) Explaining heterogeneity in meta-analysis: a comparison of methods. *Stat. Med.* **18**, 2693–2708.

Tierney L. (1996) Introduction to general state–space Markov chain theory. In *Markov Chain Monte Carlo in Practice*, eds W.R. Gilks, S. Richardson and D.J. Spiegelhalter, pp. 45–57. Chapman and Hall, London.

Tierney L. and Kadane J.B. (1986) Accurate approximations for posterior moments and marginal densities. *J. Am. Stat. Ass.* **81**, 82–86.

Torrance-Rynard V.L. and Walter, S.D. (1997) Effects of dependent errors in the assessment of diagnostic test performance. *Stat. Med.* **16**, 2157–2175.

Trimble I.M.G., West M., Knapp M.S., Pownall R. and Smith A.F.M. (1983) Detection of renal allograft rejection by computer. *Br. Med. J.* **286**, 1695–1699.

Truett J., Cornfield J. and Kannel W. (1967) A multivariate analysis of the risk of coronary heart disease in Framingham. *J. Chron. Dis.* **20**, 511–524.

Tudehope D.I., Iredell J., Rodgers D. and Gunn A. (1986) Neonatal death: grieving families. *Med. J. Aust.* **144**, 290–292.

Tudor G. and Koch G.G. (1994) Review of non-parametric methods for the analysis of crossover studies. *Stat. Meth. Med. Res.* **3**, 345–381.

Tufte E.R. (1983) *The Visual Display of Quantitative Information*. Graphics Press, Cheshire.

Tukey J.W. (1958) Bias and confidence in not quite large samples (abstract). *Ann. Math. Stat.* **29**, 614.

Tukey J.W. (1977) *Exploratory Data Analysis*. Addison-Wesley, Reading, Massachusetts.

Turnbull B.W. (1976) The empirical distribution function with arbitrarily grouped, censored, and truncated data. *J. R. Stat. Soc. B* **38**, 290–295.

Upton G.J.G. (1992) Fisher's exact test. *J. R. Stat. Soc. A* **155**, 395–402.

van Elteren P.H. (1960) On the combination of independent two-sample tests of Wilcoxon. *Bull. Inst. Int. Stat.* **37**, 351–361.

Walker N. (1998) Database systems. In *Encyclopedia of Biostatistics*, eds P. Armitage and T. Colton, pp. 1089–1093. Wiley, Chichester.

Walter S.D. (1975) The distribution of Levin's measure of attributable risk. *Biometrika* **62**, 371–374.

Walter S.D. and Day N.E. (1983) Estimation of the duration of a preclinical state using screening data. *Am. J. Epidemiol.* **118**, 865–886.

Walter S.D. and Irwig L.M. (1988) Estimation of test error rates, disease prevalence and relative risk from misclassified data: a review. *J. Clin. Epidemiol.* **41**, 923–937.

Walter S.D., Irwig L. and Glasziou P.P. (1999) Meta-analysis of diagnostic tests with imperfect reference standards. *J. Clin. Epidemiol.* **52**, 943–951.

Ware J.H. (1989) Investigating therapies of potentially great benefit: ECMO (with discussion). *Stat. Sci.* **4**, 298–340.

Ware J.H., Muller J.E. and Braunwald E. (1985) The futility index: an approach to the cost-effective termination of randomized clinical trials. *Am. J. Med.* **78**, 635–643.

Warner H.R., Toronto A.F., Veasey L.G. and Stephenson R. (1961) A mathematical approach to medical diagnosis. *J. Am. Med. Ass.* **177**, 177–183.

Weatherall J.A.C. and Haskey J.C. (1976) Surveillance of malformations. *Br. Med. Bull.* **32**, 39–44.

Wei L.J. and Durham, S. (1978) The randomized play-the-winner rule in medical trials. *J. Am. Stat. Ass.* **73**, 840–843.

Weinstein M.C. and Fineberg H.V. (1980) *Clinical Decision Analysis*. Saunders, Philadelphia.

Weiss N.S., McKnight B. and Stevens N.G. (1992) Approaches to the analysis of case–control studies of the efficacy of screening for cancer. *Am. J. Epidemiol.* **135**, 817–823.

Welch B.L. (1951) On the comparison of several mean values: an alternative approach. *Biometrika* **38**, 330–336.

Westlake W.J. (1979) Statistical aspects of comparative bioavailability trials. *Biometrics* **35**, 273–280.

Westley-Wise, V.J., Stewart B.W., Kreis I. *et al.* (1999) Investigation of a cluster of leukaemia in the Illawarra region of New South Wales, 1989–1996. *Med. J. Aust.* **171**, 178–183.

Wetherill G.B. (1981) *Intermediate Statistical Methods*. Chapman and Hall, London.

Wetherill G.B., Duncombe P., Kenward M. *et al.* (1986) *Regression Analysis with Applications*. Chapman and Hall, London.

Whitehead J. (1997) *The Design and Analysis of Sequential Clinical Trials*, revised 2nd edn. Horwood, Chichester.

Whitehead J. (1999) A unified theory for sequential clinical trials. *Stat. Med.* **18**, 2271–2286.

Whitehead R.G., Paul A.A. and Ahmed E.A. (1989) United Kingdom Department of Health and Social Service 'Present day infant feeding practice' and its influence on infant growth. In *The Physiology of Human Growth*, eds J.M. Tanner and M.A. Preece, pp. 69–79. Proc. SSHB Symp., no. 29, Cambridge University Press, Cambridge.

Whittaker J. (1990) *Graphical Models in Applied Multivariate Analysis*. Wiley, Chichester.

Whittemore A.S. (1983) Estimating attributable risk from case–control studies. *Am. J. Epidemiol.* **117**, 76–85.

WHO Collaborative Study of Neoplasia and Steroid Contraceptives (1990) Breast cancer and combined oral contraceptives: results from a multinational study. *Br. J. Cancer* **61**, 110–119.

Wilcoxon F. (1945) Individual comparisons by ranking methods. *Biometrics Bull.* **1**, 80–83.

Williams D.A. (1978) An exact confidence region for a relative potency estimated from combined assays. *Biometrics* **34**, 659–661.

Williams D.A. (1988) Tests for differences between several small proportions. *Appl. Stat.* **37**, 421–434.

Wilson P.D., Hebel J.R. and Sherwin R. (1981) Screening and diagnosis when within-individual observations are Markov-dependent. *Biometrics* **37**, 553–565.

Wilson P.W. and Kullman E.D. (1931) A statistical inquiry into methods for estimating numbers of rhizobia. *J. Bact.* **22**, 71–90.

Wishart J. (1938) Growth-rate determinations in nutrition studies with the bacon pig, and their analysis. *Biometrika* **30**, 16–28.

Woffindin C., Hoenich N.A. and Matthews, J.N.S. (1992) Cellulose-based haemodialysis membranes: biocompatibility and functional performance compared. *Nephrol. Dial. Transplant.* **7**, 340–345.

Woolf B. (1955) On estimating the relation between blood group and disease. *Ann. Hum. Genet.* **19**, 251–253.

World Health Organization (1992) *International Statistical Classification of Diseases and Related Health Problems*, 10th revision. WHO, Geneva.

Wright E.M. and Royston P. (1997) A comparison of statistical methods for age-related reference intervals. *J. R. Stat. Soc. A* **160**, 47–69.

Yates F. (1934) Contingency tables involving small numbers and the χ^2 test. *J. R. Stat. Soc., Suppl.* **1**, 217–235.

Yates F. (1948) The analysis of contingency tables with groupings based on quantitative characters. *Biometrika* **35**, 176–181.

Yates F. (1981) *Sampling Methods for Censuses and Surveys*, 4th edn. Griffin, London.

Yates F. (1982) Regression models for repeated measurements. *Biometrics* **38**, 850–853.

Yates F. (1984) Tests of significance for 2×2 contingency tables (with discussion). *J. R. Stat. Soc. A* **147**, 426–463.

Youden W.J. (1950) Index for rating diagnostic tests. *Cancer* **3**, 32–35.

Yule G.U. (1934) On some points relating to vital statistics, more especially statistics of occupational mortality. *J. R. Stat. Soc.* **97**, 1–84.

Yule G.U. and Kendall M.G. (1950) *An Introduction to the Theory of Statistics*, 14th edn. Griffin, London.

Yusuf S., Collins R. and Peto R. (1984) Why do we need some large, simple, randomized trials? *Stat. Med.* **3**, 409–420.

Yusuf S., Peto R., Lewis J., Collins R. and Sleight P. (1985) Beta-blockade during and after myocardial infarction: an overview of the randomized clinical trials. *Prog. Cardiovasc. Dis.* **27**, 335–371.

Yusuf S., Simon R. and Ellenberg S. (eds) (1987) Proceedings of the workshop on methodologic issues in overviews of randomized clinical trials. *Stat. Med.* **6**, 217–409.

Zeger S.L. (1998) Noncompliance, adjustment for. In *Encyclopedia of Biostatistics*, eds P. Armitage and T. Colton, pp. 3006–3009. Wiley, Chichester.

Zeger S.L. and Liang K.-Y. (1986) Longitudinal data analysis for discrete and continuous outcomes. *Biometrics* **42**, 121–130.

Zelen M. (1969) Play the winner rule and the controlled clinical trial. *J. Am. Stat. Ass.* **64**, 131–146.

Zelen M. (1979) A new design for randomized clinical trials. *N. Engl. J. Med.* **300**, 1242–1245.

Zelen M. (1990) Randomized consent designs for clinical trials: an update. *Stat. Med.* **9**, 645–656.

Zhang H., Crowley J., Sox H.C. and Olshen R.A. (1998) Tree-structured statistical methods. In *Encyclopedia of Biostatistics*, eds P. Armitage and T. Colton, pp. 4561–4573. Wiley, Chichester.

Zheng T., Holford T.R., Chen, Y. *et al.* (1996) Time trend and age–period–cohort effect on incidence of bladder cancer in Connecticut, 1935–1992. *Int. J. Cancer* **68**, 172–176.

Zippin C. and Armitage P. (1966) Use of concomitant variables and incomplete survival information in the estimation of an exponential survival parameter. *Biometrics* **22**, 665–672.

Author Index

Mock, P.A.   578
Moeschberger, M.L.   568, 587, 588, 590
Mohamed, S.D.   519
Molenberghs, G.   446, 447, 448
Montgomery, R.D.   519
Moon, T.E.   579
Moons, K.G.   697
Morgenstern, H.   648, 683, 698
Morley, C.J.   4
Morris, C.N.   185
Morrison, D.F.   437
Morrow, R.H.   681
Moser, C.   658
Mosha, F.   639
Moss, S.   708
MPS Research Unit   621
Mugeye, K.   639
Muller, J.E.   622
Muller, K.E.   356, 360, 368, 369, 370
Muñoz, A.   658
Murdoch, J.   745
Murray, D.M.   640
Musk, A.W.   701, 702
Mwijarubi, E.   639
Myers, M.H.   712
Myles, J.P.   536

Nachamkin, I.   697
Nagalingan, R.   642
Nam, J.   127
Naylor, A.F.   490
Naylor, J.C.   529
Nelder, J.A.   309, 376, 400, 416, 417, 485, 486, 495, 733
Newcombe, R.G.   117, 119, 122, 124, 126
Newell, D.J.   206, 574, 698
Newell, J.   639
Newey, W.K.   403
Newhouse, M.L.   512, 686
Newman, D.   225
Nicoll, A.   639
Nix, A.B.J.   452
Nizam, A.   356, 360, 368, 369, 370
Normand, S.T.   647
Nurminen, M.   125, 126, 127

O'Quigley, J.   593
O'Rourke, P.P.   604
Oakes, D.   568, 581
O'Brien, P.C.   620
O'Hagan, A.   528, 541, 542, 567
Oldham, P.D.   235
Olschewski, M.   598
Olsen, R.A.   477

O'Sullivan, M.C.   390
Ott, J.   716

Pajak, T.   614
Pan, H.Q.   406
Parad, R.B.   604
Parish, S.   741
Parker, R.A.   146
Parkins, R.A.   599
Parmar, M.K.B.   183, 533, 534, 535, 536, 568, 599, 604, 622, 642
Patel, N.R.   232, 496, 525, 526
Patterson, H.D.   423, 490
Pauker, S.G.   57
Paul, A.A.   401
Paul, S.R.   359
Pearce, N.   688
Pearce, S.C.   264
Pearson, E.S.   110, 150, 154, 176, 747, 753, 755
Pechacek, T.F.   639
Peirce, C.S.   600
Pepe, M.   593
Petkau, A.J.   602
Peto, J.   568, 575, 577, 621, 741
Peto, R.   132, 568, 575, 577, 599, 621, 643, 644, 670, 671, 741
Piantadosi, S.   592, 596, 620
Piegorsch, W.W.   737
Pike, M.C.   142, 568, 575, 577, 583, 621, 674, 681, 713, 714, 741
Pinol, A.P.Y.   146, 639
Plackett, R.L.   737
Pledger, G.   624
Plewis, I.   423, 424
Pocock, S.J.   453, 498, 590, 592, 599, 601, 613, 619, 621
Powell, I.   29
Powell, J.L.   403
Powell-Tuck, J.   599
Pownall, R.   453
Pregibon, D.   495
Prentice, R.L.   568, 575, 581, 587, 627, 671
Prorok, P.C.   710
Proskin, H.M.   643
Pullum, T.W.   667
Pygott, F.   281

Qaqish, B.   443
Quaglino, D.   482
Quenouille, M.H.   304

Radhakrishna, S.   520
Raftery, A.E.   558, 559
Räisänen, M.J.   24

Subject Index